Best Practice in Labour and Delivery

Second Edition

Edited by
Sir Sabaratnam Arulkumaran
St George's University of London, UK, University of Nicosia, Cyprus, and Institute of Global Health, Imperial College, London, UK

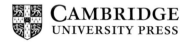

CAMBRIDGE
UNIVERSITY PRESS

CAMBRIDGE
UNIVERSITY PRESS

University Printing House, Cambridge CB2 8BS, United Kingdom

Cambridge University Press is part of the University of Cambridge.

It furthers the University's mission by disseminating knowledge in the pursuit of education, learning and research at the highest international levels of excellence.

www.cambridge.org
Information on this title: www.cambridge.org/9781107472341

© Cambridge University Press 2016

First published 2009
Second edition 2016

Printed in the United Kingdom by TJ International Ltd. Padstow Cornwall

A catalogue record for this publication is available from the British Library

Library of Congress Cataloguing in Publication data
Names: Arulkumaran, Sabaratnam, editor.
Title: Best practice in labour and delivery / edited by Sir Sabaratnam Arulkumaran.
Description: Second edition. | Cambridge, United Kingdom ; New York :
Cambridge University Press, 2016. | Includes bibliographical references and index.
Identifiers: LCCN 2016041235 | ISBN 9781107472341 (paperback)
Subjects: | MESH: Labor, Obstetric | Delivery, Obstetric–methods |
Birth Injuries–prevention & control | Obstetric Labor Complications–
prevention & control
Classification: LCC RG651 | NLM WQ 300 | DDC 618.4 – dc23
LC record available at https://lccn.loc.gov/2016041235

ISBN 978-1-107-47234-1 Paperback

Additional resources for the this publication at www.cambridge.org/
9781107472341

I dedicate this book to mothers, babies, their families and care givers who have helped us to understand the process of labour and delivery. The advanced scientific knowledge gained from studying labour and delivery has helped us to improve the safety and quality of the care we provide.

Contents

Colour plates are to be found between pages 202 and 203

Contributors

Christofides Agathoklis
Head of Obstetrics and Gynaecology, Archbishop
Makarios Hospital, Nicosia, Cyprus

Pina Amin, MBBS, FRCOG, MRCPI
Consultant Obstetrician and Gynaecologist,
University Hospital of Wales, Cardiff

Savvas Argyridis
Associate Professor, University of Nicosia, Cyprus

Sabaratnam Arulkumaran, MD, PhD, FRCS, FRCOG
Emeritus Professor of Obstetrics and Gynaecology,
St George's University of London, UK, Foundation
Professor of Obstetrics and Gynaecology, University
of Nicosia, Cyprus, and Visiting Professor, Institute of
Global Health, Imperial College London, UK

Shankari Arulkumaran
Specialist Registrar in Obstetrics and Gynaecology,
Northwick Park Hospital, London, UK

Diogo Ayres-de-Campos
Associate Professor, Department of Obstetrics and
Gynecology, Medical School, University of Porto,
S. Joao Hospital, INEB – Institute of Biomedical
Engineering, Porto, Portugal

**Edwin Chandraharan, MBBS, MS (Obs & Gyn),
DFFP, DCRM, MRCOG, FSLCOG**
Consultant Obstetrician and Gynaecologist/Lead
Clinician Labour Ward, St George's Healthcare NHS
Trust, London, UK

Laura Coleman
Specialist Registrar in Obstetrics and Gynaecology, St
Michael's Hospital, Bristol, UK

Katie Cornthwaite, BA, MBBS
Academic Clinical Fellow, Department of Women's
Health, North Bristol NHS Trust, Southmead
Hospital, Bristol and University of Bristol, Bristol, UK

Joanna F. Crofts, MRCOG, MD
School of Social and Community Medicine,
University of Bristol, Bristol, UK

**Anushuya Devi Kasi, MBBS, MD (Obs and Gyn),
DFFP, MRCOG**
Senior Registrar, St George's Healthcare NHS Trust,
London, UK

Mandish K. Dhanjal, BSc, MRCP, FRCOG
Consultant Obstetrician and Gynaecologist, Queen
Charlotte's and Chelsea Hospital, Imperial College
Healthcare NHS Trust, and Honorary Senior
Lecturer, Imperial College, London, UK

Stergios Doumouchtsis
Consultant Obstetrician, Gynaecologist and
Urogynaecologist, Department of Obstetrics and
Gynaecology, Epsom & St Helier University Hospitals
NHS Trust, UK

Leroy C. Edozien, PhD, FRCOG, FWACS
Consultant in Obstetrics and Gynaecology,
Manchester Academic Health Science Centre,
St Mary's Hospital, Manchester, UK

Jonathon Francis, MBChB, FRCA
Consultant Obstetric Anaesthetist, Norfolk and
Norwich University Hospital, Norfolk, UK

David Fraser
Consultant Obstetrician and Gynaecologist, Norfolk
and Norwich University Hospital, Norwich, UK

Kim Hinshaw, MB, BS, FRCOG
Consultant Obstetrician and Gynaecologist, Director
of Research and Innovation, City Hospitals
Sunderland NHS Foundation Trust, Sunderland, UK

Jessica Hoyle, MBBS BsC FRCA MA
Consultant Anaesthetist, Whipps Cross University
Hospital, Barts Health NHS Trust, London, UK

Guy Jackson, MBBS, FRCA
Consultant Anaesthetist, Anaesthetic Department, Royal Berkshire NHS Foundation Trust, Reading, Berkshire, UK

Jan Stener Jørgensen, MD, PhD
Professor of Obstetrics, Research Unit of Gynecology and Obstetrics, Department of Gynecology and Obstetrics, Institute of Clinical Research, Odense University Hospital, University of Southern Denmark, Odense, and Centre for Innovative Medical Technology, Odense University Hospital, Odense, Denmark

Nina Johns, MBBS, FRCOG
Consultant Obstetrician, Birmingham Women's Hospital, Birmingham, UK

Gabriel Kalakoutis, MD, MBBS, FRCOG
Senior Lecturer in Obstetrics and Gynaecology, University of Nicosia Medical School, Cyprus

Hajeb Kamali, MBChB, BSc
Obstetrics and Gynaecology Registrar, Severn Deanery, UK

Justin C. Konje, MD, FRCOG
Consultant Obstetrician and Gynaecologist, Reproductive Sciences Section, Department of Obstetrics and Gynaecology, University of Leicester, University Hospitals of Leicester, Leicester, UK, and Department of Obstetrics and Gynaecology, Sidra Medical and Research Center, Doha, Qatar

Ronald F. Lamont, PhD, FRCOG
Professor, Research Unit of Gynecology and Obstetrics, Department of Gynecology and Obstetrics, Institute of Clinical Research, Odense University Hospital, University of Southern Denmark, Odense, Denmark, and Division of Surgery, Northwick Park Institute for Medical Research Campus, University College London, London, UK

Tak Yeung Leung, MD, FRCOG
Professor, Department of Obstetrics and Gynaecology, The Chinese University of Hong Kong, Hong Kong

Tsz Kin Lo
Consultant, Department of Obstetrics and Gynaecology, Pricesss Margaret Hospital, Hong Kong, Hong Kong

Paul Mannix, MBBS, MD, MRCP, FRCPCH
Consultant Neonatologist, North Bristol NHS Trust, Southmead Hospital, Bristol, UK

K. Muhunthan, MBBS, MS, FRCOG
Head, Senior Lecturer and Consultant Obstetrician and Gynecologist, Department of Obstetrics and Gynaecology, Faculty of Medicine, University of Jaffna, Sri Lanka

Deirdre J. Murphy, MBBS, PhD, FRCOG
Professor of Obstetrics and Head of Department, Coombe Women and Infants University Hospital, Dublin, Ireland

Osric Navti, MBBS, MRCOG
University Hospitals of Leicester, Leicester, UK

Catherine Nelson-Piercy, MA, FRCP, FRCOG
Professor of Obstetric Medicine, Guy's and St Thomas' Foundation Trust, and Queen Charlotte's and Chelsea Hospital, London, UK

Daisy Nirmal, MBBS, MRCOG, MClinEd
Consultant Obstetrican and Gynaecologist, Norfolk and Norwich University Hospital, Norwich, UK

Ana Pinas Carrillo, Dip in O&G (Spain), DFM (UK)
Locum Consultant in Obstetrics and Fetal Medicine, St George's Healthcare NHS Trust, Blackshaw Road, London, UK

Mark Porter, FRCA
Consultant Anaesthetist, University Hospitals Coventry and Warwickshire, Coventry, UK

Neelam Potdar, MBBS, MD, MRCOG
University Hospitals of Leicester, Leicester, UK

Mariana Rei
Invited Lecturer, Department of Obstetrics and Gynecology, Medical School, University of Porto, S. Joao Hospital, INEB – Institute of Biomedical Engineering, Porto, Portugal

Dimitrios M. Siassakos, MD, MRCOG
Department of Women's Health, North Bristol NHS Trust, Southmead Hospital, and University of Bristol, Bristol, UK

Bryony Strachan, MBBS, MD, FRCOG
St Michael's Hospital, Bristol, UK

Abdul H. Sultan, MBBS, MD, FRCOG
Consultant Obstetrician Gynaecologist,
Croydon University Hospital, Croydon,
Surrey, UK

Vikram Sinai Talaulikar, MD, MRCOG
Clinical Research Fellow, Department of Obstetrics
and Gynaecology, St George's University of London,
London, UK

Ranee Thakar, MBBS, PhD, FRCOG
Consultant Urogynaecologists, Croydon University
Hospital, Croydon, Surrey, UK

Rosemary Townsend, MBChB
Specialist Trainee in Obstetrics and Gynaecology,
St George's Healthcare NHS Trust, London, UK

Austin Ugwumadu, MBBS, PhD, FRCOG
Clinical Director of Obstetrics and Gynaecology and
Hon. Senior Lecturer and Consultant, St George's
Healthcare NHS Trust, London, UK

Gerard H. A. Visser, MD, PhD, FRCOG(ae)
Emeritus Professor of Obstretrics, Department of
Obstetrics, University Medical Center Utrecht,
Utrecht, the Netherlands

James J. Walker, MD, FRCOG
Professor of Obstetrics and Gynaecology, University
of Leeds, Leeds, UK

Stephen Walkinshaw, BSc (Hons), MD, FRCOG
Retired Consultant in Maternal and Fetal Medicine,
Liverpool

Melissa Whitten, MD, MRCOG
Consultant in Obstetrics and Fetal Medicine,
University College London Hospitals, and Module
Lead for MBBS Women's Health and Men's Health,
University College London, UK

Steve Yentis, MD, FRCA
Consultant Anaesthetist, Chelsea and Westminster
Hospital, and Honorary Reader, Imperial College,
London, UK

Preface to the Second Edition

Best Practice in Labour and Delivery is a comprehensive textbook of 33 chapters that cover most topics of importance that one should know in labour and delivery. Starting from basic anatomy and physiology, the book covers the entire spectrum of problems encountered in labour and delivery. Special attention is paid to topics of importance that result in maternal and fetal morbidity and mortality. The layout and rational arrangement of chapters makes the book easy to navigate and read; this is made more simple by use of easy-to-assimilate tables, care pathways, suitable illustrations and pictures.

Each chapter has been contributed by nationally and internationally recognized experts. In addition to the latest evidence from guidelines published by various colleges from the UK and other countries, and the Cochrane Database, the authors have distilled the recommendations from the NICE guidelines on intrapartum care published in December 2014 and the recommendations from the UK Confidential Enquiries into Maternal Deaths, released in January 2015. Most authors have carried out original research into the topics chosen and their work blends into the respective chapters. In addition to technical aspects of labour and delivery, the important aspects of non-technical skills needed for good practice, prioritization to give care, clinical governance, risk management and objective structured assessment of technical skills are dealt with in detail. These chapters will help each and every consultant and trainee, especially those who have opted to train in advanced labour ward practice.

I am grateful to the contributors, who have sacrificed a lot of their time to provide us with the excellent chapters. Even with scrupulous proofreading there may be mistakes, and some facts may be wrong or controversial. I would be most grateful to the readers for writing to me as the editor, or to the publisher, so that we can rectify any problems in the next reprint.

Yours sincerely,

Sir Sabaratnam Arulkumaran

Preface to the First Edition

Those privileged to look after women during their labours and deliveries have a duty to practise to the highest standards. A clear understanding of what constitutes best practice will help to ensure the safety and health of mothers and babies through parturition.

Whilst the encouragement of normality is implicit, abnormality in labour must be recognized promptly and, when necessary, must be appropriately managed to ensure best outcome.

An understanding of normality and when and how to intervene are the keys to good clinical care. This textbook is an encompassing reference covering all the essential information relating to childbirth; it offers clear practical guidance across the width of labour and delivery.

We are very grateful to those well-known leading experts who, despite their busy lives, have made such excellent contributions to this definitive text. Each chapter offers a modern authoritative review of best practice with the evidence base for good clinical care necessary to optimize outcome through appropriate clinical management and justifiable intervention.

Whilst this is an ideal textbook for those training or taking examinations in labour ward practice, it offers all those professionals caring for the labouring woman a modern, evidence-based approach, which will help them understand and deliver the best possible clinical care. The importance of team working, prioritizing and the organization of maternity care receive appropriate emphasis with clear guidance and practical advice.

Guided by appropriate, clearly defined management pathways, based on national guidance, attending professionals will be best placed to improve safety and the quality of the labour process for both mother and baby.

The auditing and monitoring of standards and outcomes are vital to the organization and improvement of maternity services. The recent introduction of Clinical Dashboards (Appendix A) promises to be a major advance by facilitating the monitoring through traffic light recording of performance and governance (including clinical activity, workforce, outcomes risk incidents, complaints/women's feedback about care) against locally or nationally agreed benchmarked standards.

This book contains the most up-to-date references and evidence base, including from the Guidelines and Standards of the Royal College of Obstetricians and Gynaecologists (www.rcog.org.uk) and the National Institute for Health and Clinical Excellence (www.nice.org.uk). We believe that this textbook will be of great value for all midwives and doctors overseeing and managing childbirth.

Richard Warren
Sir Sabaratnam Arulkumaran

Acknowledgements

The editor would like to sincerely thank the authors for their excellent contributions to the second edition of the book. I thank Mrs Sue Cunningham for inviting and reminding the authors and for collating and finalizing the edited chapters. I am most grateful to Nick Dunton and Kirsten Bot of Cambridge University Press for their constant support and for their patience in producing this book.

I am indebted to Gayatri, Shankari, Nishkantha and Kailash for their kind understanding of my time away from them in doing all the writing and editing.

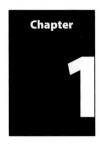
Pelvic and Fetal Cranial Anatomy and the Stages and Mechanism of Labour

K. Muhunthan

Introduction

Labour or parturition is the culmination of a period of pregnancy whereby the expulsion of fetus, amniotic fluid, placenta and membranes takes place from the gravid uterus of a pregnant woman. In a woman with a regular 28-day cycle, labour is said to take place 280 days after the onset of the last menstrual period. However, the length of human gestation varies considerably among healthy pregnancies, even when ovulation is accurately measured in naturally conceiving women [1].

Successful labour passes through three stages: the shortening and dilatation of the cervix; descent and birth of the fetus; and the expulsion of the placenta and membranes. Efficient uterine contractions (power), an adequate roomy pelvis (passage) and an appropriate fetal size (passenger) are key factors in this process.

Anatomy of the Female Pelvis

The bony pelvis consists of the two innominate bones, or hipbones, which are fused to the sacrum posteriorly and to each other anteriorly at the pubic symphysis. Each innominate bone is composed of the ilium, ischium and pubis, which are connected by cartilage in youth but fused in the adult (Figure 1.1). The pelvis has two basins: the major (or greater) pelvis and the minor (or lesser) pelvis. The abdominal viscera occupy the major pelvis and the minor pelvis is the narrower continuation of the major pelvis. Inferiorly, the pelvic outlet is closed by the pelvic floor.

The female pelvis has a wider diameter and a more circular shape than that of the male. The wider inlet facilitates engagement of the fetal head and partu-

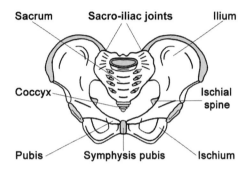

Figure 1.1 Bony female pelvis.

rition. Numerous projections and contours provide attachment sites for ligaments, muscles and fascial layers. This distinctive shape of the human pelvis is probably not only the result of an adaptation to a bipedal gait, but also a result of the need for a larger birth canal for a human fetus with a large brain [2].

The female pelvis is tilted forwards relative to the spine and described as the deviation of the pelvic inlet from the horizontal in the sagittal plane. The pelvic 'tilt' or angle of inclination is measured as an angle between the line from the top of the sacrum to the top of the pubis, and a horizontal line in a standing radiograph (Figure 1.2).

The pelvic tilt is variable between different individuals and between different races; in adult Caucasian females the pelvis is usually about 55° to the horizontal plane. It is also position-dependent and increases with growth into adulthood [3].

Based on the characteristic of the pelvic inlet, it is classified into four basic shapes: the round (gynaecoid), the wedge-shaped (android), the longitudinal oval (anthropoid) and the transverse oval (platypelloid) type of inlet (Figure 1.3). However, a large

Best Practice in Labour and Delivery, Second Edition, ed. Sir Sabaratnam Arulkumaran. Published by CAMBRIDGE UNIVERSITY Press. © Cambridge University Press 2016.

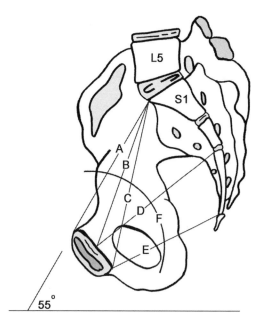

Figure 1.2 Sagittal section of the pelvis with 55° inclination. A: anatomical conjugate, B: obstetric conjugate; C: diagonal conjugate; D: mid-cavity; E: outlet; F: pelvic axis.

number of pelves appear to conform to intermediate shapes between these extreme types [4].

The true pelvis is a bony canal, through which the fetus must pass, and has three parts: the inlet, the pelvic cavity and the outlet. The pelvic inlet is bounded anteriorly by the pubic crest and spine; posteriorly by the promontory of the sacrum and ala; and laterally by the ilio pectineal line. In an adequately sized pelvis the inlet's diameter antero-posteriorly is usually more than 12 cm, and the transverse diameter is 13.5 cm.

The antero-posterior diameter of the pelvic *inlet* is also known as the true or anatomical conjugate. However, clinically the fetus must pass through the obstetric conjugate, which is the line between the promontory of the sacrum and the innermost part of the symphysis pubis, which is usually more than 10 cm. The conjugate that can be measured clinically is the diagonal conjugate, which is the line between the sacral promontory and the lowermost point of the symphysis pubis. This is about 1.5–2 cm greater than the obstetric conjugate (Figure 1.2).

The *mid-cavity* is a curved canal with a straight and shallow anterior wall which is the pubis. The posterior wall is bounded by the deep and concave sacrum and laterally by the ischium and part of the ilium. In the mid-cavity both antero-posterior (AP) and transverse diameters are usually approximately 12.5 cm.

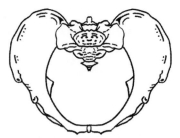

Gynaecoid pelvis
Most common and classical female pelvis.
Round inlet.

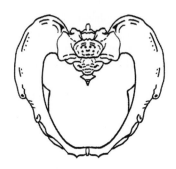

Android pelvis
Resembles human male pelvis.
Heart - shaped inlet and narrow outlet.

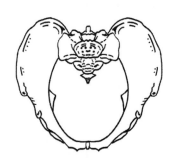

Anthropoid pelvis
Resembles pelvis of anthropoid ape.
Oval shaped inlet and wider A-P diameter.

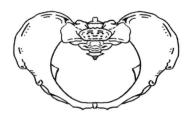

Platypelloid pelvis
Flattened inlet.
Wider transverse diameter.

Figure 1.3 Four basic shapes of pelvis.

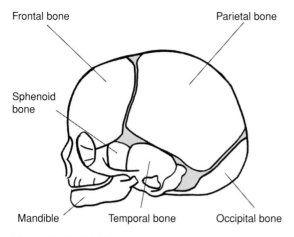

Figure 1.4 Fetal skull bones.

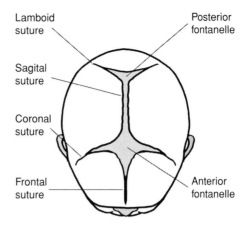

Figure 1.5 Sutures and fontanelles of the fetal skull.

The pelvic *outlet* is the lower circumference of the lesser pelvis. It is very irregular and bounded by the pubic arch anteriorly, ischial tuberosities laterally and sacrotuberous ligament and the tip of the coccyx posteriorly.

In order to have a successful delivery the fetus has to pass through this bony canal; the axis through which the fetus travels is an imaginary line joining the centre points of the planes of the inlet, cavity and outlet.

Anatomy of the Fetal Skull

The human fetal skull is considered to be the largest compared to the pelvic size of all other living primates and the most difficult part of the fetus to pass through the mother's pelvic canal, due to its hard, bony nature [5].

The skull bones encase and protect the brain, which is very delicate and subjected to pressure when the fetal head passes down the birth canal. The fetal cranium is composed of nine bones (occipital, two parietal, two frontal, two temporal, sphenoid and ethmoid). Of these, the bones that compose the skull are of clinical importance during birth (Figure 1.4).

The fetal skull bones are as follows:

1. The *frontal bone*, which forms the forehead. In the fetus, the frontal bone is in two halves which fuse (join) into a single bone after the age of eight years.
2. The two *parietal bones*, which lie on either side of the skull and occupy most of the skull.

3. The *occipital bone*, which forms the back of the skull and part of its base. It joins with the cervical vertebrae.
4. The two *temporal bones*, one on each side of the head, closest to the ear.

Sutures are joints between these bones of the skull. The *lambdoid suture* forms the junction between the occipital and the parietal bones; the *sagittal suture* joins the two parietal bones together; the *coronal suture* joins the frontal bones to the two parietal bones; and the *frontal suture* joins the two frontal bones together.

A fontanelle is the space created by the joining of two or more sutures. It is covered by thick membranes and the skin on the fetal head, protecting the brain underneath. The anterior fontanelle (also known as the bregma) is a diamond-shaped space towards the front of the fetal head, at the junction of the sagittal, coronal and frontal sutures. The posterior fontanelle (or lambda) has a triangular shape, and is found towards the back of the fetal skull. It is formed by the junction of the lambdoid and sagittal sutures.

In the fetus they permit their movement and overlap during labour under the pressure on the fetal head as it passes down the birth canal. This process, called *moulding*, can decrease the diameters of the fetal skull. The suboccipito-bregmatic diameter is more sensitive to the changes of labour force than other fetal skull diameters [6]. Significant moulding with caput can be a sign of cephalo-pelvic disproportion and this should be ruled out before attempting an instrumental vaginal delivery [7]. During early childhood, these sutures

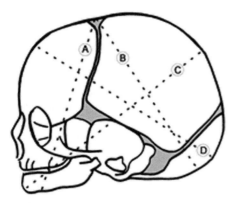

Figure 1.6 Fetal skull diameters. A: submento-bregmatic (9.5 cm); B: suboccipito-bregmatic (9.5 cm); C: mento-vertical (13.5 cm); D: occipito-frontal (11.5 cm).

harden and the skull bones can no longer move relative to one another, as they can to a small extent in the fetus and newborn.

The widest transverse diameter of the fetal skull is the biparietal diameter, which is 9.5 cm. The AP diameter of the fetal head is determined by the degree of flexion of the fetal head. This also determines which region of the fetal skull is presenting during labour, and it is described as lines that correspond to the diameter of the presenting region of the head (Figure 1.6). The suboccipito-bregmatic (fully flexed vertex) and the submento-bregmatic (face) are the narrowest AP diameters at 9.5 cm each. The widest AP diameter is 13.5 cm, and is with the fully extended head which is the mento-vertical of a brow presentation. The occipito-frontal (11.5 cm) diameter is seen with deflexed vertex presentation.

Identification of these regions and landmarks on the top of the fetal skull has particular importance for obstetric care when vaginal assessments are made during labour.

The Uterus During Pregnancy

After conception, the uterus provides a nutritive and safe environment for the embryo to develop as a fetus until delivery. The uterus undergoes extensive adaptations mainly with regards to size, shape, position, vasculature and its ability to contract.

Uterine Size

In an uncomplicated pregnancy by term, approximately the weight of the uterus increases 20-fold (from 70 g to 1000 g) and the volume by 500-fold (10 cc to 5000 cc). This increase of capacity can be expected to accommodate the fetus, placenta and amniotic fluid.

Early in gestation, uterine hypertrophy probably is stimulated by the action of mainly estrogen and also of progesterone. Later in pregnancy hypertrophy of cells of the uterus is due to response to the biological mechanical stretching of uterine walls by the growing fetus and placenta [8]. In this process of hypertrophy, stretching of muscle cells along with accumulation of fibrous and elastic tissue plays a major role, and the production of new myocytes is limited.

Uterine Shape and Position

From its original pear shape, the uterus assumes a globular shape as the pregnancy advances. It becomes palpable abdominally by 12 weeks as it is too large to remain totally within the pelvis. From this point onwards it can be measured and palpated as it is in contact with the anterior abdominal wall (Figure 1.7). By term it almost reaches the liver and this exponential enlargement of the uterus displaces the bowels laterally and superiorly. In supine position it rests on the vertebral column and the adjacent great vessels, especially the inferior vena cava and aorta. It also undergoes *dextrorotation*, which is likely caused by the recto-sigmoid

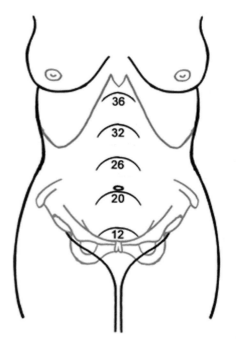

Figure 1.7 Height of the uterus at various weeks of pregnancy.

colon on the left side of the pelvis. As the uterus rises, tension is exerted on the broad and round ligaments.

Uterine Vascular Adaptations

The regulation of uterine vascular remodelling during pregnancy is part of the larger set of adaptive physiological processes required for a successful pregnancy outcome.

A multitude of physiological adaptations of the cardiovascular system takes place during pregnancy; the most notable changes are the increase in intravascular volume and cardiac output. Cardiac output increases from 3.5 to 6.0 l/min at rest, a rise of close to 40%. These changes begin as early as the first trimester of pregnancy.

The greatest changes, however, are those occurring in the uteroplacental circulation.

Haemochorial placentation in humans results in decreased downstream resistance and secretion of molecular signals. The former results in increased upstream flow velocity and initiates nitric oxide (NO) secretion as well as other effects that lead to changes in cell and matrix properties. The combination of vasodilation, changes in matrix enzymes and cellular architecture leads to an increase in lumen diameter without any change in wall thickness, decreased resistance and increased uteroplacental flow [9]. As a result, an even greater fall in vascular resistance preferentially directs some 20% of total cardiac output to this vascular bed by term, amounting to a 10-fold or greater increase over levels present in the non-pregnant state, such that, by term, uteroplacental flow may approach 1 l/min [10].

Uterine Contractility

Adaptations of human myometrium during pregnancy include cellular mechanisms that preclude the development of high levels of myosin light chain phosphorylation during contraction and an increase in the stress-generating capacity for any given level of myosin light chain phosphorylation. This process is said to be mediated through Ca^{2+} [11]. From the first trimester onward, the uterus undergoes irregular painless contraction that becomes manually detectable during the mid-trimester. These contractions vary in intensity and timing and are called *Braxton Hicks contractions* [12]. Gradually they increase in intensity and frequency during the last week or two and may cause some discomfort late in pregnancy.

Length of Pregnancy and Initiation of Labour

Length of Pregnancy

Length of pregnancy in humans averages 40 weeks. Little is known about the factors determining length of pregnancy, but it has been thought to be controlled by events occurring in late pregnancy that influence timing of parturition. Thus, preterm birth is a consequence of premature activation of parturition by a pathological process. In humans, timing of birth is associated with expression of the gene responsible for corticotrophin-releasing hormone (CRH) by the placenta. Maternal plasma concentration of CRH is a potential marker of this process. It has been postulated that a placental clock determines the timing of delivery [13].

Initiation of Labour

During pregnancy, the uterus is maintained in a state of functional quiescence through the integrated action of one or more of a series of inhibitors. Cervical ripening and myometrial contraction are main contributing factors for the initiation of labour, and they start a few weeks before the true labour. It is considered that there is an interaction between maternal and fetal factors that initiate labour in humans. Maternal endocrine and genetic factors and the influence of fetal factors play an important role.

Maternal Endocrine and Genetic Influence

The functional quiescence during pregnancy is maintained by the integrated action of one or more of a series of inhibitors, including progesterone, prostacyclin, relaxin, nitric oxide, parathyroid hormone-related peptide, calcitonin gene-related peptide, adrenomedullin and vasoactive intestinal peptide.

Change in the oestrogen:progesterone ratio, CRH, prostaglandins, oxytocin and contraction-associated proteins are some of the other factors that influence onset of labour [14]. Also it is noted that women who carried polymorphic tumour necrosis factor (*TNF α-308*) gene have a tendency to deliver preterm [15].

Fetal Influence

Initiation of labour at term or even preterm is also influenced by signals from the fetus. Its growth, resulting in uterine stretch, increased surfactant protein-A secretion by the fetal lung and increased CRH secretion by the placenta, promotes release of pro-inflammatory cytokines and activation of uterine transcription factors, such as nuclear receptor transcription factor-κB (NF-κB) and other inflammatory transcription factors. The activated NF-κB, in turn, binds to enhancers in the regulatory regions of contractile genes, such as *COX-2*, resulting in transcriptional activation and the production of prostaglandins that promote uterine contractility [16].

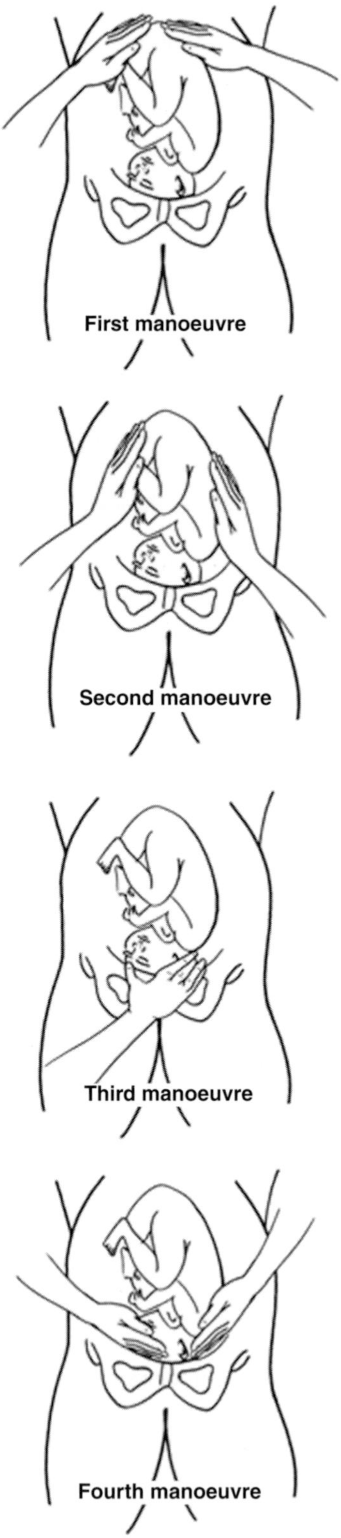

Clinical Assessment During Pregnancy and Labour

Clinical assessment of a pregnant woman plays an important role to the obstetrician. These include the general examination and some specific examinations that are done exclusively in obstetric patients. A systematic examination of the abdomen of a pregnant woman would be with the aim of establishing the symphysio-fundal height, presentation and engagement, lie, position and attitude. Pelvic examination during pregnancy is used to detect a number of clinical conditions such as anatomical abnormalities, to evaluate the size of a woman's pelvis (pelvimetry) and to assess the uterine cervix. It is usually performed when the woman is thought to be in established labour unless indicated earlier for special reasons.

Abdominal Palpation

Abdominal examination can be conducted systematically with the aim of establishing the above-mentioned components; employing the four manoeuvres described by Leopold and Spörlinin in 1894 is of great value to current practice (Figure 1.8). The mother should be supine and comfortably positioned with her abdomen bared. These manoeuvres may be of limited value and difficult to interpret if the patient is obese, if there is excessive amnionic fluid or if the placenta is anteriorly positioned.

First Manoeuvre

The uterine fundal area is palpated with both hands in order to determine what part of the fetus is occupying the fundus. The breech gives the sensation of a large, nodular mass, whereas the head feels hard and round and is more mobile and ballottable.

Figure 1.8 Leopold manoeuvres.

First manoeuvre

Second manoeuvre

Third manoeuvre

Fourth manoeuvre

Second Manoeuvre

Facing the woman, the abdomen is palpated gently using the palm of the hands placed on either side of the maternal abdomen. The fetal back will feel firm and smooth while fetal extremities feel like small irregularities and protrusions. By noting whether the back is directed anteriorly, transversely or posteriorly, the orientation of the fetus can be determined.

Third Manoeuvre

A gentle grip using the thumb and fingers of one hand are placed on the area over the symphysis pubis to determine what part of the fetal head is lying over the pelvic inlet. The differentiation between head and breech is made as in the first manoeuvre and the amount of that presenting part that is palpable abdominally is determined. This manoeuvre may be uncomfortable for the pregnant woman and, if examination is performed in this way, it must be undertaken gently.

Alternatively and in preference, the necessary clinical information may be obtained through the fourth manoeuvre.

Fourth Manoeuvre

The examiner faces the mother's feet and the fingers of both hands are moved gently down the sides of the uterus towards the pubis to confirm the presentation and on which side is the prominence of the presenting part. The side where the resistance to the descent of the fingers towards the pubis is greatest is where the brow is located. If the head of the fetus is well flexed, it should be on the opposite side from the fetal back. If the fetal head is extended, the occiput is instead felt and is located on the same side as the back.

Abdominal palpation using the above manoeuvres can be performed throughout the latter months of pregnancy and during and between the labour contractions. With experience, fetal malpresentations can be identified with high sensitivity and specificity.

Symphysio-Fundal Height

Measurement of symphysio-fundal height is simple, inexpensive and widely used during antenatal care. It can be achieved more objectively by using a tape measure in centimetres from 24 weeks onwards. When a tape measure is used, the measurement is made by identifying the variable point, the fundus, and then measuring to the fixed point of the top of the symphysis pubis, with the option of centimetre values being

hidden by keeping the non-marked side of the tape facing the examiner [17].

This can be used as a screening method for identifying fetuses that are growth restricted, unusually large and for the detection of multiple pregnancies. High detection rates can be achieved if serial measurements are plotted on customized charts for recording with standardized training and protocols to manage the patient [18].

Presentation

Fetal presentation refers to the fetal part that directly overlies the pelvic inlet. Any presentation other than cephalic (vertex) is considered malpresentation and by term or 37 completed weeks 96% of pregnancies will have cephalic presentation. Commonest malpresentation at term is breech and its incidence reduces from approximately 20% at 28 weeks to 3–4% at term.

Engagement

Engagement of the fetal head is one of the most important signs for the obstetrician to decide on mode of delivery. Engagement occurs when the widest part of the fetal head passes through the pelvic inlet. Parity, ethnicity, cephalo-pelvic disproportion, malposition and placental location are some of the factors that determine engagement of the fetal head. In different groups of the pregnant population engagement of the fetal head for primigravida and multigravida has been shown to takes place at different periods of gestation [19]. Engagement of the fetal head occurs in the majority of nulliparous women prior to labour, but not so for the majority of multiparous women. In nulliparous women, engagement usually takes place from the middle of the third trimester onwards, but in some of these women, and in most multiparous women, engagement may not take place until the onset of labour. Maternal height and birth weight of fetus also may play a significant role in determining the time at which the fetal head engages and need to be considered when assessing a patient [20]. Non-engagement at the onset of the active phase of labour is a predictor of the risk of caesarean section, which emphasizes the importance of assessing a pregnant woman for engagement of the fetal head, especially when she is in labour [21].

It is customary to describe the amount of the fetal head that is palpable outside the pelvis; when all of the fetal head is palpable above the pelvis it is described as 5/5 (five-fifths palpable). This is based on how many finger breadths are needed to cover the head above the pelvic brim. When the fetal head is engaged, it is usually two-fifths palpable, and when it is deeply engaged it is zero-fifths palpable.

Lie

Fetal lie refers to the long axis of the fetus relative to the longitudinal axis of the uterus. This can be longitudinal, transverse or oblique. Over 99% of singleton term babies have a longitudinal lie and factors such as prematurity, multiparity, multiple pregnancies, placenta praevia, polyhydramnios, uterine fibromatas, congenital uterine anomalies, intrauterine fetal death and extra uterine masses obstructing the birth canal predisposes a pregnant woman to have persistent abnormal lie.

Compared to those fetuses presenting with a longitudinal lie at the onset of labour, fetuses who are in transverse lie have been found to have a lower absolute pH, more frequent chance of developing severe acidosis, lower birth weight and are more likely to sustain birth trauma and long-term residual effects [22].

Position

Fetal position refers to the relationship of a nominated site of the fetal presenting part to a denominating location on the maternal pelvis. For example, in a cephalic presentation, the fetal site used for reference is typically the occiput (e.g. right occiput anterior). In a breech presentation, the sacrum is used as the designated fetal site (e.g. right sacrum anterior). Any fetal position that is not right occiput anterior, occiput anterior or left occiput anterior is referred to as a malposition.

Attitude

Fetal attitude describes the degree of flexion or extension of the fetal head in relation to the fetal spine. Adequate flexion (chin to chest) is necessary to achieve the smallest possible presenting diameter in a cephalic presentation. Deflexion in the early stages of labour may be corrected by the architecture of the pelvic floor and uterine contractions.

Asynclitism

Asynclitism describes the relationship of the sagittal plane of the fetal head to that of the coronal planes of the symphysis pubis and the sacral promontory. Usually the planes are not parallel and a slight degree of asynclitism is the normal. Significant asynclitism occurs with relative cephalo-pelvic disproportion, as the fetal head rocks on entering the pelvis in an attempt to make progress. If the tilt of the sagittal plane is directed towards the symphysis pubis, then more of the posterior aspect of the fetus' head is felt vaginally during examination; this is called posterior asynclitism. Anterior asynclitism occurs if more of the anterior part of the fetal head is felt on examination.

Abdominal palpation using the described manoeuvres can be performed throughout the latter months of pregnancy and during and between the labour contractions. On completion of a clinical examination it is usual to describe, in order: the symphysio-fundal height; fetal lie; presentation; and engagement. The fetal heart should be auscultated.

Pelvic Examination

Pelvic examination during pregnancy is used to detect a number of clinical conditions such as anatomical abnormalities, to evaluate the size of a woman's pelvis (pelvimetry) and to assess the uterine cervix, but it must be avoided when there is any suspicion of placenta praevia. A sterile speculum examination, allowing visual inspection, is indicated in cases of preterm labour, vaginal bleeding and suspected rupture of membranes. In addition, samples could be obtained for bacteriological tests when indicated.

Clinical Pelvimetry

Assessment of the size of a woman's pelvis (pelvimetry) can be achieved by clinical examination where the bony pelvis is digitally examined to identify prominent structures that may cause obstructed labour. The aim of pelvimetry in women whose fetuses have a cephalic presentation is to detect the possibility of cephalo-pelvic disproportion and therefore the need for caesarean section before or during labour. Other imaging techniques like X-rays, computerized tomography (CT) scanning or magnetic resonance imaging (MRI) are also used to assess the size of the pelvis. One should keep in mind that the dimensions of the pelvis and of the fetal head will change with the dynamic of labour.

During the clinical assessment, the diagonal conjugate is obtained by placing the tip of the middle finger at the sacral promontory and measuring to the point on the hand that contacts the symphysis. This is the closest clinical estimate of the obstetric conjugate and is 1.5–2.0 cm longer than the obstetric conjugate. The bi-ischial diameter is the distance between the ischial tuberosities, with a distance greater than 8 cm considered adequate. Other qualitative pelvic characteristics

Table 1.1 Bishop's score

	0	1	2	4
Dilatation of cervix (cm)	0	1–2	3–4	5+
Length of cervix (cm)	3	2	1	0
Station of vertex	–3	–2	–1,0	+1,+2
Cervical consistency	Firm	Medium	Soft	
Position	Posterior	Mid	Anterior	

include angulation of the pubic arch (more than 90° or accepts more than two fingers), prominence of the ischial spines, size of the sacrospinous notch (assessed by the sacrospinous ligament at more than three finger breadths) and curvature of the sacrum and coccyx (not being straight).

Clinical pelvimetry is not routinely practised in all pregnant women with cephalic presentation, but it is considered a useful tool in certain circumstances.

Cervical Assessment

Cervical assessment with a sterile speculum and digital vaginal examination allows the examiner to visually inspect the cervix, obtain samples for bacteriological tests and to assess certain factors of the cervix called Bishop's score (Table 1.1).

During the digital vaginal examination it is customary to start with an assessment of the effacement or cervical length, dilatation, consistency, position and the presentation and station of the presenting part relative to the ischial spines. In the 1960s Dr Edward Bishop developed a pelvic scoring system using these components, which remains the most commonly used system to assess for pre-induction readiness [23].

Currently even a simplified Bishop's score comprising dilatation, station and effacement attains a similarly high predictive ability of successful induction as the original score [24].

Cervical Effacement

The normal prelabour cervical length is 3–4 cm. The cervix is said to be 50% effaced when it shortens to approximately 2 cm, and fully effaced when there is no length and it is as thin as the adjacent lower segment of the uterus. Effacement is determined by assessing the length of the cervix from the external to the internal os. Complete cervical effacement is associated with a characteristic and profound alteration in the gene expression profile of cervical cells. The majority of these genes encode cytokines, transcription factors and cell-matrix-associated proteins [25].

The process of cervical effacement and dilatation differs between primigravida and multiparous patients. In the latter, effacement and dilatation occurs simultaneously, while in the case of primigravidae, effacement precedes dilatation.

Cervical Dilatation

During labour the cervix dilates progressively and the primary factors leading to cervical dilatation are the traction forces of the myometrial contractions, and the pressure of the fetal head or the presenting part on the cervix. From full effacement and 4 cm dilatation to full dilatation or 10 cm, the cervix usually dilates at a rate of 1 cm per hour.

Cervical Position

Cervical position describes the location of the cervix in relation to the maternal pelvis. During labour, the position progresses from posterior to mid-position and then to anterior.

Cervical Consistency

Cervical consistency ranges from firm to soft. Cervical softening during pregnancy is a unique phase of the tissue remodelling process characterized by increased collagen solubility, maintenance of tissue strength and up-regulation of genes involved in mucosal protection [26]. During this process, the junction between the fetal membranes and the decidua breaks down, and an adhesive protein – fetal fibronectin – enters vaginal fluids. This is a clinically useful predictor of imminent delivery [14].

The Station

The station of the presenting part describes the distance of the leading bony part of the fetal head relative to the ischial spines. The usual method is to measure the distance above and below the spines in centimetres, with the areas above being given a minus sign and those below the spines being given a positive sign. For example, '0' indicates that the lowest part of the fetal head is at the level of the ischial spines, while '+1' indicates that the head is 1 cm below the level of the spines (Figure 1.9).

Identifying the position of the presenting part is accomplished by identifying the bony sutures of the fetal head, following the suture until it leads to a fontanelle and then identifying the sutures radiating

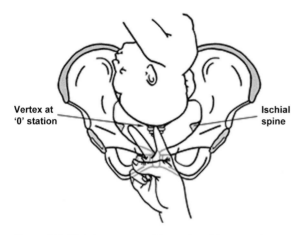

Figure 1.9 Clinical assessment of the station of the presenting part.

from it. Provided the head is low and the patient has good pain relief, it may also be possible to locate the ear of the fetus and to assess to which side it faces. The nose and mouth can usually be identified in a face presentation, while the sacrum, genitalia and anus should be identifiable with a breech presentation.

At the end of the examination the following should be described and noted: inspection of vulva and vagina to ascertain/establish the presence or absence of any liquor, blood or discharge; and palpation of the cervix to establish its length, thickness and position (anterior, mid-position or posterior).

In the active stage of labour, the clinician assesses the progress of cervical dilatation, and effacement, the station and position of the presenting part and whether there is any asynclitism, caput succedaneum and moulding.

Stages and Duration of Normal Labour

Although labour is a continuous process, it is divided into three stages to facilitate monitoring and to assist in clinical management.

First Stage

The *first stage* is said to begin with the onset of regular painful uterine contractions resulting in cervical changes, and ends when the cervix is fully dilated at 10 cm. It has been further subdivided into latent and active phases according to the rates of cervical dilatation [27].

The *latent phase* is defined as the period of time, not necessarily continuous, when there may be painful

contractions as well as cervical change, including cervical effacement and with cervical dilatation up to 4 cm. It is characterized by slow cervical dilatation and is of variable duration. The established, *active phase* of labour begins when there are regular painful contractions and there is progressive cervical dilatation from full effacement and 4 cm dilatation onwards. The length of the labour duration or curve does not differ among ethnic or racial groups, but there are significant differences between nulliparous and multiparous women [28]. The length of the active first stage of labour in nulliparous women is on average 8 hours and is unlikely to be over 18 hours. Second and subsequent labours last on average 5 hours and are unlikely to last more than 12 hours [29].

By comparing a labouring woman's rate of cervical dilatation with the normal profile described by Friedman, it is possible to detect abnormal labour patterns and identify pregnancies at risk for adverse events. This task can be facilitated by use of a partogram, which is a graphic representation of the labour curve against which a patient's progress in labour is plotted. In this way, abnormal labour patterns can be identified easily and appropriate measures taken.

Second Stage

The *second stage* starts when the cervix is fully dilated at 10 cm and is characterized by descent of the presenting part through the maternal pelvis. It ends with the delivery of the fetus. It is characterized by an increase in bloody show, maternal desire to bear down with each contraction and a feeling of pressure on the rectum accompanied by the desire to defecate.

The safe duration desirable for the second stage in the presence of an uncompromised fetus for a nulliparous patient without regional anaesthesia is said to be two hours (three hours with regional anaesthesia). For a multiparous woman the recommendation is one hour and two hours, respectively [29].

Third Stage

The third stage of labour refers to the time from delivery of the fetus to separation and expulsion of the placenta and fetal membranes. It is characterized by signs of placental separation, namely lengthening of the umbilical cord, a gush of blood from the vagina, which signifies separation of the placenta from the uterine wall, and a change in the shape of the uterine fundus from discoid to globular, with elevation of the fundal height (and lengthening of the umbilical cord at the vaginal introitus).

Though there are no uniform criteria for the normal length of the third stage of labour, it is diagnosed as prolonged if not completed within 30 minutes of the birth of the baby with active management, and 60 minutes with physiological management [29].

Mechanism of Labour

During the passages of the fetal head through the bony pelvis or birth canal, it adopts a series of changes which are traditionally described as *cardinal movements* which culminates with the delivery of the fetal head. Because of asymmetry in the shape of the fetal head and the maternal bony pelvis, such movements are required if the fetus is to negotiate the birth canal successfully. At least seven discrete movements are worth considering and they are engagement, descent, flexion, internal rotation, extension, external rotation or restitution, and expulsion.

This is followed by the delivery of the shoulders and the body of the fetus.

Engagement

Engagement occurs when the fetal head is engaged, i.e. when its maximum diameters (suboccipito-bregmatic and biparietal, when the head is well flexed) have passed the pelvic inlet. On engagement, the biparietal diameter lies at the level of the true conjugate and the vertex is 1 cm above the ischial spines. In the breech presentation, the widest diameter is the bi-trochanteric diameter. Engagement can be confirmed clinically by palpation of the presenting part abdominally when only two-fifths of the head can be palpated abdominally or vaginally, with confirmation of station at or below the ischial spines. Parity, maternal age, height and birth weight of fetus play a significant role in determining the time at which the fetal head engages, and need to be considered when assessing a patient [20].

Descent

This is the downward movement of the fetal head or the presenting part in the pelvis. Descent is usually described by the number of fifths of the presenting part still palpable above the pelvis, and by the station (the relative position of the presenting part to the ischial spines).

Descent of the fetus is not a steady, continuous process and usually starts in the late first stage and continues through the second stage. Descent is usually brought about by uterine contractions and is aided in the second stage of labour by maternal bearing down effort.

Flexion

Flexion of the fetal head initially occurs passively as the head descends. This is facilitated by the shape of the bony pelvis and the resistance of the lower segment of the uterus, the pelvic sidewalls and pelvic floor. Although some degree of flexion is present in most fetuses antepartum, complete flexion usually occurs during the course of labour as the uterus contracts. With the head completely flexed, the fetal chin coming into contact with the fetal chest, it presents the smallest diameter of its head (suboccipito-bregmatic diameter), which allows optimal passage through the birth canal.

Internal Rotation

Internal rotation is the rotation of the fetal head from its usual transverse position to the AP position as it passes through the pelvis.

This typically in more than 95% of term labours results in the fetal occiput rotating towards the symphysis pubis as it descends, which leads to the widest axis of the fetal head lining up with the widest axis of the pelvic passage. The fetal head initially descends in an asynclitic fashion, but it typically corrects itself as the head descends further (due to the curvature of the maternal sacrum). As with flexion, internal rotation is a passive movement that results from the shape of the pelvis and the resistance of the pelvic floor musculature.

Extension

As the fetal head descends to the level of the pelvic outlet, the base of the occiput will come into contact with the inferior margin of the symphysis pubis where the birth canal curves upward and forward. The head is delivered through the maternal vaginal introitus by extension from the flexed position. First to deliver is the occiput, then with further extension the vertex, bregma, forehead, nose, mouth and finally the chin.

The forces responsible for this motion are the downward force exerted on the fetus by uterine contractions and maternal expulsive efforts, along with the upward forces exerted by the muscles of the pelvic floor.

External Rotation (Restitution)

Having delivered with the sagittal suture vertical (AP) and the occiput anterior, the delivered fetal head returns to the position it occupied in the vagina. For example, if the position was left occipito-anterior (LOA), the head will 'restitute' to the left. This is followed by complete rotation of the sagittal suture to the transverse position so that the shoulders align in the antero-posterior diameter of the pelvic outlet, so facilitating their passage (i.e. one shoulder will lie behind the symphysis pubis, the other will be posterior, in front of the sacral promontory). This is again a passive movement that results from a release of the forces exerted on the fetal head by the maternal bony pelvis and its musculature, and it is mediated by the basal tone of the fetal musculature.

Expulsion

Expulsion refers to delivery of the body of the fetus. After delivery of the head and external rotation (restitution), further descent brings the anterior shoulder to the level of the symphysis pubis. The anterior shoulder rotates under the symphysis pubis, after which the rest of the body usually delivers without difficulty.

Maternal Pushing in Labour

Though the cardinal movements are largely the result of uterine contractions, the passive action of the pelvic musculature and the descending fetal head, maternal pushing, especially during the second stage, is practised frequently. This practice is said to facilitate or speed delivery, though its contribution to increasing the intrauterine pressure is said to be small even under optimal conditions [30]. The clinical significance of shortening of the duration of the second stage of labour is uncertain with active pushing, but supporting spontaneous pushing and encouraging women to choose their own method of pushing should be accepted as best clinical practice [31].

References

1. Jukic AM, Baird DD, Weinberg CR, McConnaughey DR, Wilcox AJ. Length of human pregnancy and contributors to its natural variation. *Hum Reprod.* 2013;28(10): 2848–55.

2. Lovejoy CO.The natural history of human gait and posture in Part 1: spine and pelvis. *Gait and Posture.* 2005;21: 95–112.

3. Mac-Thiong JM, Berthonnaud E, Dimar JR II, Bets RR, Labelle H. Sagittal alignment of the spine and pelvis during growth. *Spine.* 2004;29: 1642–7.

4. Caldwell WE, Moloy HC. Anatomical variation in the female pelvis and their effect in labor with a suggested classification. *Am J Obstet Gynecol.* 1933;26: 479–505.

5. Rosenberg K, Trevathan W. Birth, obstetrics and human evolution. *BJOG.* 2002;109: 1199–206

6. Pu F, Xu L, Li D, *et al.* Effect of different labour forces on fetal skull moulding. *Med Eng Phys.* 2011;33(5): 620–5.

7. Royal College of Obstetricians and Gynaecologists. Operative vaginal delivery. *Green-top Guideline No. 26.* London: RCOG Press; 2011.

8. Shynlova O, Kwong R, Lye SJ. Mechanical stretch regulates hypertrophic phenotype of the myometrium during pregnancy. *Reproduction.* 2010;139(1): 247–53.

9. Osol G, Moore LG. Maternal uterine vascular remodeling during pregnancy. *Microcirculation.* 2014;21(1): 38–47.

10. Palmer SK, Zamudio S, Coffin C, *et al.* Quantitative estimation of human uterine artery blood flow and pelvic blood flow redistribution in pregnancy. *Obstet Gynecol.* 1992;80: 1000–6.

11. Word RA, Stull JT, Casey ML, Kamm KE. Contractile elements and myosin light chain phosphorylation in myometrial tissue from nonpregnant and pregnant women. *J Clin Invest.* 1993;92(1): 29–37.

12. Hicks JB. On the contractions of the uterus throughout pregnancy: their physiological effects and their value in the diagnosis of pregnancy. *Transactions of the Obstetrical Society of London.* 1871;13: 216–31.

13. McLean M, Bisits A, Davies J, *et al.* A placental clock controlling the length of human pregnancy. *Nat Med.* 1995;1: 460–3.

14. Smith R. Parturition. *N Eng J Med.* 2007;356: 271–83.

15. Moore S, Ide M, Randhawa M, *et al.* An investigation into the association among preterm birth, cytokine gene polymorphisms and periodontal disease. *BJOG.* 2004;111: 125–32.

16. Mendelson CR. Fetal–maternal hormonal signalling in pregnancy and labour. *Mol Endocrinol.* 2009;23: 947–54.

17. Royal College of Obstetricians and Gynaecologists. Small-for-gestational-age fetus, investigation and

management. *Green-top Guideline No. 31*. London: RCOG Press; 2002.

18. Morse K, Williams A, Gardosi J. Fetal growth screening by fundal height measurement. *Best Pract Res Clin Obstet Gynaecol*. 23;2009: 809–18.

19. Weekes ARL, Flynn MJ. Engagement of the fetal head in primigravidae and its relationship to duration of gestation and time of onset to labour. *Br J Obstet Gynaecol*. 1975;82: 7–11.

20. Muhunthan K, Abarna K, Peratheepa V, Shampika R. A descriptive study on relationship between engagement of fetal head and selected maternal and fetal parameters among pregnancies in University Obstetric Unit, Teaching Hospital, Jaffna. FIGO-SAFOG-SLCOG scientific conference. *Sri Lanka J Obstet Gynaecol*. 2014;36(suppl. 1): 20–1.

21. Ann AFR. Predictors of vaginal delivery in nulliparous mothers. *Med*. 2014;13(1): 35–40. doi: 10.4103/1596-3519.126949.

22. Hankins GD, Hammond TL, Snyder RR, Gilstrap LC III. Transverse lie. *Am J Perinatol*. 1990;7: 66–70.

23. Baacke KA, Edwards RK. Preinduction cervical assessment. *Clin Obstet Gynecol*. 2006;49: 564–72.

24. Katherine Laughon S, Zhang J, Troendle J, Sun L, Reddy UM. Using a simplified Bishop score to predict vaginal delivery. *Obstet Gynecol*. 2011;117(4): 805–11.

25. Huber A, Hudelist G, Czerwenka K, *et al*. Gene expression profiling of cervical tissue during physiological cervical effacement. *Obstet Gynecol*. 2005;105: 91–8.

26. Read CP, Word RA, Ruscheinsky MA, Timmons BC, Mahendroo MS. Cervical remodeling during pregnancy and parturition: molecular characterization of the softening phase in mice. *Reproduction*. 2007;134: 327–40.

27. Friedman E. The graphic analysis of labor. *Am J Obstet Gynecol*. 1954;68(6): 1568–75.

28. Duignan NM, Studd JW, Hughes AO. Characteristics of normal labour in different racial groups. *Br J Obstet Gynaecol*. 1975;82(8): 593–601.

29. National Institute for Health and Clinical Excellence. *Intrapartum Care: Care of Healthy Women and their Babies during Childbirth*. London: NICE; 2007.

30. Buhimschi CS, Buhimschi IA, Malinow AM, *et al*. Pushing in labor: performance and not endurance. *Am J Obstet Gynecol*. 2002;186(6): 1339–44.

31. Prins M, Boxem J, Lucas C, Huttona E. Effect of spontaneous pushing versus Valsalva pushing in the second stage of labour on mother and fetus: a systematic review of randomized trials. *BJOG*. 2011;118(6): 662–70.

The First Stage of Labour

Daisy Nirmal and **David Fraser**

The perils of prolonged and often neglected labour are well known. In the developing world where there is often a lack of appropriate healthcare both in terms of provision and access, the morbidity and mortality from prolonged and neglected labour is alarming. The causes of death and morbidity include obstructed labour, sepsis, rupture of the uterus and postpartum haemorrhage. In the developed world this is extremely rare. The increasing caesarean section (CS) rate for dystocia or difficult labour contributes at least one-third to the overall CS rate, and almost 70% of those women who have a CS in their first labour will request an elective CS in subsequent pregnancies [1]. CS leads to increased maternal morbidity as well as mortality, especially when it is performed as an emergency procedure [2,3]. Furthermore, long-term risks of CS have been reported, including an increased risk of placenta praevia and ectopic pregnancy [4]. Maternal and fetal morbidity and mortality due to prolonged labour and CS for dystocia may be reduced by the proper management of poor progress in labour – especially the first labour. Care during labour should be aimed towards achieving the best possible physical, emotional and psychological outcome for the woman and baby [5].

This chapter discusses some of the physiological events of the first stage of labour and the way in which labour progress is measured, and also reviews measures that may be considered when progress in the first stage of labour is suboptimal.

Normal Labour

The precise definition of normal labour is the spontaneous onset of regular, painful uterine contractions associated with the effacement and progressive dilatation of the cervix and descent of the presenting part – with or without a 'show' or ruptured membranes. This process culminates in the birth of a healthy baby followed by expulsion of the placenta and membranes. In most cases, the outcome can be predicted prospectively by observing the progress of cervical dilatation and descent of the presenting part. Although labour is a dynamic, continuous process, it is normally divided into three functional stages for the purpose of management: the first, second and third stages of labour. Definition of the stages of labour need to be clear in order to ensure that women and the staff attending them have an accurate and shared understanding of the concepts involved, enabling them to communicate effectively.

The basis for the scientific study of the progress of labour was developed by Friedman [6]. He described the labour progress of 100 consecutive primigravid women in spontaneous labour at term. The progress was presented graphically by plotting the rate of cervical dilatation against time. The resulting graph of cervical dilatation forms the basis of the modern partogram – a pictorial representation of the key events in labour presented chronologically on a single page. The maternal and fetal parameters recorded include cervical dilatation, the level of the presenting part (in fifths of the fetal head palpable above the pelvic brim, rather than the station, which relates the level of the head to the ischial spines and is measured in centimetres above or below), the fetal heart rate (FHR), the frequency and duration of uterine contractions and the character of amniotic fluid. Other maternal parameters include temperature, pulse and blood pressure, and any drugs used in the labour. This pictorial documentation of labour facilitates the early recognition of poor progress. Plotting of the cervical dilatation at regular intervals also enables prediction of the time of onset of the second stage of labour.

Best Practice in Labour and Delivery, Second Edition, ed. Sir Sabaratnam Arulkumaran. Published by Cambridge University Press. © Cambridge University Press 2016.

Table 2.1 Summary table showing ranges for duration of stages of labour

	Lower value	Upper value
Nulliparous		
Latent phase	1.7 hours	15.0 hours
Active first stage	1.0 hours	19.4 hours
Parous		
Latent phase	Not studied	Not studied
Active first stage	0.5 hours	14.9 hours

Nomograms of Cervical Dilatation

The rate of cervical dilatation in labour has been studied in various ethnic groups in different countries. The nomograms derived show similar rates of cervical dilatation in the different ethnic groups, and comparative studies have confirmed that ethnicity has little influence on the rate of cervical dilatation or on uterine activity in spontaneous normal labour [7–12].

Observations during the first stage of labour show that the rate of cervical dilatation is composed of two phases: the 'latent' phase and the active or 'established' phase [5]:

- The 'latent' phase of the first stage of labour is defined as a period of time, not necessarily continuous, when:
  - there are painful contractions; *and*
  - there is some cervical change, including cervical effacement and dilatation up to 4 cm.
- The established first stage of labour when:
  - there are regular painful contractions; *and*
  - there is progressive cervical dilatation from 4 cm.

The first stage of labour ends at full cervical dilatation and although this is conventionally taken as 10 cm, in reality it refers to a situation when no cervix is palpable.

Pooled findings from a number of studies suggests that the range of upper limits for the duration of a normal first stage of labour are as follows: women giving birth to their first babies 8.2–19.4 hours; women giving birth to second or subsequent babies 12.5–14.9 hours (see Table 2.1) [5]. However, these figures have been challenged, and recent publications suggest that duration of spontaneous labour has increased over the last 15 years [13,14].

In order to identify women at risk of prolonged labour, a line of acceptable progress is drawn on the partogram; this is referred to as the 'alert line'. If the rate of cervical dilatation falls to the right of this line, progress is deemed unsatisfactory. Conventionally, the line of acceptable progress has been based on the slowest tenth percentile rate of cervical dilatation observed in women who progress without intervention and deliver normally; in other words, 1 cm per hour. However, a certain grace period is given before intervention and is based on a line drawn parallel and 1–4 hours to the right of this – 'the action line'. Construction of nomograms of anticipated normal progress or 'alert' lines, with the addition of 'action' lines to the right of this, reduces the likelihood of prolonged labour being overlooked, and is of considerable diagnostic and educational value (Figure 2.1). Studies looking at the efficacy of the use of the partogram, and comparison of a partogram with an action line and one without, should be carried out. Accordingly, the proportion of labours deemed to have unsatisfactory progress can vary from 5% to 50%. The World Health Organization (WHO) [15] and, more recently, the National Institute of Health and Care Excellence (NICE) recommend the use of a four-hour action line [5]. Studies using a two-hour action line seem to increase women's satisfaction without any difference in intervention rates [5].

During the peak of the active phase of labour, the cervix dilates at a rate of 1 cm per hour in both nulliparas and multiparas. Multiparas appear to dilate faster because they have shorter labours overall; not only do they seem to have a shorter latent phase resulting in a more advanced cervical dilatation on admission, they also have an increased rate of progress as full dilatation approaches.

More recent data have challenged the definition of contemporary normal labour progress [14]. In this retrospective study conducted at 19 US hospitals, the duration of labour was analysed in 62 415 parturient women, each of whom delivered a singleton vertex fetus vaginally and had a normal perinatal outcome. In this study, the 95th percentile rate of active phase dilatation was substantially slower than the standard rate derived from Friedman's work, varying from 0.5 cm/h to 0.7 cm/h for nulliparous women and from 0.5 cm/h to 1.3 cm/h for multiparous women.

The Consortium on Safe Labor data highlights two important features of contemporary labour progress. First, from 4–6 cm, nulliparous and multiparous women dilated at essentially the same rate, and more

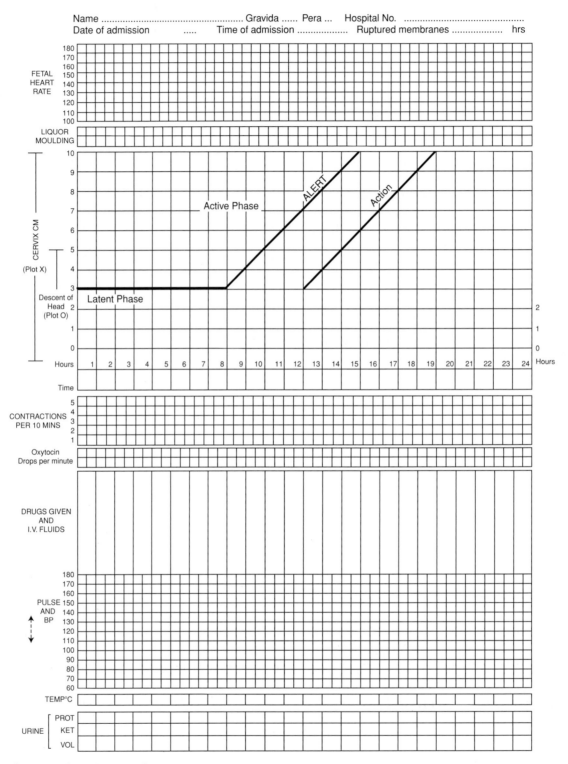

Figure 2.1 The WHO partograph.

Table 2.2 Differences between true and false labour

True labour	False labour
1. Contractions occur at regular intervals	Contractions occur at irregular intervals
2. Interval gradually shortens	Interval remains irregular
3. Intensity of pain gradually increases	Intensity of pain remains the same
4. Duration of contractions increases	Duration of contractions varies and tends to become less
5. There is progressive cervical effacement and dilatation	There is no progress in cervical effacement and dilatation
6. Progress of labour not stopped by sedation	Usually painful contractions are relieved by sedation and there is no progress in labour

slowly than historically described. Beyond 6 cm, multiparous women dilated more rapidly. Second, the maximal slope in the rate of change of cervical dilatation over time (i.e. the active phase) often did not start until at least 6 cm. The Consortium on Safe Labor data do not directly address an optimal duration for the diagnosis of active phase protraction or labour arrest, but do suggest that neither should be diagnosed before 6 cm of dilatation.

These findings may indicate that the labour process in contemporary obstetric populations may need to be re-evaluated and the definitions of normal and abnormal labour needs to be re-examined.

Diagnosis of Labour

The accurate diagnosis of labour at term may be difficult – and can be even more difficult in those labouring in the preterm period. If the contractions are painful and regular and if the cervix is >4 cm dilated (in other words, in the active phase), there is little difficulty in diagnosing labour. However, if the patient is in the latent phase of labour, it may be necessary to perform two examinations at least two hours apart (and preferably done by the same examiner) in order to detect any progressive cervical change and diagnose labour. Uterine contractions without effacement and dilatation of the cervix occur in the third trimester. They are usually termed Braxton Hicks contractions and are usually painless. These contractions may become more frequent and painful without affecting cervical changes of effacement and dilatation, and may abate spontaneously. Differentiating points between false and true labour are shown in Table 2.2.

Management of the First Stage of Labour

Good antecedents for 'natural' or 'physiological' labour and childbirth are antepartum education that eliminates fears and anxieties about labour, regular exercise to promote relaxation, muscle control and breathing without hyperventilation throughout labour. In addition, the importance of the 1:1 attention of a skilled professional attendant throughout labour to comfort the mother and give her constant reassurance has been shown to promote normal labour and good outcome.

The general principles of management are:

- initial assessment;
- observation and intervention if labour becomes abnormal;
- close monitoring of the fetal and maternal condition;
- adequate pain relief;
- emotional support; and
- adequate hydration.

Initial Assessment

On admission, eliciting a detailed history, listening to the woman and taking into account her emotional and psychological needs, should be followed by clinical examination and basic investigation. The aim is to identify high-risk pregnancies – a proportion being identified as high-risk before the onset of labour and others being identified as at-risk only at the onset, or during, labour [5].

Observations of the woman:

- Review the antenatal notes and discuss these with the woman.
- Ask her about the length, strength and frequency of her contractions.
- Ask her about any pain she is experiencing and discuss her options for pain relief.
- Record her pulse, blood pressure and temperature, and carry out urinalysis.
- Record whether she has had any vaginal loss.

Observations of the unborn baby:

- Ask the woman about the baby's movements in the last 24 hours.
- Palpate the woman's abdomen to determine the fundal height, the baby's lie, presentation, position and engagement of the presenting part, and frequency and duration of contractions.
- Auscultate the fetal heart rate for a minimum of 1 min immediately after a contraction. Palpate the woman's pulse to differentiate between the heart rates of the woman and the baby.
- Offer a vaginal examination if the woman appears to be in established labour.

General Examination

This should include the general condition of the woman and checking whether she has pallor or jaundice, the state of hydration, her blood pressure, temperature and respiratory rate. The cardiovascular status should also be assessed and any oedema noted. The frequency of bladder emptying and urinary output should be noted. In some care settings these observations may be used to ascribe a Modified Early Obstetric Warning Score (MEOWS) and used as an aid to subsequent management.

Abdominal Examination

Uterine contractions should be assessed by palpation, with relevance to their frequency and duration (every 30 min), and assessed over a 10 min period (Figure 2.2). The fundal height should be measured to identify

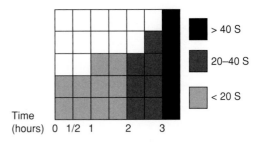

Figure 2.2 Quantification of uterine contractions by clinical palpation. Frequency per 10 min is recorded by shading the equivalent number of boxes. The type of shading indicates the duration of each contraction.

babies felt to be significantly above or below the average birth weight, and the level of the presenting part should be noted. The level of the head should be estimated in 'fifths' (Figure 2.3) – clinical estimation of descent of the head in fifths excludes variation due to excessive caput and moulding and that produced by different depths of pelvis. It is easily reproducible. The fetal heart rate should be auscultated after a contraction for a minimum period of l min, and at least every 15 min in the first stage of labour and every 5 min in the second stage. Auscultate the fetal heart rate for a minimum of 1 min immediately after a contraction and record it as a single rate [5].

Vaginal Examination

When conducting a vaginal examination:

- Be sure that the examination is necessary and will add important information to the decision-making process.

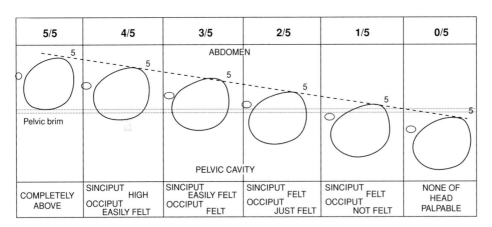

Figure 2.3 Clinical estimation of descent of head in fifths palpable above the pelvic brim.

- Recognize that a vaginal examination can be very distressing for a woman, especially if she is already in pain, highly anxious and in an unfamiliar environment.
- Explain the reason for the examination and what will be involved.
- Ensure the woman's informed consent, privacy, dignity and comfort.
- Explain sensitively the findings of the examination and any impact on the birth plan to the woman and her birth companions [5].

Tap water may be used if cleansing is required before vaginal examination. The following points should be noted during vaginal examination:

- any abnormal discharge from the vagina;
- the colour and quantity of any amniotic fluid and whether it is clear, blood-stained or contains meconium;
- the consistency, position, effacement and dilatation of the cervix;
- the presenting part in relation to the ischial spines, caput and moulding of the head; and
- the bony pelvis should be assessed with regard to its adequacy for childbirth.

Investigations

The urine should be examined for protein, ketones and sugar. Commercial dipsticks will also test for leukocytes, nitrites and blood – their presence may signify a urinary tract infection.

Oral intake is often restricted in labour to reduce the risk of gastric aspiration and Mendelson's syndrome should general anaesthesia be required. Women may drink during established labour, and isotonic drinks may be more beneficial than water [5]. The details of nutrition and hydration in labour are discussed in Chapter 7.

When rehydration is necessary in labour, it is best to give normal saline or Hartmann's solution, to maintain a more physiological fluid and electrolyte balance. This may also help to avoid water intoxication if intravenous oxytocin is used over a long period in high doses.

Observations During the Established First Stage of Labour

In most care settings it is usual practice to carry out a number of maternal and fetal observations during the first stage of labour, to detect changes in maternal or fetal health. These observations can provide an important overview of how the woman is progressing during labour and what her needs are over time. These observations should be recorded on the partogram.

The following observations should be recorded during the established first stage of labour:

- half-hourly documentation of frequency of contractions;
- hourly pulse;
- four-hourly temperature and blood pressure; and
- frequency of bladder emptying.

Offer vaginal examination four-hourly or if there is concern about progress or in response to the woman's wishes.

Mobility and Posture in Labour

It is preferable not to confine the mother to bed in early labour. She may prefer ambulation or sitting in a chair. The upright posture may increase the pelvic diameters and assist in the descent of the fetal head. Although many women prefer to be ambulatory early in labour, few remain upright for long, and they may wish to sit or adopt a reclining, lateral recumbent position or lie down as labour progresses. The dorsal position may cause aorta-caval compression and should be discouraged. The actual position the mother chooses does not appear to influence labour outcomes, and hence the mother should be encouraged and helped to adopt whatever positions she finds most comfortable throughout labour [5].

Use of Analgesia and Anaesthesia

Women should be offered support and encouraged to ask for analgesia at any point during labour. Non-pharmacological measures like labouring in water, supporting women's use of breathing/relaxation techniques, massage and music should be considered. In the UK, the four most widely used forms of pain relief for labour are transcutaneous electrical nerve stimulation (TENS), nitrous oxide (Entonox), intramuscular narcotics (e.g. Pethidine, diamorphine) and epidural analgesia. TENS may not be effective in women in well-established labour [5].

A more detailed discussion of analgesia in labour is found in Chapter 3.

Meconium

Between 15% and 20% of term pregnancies are associated with meconium staining of the amniotic fluid (MSAF), which is not a cause for concern in the vast majority of labours. Meconium may be demonstrated in the fetal gut in the first trimester, but in utero passage is rare before 34 weeks. Meconium passage usually reflects fetal gut maturity, so frequency of MSAF increases with gestation. However, the passage of meconium in labour may have a more sinister explanation. An association between meconium passage in utero and poor neonatal outcome was recorded by Aristotle. Meconium aspiration can occur with intrauterine gasping or when the baby takes its first breath, and accounts for 2% of perinatal deaths.

As part of ongoing assessment in the first stage of labour, the presence or absence of significant meconium should be documented. Significant meconium has been defined as dark green or black amniotic fluid that is thick or tenacious, or any meconium-stained amniotic fluid containing lumps of meconium [5].

The appearance of fresh meconium in labour should prompt evaluation of fetal well-being. Continuous electronic fetal monitoring should be instituted. Fetal scalp blood sampling should be considered in the presence of fetal heart rate abnormalities. This is particularly true for thick meconium, since this implies that there is little liquor to dilute the meconium, and this itself may indicate placental problems before the onset of labour. Thin meconium, on the other hand, is thin because it has been diluted with an adequate volume of liquor.

In the presence of a normal fetal heart rate, MSAF is not an indication for immediate delivery or fetal blood sampling, especially if it is thin staining. However, if the heart rate becomes abnormal in association with thick fresh meconium, early delivery should be considered, particularly in high-risk pregnancies.

Finally, if significant meconium is present in labour, healthcare professionals trained in neonatal life support should, ideally, be available for the birth [5].

Diagnosis of Poor Progress of Labour

Progress in labour is confirmed by observing the progressive effacement and dilatation of the cervix and the descent of the presenting part.

The use of a partogram for the management of labour facilitates the early detection of abnormal labour progress and identifies those women most likely to require intervention. This can be used at all levels of obstetric care by basic care providers who have been trained to assess cervical dilatation. When used properly, it helps to detect abnormal labour progress promptly, allowing timely intervention. In a WHO multi-centre trial in Southeast Asia involving over 35 000 women, the introduction of the partograph as part of an agreed labour management protocol was associated with a reduction in prolonged labour from 6.4% to 3.4%, and the proportion of labours requiring augmentation reduced from 20.7% to 9.1%. The caesarean section rates also fell from 9.9% to 8.3% and intrapartum stillbirths from 0.5% to 0.3%. There were also improvements in fetal and maternal mortality and morbidity in both nulliparous and multiparous women [15].

The term 'dystocia' or difficult labour refers to poor progress of labour and is diagnosed when the rate of cervical dilatation is slower than anticipated. When a woman is admitted in the active phase of labour, the cervical dilatation can be plotted on the partogram and an expected progress or alert line can be constructed, usually corresponding to 1 cm per hour. Another line, the action line, can be added 4 h to the right of the alert line, and parallel to it [5,11].

The outcome of spontaneous labours has been studied and three distinct patterns of abnormal progress described [16–19]. These are:

1. prolonged latent phase;
2. primary dysfunctional labour; and
3. secondary arrest of cervical dilatation.

The duration of latent phase is difficult to define. It is considered prolonged if it is greater than 15 h in a nullipara. The latent phase in parous patients has not been studied in detail [5], therefore no such figure exists for multiparas. Once established in the active phase of labour, primary dysfunctional labour is diagnosed when the progress falls to the right of the nomogram. If labour progresses normally in the early active phase but the cervix fails to dilate or dilates slowly thereafter, secondary arrest of cervical dilatation is diagnosed (Figure 2.4). More than one of these abnormal labour patterns may occur in the same patient, since they frequently share a common aetiology.

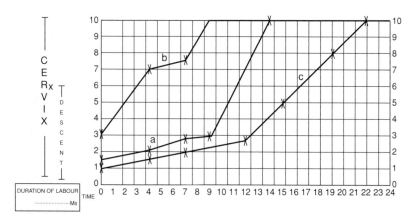

Figure 2.4 Various forms of dysfunctional labour: (a) prolonged latent phase, (b) secondary arrest of labour, (c) prolonged latent phase and primary dysfunctional labour.

The use of the partogram with the anticipated progress line for an individual patient annotated allows the prompt recognition of abnormal cervical progress. The descent of the presenting part as the proportion of the presenting part (expressed as fifths) palpable abdominally is also an integral component of the partogram, and it too is plotted at each review. A poor rate of descent may also be an indication of developing mechanical problems in the labour. If delay in the established first stage is suspected, take the following into account:

- parity;
- cervical dilatation and rate of change;
- uterine contractions;
- station and position of presenting part; and
- the woman's emotional state.

Poor progress has conventionally been related to the three 'P's, namely:

1. powers – adequacy of the uterine contractions;
2. passages – resistance of the birth canal;
3. passenger – relating to the size, position, degree of flexion, etc. of the baby.

To these may be added a fourth 'P': poor obstetric practice. Poor progress in labour does not identify the specific cause (that is, fault with the powers, passage or passenger), since they are frequently interrelated.

Primary dysfunctional labour (PDL) is the commonest abnormality of the first stage of labour, occurring in up to 25% of spontaneous primigravid labours [16] and 8% of multiparas [17]. The commonest cause is inadequate uterine activity. Secondary arrest of cervical dilatation (SACD) is much less common than the above, said to affect 6% of nulliparas and only 2% of multiparas.

Although the commonest cause of SACD (especially in nulliparas) is still inefficient uterine activity, relative disproportion is far more likely to be the explanation than with PDL. Secondary arrest does not always indicate genuine cephalo-pelvic disproportion, as inadequate uterine contractions can be corrected, resulting in spontaneous vaginal delivery [18]. However, a diagnosis of secondary arrest (especially in a multiparous woman) should prompt a search for obvious problems in the passenger (for example, hydrocephalus, brow presentation, undiagnosed shoulder presentation, large baby, malposition) and the passages (for example, a congenitally small pelvis, a deformed pelvis due to fracture following an accident or masses in the pelvis). Unfavourable pelvic diameters are rarely a cause of cephalo-pelvic disproportion in the developed world. The fetus is more commonly the cause of relative disproportion by presenting a larger diameter of the vertex due to a malposition or deflexion, or both. In such cases, the dystocia may be overcome if the flexion and rotation to an occipito-anterior position can be encouraged by optimizing the efficiency of the uterine contractions.

Management Options: Augmentation Indications

Prolonged labour is associated with high rates of maternal infection, obstructed labour, uterine rupture and postpartum haemorrhage, which may end in maternal morbidity and rarely in mortality.

In many areas of the developing world it remains a common axiom 'not to allow the sun to set twice on a woman in labour' in order to prevent such tragic outcomes. In the early 1970s, Philpott and Castle in

Table 2.3 The key components of active management of labour

- Special antenatal classes to prepare women for labour
- Strict criteria for diagnosing labour
- Routine two-hourly vaginal examination
- Early amniotomy
- Early recourse to oxytocin
- A designated midwife in constant attendance and continuous one-to-one support during labour
- A guarantee that labour would last no longer than 12 h

Harare, Zimbabwe, O'Driscoll and his colleagues in Dublin and Studd in the UK all advocated and popularized the concept of one-to-one midwifery care, use of partogram and augmentation of labour with poor progress to reduce the incidence of prolonged labour. This package of obstetric interventions is frequently referred to as the 'active management of labour'.

The active management of labour was based on the principle of anticipating and identifying that there may be a problem and then taking action. Increasing the uterine power, which was the common problem, is one of the many components of the policy of active management. It also helped to overcome any borderline disproportion by promoting flexion, rotation and moulding in vertex presentation. Each component of the active management, i.e. one-to-one midwifery care, reassurance, pain relief, hydration and feto-maternal surveillance, is essential to prevent prolonged labour in the nulliparas and to reduce the CS rate (see Table 2.3).

However, randomized control studies suggest that active management of labour shortens the length of labour but does not affect the rate of CS or maternal or fetal morbidity [20,21]. There was no assessment of pain perceived by women or neonatal outcomes. Companionship in labour and continuity of care during pregnancy and childbirth is highly recommended. The entire package of active management of labour need not be offered routinely [5].

The decision to augment labour should be governed by the rate of cervical dilatation based on the partogram, after the exclusion of gross disproportion or malpresentation. Minor degrees of disproportion due to malposition and poor flexion of the head may be overcome by oxytocin infusion. More forceful uterine contractions cause flexion at the atlanto-occipital joint and reduce the presenting diameter. This allows rotation of the occiput from a posterior to an anterior position. The increased force of contraction helps moulding, i.e. the overlapping of skull bones over the suture lines, which helps to reduce the presenting diameter of the head. It may increase the pelvic dimensions due to the descending head distending the pelvis and widening the sacro-iliac and symphysis pubic joints. The parietal, occipital and frontal bones of the skull first come together (moulding +), followed by one parietal bone going under the other. The occipital and frontal bones traverse below the parietal bones. If gentle digital pressure is adequate to reduce the overlapping of the bones, it is recorded as moulding ++, and when digital pressure does not restore the overlapping bones to their original position, it is recorded as moulding +++. Caput is the soft tissue swelling caused by the oedema of the scalp that develops as the fetal head descends in the pelvis. The degree of caput increases in prolonged labour, although it is a less reliable sign of mechanical disproportion compared to moulding.

When to Augment Labour

The mechanical 'efficiency' of uterine contractions should be defined in terms of their clinical effect (that is, the progress of cervical dilatation and descent of the head) and not in relation to the magnitude of uterine contractions, because normal labour progress is observed with a wide range of uterine activity in both nulliparas and multiparas. The more rapid the rate of progress for a given level of uterine activity, the more 'efficient' the contractions. It is also important to recognize the difference between inefficient uterine activity and 'in-coordinate' contractions. *Inefficiency* is the failure of the uterus to work in such a way that the labour progress is normal. It can be demonstrated when cervimetric progress is abnormal in the absence of disproportion (although both of these often co-exist). *In-coordinate* uterine action is a descriptive term for the tocographic tracings (Figures 2.5 and 2.6). Most records of uterine contractions will show some degree of irregularity, but they need not necessarily be associated with abnormal labour progress. Therefore the decision to augment labour should be governed primarily by the dynamic effects of the uterine activity – that is, by the rate of cervical dilatation after disproportion and malpresentation have been excluded. The issue of whether oxytocin augmentation is appropriate in the presence of slow progress but apparently normal contractions as demonstrated by intrauterine pressure measurement needs further elucidation.

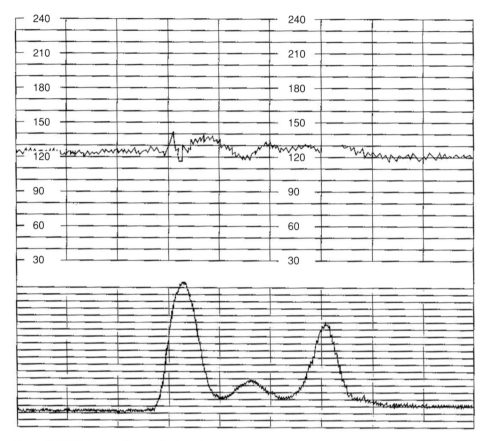

Figure 2.5 Mild degree of in-coordination of uterine contractions.

Further research is required to assess the cervical contribution to abnormal labour progress. Traditionally, the active management of labour has sought to improve the outcome by enhancing the uterine contractions with oxytocin. However, a significant proportion of labours augmented for abnormal progress still result in CS, implying that other factors are important. A recent in-vivo study suggested that cervical smooth muscle activity contributed to the duration of the latent phase [22]. Other researchers have drawn attention to the importance of the head-to-cervix relationship, linking this to the intrauterine pressures developed during labour [23,24]. Further research on this important topic is essential.

Practical Aspects of Labour Management

The diagnosis of active labour is dependent on a careful cervical assessment to define dilatation, effacement, consistency, position and station of the head. These are more important than 'soft' indicators, such as regular contractions, a show, or even amniotic membrane rupture.

On admission, the cervical dilatation should be plotted on the partogram, provided the diagnosis of labour has been made. An alert line is drawn at 1 cm/h once the active phase of labour has been reached, and an action line is then drawn parallel and to the right of this. There is no consensus as to the 'correct' placement of the action line. Recent NICE guidelines on intrapartum care recommend the action line to be drawn 4 h to the right of the alert line. Modifying factors include the level of nursing and medical care available for the supervision of labour once oxytocin has been commenced, the risk of complications associated with prolonged labour (likely to be higher in the more disadvantaged communities) and social factors.

The actual presence of the action line on the partogram is more important than the precise time interval between it and the alert line – its presence indicates that action will be necessary if labour progress falls

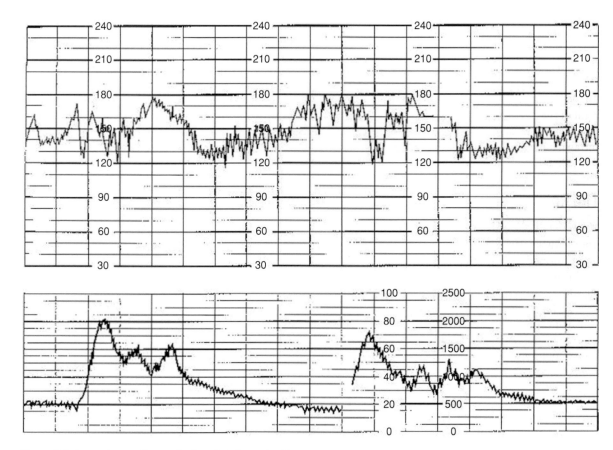

Figure 2.6 Severe degree of in-coordination of uterine contractions.

to the right of that projected. When action is needed, amniotomy alone may suffice to correct slow progress in some cases (see below), although oxytocin will be necessary if there is poor progress after amniotomy.

frequent, painful but apparently fruitless contractions for a long time, some action has to be taken. In these circumstances, augmentation may be appropriate.

Augmentation in the Latent Phase of Labour

The duration of the latent phase of labour varies widely and is a period when the diagnosis of labour can be very difficult. Appreciable proportions of women have painful contractions for long periods in the latent phase, with little cervical change. The management of the latent phase, once maternal and fetal well-being have been confirmed, consists of explanation, reassurance, hydration, nutrition and ambulation. The mainstay of management of a prolonged latent phase is to avoid unnecessary intervention. The decision to augment in the latent phase should be based on clear medical or obstetric indications, since augmentation with an unfavourable cervix is associated with a high risk of CS. However, when the woman has been experiencing

Augmentation in the Active Phase of Labour

Most patients are admitted in the active phase with cervical dilatation >3 cm. The expected progress line or 'alert line' can be drawn at 1 cm/h on the partogram. Proponents of active management of labour augment labour when the progress is to the right of this alert line, whereas most advocate augmentation only when the progress has deviated to the right of the 'action line' drawn 1–4 h parallel to the alert line. By allowing a 'period of grace', fewer patients will require augmentation: 55% of nulliparas with no period of grace [7] compared to 19% of women given a 2 h period of grace [18]. Both methods of management yield comparable results, although prompt intervention does decrease the duration of labour and may be more appropriate when labour ward staffing is inadequate and/or number of beds is limited. However, 'natural childbirth' should be encouraged, and hoping to avoid intervention, the action line may be drawn 4 h to the right of the alert line, since the obstetric outcomes are similar. The WHO study with the action line drawn 4 h to the right of the alert line showed a reduction in prolonged labour and CS rates [15]. Recent NICE guidelines on intrapartum care also support the use of the 4 h action line [5].

The Role of Artificial Rupture of the Membranes (Amniotomy – or ARM)

The artificial rupture of the membranes need not be performed as a routine [5]. However, if delay in established first stage of labour is suspected, artificial rupture of membranes or amniotomy should be considered for all women with intact membranes, after explanation of the procedure and advice that it will shorten her labour by about an hour and may increase the strength and pain of her contractions [5]. However, it does not lower the rate of CS or operative vaginal deliveries, and in normally progressing labour amniotomy should not be performed routinely [25]. Although not routinely recommended, there are some occasions when it is indicated:

- to enhance the strength of contractions when labour progress is abnormal;
- to assess the volume and nature of the liquor in a high-risk labour, especially if the FHR pattern is abnormal; and
- to attach a fetal scalp electrode or to insert an intrauterine pressure catheter.

Amniotomy does have some drawbacks. When the presenting part is high, there is a chance of cord prolapse, and if labour becomes unduly prolonged the risk of intrauterine infection is increased. Furthermore, there is also an increased rate of fetal heart abnormalities possibly due to cord compression as a consequence of reduced amiotic fluid.

Oxytocin Dosage and Time Increment Schedules

For women making slow progress in spontaneous labour, treatment with oxytocin as compared with no treatment was associated with a reduction in the time of delivery of approximately two hours, but did not increase the normal delivery rate [26]. Women should be informed that oxytocin usage will bring forward the time of birth but will not influence the mode of birth or other outcomes [5].

Oxytocin receptors in the uterus increase during pregnancy and labour, so that the uterus may be sensitive to very small doses of administered oxytocin. The drug is best titrated in an arithmetical or geometric manner starting from a low dose. Oxytocin should not be administered by gravity-fed drips, because they are unreliable and potentially unsafe. Overdosage may lead to uterine hyper-stimulation and fetal distress, while a suboptimal dose may lead to failure to progress in labour, resulting in unnecessary intervention. The dangers of uncontrolled infusions include severe fetal hypoxia and uterine rupture. Ideally, intravenous oxytocin should be administered using a peristaltic infusion pump.

Published protocols vary widely in terms of the oxytocin dilution. Higher-dose regimens of oxytocin (4 mU per minute or more) were associated with a reduction in the length of labour and in CS, and an increase in spontaneous vaginal birth. However, there is insufficient evidence to recommend that high-dose regimens are advised routinely for women with delay in the first stage of labour [27]. A more detailed discussion of oxytocin administration for augmenting labour may be found in Chapter 19, relating to induction and augmentation of labour.

Achievement of Optimal Uterine Activity

There remains a dearth of literature regarding the level of uterine activity that should be produced by oxytocin titration to produce a good obstetric outcome. It has been suggested that the use of intrauterine pressure catheters may identify those who are most likely to need a CS for failure to progress. It is known that active contraction area measurements using an intrauterine pressure catheter correlate better with the rate of cervical dilatation than do the individual components of frequency or amplitude of contractions. Despite this, there is little evidence that using an intrauterine pressure catheter to measure uterine activity or using oxytocin titration to achieve a preset active contraction area profile is associated with a better obstetric outcome in augmented labours, compared with an oxytocin infusion titrated against the frequency of contractions [28].

In most centres, facilities to monitor the uterine activity with pressure catheters are not available. The uterine activity has to be judged clinically, on the basis of the frequency and duration of the palpated contractions. As a guide, three contractions in 10 min is an appropriate target uterine activity with oxytocin titration, but if there is no progress with this frequency of contractions, the oxytocin dose may be increased to achieve a frequency of four or five in 10 min, provided the FHR pattern is normal.

The Measurement of Uterine Contractions

The frequency of contractions can be assessed by either external or internal tocography. Some centres use intrauterine pressure catheters when oxytocin is administered because they feel that hyper-stimulation of the uterus can be identified early and the oxytocin infusion rate adjusted accordingly, in the hope that this will improve the neonatal outcome. However, excessively frequent contractions can also be identified by external tocography. Internal tocography for augmented labour does not give rise to a better obstetric outcome when compared with external tocography. Therefore, in a busy clinical practice it is far easier, less invasive, cheaper and perfectly appropriate to assess uterine contractions using external tocography. On the other hand, in certain high-risk cases (such as pregnancies complicated by intrauterine growth restriction, or in those practices where medico-legal concerns are important) there are theoretical advantages to using intrauterine pressure catheters. In addition, internal tocography can be valuable in very obese women, where external tocography is less reliable. The use of intrauterine pressure catheters has also been recommended in women with a previous CS who are being augmented for poor labour progress. A sudden decline in uterine activity may precede any clinical signs of scar rupture, such as scar pain, vaginal bleeding or maternal collapse. Overall, there is only a limited place for intrauterine pressure measurement outside a research setting.

Duration of Augmentation

There is general agreement that the use of the partogram and oxytocin augmentation for the management of abnormal labour progress is valuable. However, there is far less consensus regarding how long augmentation should continue before performing a CS for 'failure to progress'.

Recent recommendations advise that women have a vaginal examination four hours after starting oxytocin in established labour:

- If cervical dilatation has increased by less than 2 cm after four hours of oxytocin, further obstetric review is required to assess the need for CS.
- If cervical dilatation has increased by 2 cm or more, advise four-hourly vaginal examinations [5].

Fetal and maternal surveillance and monitoring of the progress of labour are essential to avoid iatrogenic fetal morbidity.

Summary

Labour is a natural physiological phenomenon leading to childbirth. Many women have the rewarding experience of a safe vaginal birth of a healthy baby, while a small proportion continue to suffer from the complications of prolonged labour and its sequelae. In an attempt to minimize the risks of adverse outcomes, obstetric interventions in labour have become more common. However, a perception of the widespread use of what are seen as unnecessary interventions has caused a healthy degree of scepticism among patients and some clinicians. These concerns, expressed by the general public in recent years, are perfectly valid and will continue to increase if obstetric practice is not continually scrutinized and subjected to rigorous scientific evaluation wherever possible.

This is one of the many challenges currently faced by those with an interest in the welfare of pregnant and labouring women and their babies.

References

1. Thomas J, Paranjothy S. *The National Sentinel Caesarean Section Audit Report*. London: RCOG Press; 2001.
2. Bewley S, Cockburn J. The unfacts of 'request' caesarean section. *Br J Obstet Gynaecol*. 2002; 109: 597–605.
3. Villar J, Carroli G, Zavaleta N, *et al.* Maternal and neonatal individual risks and benefits associated with caesarean delivery: multicentre prospective. *Br Med J*. 2007; 335: 1025.
4. Hemminki E, Merilainen L. Long term effects of cesarean section: ectopic pregnancies and placental problems. *Am J Obstet Gynecol*. 1996; 174: 1569–74.

5. NICE. *Intrapartum Care: Care of Healthy Women and their Babies during Childbirth*: NICE Clinical Guideline 190. London: NICE; 2014.

6. Friedman E. The graphic analysis of labor. *Am J Obstet Gynecol.* 1954; 68(6): 1568–75.

7. Philpott RH. Graphic records in labour. *Br Med J.* 1972; IV: 163–5.

8. O'Driscoll K, Stronge JM, Minogue M. Active management of labour. *Br Med J.* 1973; III: 135–8.

9. Studd JWW. Partograms and nomograms in the management of primigravid labour. *Br Med J.* 1973; IV: 451–5.

10. Ilancheran A, Lim SM, Ratnam SS. Nomograms of cervical dilatation in labour. *Sing J Obstet Gynecol.* 1977; 8: 69–73.

11. Duignan NM, Studd JWW, Hughes AO. Characteristics of labour in different racial groups. *Br J Obstet Gynaecol.* 1975; 82: 593–601.

12. Arulkumaran S, Gibb DMF, Chau S, Singh P, Ratnam SS. Ethnic influences on uterine activity in spontaneous labour. *Br J Obstet Gynaecol.* 1989; 96: 1203–6.

13. Laughton K, Branch W, Beaver J, *et al.* Changes in labor patterns over 50 years. *Am J Obstet Gynecol.* 2012; 206: 419–21.

14. American College of Obstetricians and Gynecologists Obstetric Care Consensus Series. *Safe Prevention of the Primary Cesarean Delivery.* March 2014.

15. World Health Organization Maternal Health and Safe Motherhood Programme. World Health Organization partograph in management of labour. *Lancet.* 1994; 343: 1399–404.

16. Studd J, Clegg DR, Saunders RR, Hughes AO. Identification of high risk labours by labour nomogram. *Br Med J.* 1975; II: 545–7.

17. Cardozo LD, Gibb DMF, Studd JWW, Vasant RV, Cooper DJ. Predictive value of cervimetric labour patterns in primigravidae. *Br J Obstet Gynaecol.* 1982; 89: 33–8.

18. Gibb DMF, Cardozo LD, Studd JWW, Magos AL, Cooper DJ. Outcome of spontaneous labour in multigravidae. *Br J Obstet Gynaecol.* 1982; 89: 708–11.

19. Arulkumaran S, Koh CH, Ingemarsson I, Ratnam SS. Augmentation of labour: mode of delivery related to cervimetric progress. *Aust NZ J Obstet Gynecol.* 1987; 27: 304–8.

20. Lopez-Zeno JA, Peaceman AM, Adashek JA, Socol ML. A controlled trial of a program for the active management of labor. *N Eng J Med.* 1992; 326: 450–4.

21. Frigoletto FD, Lieberman E, Lang JM, *et al.* A clinical trial of active management of labor. *N Eng J Med.* 1995; 333: 745–50.

22. Pajntar M, Leskosek B, Rudel D, Verdenik I. Contribution of cervical smooth muscle activity to the duration of latent and active phases of labour. *Br J Obstet Gynaecol.* 2001; 108: 533–8.

23. Gough GW, Randall NJ, Genevier ES, Sutherland IA, Steer PJ. Head to cervix pressure and their relationship to the outcome of labour. *Obstet Gynecol.* 1990; 75: 613–18.

24. Allman ACJ, Genevier ESG, Johnson MR, Steer PJ. Head-to-cervix force: an important physiological variable in labour. *Br J Obstet Gynaecol.* 1996; 103: 763–8.

25. Smyth RMD, Markham C, Dowswell T. Amniotomy for shortening spontaneous labour. *Cochrane Database Syst Rev.* 2013; 4.

26. Bugg GJ, Siqqiqui F, Thornton JG. Oxytocin versus no treatment or delayed treatment for slow progress in the first stage of spontaneous labour. *Cochrane Database Syst Rev.* 2013; 6.

27. Kenyon S, Tokumasu H, Dowswell T, *et al.* High dose versus low dose oxytocin for augmentation of delayed labour. *Cochrane Database Syst Rev.* 2013; 7.

28. Arulkumaran S, Yang M, Ingemarsson I, Piara S, Ratnam SS. Augmentation of labour: does oxytocin titration to achieve preset active contraction area values produce better obstetric outcome? *Asia Oceania J Obstet Gynecol.* 1989; 15: 333–7.

Chapter 3

Analgesia and Anaesthesia in Labour

Mark Porter

Labour hurts; women's experience of this pain, and their choices about methods to ameliorate and control that pain, vary between women and as each woman progresses through labour. In this chapter I discuss why labour hurts, how to prepare for childbirth, the different methods available and the evidence for and against their use, and their effect on the course of labour. The midwife uses techniques such as relaxation, TENS (transcutaneous electrical nerve stimulation), nitrous oxide and pethidine. The anaesthetist uses techniques such as intravenous opioids (remifentanil) and lumbar epidurals. I also discuss the operative interventions that may be required in labour and current best practice in anaesthesia for those operations with epidurals, spinal anaesthesia and general anaesthesia.

The Pain of Labour

Labour is painful; the extent, nature and purpose of that pain is a subject of contested debate, indeed whether it has a purpose at all, as is the proper response of the mother and the proper response of healthcare practitioners, whether midwives or physicians. Each woman's experience of labour pain is different and is the summation of her experiences, knowledge and beliefs, overlaid by societal and cultural expectations and modified by preparation, coping strategies and analgesic techniques. This experience also bears on her acceptance of the techniques she may wish to use to make the pain bearable.

Why Labour Hurts

The fetal head is a tight fit in the female birth canal through the opposing actions of two evolutionary trends in our ancestors [1]. The first is the develop-

ment of bipedalism and the associated smaller pelvis in australopithecines; the second is the increase in brain size in humans. The fetal head at term takes up most of the space inside the pelvis, and to undergo childbirth the uterus has to push and rotate the fetus through the cervix and then the birth canal. The difficulty and tight fit of this process is the probable cause of the length of labour and the associated pain that marks human childbirth.

The onset of labour is marked by the development of uterine contractions that become more frequent, more regular, stronger and more painful, in order to present the fetus to the cervix for dilation and delivery. Tonic uterine contractions cause ischaemic pain that is transmitted to the spinal cord in the T10–L1 nerve roots, and thence in the spinothalamic tracts to the brain for distribution to the sensory cortex and the cardiovascular centre, among other centres. Pain is usually defined as an unpleasant sensory and emotional experience associated with actual or potential tissue damage, or described in terms of such damage, and the pain of uterine contractions are felt by the mother to be in the corresponding dermatomes, typically referred to the anterior abdomen. As full dilatation is reached and the fetal presenting part descends through the birth canal, the stretching and pressure causes pain that is transmitted to the spinal cord in the sacral nerve roots, and thence to the brain. This pain is felt as distinctly different and assumes a more constant character, sometimes prompting the mother to undertake voluntary pushing at a too-early stage.

The extent of the mother's unpleasant sensory and emotional experience is determined by further factors such as exhaustion, fatigue, fear and anxiety, or conversely the fortitude that can come from a positive expectation combined with good support from her

Best Practice in Labour and Delivery, Second Edition, ed. Sir Sabaratnam Arulkumaran. Published by CAMBRIDGE UNIVERSITY Press. © Cambridge University Press 2016.

partner, a birth companion or a midwife or physician. As plans are made and changed, as the hard work of labour tires the woman, as she becomes anxious with changing plans and her inability to control the progress of childbirth, as her reserves lessen and the physical pain signals become more intense and arrive from a wider range of nerve roots, her needs may change markedly. Her midwife's skill and those of the physicians rest not only in the technical procedures, but also more importantly the recognition of this process and the support that can be given to the woman according to her needs and desires.

Accordingly, medical interventions to deal with the pain cover a spectrum across systemic and localized interventions. All should be built on the pain management strategy of a skilled midwife.

The Effects of Pain and Pain Relief

Aside from the unpleasant suffering, labour pain can lead to a number of undesirable outcomes through the sympathetic nervous outflow stimulated by the pain and the neuroendocrine response to labour. These include:

- catecholamine release;
- haemodynamic changes – tachycardia, hypertension and increased cardiac output;
- delayed gastric emptying;
- increased adrenocortical activity – stress response;
- impaired uterine contraction;
- decreased uteroplacental blood flow; and
- maternal and fetal acidosis.

Effective relief of pain, particularly using regional techniques, may resolve these challenges (though these techniques may bring their own complications). Reducing stress is not just a humane outcome, as the woman's ability to cooperate with the midwife in delivering her baby may be enhanced. Management of some co-morbidities such as diabetes mellitus and cardiovascular compromise will also be facilitated, and the fetus will be protected from fetal acidosis. In some women these benefits may themselves amount to a positive indication for epidural pain relief.

Supporting Women's Choices During Childbirth

As labour ward practitioners it is our fundamental responsibility to present information to a woman in order to allow and encourage her to make her own choices about what she wishes to do in labour. Her ability to be informed, to participate in the decisions about her care and techniques that work all contribute to maternal satisfaction. A successful outcome does not necessarily require absence of pain or loss of sensation; the point is to reduce the pain to the point where she is happy that the right balance has been reached, and augment her ability to cope with the pain of labour.

To do this, we should reflect on our own values and beliefs and how they inform our own attitudes to coping with the pain of labour. Our care should support the woman's choice [2]. Most of the time we do not need to make an active recommendation on which method of pain relief to use, as in only a small number of cases is a specific method indicated strongly. That being said, the recent increase in availability of midwife-led delivery units and the promotion of normality have limited the analgesia options available to those women who choose to give birth in lower-intervention environments. Information on appropriate options must be made available to women as part of their informed choices on the place of delivery.

The Obstetric Anaesthetists Association has a website with resources for such use, containing written materials to reinforce the verbal dialogue with the woman [3].

Preparing for Childbirth

Women should be helped to prepare for childbirth by being provided with opportunities to learn about the experience and the support available. Antenatal classes are usually provided by midwives and cover this, among many other things. Some classes provide written information about pain relief including invasive methods, but others prefer not to assume a medical model of delivery for all women, providing information when required and if the woman is going to have an obstetrician-led delivery. Some women will benefit from a consultation with an obstetric anaesthetist. This will include:

- women whose body mass index is above a threshold level, locally determined at 35–40 kg/m^2;
- women with a history of unsatisfactory pain relief in labour, or complications with analgesia techniques;
- unusual medical conditions that may interfere with choices in labour, such as previous back

surgery, injury or congenital anomaly, coagulation disorders, allergies to medication or neurological disorders.

Obstetric anaesthetists should make themselves available for such referrals from midwives or obstetricians, whether on an occasional basis or, better, through a specifically arranged clinic.

Midwife-led Pain Relief

Midwives are the main carers for women in labour and their care makes a profound difference to the woman's experience of pain. The active use of postural coping strategies during the first stage of labour is associated with providing some pain relief and also helping a woman to cope with pain; use of the upright position and walking in labour are associated with reductions in the length of the first stage and the use of epidural analgesia [4]. While these benefits are real, they are unlikely to provide the entirety of pain relief needed by most women.

Relaxation Techniques

Labour pain can cause positive feedback into anxiety, fear and bodily tension, which in turn can exacerbate the pain and the fear of pain. Use of relaxation techniques including mindfulness, meditation, visualization and yoga may help a woman to manage her pain, with some women reporting very positive benefits, such as a sense of calm empowerment [5]. Rigorous evidence of benefit is harder to find [6], though this may reflect varying techniques, the individual ability to maintain control and the variance of individual response to the feeling of being in control. Women should be supported in their personal choices [2]. Breathing exercises, immersion in water and massage may reduce pain during the latent first stage [2]. If labouring in water, the temperature of the water and the woman must be monitored at least hourly to guard against fever.

TENS (Transcutaneous Electrical Nerve Stimulation)

TENS units are available in many hospitals and also in pharmacy retail outlets. Mothers apply the units themselves, typically over the lower back, and thereby receive low-voltage electrical impulses in various frequency and intensity. They appear to work satisfactorily for some women in the third trimester (for back pain and Braxton Hicks or prodromal contractions) and at home in early labour. This may be related to the physiological basis of pain transmission in the spinal cord; more likely it gives a sense of control to the mother that helps her to control the pain. Although TENS lacks serious side-effects in women and babies, evidence for efficacy in established labour is weak [7] and it should not be offered [2].

Inhaled Analgesia

The most ubiquitous and popular agent for self-administration is nitrous oxide in oxygen, utilizing the Poynting effect in which combining nitrous oxide and oxygen at high pressure allows both components to remain in gaseous form. Premixed cylinders such as Entonox, stored and used between 10 °C and room temperature, will reliably deliver 50% nitrous oxide (a potent analgesic and weak anaesthetic at that concentration) with 50% oxygen (to prevent hypoxia). It crosses the lungs swiftly, whether being breathed in or out, and so mothers should be instructed to commence inhalation as the contraction pain starts and to remove the mouthpiece as the contraction starts to fade. In this way she will have an adequate period between inhalations to allow nitrous oxide levels to subside and minimize side-effects. She should remain awake throughout and retain protective laryngeal reflexes.

Entonox is effective in reducing pain intensity and giving relief, albeit with a side-effect profile including nausea, vomiting, dizziness and drowsiness [8]. NICE requires that it is available in all birth settings. Adding low-dose flurane derivatives such as isoflurane 0.25% may reduce side-effects by enhancing analgesia while not producing sedation.

Pethidine (Meperidine) and Other Intramuscular Opioids

NICE requires that intramuscular opioids should be available in all birth settings [2]. Opioid injections have been used for many decades and have a traditional place in labour, with UK midwives able to prescribe pethidine independently. It is important to remember that evidence for efficacy of pethidine or other opioids in relieving pain is very limited and that the main benefit felt by women may be in promoting relaxation and dissociation [9]. However, some women report dissatisfaction as that dissociation is not only from the pain but also from the experience of childbirth. These drugs cannot be used in synchrony with labour contractions, but their effects are present whether needed or not.

Complications include nausea, vomiting, maternal and neonatal drowsiness, and short-term neonatal respiratory depression and drowsiness. Administer concurrent antiemetics. Opioids may interfere with breastfeeding. Women should not enter water for two hours after administration or if they feel drowsy.

Methods Not Based in Evidence

Enthusiasts have advocated a variety of other pain relief methods, some of which are listed here. These methods lack rigorous evidence of their efficacy, and the future acquisition of such evidence seems unlikely given their questionable basis in human physiology [10]. They are also generally associated with an absence of significant harm, and so appear to be safe for mother and baby. The best-studied methods are acupuncture and hypnosis, but the studies remain small and the evidence elusive [11].

The methods described below have value for some women; these techniques should not be offered or recommended, though choices for acupressure, acupuncture and hypnosis should be respected [2]:

- intracutaneous or subcutaneous sterile water injections [12];
- electromyographic biofeedback [13];
- antenatal hypnotherapy – this method is handicapped by lack of consistent technique and while it shows some early promise, evidence of efficacy is lacking [14];
- massage, reflexology and other manual methods [15];
- acupuncture and acupressure [16];
- aromatherapy [17]; and
- moxibustion, with or without needles.

Invasive Methods for Pain Relief

The strength of demand for better-quality analgesia in what can be the very extremes of a painful experience has driven the development and provision of invasive methods. These techniques should only be undertaken on labour wards that have immediate access to an anaesthetist. All women should be informed about and have timely access to transfer to an obstetric unit

Table 3.1 Indications and contraindications for epidural analgesia

Indications for epidural analgesia	Contraindications
Maternal request	Unwilling patient
Multiple pregnancy	Coagulopathy
Pre-eclampsia	Local or generalized sepsis
Diabetes mellitus	Elevated intracranial pressure
Cardiorespiratory disease	Uncorrected hypovolaemia
Other high risks	Inadequate unit staffing

from home or a midwifery unit, should they wish to request regional analgesia [2].

Lumbar Epidurals

A lumbar epidural is a targeted central neuraxial block by which the anaesthetist intends not to abolish sensation, but to dial down the intensity of the abdominal and pelvic pain so that it becomes bearable and tolerable, even comfortable. While every woman will have her own concept of what the ideal of pain relief amounts to, and that concept will change during the progress of her labour, very few will want or even benefit from the complete abolition of sensation, particularly where that is accompanied by increasing side-effects such as leg weakness. While lumbar epidurals are the most effective form of pain relief in labour that we know, with maternal satisfaction rates more than 80%, the search for a means by which to better deliver this ideal level of analgesia continues to keep anaesthesia practice and research a vigorous area.

About 20% of women giving birth in England do so with an epidural in place, predominantly first-time mothers [18].

Epidural placement should be offered for severe pain in the latent first stage of labour [2] and throughout the first stage, with no time limitations (Table 3.1). If undertaking a lumbar epidural where delivery may not be far away, it is prudent to do so with the woman in the lateral position as the midwife can still deliver the baby if it arrives during the procedure.

Technique for Lumbar Epidural

Epidurals are inserted and maintained by anaesthetists. While the technical skills associated with it can be taught to other staff, anaesthetists best undertake integrating epidurals into an overall anaesthesia service and managing potential complications. One of the most important components of the technique for establishing a lumbar epidural is cooperation of the woman and her positioning; the midwife is the key to this and thus central to successful blockade. A catheter is placed into the epidural space surrounding the spinal cord: a space containing fibrous tissue, blood vessels, fat and the nerve roots entering and exiting the spinal cord. Drug solutions infused into this space will affect the nerve roots with a minor effect through diffusing into the intrathecal space and being directly applied to the spinal cord.

With an epidural catheter placed and securely fastened, modern practice is to use dilute solutions of local anaesthetic augmented with fentanyl. This reduces the motor effect of the epidural, which largely depends on the mass of local anaesthetic administered to the epidural space, by adding synergistic opioids. Bupivacaine in concentrations of 0.0625–0.1% is commonly used with fentanyl 2 mcg/ml. A dose of 10 ml is not very likely to establish satisfactory analgesia; 15 ml is more likely but more may be needed. Contraction pains will generally indicate block to T10.

The dose is titrated against the woman's pain, which although is the more pronounced the further along labour is, is also affected markedly by her tolerance level, by the presence of labour augmentation with oxytocin infusion, by descent of the fetal head into the birth canal and by the position of the fetal head. Any presentation or position other than cephalic and occipito-anterior is likely to be associated with greater maternal pain. In general the more pelvic the pain the more useful is fentanyl; a concentration of 5 mcg/ml, to a dose of up to 100 mcg, will benefit a woman whose fetus is in the not uncommon occipito-posterior position.

Pain relief can be maintained by a continuous infusion, or better by repeated bolus doses, whether administered by the mother using a PCEA device (patient-controlled epidural analgesia) or by the midwife [2]. The most effective option is bolus dosing with a bupivacaine concentration of no more than 1 mg/ml, probably because this gives the widest nerve root spread of analgesia, and is the most satisfactory for the mother where it is under her control with a PCEA.

Effect on the Progress and Outcome of Labour

Discontinuing epidural analgesia late in labour is sometimes advocated in order to allow motor strength to return for pushing. With dilute solutions of local anaesthetic there is no longer a justification for this and routine discontinuation leads to an increase in inadequate analgesia [19]. With an epidural, a woman should delay pushing for one hour after full cervical dilation unless there is an urge to push or the fetal head is visible, though delivery should take place within four hours regardless of parity. Regional analgesia should be continued until after the third stage of labour [2].

Nevertheless, women receiving epidural analgesia experience a longer second stage of labour and a 40% higher rate of operative vaginal delivery, with the 95% confidence interval running from 28% to 57% [20]. This may be in part due to the increased monitoring, including CTG (cardiotocography), that a woman will receive while she has a lumbar epidural. CTG monitoring is itself associated with significant increases in caesarean section and operative vaginal delivery [21]. However, epidural analgesia does not lead to a longer first stage of labour or an increased chance of delivery by caesarean section.

Neuraxial analgesia is associated with better fetal outcome. Neonatal acid–base status is not only better with epidural than with systemic opioid analgesia, it is also better than with no analgesia [22].

PDPH (Post-Dural Puncture Headache)

The commonest serious complication is a slow leak of CSF (cerebrospinal fluid) caused by accidental puncture of the dural membrane around the intrathecal space. When done with a large epidural needle this leak will overwhelm the body's ability to replace CSF, producing a low-pressure headache from front to back of the head and into the neck that worsens considerably with an upright posture. About 1:150 epidurals will be followed by PDPH. This will delay discharge or, as it commonly becomes serious about 24 hours after delivery, will bring a new mother back into hospital with a headache that is extremely limiting to her ability to care for herself or her baby, and warrants prompt and effective treatment. There are small long-term risks of chronic headache and subdural haemorrhage if untreated.

Traditional treatments are to encourage bed rest, hydration and caffeine intake, and prescribe NSAIDs (non-steroidal anti-inflammatory drugs). They are effective only for mild headaches. The standard treatment is epidural blood patch [23], whereby the anaesthetist will replace an epidural needle and slowly inject about 20 ml of the patient's own blood, taken aseptically. The immediate effect is to squeeze the epidural space and transfer the same volume of CSF into the head, resolving almost all headaches and allowing mobilization, and in the longer term is thought to help seal the dural puncture. NSAIDs will still be required and about one in four women will come back in a day or two for a repeat blood patch.

Intrapartum Fever

Epidural analgesia in labour is associated with the development of maternal fever, the risk increasing with duration of the epidural and being higher in primigravid mothers at between 13% and 33% [24]. Although some biochemical markers of inflammation are found, the cause, best prevention and best treatment of the fever are not known with certainty. Maternal fever, especially if combined with neonatal acidosis, is highly associated with neonatal encephalopathy. The questions are whether the link from choosing an epidural through fever to impaired fetal neurodevelopment is causative, whether it is statistically significant and what is the magnitude of the risk. Recent research appears to indicate that the link is not direct and that mothers at higher risk (e.g. prolonged rupture of membranes) may also choose epidurals [25].

Other Complications

Probably the most profound complication is the change in the character of the mother's labour. She may have planned for a low-intervention delivery at home or in a midwife-led unit; even if in an acute hospital this can still feel close to natural. Her change of plan might require transfer of location and brings with it an increase in medical intervention, with intravenous access, blood samples, intravenous infusions, blood pressure and sensory level monitoring, mandatory CTG monitoring and a concomitant reduction in mobility. This can not only limit mobility, but may be profoundly demoralizing to a woman who planned to control her own low-intervention delivery, and she may need support to validate her choices.

Maternal hypotension occurs commonly after epidural analgesia [20]. Intravenous preloading is a traditional practice whereby up to 1000 ml of an isotonic saline solution is infused before establishing epidural analgesia. While it may have been of use in the past to prevent maternal hypotension, it is not effective where low-concentration local anaesthetics (such as bupivacaine 1 mg/ml) are used in conjunction with

opioids [26]. Better advice is to avoid high-dose epidurals and to make sure that women receiving any bolus administration to their epidural catheter have their uterus displaced leftwards using left tilt or the full left lateral position. Administering boluses in the full left lateral position is also more likely to achieve a greater dermatomal spread of analgesia.

Motor blockade also occurs commonly [20] and is particularly associated with the dose of local anaesthetic given to the woman, whether in high concentration (e.g. bupivacaine 0.25% for bolus dosing) or in high volume, with epidural infusions left running instead of a bolus dose being delivered on maternal request, either electronically or by a practitioner. A high concentration of local anaesthetic or continuous infusion should not be used routinely for establishment or maintenance of epidural analgesia [2].

The association of epidural analgesia with long-term backache has long been shown to be just that, an association and not causative. Women can be reassured that (except in the rarest of circumstances, e.g. chronic adhesive arachnoiditis) epidurals do not cause backache other than short-term bruising due to the injection.

Combined Spinal-Epidural

The basic idea is to gain control of the labour pain by using a small intrathecal component alongside the epidural, thereby obviating the need for a loading epidural dose and preserving mobility. The 'walking epidural' has been limited by the lack of evidence of a difference in maternal satisfaction to offset the higher resources used and the concerns over a very low but still significantly higher incidence of serious and permanent nerve and cord damage to the mother when compared with low-dose epidurals [27].

Intravenous Opioids

Opioids given intravenously will act more rapidly and more potently than when given intramuscularly. Most are useless in labour due to their durations of action not matching contraction pains, and the high potential for maternal and neonatal complications. The recent invention of remifentanil has spurred new developments.

Remifentanil

Remifentanil is an ultra-short-acting agonist at the mu-receptor, with a context-sensitive half-life of three minutes. It has a rapid onset of activity and undergoes almost equally rapid enzymatic degradation to inactive metabolites. These properties raised the possibility that intravenous remifentanil might be used in a patient-controlled device to provide pulsatile analgesia for the pain of a single contraction, and be relied upon to wear off between contractions: an intravenous and more potent alternative to nitrous oxide. This promise has been tempered in experience by imperfect timing and occasional serious complications. The risk of respiratory depression mandates a dedicated intravenous cannula, rigorous 1:1 care while in use from a midwife with specific training, and availability of oxygen supplementation along with pulse oximetry and CTG monitoring. A very small number of UK obstetric units use it widely in labour, and in a larger number of units it is used for a very small number of women desiring potent analgesia but in whom neuraxial analgesia is either unsuitable (e.g. coagulation disorder) or not wanted by the woman.

Other Opioids

Morphine, possibly by infusion but more likely by a PCA (patient-controlled analgesia) device, is too sedating and has too long a duration of action for both mother and neonate to be useful in normal labour. However, it has a place in labour analgesia in the case of intrauterine fetal death, where sedation is often desirable.

Anaesthesia in Labour

This is most commonly needed for caesarean section, with approximately one in six women going into labour being delivered by caesarean section (including elective cases, the overall caesarean rate in England is about 25%), but may also less often be needed for other operative procedures.

Operative interventions in labour are marked by urgency and sometimes by confusion as to what is the required urgency in this particular case. The Lucas classification of urgency in caesarean section is now well established and should be embedded into clinical practice as a communication tool [28]. There are no time thresholds built in: any such thresholds have utility as audit standards but must not be allowed to dictate clinical practice, as undue haste can introduce surgical and anaesthetic risks with the potential for maternal and neonatal harm arising from the haste itself.

Table 3.2 Classification relating the degree of urgency to the presence or absence of maternal or fetal compromise. See the colour plate section for a colour version of this table

	Urgency	Definition	Category
Most urgent	Maternal or fetal compromise	Immediate threat to life of woman or fetus	1
		No immediate threat to life of woman or fetus	2
	No maternal or fetal compromise	Requires early delivery	3
Least urgent		At a time to suit the woman and maternity services	4

Close and effective communication between all team members is important, but critically so over the degree and category of urgency, and the associated plans for anaesthesia.

Choice of Technique and Preparation

The broad choice for a woman is 'awake or asleep?' Most women today will prefer to be awake, having been prepared that way by custom and expectation overlaid with the desire to be awake with their birth partner at their baby's delivery. Most anaesthetists appreciate the concomitant reduction of the risk of difficult intubation or pulmonary aspiration, and lower postoperative analgesia requirements. Regional anaesthesia is the default method for most caesareans, with spinal anaesthesia considered the gold standard by anaesthetists, including for most cases complicated by severe pre-eclampsia [24] or placenta praevia. General anaesthesia (GA) is usually reserved for mothers with severe fetal distress where a reliable short decision to delivery interval is required, for haemorrhage or for anticipated bleeding so heavy that avoidance of heavy sympathetic blockade is required; and for those few women who choose it. As long as she is properly informed, her choice on this must be respected; there is little or no evidence that there is a real difference in long-term outcomes for either mother or neonate dependent on the anaesthesia method chosen, all other things being equal [29]. If there were it might be unethical to offer GA at all. A potential trap for an anaesthetist is to persuade a woman that GA carries greater potential for risk and harm, only to have to recommend it as a technique following the failure of a regional anaesthetic.

Particularly in category 1 and 2 caesarean sections, the anaesthetist's interview of the mother takes place against the backdrop of changing maternal expectations, possibly serious disappointment and anxiety, and clinical urgency. Information and consent remains essential despite these challenges. Antacid prophylaxis with oral ranitidine 150 mg is standard (50 mg intravenously if less than an hour to theatre), and if the patient is to have GA then 30 ml of sodium citrate solution immediately prior to induction. Metoclopramide 10 mg intravenously just before induction whatever the anaesthetic type will promote gastric emptying, raise lower oesophageal tone and may contribute to antiemesis.

Lumbar Epidural Anaesthesia

Most epidurals for theatre cases will be current labour epidurals that are assessed as being suitable for bolus top up. Having confidence in the epidural requires judgement that the block was successful in relieving labour pain, that high levels of maintenance such as repeated visits by the anaesthetist were not required, that there are no missed segments or inadequate laterality and that the results of testing the sensory extent of the block are compatible with the amount of drug administered.

If the epidural is considered suitable then a typical bolus dose to convert to caesarean anaesthesia will be 20 ml 2% lidocaine (with adrenaline 5 mcg/ml) or 0.5% levobupivacaine. This should be given in divided doses to check catheter positioning, but also to make sure that the upper level of the anaesthetic does not overshoot into high block (see below). Diamorphine 2.5–5 mg should be added for postoperative analgesia.

Spinal Anaesthesia

Applying the anaesthetic drugs in the right dose directly to the spinal cord gives rapid and profound anaesthesia. Smaller needles (24–27 gauge) with pencil point tips have reduced PDPH to less than 1%. The standard spinal drug is bupivacaine 5 mg/ml, with dextrose 80 mg/ml to make the solution hyperbaric and thus controllable with posture. The dose is subject to much debate, with volumes from 2.4 ml to 3 ml being used for caesarean section. Administering 3 ml will produce more consistent anaesthesia and almost eliminate the need for supplemental analgesia or anaesthesia during surgery, but will be associated with a greater degree of spinal hypotension (see below).

An opioid should be added: a lipid-soluble opioid such as fentanyl will give better intra-operative analgesia but almost no postoperative effect, while a more water-soluble drug such as diamorphine will give good postoperative analgesia for 12–24 hours. Experience with diamorphine has grown and initially high rates of postoperative pruritus and nausea may be reduced by measures such as feeding the patient immediately after surgery rather than leaving her on an intravenous drip. Diamorphine is now the recommended drug in the UK, a typical dose being 300–400 mcg [30].

Spinal hypotension will develop with thoracolumbar sympathetic blockade, and should be avoided so as to protect the fetus from the potential of metabolic acidosis, as well as the mother from severe nausea. Tilting the gravid mother to the left will decompress the inferior vena cava and is essential, but a vasoconstrictor will be needed. Traditional use of prophylactic intravenous fluids or bolus ephedrine after the hypotension develops has given way to the prophylactic use of alpha adrenoreceptor agonists such as phenylephrine or metaraminol, which are more effective in preventing hypotension while not inducing relative fluid overload, maternal tachycardia or fetal acidosis [24]. A typical dose will be metaraminol 10 mg/h (167 mcg/min) started immediately after the block insertion and running for up to 20 minutes, with cardiovascular monitoring using the maternal pulse rate as the most immediate indicator of the correct dosing.

Height of Block Required

Any operative procedure indicates the lower extent of the block to cover the sacral segments in order to anaesthetise the birth canal, and the indicated upper extent of the block and thus the dose of heavy bupivacaine varies with the procedure (Table 3.3).

Principal Complications of Regional Anaesthesia

Pain

Pain, due to an inadequate block for the survey undertaken, is a serious complication and indeed may be seen as failure to achieve appropriate anaesthesia. Thorough checking of the block by different modalities is a preventive measure. Although clinical monitoring of the patient during block development is mandatory, it is unlikely that a caesarean block will be achieved in

Table 3.3 Considerations for different operations

	Block required	0.5% heavy bupivacaine	Opioids
Operative vaginal delivery	T8–sacral (see below)	2.0 ml	Epidural or spinal diamorphine in case of caesarean section
Manual removal of placenta	T8–sacral	2.0 ml	Not needed; fentanyl 20 mcg possible
Repair of perineal tear (first and second degree)	Perineal local anaesthetic infiltration	–	–
Repair of perineal tear (third and fourth degree)	T8–sacral	2.0 ml	Diamorphine (epidural 2.5–5 mcg or spinal 300–400 mcg) for extensive perineal tear
Caesarean section	T4–sacral	3.0 ml	Diamorphine 300–400 mcg

With a trial of operative vaginal delivery using epidural top up, the procedure can start when the upper end of the block has reached T8 and with successful delivery the anaesthetic will not need extending to T4. If there is no epidural in place and caesarean section is not expected, then pudendal block along with perineal local anaesthetic should be offered [2].

less than ten minutes for a spinal or 20 minutes for an epidural, and so appropriate time should be allowed to pass for the block to develop. Early signs of leg weakness should be observed to give way to a complete inability to undertake straight leg raising; motor block will precede sensory block. Check the sensory block with both loss of sensation to cold (ice or ethyl chloride spray) and sharp sensation (cocktail stick or pinch). Light touch can also be used but seems to be more operator-dependent. The T4 level is at the level of the fourth intercostal space: usually the nipples but beware variability in breast positioning. The sacral end should be checked on the inner posterior thigh (S3) and that the ankle can no longer move. If the block does not develop at the expected time then positioning the patient head down, undertaking a Valsalva manoeuvre and raising the patient's legs can all help to raise the block.

Treatment should not be required in most cases, except where the surgical time exceeds 100 minutes after the spinal insertion. Pain during uterine manipulation has diminished as a problem with opioids in the spinal and with higher dose spinals. Entonox administration or intravenous alfentanil will help with this. If close to the end of surgery then surgical infiltration into the skin will allow the last few stitches in.

High Block

This is a central neuraxial block that not only rises above the desirable level of T4 but is also associated with respiratory, or much more rarely, cardiovascular complications. It is a risk at about the 1% level when any form of central neuraxial block is used on top of an existing labour epidural. Whether this is adminis-

tering a high-concentration bolus dose to achieve caesarean anaesthesia, or a spinal anaesthetic because the epidural does not inspire confidence for topping up, the effects of a subsequent block are less predictable and vigilant clinical observation is required. A mother may complain of feeling unable to breathe. This must be distinguished from the normal such feeling caused by the loss of muscular tone in most of the intercostal muscles, in which case the woman will be able to talk normally when calmed and will be able to squeeze the anaesthetist's fingers in her fist. With weakened hand muscles the block is ascending into cervical root levels and may impair the accessory muscles of respiration and the diaphragm.

If either of those reassuring signs is absent then the block may be ascending too rapidly, reassurance may not suffice and airway control may be needed. The pathological effects of the ascending block will be exacerbated by an acute sense of severe distress in the mother, making this one of the most challenging scenarios to manage anaesthetically, with the decision as to whether to intubate or not. Intubation will require the anaesthetist to induce GA rapidly, with excellent communication to the patient, her birth partner and the rest of the theatre team. The anaesthetist should summon help rapidly when faced with such a challenge.

General Anaesthesia (GA)

General anaesthesia is done rarely in labour ward theatres today: perhaps 10–15% of caesarean sections and few other cases. Its retreat as spinal anaesthesia has become the default and has accompanied improvements in its safety with better SADs (supraglottic airway devices) such as next-generation LMAs (laryngeal mask airways) for airway control and videolaryngoscopy for predicted difficult intubation.

Although debate remains over whether it is still necessary, the standard method is to pre-oxygenate the mother and undertake a rapid sequence induction with thiopental and suxamethonium, applying cricoid pressure until intubation.

Intubation may be unexpectedly difficult. Focusing on basic anaesthesia practice can prevent this: sometimes the patient may be put rapidly on the operating table and the theatre filled with a sense of urgency and haste. The anaesthetist must create a safe zone around the patient in which they can reduce interruption and distraction, positioning the patient properly: at the appropriate height for them, and for all but morbidly obese patients, with the neck flexed on the body and the head extended on the neck with a pillow under the occiput. Traditional drills for difficult intubation had intubation as the desired end point, whereas the development of better SADs such as LMA Supreme has allowed recognition that it is safer to rapidly insert one of these than to persist in attempting to intubate the patient. Authoritative new guidelines in 2015 include this [31].

Postoperative patients are often recovered in labour ward theatres rather than main theatre suites. If so, those staff caring for mothers who have had GA must be skilled or trained in postoperative recovery, including airway care; the labour ward anaesthetist must also be close by during the immediate phase.

Caesarean Section Considerations

Modern practice balances traditional medical care models with the imperative to treat the woman as someone having a baby by the abdominal route, rather than a patient having a laparotomy. A multidisciplinary approach, devising guidelines with the midwives, as well as following new evidence is essential.

NICE has emphasized doing fewer routine blood tests specifically for caesarean section [30]. However, as caesarean section in labour is a specific haemorrhage risk, all women undergoing such surgery should have blood group serology undertaken.

Supplemental oxygen for the mother during regional anaesthesia results in measurably higher oxygen levels but this does not translate to benefits for mother or neonate [32].

Fluid management should be directed towards early postoperative oral intake. Reducing intravenous fluids and using syringe drivers for prevention of spinal hypotension and oxytocin infusions, and recognizing that volume lost in theatre should only be replaced in theatre, allows most women to sit up in recovery, feeding their baby and taking oral fluids; this is likely to facilitate early discharge from hospital care.

Antibiotics were traditionally given after cord clamping, but prevention of surgical infection now mandates delivery of the hospital's recommended prophylaxis before skin incision [30].

Effective uterotonic treatment is in the hands of the anaesthetist. Oxytocin 5 units intravenously at cord clamping will assist, although lower slow doses should be used in massive haemorrhage or cardiac insufficiency due to the profound vasodilator effect. The effect will need to be maintained in immediate recovery; conventional treatment is with oxytocin infusion at 6 units per hour, reducing over a couple of hours. Delivering this from a syringe driver rather than an infusion bag will better control the dose and maternal fluid intake. Ergometrine is a good second line treatment at 50–100 mcg slow intravenous bolus.

Intra-operative cell salvage is a technique for collecting the mother's blood lost at caesarean section. With blood loss approaching 1000 ml, salvaged blood can be successfully processed in order to commence returning maternal (and some fetal) red cells to the mother. All units should have access to this for major haemorrhage, but debate continues over whether it should be reserved for such cases or be applied in all caesarean sections due to the difficulty of predicting each case of massive haemorrhage. Some units use cell salvage as a perioperative blood conservation strategy in all cases, but overall benefits in reducing red cell use or length of stay remain controversial [33].

Following up Mothers After Regional Blocks or GA

Most obstetric units have women on postnatal wards that are relatively close to labour wards, allowing the anaesthetists to interview the women postoperatively to discuss satisfaction, adjust medication if required and detect complications. Post-dural puncture headache and inadequate analgesia are important to diagnose and manage in order to facilitate the woman going home. Nerve injuries are more rare and while most apparent injuries are due to obstetric palsy (typical signs are in the distribution of a nerve or plexus), rarely they will be due to complications of anaesthesia (typical signs are in the distribution of a dermatome). All units should have in place procedures for such review.

Further Reading

The reader who is interested in learning more will find a rich selection of textbooks and other publications which augment this chapter, which can only summarize the field. The following are recommended.

- Steve Yentis and Surbhi Malhotra (2012) *Analgesia, Anaesthesia and Pregnancy: A Practical Guide*, 3rd edition (Cambridge University Press).
- Paul Clyburn, Rachel Collis, Sarah Harries and Stuart Davies (2008) *Obstetric Anaesthesia* (Oxford Specialist Handbooks in Anaesthesia).
- Rachel E. Collis, Felicity Plaat and John Urquhart (2011) *Textbook of Obstetric Anaesthesia*, reissue edition (Cambridge University Press).

References

1. Steer P, Flint C. Physiology and management of normal labour. *Br Med J*. 1999;318: 793–6.

2. National Institute for Health and Care Excellence. Intrapartum care: clinical guideline 190; 2014. www.guidance.nice.org.uk/cg190 (accessed 15 May 2016).

3. Obstetric Anaesthetists Association. Information about pain relief and anaesthesia by doctors for you. www.LabourPains.com (accessed 1 September 2014).

4. Royal College of Midwives. Positions for labour and birth; 2012. www.rcm.org.uk/sites/default/files/Positions%20for%20Labour%20and%20Birth.pdf (accessed 15 May 2016).

5. Fletcher S. *Mindful Hypnobirthing: Hypnosis and Mindfulness Techniques for a Calm and Confident Birth*. London: Vermilion; 2014.

6. Smith CA, Levett KM, Collins CT, Crowther CA. Relaxation techniques for pain management in labour. *Cochrane Database Syst Rev*. 2011;12. CD009514. doi: 10.1002/14651858.CD009514.

7. Dowswell T, Bedwell C, Lavender T, Neilson JP. Transcutaneous electrical nerve stimulation (TENS) for pain management in labour. *Cochrane Database Syst Rev*. 2009;2. CD007214. doi: 10.1002/14651858.CD007214.pub2.

8. Klomp T, van Poppel M, Jones L, *et al*. Inhaled analgesic for pain management in labour. *Cochrane Database Syst Rev*. 2012;9. CD009351. doi: 10.1002/14651858.CD009351.pub2.

9. Olofsson C, Ekblom A, Ekman-Ordeberg G, Granstrom L, Irestedt L. Lack of analgesic effect of systemically administered morphine or pethidine on labour pain. *Br J Obstet Gynaecol*. 1996;103: 968–72.

10. Jones L, Othman M, Dowswell T, *et al*. Pain management for women in labour: an overview of systematic reviews. *Cochrane Database Syst Rev*. 2012;3. CD009234. doi: 10.1002/14651858.CD009234.pub2.

11. Smith CA, Collins CT, Cyna AM, Crowther CA. Complementary and alternative therapies for pain management in labour. *Cochrane Database Syst Rev*. 2006;4. CD003521. doi: 10.1002/14651858.CD003521.pub2.

12. Derry S, Straube S, Moore RA, Hancock H, Collins SL. Intracutaneous or subcutaneous sterile water injection compared with blinded controls for pain management in labour. *Cochrane Database Syst Rev*. 2012;1. CD009107. doi: 10.1002/14651858.CD009107.pub2.

13. Barragán Loayza IM, Solà I, Juandó Prats C. Biofeedback for pain management during labour. *Cochrane Database Syst Rev*. 2011;6. CD006168. doi: 10.1002/14651858.CD006168.pub2.

14. Madden K, Middleton P, Cyna AM, Matthewson M, Jones L. Hypnosis for pain management during labour and childbirth. *Cochrane Database Syst Rev*. 2012;11. CD009356. doi: 10.1002/14651858.CD009356.pub2.

15. Smith CA, Levett KM, Collins CT, Jones L. Massage, reflexology and other manual methods for pain management in labour. *Cochrane Database Syst Rev*. 2012;2. CD009290. doi: 10.1002/14651858.CD009290.pub2.

16. Smith CA, Collins CT, Crowther CA, Levett KM. Acupuncture or acupressure for pain management in labour. *Cochrane Database Syst Rev*. 2011;7. CD009232. doi: 10.1002/14651858.CD009232.

17. Smith CA, Collins CT, Crowther CA. Aromatherapy for pain management in labour. *Cochrane Database Syst Rev*. 2011;7. CD009215. doi: 10.1002/14651858.CD009215.

18. Health and Social Care Information Centre. NHS maternity statistics: England, 2012–13; 2013. www.hscic.gov.uk/catalogue/PUB12744 (accessed 15 May 2016).

19. Torvaldsen S, Roberts CL, Bell JC, Raynes-Greenow CH. Discontinuation of epidural analgesia late in labour for reducing the adverse delivery outcomes associated with epidural analgesia. *Cochrane Database Syst Rev*. 2004;4. CD004457. doi: 10.1002/14651858.CD004457.pub2.

20. Anim-Somuah M, Smyth RMD, Jones L. Epidural versus non-epidural or no analgesia in labour. *Cochrane Database Syst Rev.* 2011;12. CD000331. doi: 10.1002/14651858.CD000331.pub3.

21. Alfirevic Z, Devane D, Gyte GML. Continuous cardiotocography (CTG) as a form of electronic fetal monitoring (EFM) for fetal assessment during labour. *Cochrane Database Syst Rev.* 2013;5. CD006066. doi: 10.1002/14651858.CD006066.pub2.

22. Reynolds F. Labour analgesia and the baby: good news is no news. *Int J Obstet Anesth.* 2011;20(1): 38–50.

23. Butwick AJ. 2012 Gerard W. Ostheimer Lecture: what's new in obstetric anesthesia? *Int J Obstet Anesth.* 2012;21: 348–56.

24. Hawkins JL. The 2013 SOAP/FAER/Gertie Marx Honorary Lecture 2013: from print to practice – the evolving nature of obstetric anaesthesia. *Int J Obstet Anesth.* 2014;23: 376–82.

25. Palanisamy A. The 2013 Gerard W. Ostheimer Lecture: what's new in obstetric anesthesia? *Int J Obstet Anesth.* 2014;23: 58–65.

26. Hofmeyr GJ, Cyna AM, Middleton P. Prophylactic intravenous preloading for regional analgesia in labour. *Cochrane Database Syst Rev.* 2004;4. CD000175. doi: 10.1002/14651858.CD000175. pub2.

27. Simmons SW, Taghizadeh N, Dennis AT, Hughes D, Cyna AM. Combined spinal-epidural versus epidural analgesia in labour. *Cochrane Database Syst Rev.* 2012;10. CD003401. doi: 10.1002/14651858. CD003401.pub3.

28. Royal College of Obstetricians and Gynaecologists and the Royal College of Anaesthetists. Classification of urgency of caesarean section: a continuum of risk. *Good Practice No. 11*, April 2010.

29. Afolabi BB, Lesi FEA. Regional versus general anaesthesia for caesarean section. *Cochrane Database Syst Rev.* 2012;10. CD004350. doi: 10.1002/14651858. CD004350.pub3.

30. National Institute for Health and Care Excellence. Caesarean section: clinical guideline 132; 2014. www. nice.org.uk/guidance/cg132 (accessed August 2012).

31. Mushambi MC *et al.* Obstetrics Anaesthetists' Association and Difficult Airway Society guidelines for the management of difficult and failed tracheal intubation in obstetrics. *Anaesthesia.* 2015;70(11): 1286–306. doi: 10.1111/anes.13260.

32. Chatmongkolchart S, Prathep S. Supplemental oxygen for caesarean section during regional anaesthesia. *Cochrane Database Syst Rev.* 2013;6. CD006161. doi: 10.1002/14651858.CD006161.pub2.

33. Ralph CJ, Sullivan I, Faulds J. Intraoperative cell salvaged blood as part of a blood conservation strategy in caesarean section: is fetal red cell contamination important? *Br J Anaes.* 2011;107(3): 404–8.

Intrapartum Fetal Monitoring

Savvas Argyridis and Sabaratnam Arulkumaran

Introduction

The fetus receives its oxygen and nutrition through the umbilical cord from the placenta that floats in the amniotic fluid. The placenta receives oxygen and nutrition from the maternal blood and excretes its waste products into the maternal side. Uterine contractions of labour reduce or intermittently cut off the blood perfusion into the retro-placental area, thus reducing the exchange of gases and essential nutrition to the fetus. Contractions may also compress the umbilical cord and prevent or reduce gas and nutrition exchange by reducing or obstructing the flow of blood to the placenta.

While waiting for labour to progress, the uterine contractions and fetal heart rate are observed to identify any fetal compromise caused by uterine contractions. Fetal heart rate (FHR) monitoring is done by intermittent auscultation every 15 min for a period of 1 min immediately after contraction in the first stage and every 5 min in the second stage of labour in low-risk pregnancy. Pregnancies known to be at high risk (e.g. diabetes, hypertension, intrauterine growth restriction, prolonged pregnancy, etc.) have continuous observation of the FHR and uterine contractions, i.e. cardiotocography (CTG), which is done electronically and is termed electronic fetal monitoring (EFM).

During this process of labour and delivery, the fetus may be subjected to insults of hypoxia, infection and trauma. Although most labours are not associated with complications, they may arise at any time and may cause compromise to mother, baby or both. Some complications may be anticipated and managed appropriately to avoid injury to fetus or mother.

Cardiotocography is sensitive in picking up any stress to the fetus, like cord compression (variable decelerations), head compression (early deceler-

ations) or reduced retro-placental pool of blood (late decelerations). When the baby is distressed due to hypoxia it tends to show rise in the baseline rate and reduced baseline variability along with decelerations. Prolonged decelerations with FHR <80 bpm lasting greater than 3 min can indicate acute stress, and acidosis can develop rapidly if the FHR does not recover within 6–10 min, depending on the physiological reserve of the fetus. The lower the FHR and the longer the duration of deceleration, the greater the degree of acidosis. Such prolonged decelerations are usually transient and if they recover back to the baseline rate with normal baseline variability and accelerations it is unlikely that there will have been any hypoxic injury to the fetus because of such episodes.

An FHR of concern may necessitate measures to alleviate the factor causing the problem (e.g. hydration, maternal position change, cessation of oxytocin, transient tocolysis), fetal scalp blood sampling (FBS) to assess the fetus or delivery of the baby by caesarean section (CS) in the first stage of labour and by forceps or vacuum delivery in the second stage of labour. Such operative delivery is rarely associated with complications. The trauma, if any, are usually of a minor nature, but exceptionally they can give rise to severe morbidity or mortality. Attention and care in labour are required to anticipate, avoid and manage these problems; but despite the utmost and advanced care, fetal and maternal morbidity do occur.

Monitoring During Initial Assessment

Intermittent Auscultation

The following recommendations are made by the National Institute of Care Excellence (NICE) [1] as regards intermittent auscultation (IA) during labour:

Best Practice in Labour and Delivery, Second Edition, ed. Sir Sabaratnam Arulkumaran. Published by Cambridge University Press. © Cambridge University Press 2016.

offer IA with a fetal stethoscope (Pinard) or Doppler device. Auscultate the FHR at the first contact and at each further assessment. Auscultate for a minimum of 1 min immediately after a contraction, every 15 min in the first stage and every 5 min in the second stage of labour, and record the value as a single rate. Simultaneously palpate the maternal pulse in order to differentiate between maternal and fetal heart rate. Record accelerations (*listen with fetal movements*) and decelerations (*listen soon after contractions*) if heard. Do not offer admission CTG for low-risk women in suspected or established labour in any birth setting as part of initial assessment. Offer CTG if intermittent auscultation indicates possible FHR abnormalities, and explain why. Discontinue the CTG in 20 minutes if the trace is normal.

Meconium-stained Amniotic Fluid

The fetus passes meconium as a function of maturity and it is seen by about 5% incidence at 39–40 weeks, and increases to 10–15% by 41 weeks and 25% by 42 weeks. Passage of meconium may indicate infection, especially in the preterm, and is well known with listerial infections. In a breech presentation in labour, squeezing of the abdomen and pelvis as the fetus descends will reveal meconium. Use of misoprostol (prostaglandin E1) for induction of labour causes fetal intestinal motility and higher incidence of meconium-stained amniotic fluid.

Meconium is also considered to signify possible hypoxia if thick meconium is present with scanty fluid. Scanty fluid indicates reduced amniotic fluid, which is mostly the baby's urine, and hence it may signify less blood flow through fetal kidneys to redirect blood to the fetal brain and heart. Appearance of fresh meconium may also signify possible hypoxia. Recent NICE guidelines [1] suggest that the presence or absence of meconium should be documented. Significant meconium, defined as dark green or black fluid with thick clumps of meconium, or tenacious or gelatinous type of meconium needs continuous monitoring and facilities for neonatal resuscitation.

Meconium aspiration is not linked to acidosis but more to gasping movements associated with prolonged decelerations. Such decelerations may be more linked to uterine hyper-stimulation with oxytocin and hence caution should be exercised in monitoring the FHR and contractions, and control of oxytocin infusion. Maternal temperature may suggest possible infection/chorioamnionitis. Aspiration of infected meconium may cause infective pneumonitis, in addition to the chemical pneumonitis. Hence careful management of labour is needed with a low threshold for delivery in the presence of significant meconium, maternal temperature and the need for oxytocin augmentation.

Intermittent Electronic Fetal Monitoring

A randomized controlled trial (RCT) that compared intermittent EFM versus continuous EFM during the first stage of labour showed no significant difference in CS rates or neonatal outcomes such as umbilical cord pH, Apgar score or admissions to neonatal units [3]. In this study, intermittent EFM was done at every two hours for 15–30 min and in between IA was carried out every 15 min during the first stage of labour.

Admission Test (AT) Cardiotocography

Upon admission to the delivery unit, use of a 20 min CTG is called the admission test (AT). The AT was introduced as a screening method for identifying a high-risk fetus for hypoxia in an otherwise 'low-risk population' based on prospective studies [4,5]. However, RCTs did not show improvement in neonatal outcome when the AT was compared with intermittent auscultation [6,7]. On the other hand, there was significant difference in the use of epidural analgesia, augmentation of labour and operative delivery rates [7]. The duration of the admission CTG seems to affect the operative delivery rate, and units that offered a one-hour CTG have higher rates [8]. Poor predictive value and low sensitivity of the test was suggested in another trial that assessed inter-observer agreement among healthcare professionals in the clinical and non-clinical setting [9]. A large systematic review of more than 13 000 pregnancies that compared the effects of admission CTG with IA in low-risk pregnancies concluded that there was no statistically significant difference in operative delivery rates or fetal and neonatal outcomes, but there was a difference in continuous FMR and FBS in the groups having admission CTG compared with IA on admission. Data suggest that there is a non-significant increase in CS rate among the admission CTG groups [10].

Continuous Electronic Fetal Monitoring

Several trials compared IA with EFM in order to assess whether the neonatal outcome was better with EFM. Earlier trials showed similar rates of poor Apgar scores at birth and intensive care unit admissions. However, there was significant reduction in neonatal seizures among those monitored by EFM [11–13]. An RCT of over 13 000 pregnancies [14] concluded that the reduction of neonatal seizures reached almost 55%, but there was no difference in long-term outcome such as cerebral palsy. A meta-analysis of nearly 19 000 pregnancies [15] showed a significant increase of operative delivery and CS rates, but a significant decrease of perinatal mortality due to hypoxia in the EFM group. A systematic review of most trials comparing IA with EFM in low-risk pregnancies [16] concluded that there is no significant difference in perinatal mortality or cerebral palsy, but there is significant decrease in neonatal seizures among the EFM group of pregnancies. There is also an increase of CS rate and an increased risk of operative delivery among those monitored by continuous EFM.

Despite evidence from various RCTs regarding the dubious performance of EFM, there is continued reliance by healthcare professionals on this modality on medical and legal grounds. Hence the proper understanding of the use of this fetal surveillance method is vital to ensure safe practice. Table 4.1 provides the indications for continuous EFM.

At the commencement of EFM, the patient's name, hospital number, date of birth, date and time of recording should be recorded. Maternal vital signs should be checked and recorded before the start of the recording. The accuracy of the time that is automatically recorded on the trace should be checked. If the CTG trace is extended beyond one pack of paper, each pack should have a serial number. With the wide-beam ultrasound transducer the maternal heart rate (MHR) may be picked up and misconstrued as the FHR. Hence it is

Table 4.1 Indications for continuous EFM [1,17]

1. Labour abnormalities	Induction of labour Augmentation of labour Prolonged first or second stage of labour Prolonged rupture of membranes Regional analgesia Previous caesarean section Abnormal uterine activity/use of oxytocin
2. Suspected fetal compromise in labour	Presence of significant meconium staining Suspicious fetal heart rate on intermittent auscultation (FHR <110 or >160 bpm) or decelerations Abnormal admission CTG Vaginal bleeding in labour Intrauterine infection/chorioamnionitis/temperature >38 °C
3. Fetal problems	Multiple pregnancies Fetus with growth restriction or macrosomia Reduced fetal movements in the previous 24 hours Preterm fetus Breech presentation Poly-, oligo- or anhydramnios Postterm pregnancy Rhesus isoimmunization
4. Maternal medical disease	Moderate to severe hypertension/pre-eclampsia Diabetes, renal disease Cardiac disease Haemoglobinopathy, severe anaemia Hyperthyroidism Collagen disease

Box 4.2

The woman should have an explanation regarding the recommendations for the use of continuous CTG. Amniotomy alone is not an indication for EFM. The woman should be informed that if there is a normal trace that it is reassuring, while an abnormal trace is reason for further EFM, and if needed this may necessitate additional tests. She should also have the understanding that decisions concerning further action are based on assessment of several factors, one of which is the finding of the EFM.

good practice to auscultate the FHR and then to place the transducer. A sudden shift in the baseline rate from fetus to mother may occur and is due to slippage of the transducer (Figure 4.1); this should be noted and recorded.

If FHR cannot be obtained with an ultrasound transducer, listen with a stethoscope and if still not audible establish whether FHR is present using a

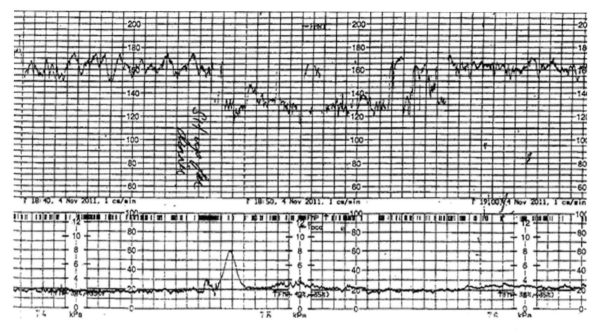

Figure 4.1 The FHR recording is seen initially followed by MHR recording; the transducer is readjusted to get the FHR.

portable ultrasound machine. Once it is established that the FHR is present, a scalp electrode may be employed to obtain EFM.

FHR changes are known to occur with vaginal examination, artificial rupture of membranes, sitting up, insertion of epidural, fetal scalp blood sampling, etc. The events that lead to these changes should be noted on the CTG paper. The interpretation of the trace at regular intervals should be recorded on the notes and, if significant, on the trace, and the health-care personnel should sign and indicate the date and time.

If CTG is discontinued the reason for this should be recorded on the trace, e.g. birth of the baby – in this case the time and condition of the baby at birth should be noted. It is not uncommon to see that either the FHR or contractions are not recorded satisfactorily, especially with the use of oxytocin towards the late first and second stage of labour when there is maximal stress to the fetus. Every effort should be made to obtain optimal recordings that could help with meaningful interpretation. A central system with display of CTG recordings in all labour rooms acts as a 'neighbourhood watch' to identify abnormal traces and for staff to help each other, but also when suitably connected to a server will help archive information for up to 25 years, which is a medico-legal requirement.

Interpretation of CTG

A systematic approach is required when interpreting an FHR pattern. This should include review of the baseline heart rate, baseline variability and presence or absence of accelerations and decelerations.

Baseline Rate

The baseline rate is the mean FHR after exclusion of accelerations and decelerations determined over a period of 5–10 min and expressed in beats per minute (bpm). A normal baseline rate is considered between 100 and 160 bpm [1]. Tachycardia is defined as a mean FHR of above 160 bpm for 10 min or more and is further classified as moderate (160–179 bpm) and severe (>180–199 bpm). Causative factors of fetal tachycardia include maternal or fetal infection (chorioamnionitis), maternal hyperthyroidism, excessive catecholamine secretion due to stress, fetal hypoxia and tachyarrhythmias [18]. Tachycardia may not have strong association with fetal acidaemia or umbilical cord pH less than 7.20, but if it is associated with infection, minimal or absent variability and/or late, recurrent decelerations, the risk is increased [19,20].

The terms bradycardia and prolonged deceleration are used interchangeably. If we consider that the baseline rate is assessed over a 10 min period, the term

Box 4.3

A baseline rate of 110–160 bpm is considered to be normal, while a rate of 100–109 bpm with normal baseline variability and no variable or late decelerations is normal and should not prompt further actions [1]. A baseline rate between 90 and 99 bpm with normal baseline variability may be a normal variant if the other CTG features are normal and that the trace is maternal has been excluded. However, a second opinion in these cases would be useful.

If the baseline rate is between 100 and 109 bpm or above 160 bpm and there is one more non-reassuring feature, start conservative measures.

A baseline rate between 161 and 180 bpm with reassuring features of accelerations and normal baseline variability in the absence of decelerations is of no concern. If it has no other non-reassuring features other than the rate, the possible underlying cause may be an infection and appropriate investigation should be instituted, including observation of maternal vital signs of pulse and temperature. If raised, paracetamol and fluids should be given and the temperature lowered.

If the baseline rate is above 180 bpm with no other non-reassuring features, possible underlying causes (such as infection) should be considered and appropriate investigation should be commenced, including observations of maternal vital signs (pulse, temperature). If temperature is raised, the mother should be given paracetamol and fluids. It may be advisable to offer fetal scalp blood sampling to measure lactate or pH if the rate remains above 180 bpm despite conservative measures.

With prolonged deceleration when the FHR is below 100 bpm for 3 min or more, conservative measures of positioning the woman to left lateral and stopping the use of oxytocin should be started, along with summoning urgent obstetric help with the view that urgent birth may be warranted. If bradycardia persists for more than 9 min, birth should be expedited. If the FHR recovers within 9 min, the case should be re-evaluated as to the best management.

Box 4.4

Fluctuations of the baseline rate between 6 and 25 bpm amplitude that is irregular and abrupt, occurring at 3–5 cycles per minute (frequency) is defined as baseline variability [25,26]. The baseline variability is calculated by assessing the bandwidth between the topmost and the lowest FHR within a centimetre segment. The baseline variability differs minute to minute and the best segment during the last 10 min may be indicative of the integrity of the autonomic nervous system. Maintaining normal variability (6–25 bpm) is a sign that fetal compensatory mechanisms provide adequate oxygen to the fetal brain. Variability of 0–5 bpm is classified as reduced and that with undetectable amplitudes termed absent. The normal fetal sleep cycle lasts approximately 30 min [1]. Some studies suggest that it may last up to 90 min [27], although interventions may be required by that time if associated with other non-reassuring features of decelerations and/or tachycardia. Central nervous system (CNS) depressants such as magnesium sulphate or opioids can cause reduced baseline variability. Central nervous system congenital abnormalities like anencephaly and some chromosomally abnormal fetuses may exhibit reduced or absent baseline variability. Drugs that influence the heart rate such as atropine or cardiac abnormalities (complete heart block) may also cause minimal variability. Fetal hypoxia is the most likely aetiology if other features such as late or variable recurrent decelerations, bradycardia or sinusoidal pattern are present. In such situations there is high probability of fetal acidaemia [19,28]. An adverse neonatal outcome in such an event has been estimated at 16.9% of cases [29]. If minimal or absent variability lasts for more than one hour with recurrent abnormal decelerations, the probability of significant fetal acidaemia (pH less than 7.00) is estimated at 12–31%. It is considered as the most significant intrapartum parameter for prediction of acidaemia [30].

bradycardia should be for those who have a mean FHR of below 100 bpm. If bradycardia is associated with minimal or absent variability and/or late, recurrent decelerations, there is higher risk of fetal acidosis [20,21]. When the baseline heart rate is 130–140 bpm and then drops to <100 bpm it should be termed prolonged deceleration. Causative factors for prolonged decelerations include fetal descent, uterine rupture, hypotension, cord prolapse and abruption [21]. According to various prospective observational studies, the commonest non-reassuring FHR that resulted in CS was prolonged decelerations [22,23]. Prolonged and late decelerations during second stage of labour are independently associated with fetal acidosis (umbilical arterial pH < 7.20) [24].

Accelerations

Accelerations are defined as abrupt increases of the baseline rate of more than 15 bpm that last for at least 15 sec, but less than 2 min (Figure 4.2). If a pregnancy is less than 32 weeks, an increase of 10 bpm for at least 10 sec is considered as an acceleration [32]. In a 20 min period, if two or more accelerations are recorded, the trace is considered as reactive, with a sensitivity of 97% for an Apgar score greater than 7 in 5 min [33,34]. If accelerations are present it is indicative of a non-acidotic fetus, especially when accompanied by normal baseline variability [35], and if absent and combined with minimal variability there is an increased rate of adverse neonatal outcome [36]. Absence of accelerations in a normal CTG does not indicate acidosis. During quiet epochs of the FHR cycles there may be absence of accelerations and reduced baseline variability (Figure 4.3).

Decelerations

Early Decelerations

There is a gradual fall of the FHR and return to baseline rate in parallel with uterine contractions (Figure 4.4). They are uniform and repetitive, with the nadir of FHR and peak of contraction occurring at the same time, i.e. decelerations are the mirror image of the contractions [32]. The drop is not usually more than 40 bpm

---

Box 4.5

If baseline variability less than 5 bpm with no other non-reassuring features is present and persists for more than 30 min, conservative measures should be taken. Fetal blood sampling for lactate or pH measurement should be considered if it persists for more than 90 min but had no reactive trace from the onset of labour or has developed non-reassuring features of decelerations or increase in FHR. If decelerations are absent, the reduced baseline variability may be due to causes other than hypoxia, e.g. infection.

With baseline variability less than 5 bpm for over 30 min, with one or more features of tachycardia, bradycardia or decelerations (variable, late), if conservative measures do not improve the FHR trace, FBS for lactate or pH measurement should be considered based on the clinical situation.

Baseline Variability

Markedly increased or saltatory variability is defined as an amplitude of more than 25 bpm and is also considered as an FHR abnormality [31]. It may be indicative of acute hypoxia and the increased variability may be due to an overreaction of the autonomic nervous system. Pseudo-sinusoidal patterns such as amplitude of 5–15 bpm are not significant.

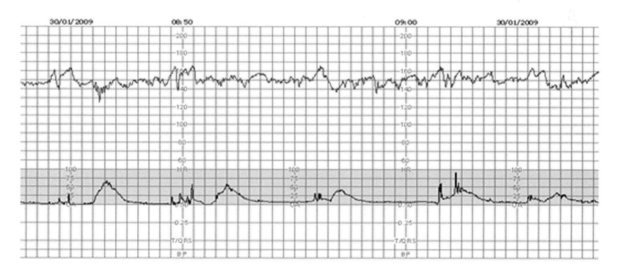

Figure 4.2 Presence of accelerations – sign of a fetus with no acidosis [1].

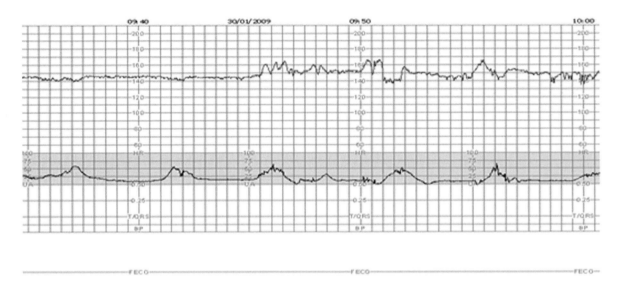

Figure 4.3 Quiet (minimal or no accelerations and reduced baseline variability) epoch alternating with an active (accelerations with normal baseline variability) epoch ('cycling'), suggestive of a healthy fetus at term.

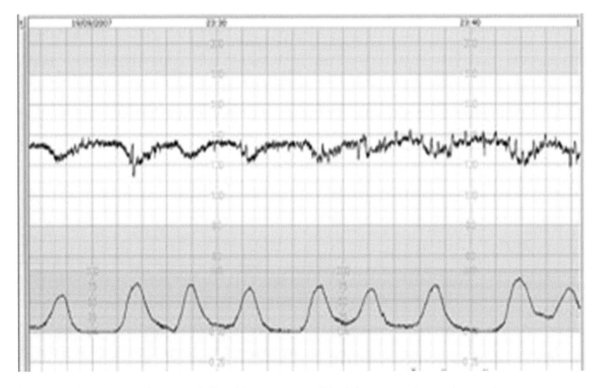

Figure 4.4 Early decelerations: the onset and offset of the contractions and decelerations occur almost at the same time.

from the baseline rate and is not associated with fetal acidosis or adverse neonatal outcome [37,38]. They are mostly attributed to head compression during late first stage and second stage of labour [39].

Late Decelerations

The drop in the FHR is gradual in onset and appears later than 30 sec from the onset of contractions. The FHR gradually decreases and has a slow return to

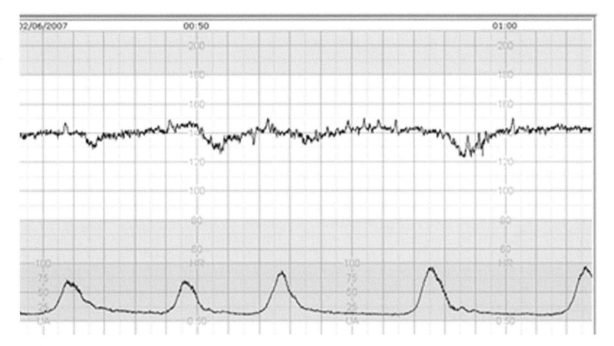

Figure 4.5 Late decelerations: the nadir of the deceleration is >30 sec from the acme of the contraction.

baseline rate. They are uniform and repetitive, with the nadir of FHR after the peak of contraction [32] (Figure 4.5). There is association between late decelerations and reduced Apgar score at 5 min [37,40]; umbilical pH less than 7.00 [39] and increased risk of cerebral palsy [19].

When accompanied by minimal variability and absence of accelerations, recurrent late decelerations are associated with metabolic acidosis in more than 50% of cases [41] (Figure 4.6).

As a solitary finding, late decelerations have a low predictive value, with a high false-positive rate [19,42], not correlating well with an adverse neonatal outcome [43]. Aetiologies responsible for late decelerations include uterine tetany, maternal hypotension and placental insufficiency. It is a reflex CNS response to hypoxia and/or metabolic acidosis [44]. The mechanism responsible is primarily hypoxaemic hypoxia, i.e. decreased availability of oxygen [45–47]. If there is association with a rising baseline rate and reduction in variability, the hypoxia is gradual. The FHR may reach a maximal rate, after which the baseline variability is reduced and the fetus might tolerate this for up to 60 min, but FBS is required to determine the fetal status [47].

Variable Decelerations

These are abrupt and the onset is in less than 30 sec of the start of a contraction. The FHR decreases precipitously and returns to baseline rate quickly; it has a variable relationship to uterine contractions [32]. They are further categorized into uncomplicated [32] or <60 sec and <60 beats [1] and complicated [32] or >60 sec or >60 beats, or both [1]. Uncomplicated decelerations are characterized by small depth and short duration, with primary and secondary slight rises in the baseline rate i.e. 'shoulders'. They show quick recovery to the baseline rate in the presence of normal variability and lack of late decelerations [48]. They are well tolerated by the fetus and are not consistently associated with a poor neonatal outcome [49] (Figure 4.7).

If recurrent with more than 50% of contractions over a 90 min period, there is an increased risk of adverse neonatal outcome [50]. However, before the fetus is compromised there is likely to be a rise in the baseline rate, increase in depth and duration of decelerations and reduction in baseline variability. Complicated decelerations are characterized by greater depth (>60 beats) and duration (>60 sec), lack of 'shoulders', late recovery, minimal variability and presence of late decelerations. They are associated with

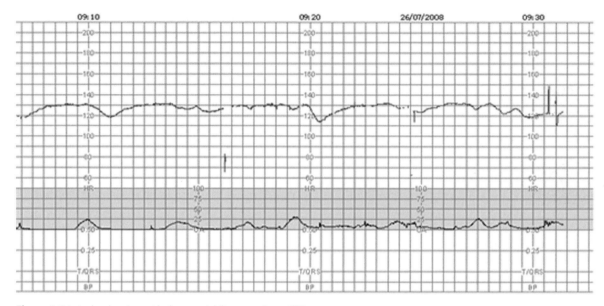

Figure 4.6 Late decelerations with absent variability: an ominous CTG trace.

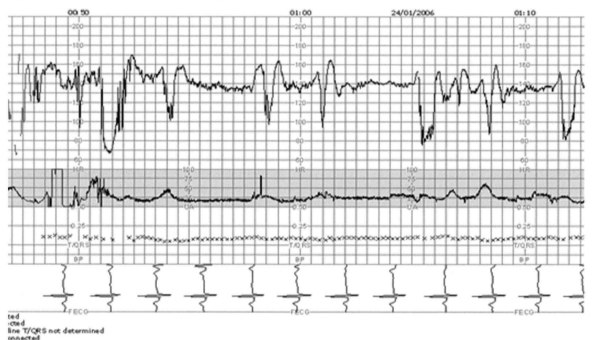

Figure 4.7 Recurrent variable decelerations with 'shoulders' (<60 beats and <60 sec with some which are >60 beats or >60 sec).

an adverse neonatal outcome [28,51,52]. Aetiologies include umbilical cord compression, especially in the presence of oligo- or anhydramnios (at rupture of membranes) or a nuchal cord. The hypoxia mechanism is interference with blood flow and oxygen availability, i.e. ischaemic hypoxia [45–47].

Prolonged Decelerations

A decrease of FHR below 15 bpm from baseline rate and lasting for more than 2 min but less than 10 min is considered as a prolonged deceleration [32]. This has been described in brief in the section on baseline FHR. If the FHR remains less than 80 bpm and lasts for

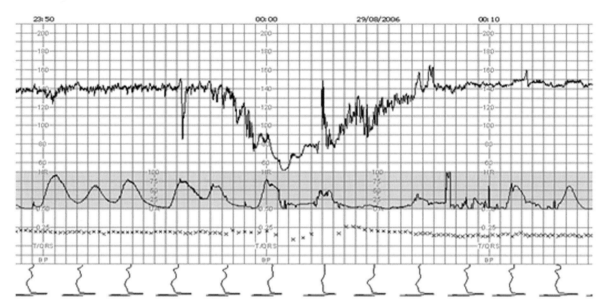

Figure 4.8 Prolonged deceleration (acute hypoxia) reversed by stopping oxytocin infusion.

more than 3 min, it is considered abnormal [25] and is associated with fetal acidosis, especially in the presence of minimal variability [53]. Immediate delivery is indicated if the FHR fails to recover by 9 min with conservative measures. Aetiologies that need prompt delivery based on clinical assessment include placental abruption, uterine scar rupture and cord prolapse. Dorsal position, hyper-stimulation with oxytocin or prostaglandin, vaginal examination, amniotomy and administration of epidural can give rise to prolonged decelerations that are likely to recover with conservative measures of correcting position to left lateral, fluid administration, stopping oxytocin and acute tocolysis (Figure 4.8).

Current NICE recommendations suggest that decelerations should be described in terms of depth, duration, timing in relation to contractions, return or not to baseline rate, persistence and occurrence with less or more than 50% of contractions [1]. The terms 'early', 'late' and 'variable' are used. With variable decelerations, NICE recommends that instead of 'typical' and 'atypical' variable decelerations, to use the terms of greater or less than 60 sec in duration or greater or less than 60 beats in depth.

The following considerations and actions are recommended in the presence of decelerations.

Early deceleration assessment should take into account that they are uncommon, benign and associated with head compression, and hence should be

seen only in the late first and second stage of labour. If not accompanied with non-reassuring features they should not prompt further action.

Variable decelerations that begin with onset of contraction are very common and are a normal feature in an uncomplicated birth and are usually the result of cord compression. Manage by change of position or mobilization.

Conservative measures should be undertaken if variable decelerations are present with normal baseline rate and normal variability and the drop from the baseline rate is <60 bpm or less, takes 60 sec or less to recover and is present for over 90 min, occurring with over 50% of contractions.

Conservative measures are appropriate if variable decelerations with normal baseline rate and normal variability are present with decelerations with a drop from baseline rate by more than 60 bpm or taking over 60 sec to recover, and are present for up to 30 min, occurring with over 50% of contractions. Fetal blood sampling for pH or lactate measurement should be considered if variable decelerations are non-reassuring, i.e. there is no change after 30 min of conservative measures or the FHR is accompanied by tachycardia and/or reduced variability.

In the presence of late decelerations, conservative measures should be tried if they occur with over 50% of contractions in a 30 min window. If there is no improvement and it persists for >30 min and with over

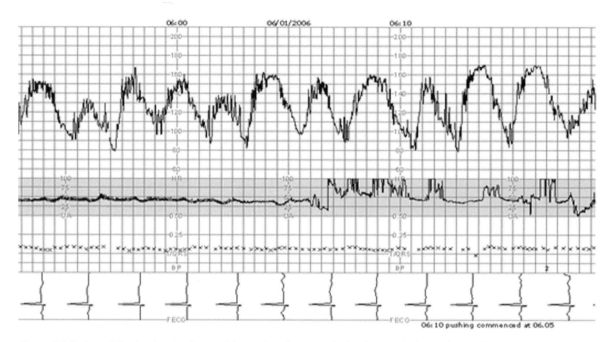

Figure 4.9 Prolonged decelerations that last much longer than the time at the baseline rate ('sub-acute hypoxia')

50% of contractions, consider fetal blood sampling to measure lactate or pH and/or actions to expedite birth. These actions should be sooner if they are accompanied by abnormal baseline rate and/or reduced variability.

If decelerations are longer, later and deeper, with less time at the baseline rate compared with during the deceleration, development of fetal acidosis is rapid and action should be taken sooner than 30 min ('sub-acute hypoxia') (Figure 4.9).

Sinusoidal Pattern

A sinusoidal pattern is a smooth sine wave that is periodical (3–5 cycles per minute), has an amplitude of 5–15 bpm above and below the baseline, lasting for 10–20 minutes [35]. There is also a lack of accelerations or decelerations in response to stimuli. It is believed to be a response mechanism to fetal hypoxia, with small beat-to-beat alterations. The most severe associated condition is fetal anaemia, which may be due to alloimmunization, parvovirus infection, placental abruption or vasa praevia, and is believed to be preterminal [54]. Other aetiologies associated with this pattern are fetal sucking movements or narcotic administration [55]. In order to determine the aetiology and risk of fetal acidosis and adverse neonatal outcome, fetal scalp stimulation or FBS may be helpful [56]. Depending on the

period of gestation, prompt delivery or therapy in a fetal medicine unit may be needed if fetal anaemia is suspected.

Categorization of CTGs Based on the Features of the Trace

Based on the above description of individual features of the CTG, the traces can be categorized as normal/reassuring, non-reassuring and abnormal, and are described in Table 4.2.

Depending on the FHR pattern, there are several measures that need to be taken in order to identify potential fetal compromise, improve oxygenation and placental perfusion, as well as expedite delivery in order to prevent perinatal and neonatal morbidity or mortality [57].

Conservative Measures

If a trace is categorized as suspicious, conservative measures are required.

Mobilization or obtain a left lateral position. This position improves placental perfusion and may reduce cord compression.

Oral or intravenous fluids bolus (500–1000 ml of Ringer's lactate or normal saline). This may be effective in cases of dehydration, hypovolaemia or hypotension

Table 4.2 Categorization of FHR patterns [1]

Feature	Baseline rate	Baseline variability	Decelerations
Normal/reassuring	100–160 bpm	≥5 bpm	None Early
Non-reassuring	161–180 bpm	<5 for 30–90 min	*1. Variable:* Drop by ≤60 bpm and taking ≤60 sec to recover Present for >90 min Occurs >50% of contractions; or *2. Variable:* Drop >60 bpm or taking >60 sec to recover Present for >30 min Occurs >50% of contractions; *or* *3. Late:* Present for ≤30 min Occurs >50% of contractions
Abnormal	>180 or <100 bpm	<5 for >90 min	*1. Variable:* Present 30 min after conservative measures Occur >50% of contractions; *or* *2. Late:* Present >30 minutes No improvement with conservative measures Occur >50% of contractions; *or* *3. Prolonged* Deceleration for ≥3 min

Some hospitals may use the previous classification produced by the RCOG [25] or that recommended by the NICHD [32], given in Tables 4.3 and 4.4.

due to epidural analgesia administration. With fluids there is improvement of placental perfusion [58]. Caution is needed in pregnancies complicated with preeclampsia, chorioamnionitis or when using tocolytics, in which case there is a risk of overload.

Paracetamol and fluids should be given if there is raised maternal temperature with fetal tachycardia. Discontinuation of oxytocin infusion is essential in cases of uterine tetany or too frequent contractions to avoid placental blood flow disruption during contractions. Tocolytic administration such as terbutaline 0.25 mg subcutaneously helps to relax the uterus and to improve retro-placental perfusion and/or to avoid cord compression. Oxygen administration at a rate of

8–10 l/min in order to improve fetal oxygenation is controversial since there are conflicting data regarding efficacy of this practice in reducing fetal acidosis [59,60], because the underlying cause of the fetal distress is due to reduction of placental perfusion and this cannot be corrected by oxygen supplementation

Table 4.3 Categorization of FHR patterns by the RCOG [25]

Category	Definition
Normal	All features are reassuring
Suspicious	One feature is non-reassuring Remaining features reassuring
Pathological	Two or more features are non-reassuring One or more feature is abnormal

Table 4.4 Categorization of FHR patterns by the NICHD [32]

Category	Baseline rate	Variability	Decelerations
Category I	110–160 bpm	6–25 bpm	None Early, may be present Variable absent Late absent
Category II	Tachycardia (>160 bpm)	6–25 bpm	Variable present + variability present Late present + variability present
Category III	Bradycardia (<100 bpm)	Absent	Variable recurrent Late recurrent *or* Sinusoidal pattern

Actions on (a) suspicious/non-reassuring/Category II; or (b) pathological/abnormal/Category III CTG trace.

only. Amnioinfusion is practised in some centres, but evidence for such practice is lacking and is not recommended for intrauterine resuscitation [1].

Testing Fetal Well-being by Adjunct Technology

Fetal Stimulation

If accelerations are present with fetal scalp stimulation during a vaginal examination, the risk of fetal acidosis is unlikely. If absent there is a significant risk. It is useful when facilities for FBS are not available [1]. In some countries fetal vibro acoustic stimulation (FAST) is used to elicit accelerations.

Fetal Scalp Blood Sampling

This method is used in cases of abnormal/pathological traces, in order to evaluate fetal acidosis by measuring fetal pH and lactate. It is good practice to explain to the woman why FBS is advised. You must state that the procedure is to measure the acid in the baby's blood, and that it requires a vaginal examination followed by a small scratch on the baby's scalp. The mother should be made to understand that it might help to reduce the need for further interventions. She must also be told that different actions may follow the result, such as caesarean section or instrumental birth.

The woman should be in the left lateral position. An amnioscope is introduced through the vagina and cervix to expose the fetal head. The amnioscope is held against the scalp with pressure to create a 'cofferdam' effect that prevents amniotic fluid soiling the area of sampling. The area is cleaned and dried with cotton swabs. Ethyl chloride is sprayed on the testing site to 'arterialize' the capillaries and the area is gently smeared with silicone gel so that blood will come out as drops. A small puncture 2 mm in depth is made by a special blade for blood collection. Contraindications for this procedure are risk of infection that may give rise to immediate and long-term problems for the fetus (hepatitis, HIV, herpes), prematurity (gestational age less than 34 weeks) and fetal bleeding diathesis (haemophilia). In such cases and where the cervix is less than 3 cm dilated, making it difficult to do an FBS, it may be best to expedite delivery.

Technical problems associated with this procedure include insufficient blood quantity, air bubbles and blood clots. Failure to obtain results for acid–base balance is reported to be as high as in 20% of cases [61].

Table 4.5 Interpretation of scalp blood pH values

Interpretation	pH	Lactate
Normal	≥7.25	≤4.1
Borderline	7.21–7.24	4.2–4.8
Abnormal	≤7.20	≥4.9

Box 4.6

Following a normal result, repeat measurement is advised at one-hour intervals if the CTG is non-reassuring, or earlier if there are additional non-reassuring or abnormal features, e.g. rise in the baseline rate, increase in the depth and/or duration of deceleration, reduction of baseline variability. After a borderline result, repeat sampling in 30 min is recommended, unless there are additional non-reassuring or abnormal features. Take into account the time needed to take the sample if the plan is to repeat. Stable results (unchanged pH and lactate) after a second sample indicate that there is no need for a third sample, unless additional non-reassuring or abnormal features evolve.

Results are classified according to pH value and lactate concentration and should be informed as such [1] (see Table 4.5).

Following an abnormal or third result, consultant obstetric advice should be requested [1]. If a sample cannot be obtained and scalp stimulation results in accelerations, decide whether to continue labour or expedite birth. If a sample cannot be obtained and the CTG has not improved, consideration should be given to an expedited birth.

Lactate and pH has poor sensitivity in predicting long-term neurological outcomes [62]. When measuring umbilical artery blood gases at a pH less than 7.00, base deficit is a good indicator of fetal tissue oxygen debt. A base deficit of >8 mmol/l is considered moderate, while >12 mmol/l is considered to indicate severe metabolic acidosis [63]; these are the limits at which neonatal complications have been reported [64].

Lactate measurement is performed via a similar method as that for scalp pH. Due to the requirements of smaller blood samples (5 μl instead of 35 μl for pH and base excess), failure rates are lower compared with testing for pH and base excess and the time taken for sampling to result is reduced [61]. Caput formation does not alter the correlation between scalp and

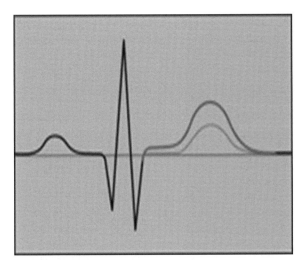

Figure 4.10 Fetal ECG with rises in the ST segment and increase in height of the T wave.

circulatory values [65]. Maternal and fetal lactate production are increased with the duration of active bearing down efforts in the second stage of labour. It is estimated that with every 30 min of pushing, there is an increase of lactate by 1 mmol/l [66]. A good correlation has been shown between scalp and umbilical cord blood lactate [67].

Fetal Electrocardiogram (ECG): ST Waveform Analysis

This method involves the detection of changes in the ST segment of the fetal ECG with hypoxic stress. The ST waveform provides information on the ability of the fetal heart muscle to respond to the stress of labour. If the ST segment is elevated and T wave increased, this is indicative that the myocardium is responding to hypoxia. This is brought about by the increase of catecholamines that mobilizes the stored myocardial glycogen. The ingress of glucose with potassium ions into the myocardial cells brings about the changes in the ST segment and the T wave (Figure 4.10).

The changes in the T/QRS ratio due to hypoxia can be in the form of a steady increase, i.e. 'baseline rise', or transient increase with the contractions, i.e. 'episodic increase'. Other aetiologies for ST elevation include fetal infection, anaemia and hypotension. These changes occur well in advance of any CNS failing function. An ST depression with negative T waves indicates that the myocardium is not fully responding to the hypoxic stress [68]. If the ST segment distortion is above the isoelectric line set along the base of the P wave then it is termed biphasic T/QRS – grade

1 change. If the ST distortion cuts the isoelectric line it is called biphasic grade 2, and if the ST distortion is below the isoelectric line it is called biphasic grade 3 (Figure 4.11). The ST distortion may be a feature in cases of initial hypoxia and long-term reduction in oxygen and nutritional supply. The pathophysiological mechanism behind this is an uncoordinated repolarization within the myocardium, with prolonged repolarization of the endocardium [68]. However, these changes are best considered in the context of the clinical situation and the CTG.

A ST analyser or STAN machine (Neoventa Medical, Sweden) developed for FHR and ST waveform assessment identifies ECG changes by computer technology and provides guidelines on clinical action that should be taken. The fetal ECG signal is obtained by a single spiral electrode attached to the fetal scalp during labour. A maternal skin reference electrode should be applied on the upper thigh of the mother. Studies report sensitivity and specificity of 38–90% and 83–100% respectively for the prediction of fetal acidosis [69,70].

Meta-analysis shows that when fetal ECG is used with continuous CTG there is significant reduction of FBS, fetal acidosis and operative delivery rates [71]. For application of the electrode, the cervix should be sufficiently dilated, membranes should be ruptured and there should be no contraindication for using an internal fetal electrode. Staff training on interpretation of the CTG and the use of the automated ECG readings is a must for this method to be successful (Figure 4.12). In many centres FBS is performed in rare cases where the CTG abnormality shows tachycardia and absent baseline variability, with decelerations longer than one hour and in cases where CTG abnormalities are present before the commencement of ECG monitoring. In some ways the readings of the CTG reflects the activity of the CNS (accelerations reflecting the somatic and baseline variability of the autonomic nervous system) while ECG changes reflect the response of the heart to the stress and catecholamine surge.

Fetal Pulse Oxymetry (FPO)

Fetal arterial oxygen saturation ($FSpO_2$) has been studied in order to assess its correlation to fetal acidaemia and possible applications during labour in order to predict hypoxic events of concern. Studies suggest a threshold of SpO_2 of >30% is equivalent to pH >7.13

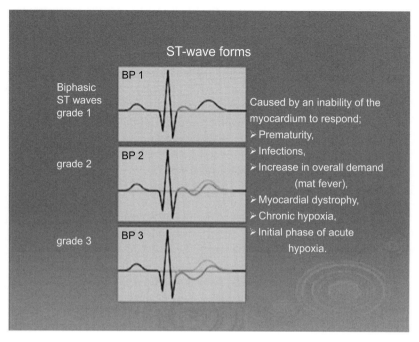

Figure 4.11 ECG complexes showing biphasic ST waves and possible causations.

[72,73] and if SpO$_2$ remains less than 30% for more than 10 min there is an increased risk of fetal acidosis [74,75]. The mean fetal SpO$_2$ during the first and second stage of labour is 59% and 53% respectively [76]. The clinical utility of this method remains controversial. A large RCT concluded that the overall CS rate was not reduced despite a reduction in CS rate for non-reassuring FHR patterns [77]. A systematic review and meta-analysis in 2014 concluded that the CS rate, maternal and neonatal outcomes were similar with or without the use of FPO [78]. The American College of Obstetricians and Gynecologists (ACOG), stated that the adoption of this device could not be endorsed because it would increase the cost of care without necessarily improving the clinical outcome [79].

Conclusion

The expected results from different methods of intrapartum fetal surveillance are less than optimal. A recent review of cases by the National Health Service Litigation Authority on adverse outcomes of intrapartum mortality and morbidity [80] points to the same issues that were identified in the fourth *Confidential Enquiry into Stillbirths and Deaths in Infancy* (CESDI) report [81]. The areas that were highlighted were: the inability to interpret the CTG; failure to incorporate the clinical situation; delay in taking action; and poor communication and teamwork. Attempts have been made to improve education by day master classes and computerized e-learning packages such as one produced by the Royal College of Midwives and Royal College of Obstetricians and Gynaecologists

Table 4.6 STAN clinical guidelines [68]

ST	Intermediate CTG	Abnormal CTG	Preterminal CTG
Episodic T/QRS rise	Increase >0.15 from baseline	Increase >0.10 from baseline	Immediate delivery regardless of ST
Baseline T/QRS rise	Increase >0.10 from baseline	Increase >0.05 from baseline	Delivery regardless of ST changes
Biphasic ST (a component of ST below baseline)	Continuous >5 min or >2 episodes of coupled biphasic ST type 2 or 3	Continuous >2 min or >1 episode of coupled biphasic ST type 2 or 3	

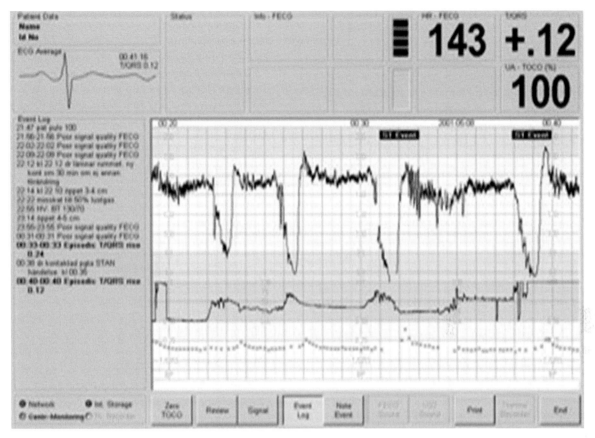

Figure 4.12 A screen display of combined CTG and STAN recording. The T/QRS ratio is displayed at the right upper corner as +.12. The computerized detection of ECG changes are shown on the event log and on the trace – in this case it shows episodic rise of T/QRS, which is seen at the T/QRS plot at the base of the trace.

with the help of NHS e-learning [82]. These are in addition to the in-house weekly CTG meetings. Despite these efforts, in the authors' opinion the expected outcomes of mothers, babies and care givers are unlikely to be realized unless compulsory testing on CTG pattern recognition, the pathophysiology behind the changes, and situational analysis and escalation are tested. It is mind boggling that we expect and have certification in other areas of our practice, such as different levels of competence for performing endoscopic surgery, but yet do not have competency testing for interpreting CTG and taking appropriate actions. Cardiotocography may be an inaccurate science, but improvements can be made although it may not become 100% perfect. Those who do not reach an optimal standard need not be stopped from practice but could be required to ask for a second opinion at regular intervals when they are faced with an abnormal trace until such a time as they reach an optimal

level of competence. These tests should be done at regular intervals to keep up this competence. The responsibility of training, testing and helping should fall to professional bodies who certify competence, the trusts that provide the clinical services and the individuals who practice.

Attempts have been made to use computer technology to automatically interpret CTGs and highlight risk factors. The results of the INFANT study that recruited 45 000 women are anxiously awaited. This is a powerful RCT with end points of intrapartum deaths and severe neonatal morbidity. The fetal ECG combined with CTG (STAN technology) has proven to be useful in some centres and not in others. The FM Alert RCT with 6000 women recruited has the CTG and the ECG analysed by the computer as opposed to the standard STAN technology of clinician interpretation of CTG and computerized interpretation of ECG. The end point is the incidence of metabolic acidosis. If the computerized CTG–ECG analysis shows significant reduction, a large RCT is warranted to examine the end points of intrapartum mortality and severe morbidity. Until such time as the technology improves, the following points, put together by a group of experts, may be useful for CTG interpretation [83]:

- Accelerations and baseline variability are hallmarks of fetal health.
- Accelerations without baseline variability should be considered suspicious.
- Periods of decreased variability without decelerations may represent quiet sleep.
- Hypoxic fetuses may have a normal baseline FHR of 110–160 bpm with no accelerations and baseline variability of <5 for >40 minutes.
- In the presence of baseline variability <5 bpm, even shallow late decelerations <15 bpm are ominous in a non-reactive trace.
- Abruption, cord prolapse and scar rupture can cause acute hypoxia and should be suspected and managed clinically (may give rise to prolonged decelerations/bradycardia).
- Fetal hypoxia and acidosis may develop faster with an abnormal trace when there is scanty fluid with thick meconium, intrauterine growth restriction, intrauterine infection with pyrexia, bleeding and/or pre- or postterm labour.
- In preterm fetuses (especially <34 weeks), hypoxia and acidosis can increase the likelihood of respiratory distress syndrome and may contribute to intraventricular haemorrhage, warranting early intervention in the presence of an abnormal trace.
- Hypoxia can be made worse by oxytocin, epidural analgesia and difficult operative deliveries.
- During labour, if decelerations are absent, asphyxia is unlikely, although it cannot be completely excluded.
- Abnormal patterns may represent the effects of drugs, fetal anomaly, fetal injury or infection, and not only hypoxia.

References

1. NICE, Intrapartum care: care of healthy women and their babies during childbirth: clinical guideline 190; 2014. www.nice.org.uk.

2. Mahomed K, Nyoni R, Mulambo T, Kasule J, Jacobus E. Randomised controlled trial of intrapartum fetal heart rate monitoring. *BMJ.* 1994; 308: 497–500.

3. Herbst A, Ingemarsson I. Intermittent versus continuous electronic monitoring in labour: a randomised study. *Br J Obstet Gynaecol.* 1994; 101: 663–8.

4. Ingemarsson I, Arulkumaran S, Ingemarsson E, TambyRaja RL, Ratnam SS. Admission test: a screening test for fetal distress in labour. *Obstet Gynecol.* 1986; 68: 800–6.

5. Ingemarsson I, Arulkumaran S, Paul RH, Ingemarsson E, TambyRaja RL, Ratnam SS. Fetal acoustic stimulation in early labour in patients screened with the admission test. *Am J of Obstet Gynecol.* 1988; 158: 70–74.

6. Impey L, Reynolds M, MacQuillan K, *et al.* Admission cardiotocography: a randomised controlled trial. *Lancet.* 2003; 361: 465–70.

7. Mires G, Williams F, Howie P. Randomised controlled trial of cardiotocography versus Doppler auscultation of fetal heart at admission in labour in low risk obstetric population. *BMJ.* 2001; 322(7300): 1457–60.

8. Mitchell K. The effect of the labour electronic fetal monitoring admission test on operative delivery in low-risk women: a randomised controlled trial. *Evidence Based Midwifery.* 2008; 6(1): 18–26.

9. Bix E, Reiner LM, Klovning A, Oian P. Prognostic value of the labour admission test and its effectiveness compared with auscultation only: a systematic review. *Br J Obstet Gynaecol.* 2005; 112: 1595–604.

10. Devane D, Lalor JG, Daly S, McGuire W, Smith V. Cardiotocography versus intermittent auscultation of fetal heart on admission to labour ward for assessment of fetal wellbeing. *Cochrane Database Syst Rev.* 2012; 15 (2). CD005122. doi: 10.1002/14651858.CD005122. pub4.

11. Wood C, Renou P, Oats J, Farrell E, Beischer N, Anderson I. A controlled trial of fetal heart rate monitoring in a low-risk obstetric population. *Am J Obstet Gynecol.* 1981; 141(5): 527–34.

12. MacDonald D, Grant A, Sheridan-Pereira M, Boylan P, Chalmers I. The Dublin randomized controlled trial of intrapartum fetal heart rate monitoring. *Am J Obstet Gynecol.* 1985; 152(5): 524–39.

13. Thacker SB, Stroup DF, Peterson HB. Efficacy and safety of intrapartum electronic fetal monitoring: an update. *Obstet Gynecol.* 1995; 86(4 Pt 1): 613–20.

14. Grant A, O'Brien N, Joy MT, Hennessy E, MacDonald D. Cerebral palsy among children born during the Dublin randomised trial of intrapartum monitoring. *Lancet.* 1989; 2(8674): 1233–6.

15. Vintzileos AM, Nochimson DJ, Guzman ER, Knuppel RA, Lake M, Schifrin BS. Intrapartum electronic fetal heart rate monitoring versus intermittent auscultation: a meta-analysis. *Obstet Gynecol.* 1995; 85(1): 149–55.

16. Alfirevic Z, Devane D, Gyte GM. Continuous cardiotocography (CTG) as a form of electronic fetal monitoring (EFM) for fetal assessment during labour. *Cochrane Database Syst Rev.* 2013; 31(5). CD006066. doi: 10.1002/14651858.CD006066.pub2.

17. Steer P. ABC of labour care: assessment of mother and fetus in labour. *BMJ.* 1999; 318(7187): 858.

18. Krebs HB, Petres RE, Dunn LJ. Intrapartum fetal heart rate monitoring. V. Fetal heart rate patterns in the second stage of labor. *Am J Obstet Gynecol.* 1981; 140(4): 435–9.

19. Nelson KB, Dambrosia JM, Ting TY, Grether JK. Uncertain value of electronic fetal monitoring in predicting cerebral palsy. *NEJM.* 1996; 334(10): 613–19.

20. Gilstrap LC III, Hauth JC, Toussaint S. Second stage fetal heart rate abnormalities and neonatal acidosis. *Obstet Gynecol.* 1984; 63: 209–13.

21. Cahill AG, Caughey AB, Roehl KA, Odibo AO, Macones GA. Terminal fetal heart decelerations and neonatal outcomes. *Obstet Gynecol.* 2013; 122(5): 1070–6.

22. Roy KK, Baruah J, Kumar S, *et al.* Cesarean section for suspected fetal distress, continuous fetal heart monitoring and decision to delivery time. *Ind J Pediatr.* 2008; 75(12): 1249–52.

23. Gilstrap LC III, Hauth JC, Hankins GD, Beck AW. Second-stage fetal heart rate abnormalities and type of neonatal acidemia. *Obstet Gynecol.* 1987; 70(2): 191–5.

24. Sheiner E, Hadar A, Hallak M, *et al.* Clinical significance of fetal heart rate tracings during the second stage of labor. *Obstet Gynecol.* 2001; 97(5): 747–52.

25. NICE. Intrapartum care: care of healthy women and their babies during childbirth; 2007. www.publications.nice.org.uk/intrapartum-care-cg55. This guideline is an update of 'The use of electronic fetal monitoring: the use and interpretation of cardiotocography in intrapartum fetal surveillance' (Guideline C) issued in May 2001.

26. Samueloff A, Langer O, Berkus M, *et al.* Is fetal heart rate variability a good predictor of fetal outcome? *Acta Obstet Gynecol Scand.* 1994; 73(1): 39–44.

27. Spencer JA, Johnson P. Fetal heart rate variability changes and fetal behavioral cycles during labour. *Br J Obstet Gynaecol.* 1986; 93(4): 314–21.

28. Cahill AG, Roehl KA, Odibo AO, Macones GA. Association and prediction of neonatal acidemia. *Am J Obstet Gynecol.* 2012; 207(3): 206-e1–8.

29. Maso G, Businelli C, Piccoli M, *et al.* The clinical interpretation and significance of electronic fetal heart rate patterns 2 h before delivery: an institutional observational study. *Arch Gynecol Obstet.* 2012; 286(5): 1153–9.

30. Williams KP, Galerneau F. Intrapartum fetal heart rate patterns in the prediction of neonatal acidemia. *Am J Obstet Gynecol.* 2003; 188(3): 820–3.

31. Schifrin BS. The CTG and the timing and mechanism of fetal neurological injuries. *Best Pract Res Clin Obstet Gynaecol.* 2004; 18(3): 437–56.

32. NICHD. Electronic fetal heart rate monitoring: research guidelines for interpretation. National Institute of Child Health and Human Development Research Planning Workshop. *Am J Obstet Gynecol.* 1997;177(6): 1385–90.

33. Krebs HB, Petres RE, Dunn LJ, Smith PJ. Intrapartum fetal heart rate monitoring. VII. The impact of mode of delivery on fetal outcome. *Am J Obstet Gynecol.* 1982; 143(2): 190–4.

34. Powell OH, Melville A, MacKenna J. Fetal heart rate acceleration in labor: excellent prognostic indicator. *Am J Obstet Gynecol.* 1979; 134(1): 36–8.

35. Macones GA, Hankins GDV, Spong CY, Hauth J, Moore T. The 2008 National Institute of Child Health and Human Development workshop report on electronic fetal monitoring: update on definitions, interpretation, and research guidelines. *J Obstet Gynecol Neonatal Nurs.* 2008; 37(5): 510–15.

36. Spencer JAD, Badawi N, Burton P, *et al.* The intrapartum CTG prior to neonatal encephalopathy at term: a case-control study. *BJOG.* 1997; 104(1): 25–8.

37. Cibils LA. Clinical significance of fetal heart rate patterns during labor. II. Late decelerations. *Am J Obstet Gynecol.* 1975; 123(5): 473–94.

38. Krebs HB, Petres RE, Dunn LJ, Jordaan HV, Segreti A. Multifactorial analysis of intrapartum fetal heart rate tracings. *Am J Obstet Gynecol.* 1979; 133(7): 773–80.

39. Low JA, Victory R, Derrick EJ. Predictive value of electronic fetal monitoring for intrapartum fetal asphyxia with metabolic acidosis. *Obstet Gynecol.* 1999; 93(2): 285–91.

40. Ellison PH, Foster M, Sheridan-Pereira M, MacDonald D. Electronic fetal heart monitoring, auscultation, and neonatal outcome. *Am J Obstet Gynecol.* 1991; 164(5): 1281–9.

41. Sameshima H, Ikenoue T. Predictive value of late decelerations for fetal acidemia in unselective low-risk pregnancies. *Am J Perinatol.* 2005; 22(1): 19–23.

42. Skupski DW, Rosenberg CR, Eglinton GS. Intrapartum fetal stimulation tests: a meta-analysis. *Obstet Gynecol*. 2002; 99(1): 129–34.

43. Roy KK, Baruah J, Kumar S, *et al*. Cesarean section for suspected fetal distress, continuous fetal heart monitoring and decision to delivery time. *Indian J Pediatr*. 2008; 75(12): 1249–52. doi: 10.1007/s12098-008-0245-9.

44. Westgate JA, Wibbens B, Bennet L, *et al*. The intrapartum deceleration in center stage: a physiologic approach to the interpretation of fetal heart rate changes in labor. *Am J Obstet Gynecol*. 2007; 197(3): 236-e1–11.

45. Aldrich CJ, D'Antona D, Spencer JAD, *et al*. Fetal heart rate changes and cerebral oxygenation measured by near infrared spectroscopy during the first stage of labour. *Eur J Obstet Gynaecol Reprod Biol*. 1996; 64(2): 189–95.

46. Ball RH, Parer JT. The physiologic mechanisms of variable decelerations. *Am J Obstet Gynecol*. 1992; 166(6): 1683–9.

47. Fleischer A, Schulman H, Jagani N, Mitchell J, Randolph G. The development of fetal acidosis in the presence of an abnormal fetal heart rate tracing. I. The average for gestational age fetus. *Am J Obstet Gynecol*. 1982; 144(1): 55–60.

48. Gaziano EP. A study of variable decelerations in association with other heart rate patterns during monitored labor. *Am J Obstet Gynecol*. 1979; 135(3): 360–3.

49. Tortosa MN, Acien P. Evaluation of variable decelerations of fetal heart rate with the deceleration index: influence of associated abnormal parameters and their relation to the state and evolution of the newborn. *Eur J Obstet Gynaecol Reprod Biol*. 1990; 34(3): 235–45.

50. Morris RK, Malin G, Robson SC, *et al*. Fetal umbilical artery Doppler to predict compromise of fetal/neonatal wellbeing in a high-risk population: systematic review and bivariate meta-analysis. *Ultrasound Obstet Gynecol*. 2011; 37(2): 135–42.

51. Hamilton E, Warrick P, O'Keeffe D. Variable decelerations: do size and shape matter? *J Matern Fetal Neonatal Med*. 2012; 25(6): 648–53.

52. Özden S, Demirci F. Significance for fetal outcome of poor prognostic features in fetal heart rate traces with variable decelerations. *Arch Gynecol Obstet*. 1999; 262(3–4): 141–9.

53. Parer JT, Livingston EG. What is fetal distress? *Am J Obstet Gynecol*. 1990; 162(6): 1421–7.

54. Katz M, Wilson SJ, Young BK. Sinusoidal fetal heart rate. II. Continuous tissue pH studies. *Am J Obstet Gynecol*. 1980; 136(5): 594–6.

55. Johnson TR Jr, Compton AA, Rotmensch J, Work BA Jr, Johnson JW. Significance of the sinusoidal fetal heart rate pattern. *Am J Obstet Gynecol*. 1981; 139(4): 446–53.

56. Young BK, Katz M, Wilson SJ. Sinusoidal fetal heart rate. I. Clinical significance. *Am J Obstet Gynecol*. 1980; 136(5): 587–93.

57. Winkler CL, Hauth JC, Martin Tucker J, Owen J, Brumfield CG. Neonatal complications at term as related to the degree of umbilical artery acidemia. *Am J Obstet Gynecol*. 1991; 164(2): 637–41.

58. Thorp JA, Trobough T, Evans R, Hedrick J, Yeast JD. The effect of maternal oxygen administration during the second stage of labor on umbilical cord blood gas values: a randomized controlled prospective trial. *Am J Obstet Gynecol*. 1995; 172(2): 465–74.

59. Fawole B, Hofmeyr GJ. Maternal oxygen administration for fetal distress. *Cochrane Database Sys Rev*. 2012; 12. CD000136. doi: 10.1002/14651858.CD000136.pub2.

60. McNamara H, Johnson N, Lilford R. The effect on fetal arteriolar oxygen saturation resulting from giving oxygen to the mother measured by pulse oximetry. *BJOG*. 1993; 100(5): 446–9.

61. Westgren M, Kruger K, Ek S, *et al*. Lactate compared with pH analysis at fetal scalp blood sampling: a prospective randomised study. *BJOG*. 1998; 105(1): 29–33.

62. Kruger K, Hallberg B, Blennow M, Kublickas M, Westgren M. Predictive value of fetal scalp blood lactate concentration and pH as markers of neurologic disability. *Am J Obstet Gynecol*. 1999; 181(5): 1072–8.

63. Herbst A, Wölner-Hanssen P, Ingemarsson I. Risk factors for acidemia at birth. *Obstet Gynecol*. 1997; 90(1): 125–30.

64. Low JA. Intrapartum fetal asphyxia: definition, diagnosis, and classification. *Am J Obstet Gynecol*. 1997; 176(5): 957–9.

65. Nordström L. Fetal scalp and cord blood lactate. *Best Pract Res Clin Obstet Gynaecol*. 2004; 18(3): 467–76.

66. Nordström L, Achanna S, Naka K, Arulkumaran S. Fetal and maternal lactate increase during active second stage of labour. *BJOG*. 2001; 108(3): 263–8.

67. Krüger K, Kublickas M, Westgren M. Lactate in scalp and cord blood from fetuses with ominous fetal heart rate patterns. *Obstet Gynecol*. 1998; 92(6): 918–22.

68. Rosén KG, Amer-Wåhlin I, Luzietti R, Norén H. Fetal ECG waveform analysis. *Best Pract Res Clin Obstet Gynaecol*. 2004; 18(3): 485–514.

69. Mansano RZ, Beall MH, Ross MG. Fetal ST segment heart rate analysis in labor: improvement of

intervention criteria using interpolated base deficit. *J Matern Fetal Neonatal Med.* 2007; 20(1): 47–52.

70. Vayssiere C, Haberstich R, Sebahoun V, *et al.* Fetal electrocardiogram ST-segment analysis and prediction of neonatal acidosis. *Int J Gynecol Obstet.* 2007; 97(2): 110–14.

71. Olofsson P, Ayres-de-Campos D, Kessler J, *et al.* A critical appraisal of the evidence for using cardiotocography plus ECG ST interval analysis for fetal surveillance in labor. Part II: the meta-analyses. *Acta Obstet Gynecol Scand.* 2014; 93(6): 571–86.

72. Dildy GA. Fetal pulse oximetry. *Clin Obstet Gynecol.* 2011; 54(1): 66–73.

73. Kühnert M, Seelbach-Göebel B, Butterwegge M. Predictive agreement between the fetal arterial oxygen saturation and fetal scalp pH: results of the German multicenter study. *Am J Obstet Gynecol.* 1998; 178(2): 330–5.

74. Seelbach-Göbel B, Heupel M, Kühnert M, Butterwegge M. The prediction of fetal acidosis by means of intrapartum fetal pulse oximetry. *Am J Obstet Gynecol.* 1999; 180(1): 73–81.

75. Nonnenmacher A, Hopp H, Dudenhausen J. Predictive value of pulse oximetry for the development of fetal acidosis. *J Perinatal Med.* 2010; 38(1): 83–6.

76. Dildy GA, van den Berg PP, Katz M, *et al.* Intrapartum fetal pulse oximetry: fetal oxygen saturation trends during labor and relationship to delivery outcome. In Knitza R (ed.), *Hypoxische Gefährdung des Fetus sub partu* (pp. 185–93). Darmstadt: Steinkopff; 1994.

77. Garite TJ, Dildy GA, McNamara H, *et al.* A multicenter controlled trial of fetal pulse oximetry in the intrapartum management of non-reassuring fetal heart rate patterns. *Am J Obstet Gynecol.* 2000; 183(5): 1049–58.

78. East CE, Dunster KR, Colditz PB, Nath CE, Earl JW. Fetal oxygen saturation monitoring in labour: an analysis of 118 cases. *Aust N Z J Obstet Gynaecol.* 1997; 37(4): 397–401.

79. ACOG Committee. Fetal pulse oximetry: American College of Obstetricians and Gynecologists Committee on Obstetric Practice. *Obstet Gynecol.* 2001; 98(3): 523–4.

80. NHS Litigation Authority. *Ten Years of Maternity Claims: An Analysis of NHS Litigation Authority Data.* London: NHSLA; 2012.

81. Confidential Enquiry into Stillbirths and Deaths in Infancy. *4th Annual Report.* London: Maternal and Child Health Research Consortium; 1997.

82. Electronic Fetal Monitoring. www.e-lfh.org.uk/ projects/electronic-fetal-monitoring.

83. Arulkumaran S, Ingemarsson I, Montan S, *et al. Traces of You: Fetal Trace Interpretation.* Netherlands: Philips Medical Systems; 2002.

Uterine Contractions

Christofides Agathoklis and Sabaratnam Arulkumaran

Introduction

The uterus acts as a receptacle providing the home for the growing fetus from conception to the time of delivery. Globally the majority of women deliver vaginally. The mechanism of onset of labour is still a speculation. Current theory is that hormonal change brought about by the hypo-thalamo-pituitary axis lowers progesterone, which is a muscle relaxant. This is followed by local changes in the chorioamnion that result in the production of prostaglandins (PGs). Prostaglandins cause softening and effacement of the cervix and uterine contractions that are key elements for the onset and progress of labour. In the absence of mechanical difficulties, uterine contractions bring about the process of cervical dilatation and descent of the head, resulting in spontaneous expulsion of the fetus, placenta, and membranes. The main reasons for slow progress are inefficient uterine contractions (P-power), relative disproportion due to malposition, or cephalo-pelvic disproportion either due to a large baby and head (P-passenger) or a relatively small or non-gynaecoid pelvis (P-passage). These three Ps influence labour outcome. In the second stage of labour, i.e. after full dilatation of the cervix, maternal expulsive efforts assist in the process of birth.

In most settings uterine contractions are assessed by palpation and are noted in terms of frequency and duration. The intensity of the contraction is difficult to assess by palpation. Most labours assessed by palpation progress normally and deliver vaginally; some have slow progress and a difficult labour, i.e. dysfunctional labour. Depending on the acceptable norms set for progress of labour, the percentage of women who are diagnosed to have dysfunctional labour would vary and is more common in nulliparous women compared with multiparas [1,2]. In the past, a rate of progress of 1 cm/h was thought to be the norm. Recent studies dispute this and state that the progress is slower than we learned a few decades ago [3]. This is attributed to increases in obesity rates and size of the fetus and possible change in shape of the pelvis. Management of dysfunctional labour has been by the use of oxytocin infusion to correct inefficient uterine activity and to correct malposition or overcome minor disproportion by moulding of the head and increasing pelvic capacity. Suboptimal management of labour, especially in the nulliparas, despite use of invasive intrauterine monitoring, has given rise to an increase in caesarean section (CS) rate and cost of healthcare delivery [4]. This chapter will discuss the molecular mechanisms of contractions, the different techniques used to measure contractions, their reliability and how the monitoring should help us to manage spontaneous, augmented, induced women in labour with a previous CS.

Physiological Basis of Uterine Contractions

Studies on human or animal models have not been able to demonstrate physiological, anatomical or pharmacological evidence of a uterine pace maker [5]. Unlike the myocardium in the heart, which is a syncytium of muscle cells with efficient electrical conductivity, the conduction of the electrical stimulus through the myometrial cells may not be uniform and thus in some cases do not bring about the desired synchronized contraction [6]. The basis of muscle contraction is the interaction of myosin and actin fibrils brought about by the phosphorylation of serine 19 on the light chain myosin. This interaction is dependent on the membrane permeability and calcium channels that help to bind to calmodulin [7]. The uterine activity generated

Best Practice in Labour and Delivery, Second Edition, ed. Sir Sabaratnam Arulkumaran. Published by Cambridge University Press. © Cambridge University Press 2016.

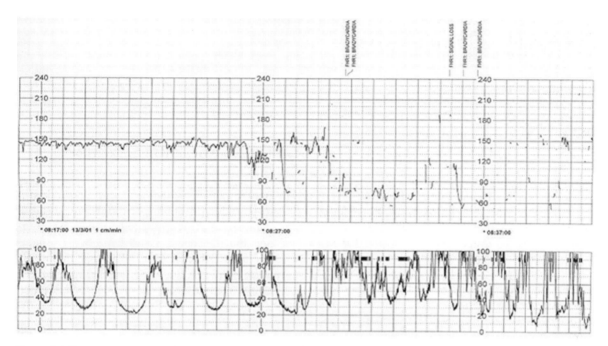

Figure 5.1 The uterine contractions that were one in every 2–2.5 min become one in every minute without any escalation of the oxytocin infusion precipitating prolonged deceleration. This is due to increasing sensitivity of the uterus to the same dose of oxytocin with advancing cervical dilatation.

(amplitude and duration) would be dependent on the total muscle mass recruited synchronously during each contraction. The frequency will depend on the electrical activity generated [8]. Despite the absence of a defined pace maker, medications are used to modulate uterine contractions. This mechanism is exploited to inhibit preterm labour by administering calcium channel blockers or beta mimetics, or to enhance uterine activity with the administration of oxytocin. There is an inherent sensitivity of the uterus to have increased frequency of contractions with the use of oxytocin with advancing cervical dilatation, despite no increase in the infusion dosage. Hence it is important to monitor uterine contractions and stop or reduce the dose of oxytocin if one is to avoid hyper-stimulation and fetal compromise (Figure 5.1). In addition to stopping oxytocin, acute tocolysis or delivery may become necessary at times.

Measurement of Uterine Activity: The Need and the Methods

Uterine activity has four components: resting uterine tone, frequency, amplitude and duration (Table 5.1). For clinical purposes, information about resting uter-

ine tone is not needed in almost all cases other than in a few high-risk situations. With a uterine rupture the tone may be lost and with abruption there may be an increase. In these situations the clinical evaluation will point to the problem, in addition to the information on uterine tone. Prostaglandin or oxytocin use may also raise the resting tone but usually they are associated with markedly increased frequency of contractions. The presence of contractions and whether there is an increase in frequency and duration and whether they are regular is of value to manage preterm labour,

Table 5.1 Definition of contraction parameters

Parameter	Definition
Relaxation time	Time in seconds between offset of one contraction and onset of the next
Contraction duration	Duration in seconds between onset and offset of contractions
Contraction amplitude	Maximum uterine pressure above basal tone in mmHg
Contraction area	Area of contraction above baseline pressure in mmHg seconds
Contraction frequency	Number of contractions in a 10 min period

i.e. to decide to inhibit contractions. In term labour, if there is slow progress of labour and there is inadequate uterine activity with no evidence of fetal compromise, augmentation of contractions may help with progress of labour and vaginal delivery.

In addition to the usefulness in inhibiting or augmenting contractions, it is of value to identify whether the fetus is likely to be compromised by the contractions that reduce or cut off the blood supply to the retro-placental area that produce late decelerations or compress the umbilical cord which cause variable decelerations. Monitoring the fetal heart rate (FHR) during and soon after contractions could pick up these decelerations. Identifying such compromise related to uterine contraction would prompt us to stop oxytocin infusion or to give tocolytic drugs.

Maternal Perception

All women feel painful uterine contractions during labour, although how they perceive the intensity may vary. Mothers in different cultures and women in the same culture react differently to pain. Obese women may have difficulties feeling the uterine contractions and parous women may feel the contractions to be less painful [9]. Maternal perception of the frequency of contractions can be relied upon, the duration is an approximation, but their assessment of intensity may not have any relationship to measured amplitude of uterine contractions. It is known that contractions with amplitudes of greater than 15 mmHg from the baseline is associated with pain and is also effective in bringing about cervical effacement and dilatation.

Contraction Assessment by Manual Palpation

Globally the commonest method of uterine contraction assessment is by palpation. Palpation provides a reliable assessment of frequency, but an approximation of the duration as the very start and end of contractions may be difficult to palpate [10]. Palpation will not be able to provide information on the strength or intensity, although in many centres the care givers make comments stating that the contractions are strong, moderately strong or weak – this has no scientific basis. The advantage of palpation is that it promotes the rapport between the care giver and the woman, does not need expensive technology and is adequate to manage most labours. Palpation can be done in any position adopted by the mother, i.e. lying, sitting, standing or in the water pool. Palpation is performed over a 10 min period, is assessed every 30 min and is plotted on the partogram (see Figure 2.2 in Chapter 2). The plotting in the partogram provides the frequency of contractions in 10 min and the average duration shaded differently for <20 sec, 20–40 sec and >40 sec.

Contraction Assessment by External Tocography

Uterine contractions cause the uterus to expand in an antero-posterior direction that causes protrusion of the abdomen in the uterine fundal region. An external pressure transducer placed between the fundus and the umbilicus perceives this change due to the thrust on the button or diaphragm of the transducer. This helps to monitor contraction frequency, duration and amplitude. Most fetal monitors provide for adjustment of baseline tone or pressure that is usually set at 20 mmHg. When applied properly, this non-invasive method of monitoring provides accurate assessment of the frequency, near accurate measurement of the duration, but only a relative assessment of the amplitude. The amplitude is much less accurate in obese women, in a restless woman or when the belt is loose [11]. External tocography does not assess the baseline pressure, which can be increased on the recording by tightening the toco transducer belt or by manipulating the toco button on the machine. The continuous display of contractions in relation to the fetal heart rate, i.e. cardiotocography (CTG), is useful to monitor high-risk labours [12]. More accurate assessment of baseline pressure, frequency, duration and amplitude can be obtained by internal tocography [13].

Contraction monitoring in the second stage of labour should be meticulous as the contraction frequency is maximal with risks to the fetus, especially when a woman is on oxytocin infusion (Figure 5.1). Medical negligence cases point to poor or no monitoring of contractions in the second stage and this may be due to the woman squatting or in the pool, or flicking the transducer to make the sensor face upwards, or loosening it due to discomfort. In such situations the contractions should be assessed by external palpation and a mark made on the CTG recording to indicate when the contractions occurred.

At times the ultrasound transducer can display the maternal heart rate (MHR) on CTG, especially in the second stage when the FHR is bradycardic. Normally

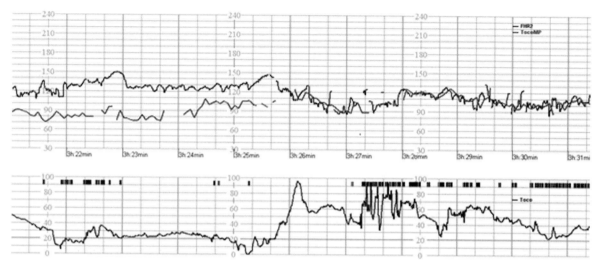

Figure 5.2 CTG recording that shows contractions, FHR and MHR. See the colour plate section for a colour version of this figure.

the MHR accelerates coinciding with contractions in the second stage, while the FHR decelerates due to head compression. Despite these physiological differences that should alert the care giver, mistakes are made by continuing to monitor the MHR, thinking it is the FHR. To overcome this problem some toco transducers have inbuilt optical sensors which would identify the MHR from the maternal abdominal skin and record it separately on the CTG paper (Figure 5.2).

Contraction Assessment by Internal Tocography

Intrauterine pressure measurement provides an accurate measure of resting tone, frequency, duration and amplitude [14]. It is used almost routinely in some centres/countries but is not popular universally because of the invasive nature of placing an intrauterine catheter in utero via the cervical canal and due to lack of clear evidence of benefit in clinical practice. The advantages are that pressure recordings are not influenced by the position of the mother and some catheters have ports for amnioinfusion when there is meconium-stained amniotic fluid or variable decelerations. Intraamniotic placement provides more reliable readings compared with catheters placed in the extra amniotic space [15]. Complications of intrauterine pressure measurements are rare but include intrauterine infection, exceptionally perforation of fetal or placental vessels and injury to the fetus or the uterus [16,17].

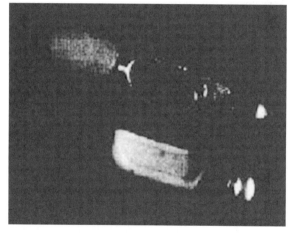

Figure 5.3 The tip of a fibre-optic catheter with a smooth dome and distal fenestration housing the mirror arrangement is shown alongside the tip of the Gaeltec catheter with a recessed area behind the rounded tip.

Different types of catheters (fluid-filled, fibre-optic, pressure transducer-tipped) are available and provide reliable readings, but solid-tipped catheters are preferred as fluid-filled catheters may require more frequent adjustment and have an increased tendency for artefacts due to air bubbles, kinked cables and catheter occlusion by meconium, blood or fetal parts [18]. Figure 5.3 shows the transducer-tipped catheter with a bridge strain gauge deposited on a thin metal pressure-sensing surface at the end of a 90 cm catheter. The sensing area is recessed to minimize damage and lateral pressure measurements. Placement of flexible fibre-optic catheters is associated with hardly any placental or fetal injury. These catheters do not get damaged and can be used in the second stage of labour [19]. New dual-channel, multifunctional uterine probes and balloon probes were introduced for accurate FHR monitoring in addition to measurement of uterine activity, but are not readily available for clinical use [20].

Since there are possibilities of different pockets of fluid in the uterine cavity with little connection, the pressure measurement in one pocket of fluid may be different from another. When two catheters were placed in different sections of the uterus, small differences in the amplitude of contractions were observed but cumulative uterine activity was not so different as to influence clinical management [21,22]. The slight differences in pressure may be due to mechanical (direct force) rather than fluid pressure acting on the transducer.

Randomized controlled trials (RCTs) comparing external to internal tocography have failed to show any benefit in clinical outcome in terms of reduction of CS, operative vaginal delivery or better neonatal outcome in augmented labour [23,24]. This may be due to the fact that labour is managed by considering mainly the frequency of uterine contractions that are assessed reasonably well by external tocography even in the moderately obese. Studies have also shown no advantage of internal monitoring in induced labour [25]. There may be a special group of women who may benefit by internal tocography, i.e. where external tocography is not providing the needed information of frequency and duration of contractions due to severe obesity or restlessness. It is postulated that intrauterine pressure monitoring may be of value in women who are in labour with a previous CS scar, but there is no evidence to recommend such use.

Uterine Electromyography (EMG)

Measurements of uterine activity by EMG obtained by external abdominal probes provide nearly as accurate readings as those obtained by intrauterine pressure catheters [26,27]. Early studies suggested the possibility of detecting contractions that may lead to preterm labour from those that are unlikely to progress to labour by looking at the synchronous wave patterns from various parts of the uterus using a multi-channel myographic recording [28]. The complexity of equipment needed for EMG measurement that would meas-

ure the synchronization and concordance of contractions is constantly being improved and may find clinical usefulness in the future [29].

Quantification of Uterine Activity

Uterine activity has been expressed simply based on the baseline tone, frequency, duration and amplitude of contractions. Efficiency of contractions is not judged by the measurements but by what they are expected to achieve, i.e. cervical effacement and dilatation of the cervix, followed by descent of the head and delivery of the fetus, followed by the placenta and membranes. If a woman has few contractions that are of short duration but labour is progressing well, then she would not need augmentation of labour. Similarly, contractions may be in-coordinate (Figures 2.5 and 2.6), i.e. a few contractions together followed by single contractions every few minutes followed by another series of contractions together. Hence the description of in-coordinate contractions is based on what is seen on tocography. However, in-coordinate contractions do not mean that these contractions are inefficient.

In order to improve assessment of uterine activity by making maximum use of the measurements obtained, individual elements of the tocograph are considered and combined in different ways, e.g. multiplying mean amplitude of contractions over 10 min by the frequency of contractions, i.e. Montevideo units. Total contraction area is considered by calculating the area under a contraction, including the resting pressure. The basal intrauterine pressure is the pressure at the lowest point of the tracing between contractions, due to atmospheric pressure, hydrostatic pressure and elastic recoil of the uterus and surrounding tissues, and is unlikely to contribute to cervical dilatation or descent of the head [5]. Hence this pressure is excluded from quantitative measures because it is affected by variables that are not related to uterine activity. The refined measure is to calculate the active contraction area by considering only the area above the resting pressure and hence considering the active pressure, which is the difference between the maximum intrauterine pressure and the resting intrauterine pressure (Figure 5.4). In order to capture all the activity of the uterus in a continuous manner including that due to in-coordinate contractions, i.e. to calculate the total work done, continuous measurement of activity every 15 min was introduced as kPa secs/15 minutes, and this can be automatically calculated and reflected

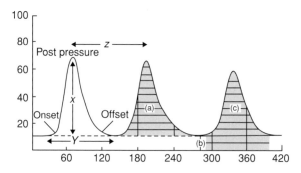

Figure 5.4 Terms used in describing the different elements of uterine contractions. *X*: active pressure or amplitude; *Y*: duration; *Z*: contraction interval related to frequency; (a) active contraction area; (b) baseline pressure or basal tone; (c) total contraction area.

on the CTG paper as a horizontal mark read against a vertical axis of 0–2500 kPa secs (Figure 5.5) [11].

The clinical situations of sudden change in posture, e.g. sitting up or squatting, uterine hyper-stimulation by PG or oxytocin infusion, irritation of the uterus due to blood seeping into the myometrium in cases of abruption, can increase the baseline pressure and need

to be recognized [30,31]. The shape of the contraction may be related to dysfunctional labour. The shape is measured by the F:R ratio, where the F (fall) is the time for a contraction to return to baseline from its peak and the R (rise) is the time for a contraction to rise to its peak [32]. An increased F:R ratio is associated with a higher need for caesarean delivery, although this concept needs further study [33]. The total amount of uterine activity per unit time can be described in different ways (see Table 5.2).

Uterine Activity Measurement

The cumulative work done by the uterus has been expressed by taking different elements of the components of the uterine contractions (Table 5.2).

Uterine activity measurements may concentrate on the work done by the uterus, but one needs to remember that too frequent contractions of low amplitude may be reflected as low uterine activity but may compromise the fetus especially if one increases the oxytocin infusion to achieve a higher uterine activity. Hence it is important not to increase the oxytocin

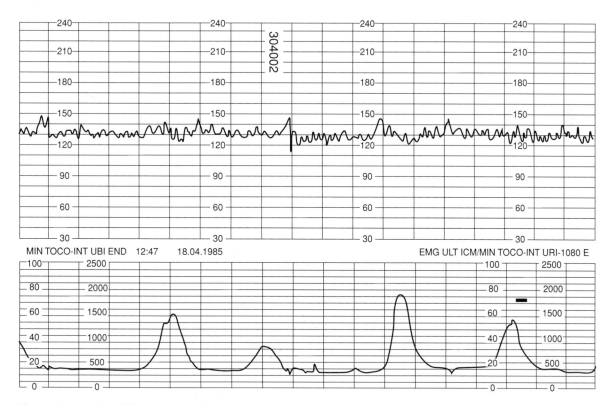

Figure 5.5 Recording of UAI as a short dark line against a vertical axis from 0 to 2500 kPa secs and the numerical printout of the UAI in addition to mode of recording, paper speed and time.

Table 5.2 Uterine activity by considering different components of the contractions

Unit of measurement	Components considered	Comments
Montevideo unit [34]	Mean amplitude × mean frequency over 10 min	The duration and shape of the contractions not considered
Alexandria unit [35]	Montevideo × unit mean duration over 10 min	Shape not considered. Incorporating duration showed longer duration was associated with shorter labour
Uterine activity unit (UAU) [36]	Area under the pressure curve (Torr-min) over 1 min – 1UAU = 1 Torr-min (included frequency, duration and amplitude)	Included baseline pressure which did not actively contribute to uterine work
Uterine activity integral (UAI) or active contraction area [37]	Active area under the pressure curve over 15 min (intrauterine pressure minus the baseline pressure) (Figure 5.5)	Active pressure measurements may include maternal efforts, in the second stage
Mean active pressure (MAP) [38]	UAI divided by 900 (kPa), measuring over 1 sec (15 min × 60 = 900 sec)	Complex measurement but is independent of duration
Mean contraction active pressure (MCAP) [38]	UAI/total duration of contraction	When the integration period is with respect to one contraction

infusion to achieve more than four or five contractions in 10 min while trying to increase the uterine activity measurements performed by Montevideo units or UAIs. The in-coordinate nature and shape of contractions are not considered with area measurements. Despite sophistication in equipment and technology and different methods of quantifying, internal tocography and quantifying uterine activity has not improved the clinical outcome in spontaneous, augmented or induced labour [39,40].

Uterine Activity in Normal Labour

A healthy, well-grown fetus with normal amniotic fluid and no medical or obstetric disorder is not easily compromised by uterine contractions of spontaneous normal labour. The contractions of labour start infrequently from about one in ten minutes. Gradually it increases in frequency, duration and amplitude. The uterine activity peaks towards the end of the first stage due to the 'Ferguson reflex', which is due to the reflex release of oxytocin due to the presenting part stretching the almost fully dilated cervix and the upper vagina. Towards the end of the first stage of labour the contraction frequency may be 3–5 in 10 min, with each contraction lasting longer than 60 sec and with amplitudes of >50 mmHg. In cases with slow progress of labour, oxytocin titration to achieve a contraction frequency of four in 10 min leads to satisfactory progress [41]. A contraction frequency greater than 5 min may reduce the uterine relaxation time. It has been shown that if this time is less than 51 sec in the first stage and

36 sec in the second stage it may lead to fetal compromise [42]. It is simple to understand that increase in the contraction frequency and a decrease in relaxation time would be associated with lower umbilical artery pH. Infrared spectroscopic studies have shown that fetal cerebral oxygen saturation remains stable or even increases if the contractions are every 2–3 min or longer [43].

Uterine Contractions and Parity

Studies on oxytocin-induced labour evaluated the total uterine activity needed to achieve full dilatation of the cervix. The total uterine activity needed is influenced by the parity and cervical score and reflects the work needed to overcome the cervical and pelvic tissue resistance [44].

If a woman has not reached full dilatation despite the uterine activity exceeding the total uterine activity which is the norm for that cervical score and parity, and there are associated clinical signs of failure in cervical dilatation, increasing caput and moulding with no progress, then it suggests cephalo-pelvic disproportion. Since some women in the same parity group progress normally with low levels of uterine activity and there is a broad spectrum of uterine activity associated with normal progress of labour, it is difficult to prognosticate possible labour progress based on uterine activity [45,46] (Figure 5.6). Hence labour progress needs to be monitored by assessing the progress of cervical dilatation. If partographic progress is normal, then uterine activity measurements would not be of

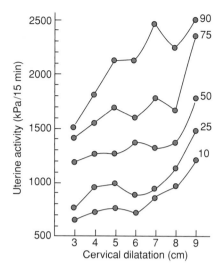

Figure 5.6 Cervical dilatation-specific uterine activity in kPa/15 min in nulliparous spontaneous normal labour.

great value. The parous uterus needs to expend significantly less effort to affect normal vaginal delivery than its nulliparous counterpart until the late first stage, suggesting that parity may have a greater influence on the resistance offered by the cervix than the pelvic tissues [47].

Maternal Characteristics that Affect Uterine Contractions

Increasing body mass index in our population, especially in the reproductive age group, is partly to blame for slow and prolonged labour and the cause for increasing CSs. This may be due to poor uterine contractility or larger babies, or decreased available space in the pelvis or for a combination of all three [48]. The poor contractility is attributed to the in-vitro findings that relate to elevated cholesterol in obese women that may disrupt the signalling mechanisms that impair contractions [49]. Intracellular acidification decreases and alkalization increases contractility [50]. In recent times, amniotic fluid lactate is measured to identify myometrial hypoxia and lactic acidosis associated with dysfunctional labour [51]. Early research of preloading the mother with bicarbonate solutions suggests this appears to reduce the incidence of intrauterine lactic acidosis, just as with muscles in athletes, but this aspect needs further study. Such interventions may help to reduce the incidence of dysfunctional labour.

Uterine Contractions and Previous Caesarean Section (CS)

The main concern in labour with a previous CS scar is the possibility that the scar may give way and cause morbidity to the mother and severe morbidity or mortality to the fetus and the newborn. Aspects of vaginal birth after previous CS are discussed in detail in Chapter 23. In terms of prognostication for possible vaginal delivery it is known that women who had a previous normal labour and vaginal delivery either before or after the CS have a better chance of achieving vaginal delivery. It is also reassuring to know that the uterine activity in these women is much lower than in those who had no vaginal delivery, which in some way reassures that the chance of rupture may be less because of less total uterine activity on the scar [52]. Previous labour and delivery reduces the uterine work done to overcome the cervical and pelvic tissue resistance compared with women who had elective CS or CS in the latent phase of labour. When labour is not progressing adequately, oxytocin augmentation is used to increase the uterine activity. The augmented uterine activity is higher than that observed in normal labour. Augmentation improves poor uterine activity and helps to overcome any minor disproportion due to malposition. In the cohort of women with augmented labour, if the labour progresses normally, i.e. 1 cm/h, then the uterine activity is less than those who have a slow or no progress of labour despite augmentation, indicating that it may be wise to consider delivery by CS if the progress of labour is not optimal in the first four hours of augmentation. Those who have satisfactory progress of labour during the first four hours of augmentation are likely to deliver vaginally. Others can be given more time, but with a longer duration of augmented labour with higher levels of uterine activity the risk of scar rupture is likely to increase. Hence careful monitoring of the mother, fetus and labour is needed, with ready recourse to CS in cases where labour is managed with a previous CS; signs of scar rupture may be first noted as abnormalities of the FHR pattern [53,54].

Scar rupture is dependent on (a) the integrity of the scar and (b) the force of uterine activity on the scar, which is dependent on the intensity and duration of uterine contractions. Based on such a hypothesis, quantifying uterine activity at 15 min intervals or cumulative uterine activity calculations should help to predict the possibility of scar rupture, but this has not been found to be the case. One or two strong contractions due to hyper-stimulation in a case with otherwise normal uterine activity may also rupture the scar. Hence the evidence for the use of intrauterine catheters to measure pressures or uterine activity to predict or diagnose scar rupture is not that strong [55,56].

In the intact uterus, the head forms a seal at the cervix and pelvis and the intrauterine pressure builds up with contractions. If the scar gives way then the liquor will leak out and the fetus may also be extruded with early loss of integrity of the scar. This should lead to reduction in the resting uterine pressure or tone. The reduction of the uterine tone and amplitude of contractions or absence of recording contractions should alert to the possibility of scar rupture [57]. The expected reduction of baseline resting pressure or the amplitude may not be affected if the catheter tip lies in a localized well-enclosed pocket of amniotic fluid. The presence of contractions may also be seen in cases of scar dehiscence where the visceral peritoneum is intact and helps to maintain the resting tone and also the build-up of contraction pressure, but these contractions may stretch the dehisced scar and lack of pull on the cervix to make it dilate [58]. Loss of uterine contraction recording with external tocography is common and is due to the loosening of the toco belt or change in position of the mother. Sudden loss of uterine contractions with intrauterine pressure measurement should suggest scar dehiscence unless the catheter has slipped out or has become blocked (with fluid-filled catheters). More often than not, the first sign is the sudden appearance of prolonged deceleration or repeated profound decelerations.

Uterine Contractions and Induced Labour

Induction of labour for maternal or fetal risk factors has increased in most centres; figures of 20–30% are quoted in many countries. The use of oxytocin or PG causes the uterine contractions to become more frequent, of a higher amplitude and greater duration, leading to higher uterine activity in induced labour [59]. Many women who had normal and induced labour with different pregnancies claim that induced labour was more painful and this may have some relationship to the increased uterine activity in induced labour. The incidence of tachysystoles or polysystoles (more than five contractions in 10 min) is greater due to the increasing doses of the medication and the

increasing sensitivity of the uterus to the same dose of oxytocin with advancing cervical dilatation. Induction with oxytocin reduces the inter-contraction interval and increases the contraction regularity, and can be used as a predictor for likely progress of labour [60]. The use of oxytocin increases the frequency of contractions and then the duration and the amplitude for a while until it reaches a stable phase when the uterine activity remains the same [61]. Any attempt to increase the uterine activity by increasing the oxytocin may result in hyper-stimulation with reduction in amplitude which follows the simple physiological principle that the uterus contracts better with a higher amplitude when it has relaxed adequately rather than stimulating it again before it has reached a resting tone. In addition, such action can cause compromise to the fetus because of reduced inter-contraction intervals. Measuring the uterine contraction area was postulated to be useful and was expected to decrease the number of cases of inadequate stimulation and to prevent hyper-stimulation. However, oxytocin titration to achieve four or five contractions in 10 min compared with the goal of achieving the 75th centile of uterine activity expected in normal labour according to parity, using automated pumps, did not show better maternal or fetal outcome in induced labour [62]. It was also postulated that measurement of uterine activity may be helpful to identify true active phase arrest, but its clinical usefulness is yet to be proven [63].

Each uterus has a different level of sensitivity to oxytocin and PGs, depending on parity, gestation and cervical score. The dose, route of administration and the type of drug used will also exert an influence [64]. The PGE1 compound misoprostol is associated with a greater incidence of polysystoles. Prostaglandin E2 – dinoprostone pessaries or gel – can cause hyper-stimulation and is dependent on the rapidity of absorption in the vagina, which may be influenced by the moisture content of the vagina, pH, temperature and presence or absence of inflammation. With repeated doses of the drug there is a greater tendency to cause hyper-stimulation [65]. With vaginally administered PG, especially with FHR abnormalities, acute tocolysis (e.g. terbutaline 0.25 mg SC or slow IV in 5 ml saline over 5 min) should be the mainstay of management. If uterine hyper-stimulation is due to oxytocin infusion, stopping oxytocin may not be adequate and acute tocolysis may be needed to quickly reduce the uterine activity [66].

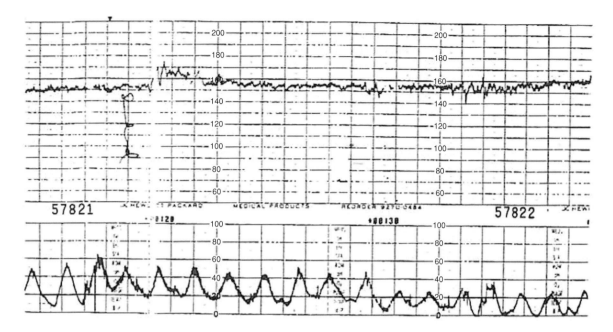

Figure 5.7 Polysystolic contractions of low amplitude due to abruptio placenta in a patient who presented with continuous abdominal pain and bleeding per vaginum with the cervix 1 cm dilated. There is associated fetal tachycardia.

Abnormal Contraction Patterns (In-Coordinate Uterine Contractions)

Due to the lack of coherent recruitment of uterine muscles, different types of in-coordinate contractions may be seen in multiparous and nulliparous spontaneous labour with normal progress [67]. In-coordinate contractions can be effective in causing cervical dilatation and descent of the head, and on its own is not an indication for the use of oxytocin. The use of oxytocin may not correct the in-coordination, but may improve the efficacy in cases of slow progress of labour. Various degrees of in-coordinate uterine activity are described in Chapter 2.

Intrauterine pressure reaches up to 60 mmHg in normal labour, with relaxation in between to replenish the intervillous space. Spiral arterioles are completely compressed with an intrauterine pressure of 30 mmHg. Contraction frequency of greater than seven in 10 min may appear as a single contraction with several peaks and raised baseline pressure, and is termed polysystole (Figure 5.7), i.e. the baseline tone in between the peaks does not reach the original baseline. The term 'tetanic contractions' is used if the merged contractions last for more than three minutes. Such contractions have the tendency to reduce uterine per-

fusion and increase fetal compromise. Hence continuous FHR monitoring may be needed in cases where it recurs frequently. If the mother was on oxytocin, consideration should be given to reducing the oxytocin and certainly to stop it if there is a prolonged deceleration of the FHR. Such contractions are unusual in spontaneous normal labour; they are mainly seen with the use of oxytocin (Figure 5.8). When contractions do not merge but the baseline pressure is elevated by more than 20 mmHg for more than 3 min, they are called hypertonic contractions (Figure 5.9). Tetanic contractions will cut off perfusion to the retro-placental pool of blood, while hypertonic activity will reduce perfusion.

Conclusion

Uterine contraction monitoring is an essential part of management of labour. This could be by palpation, or external or internal tocometry. As yet there is no convincing evidence to resort to intrauterine pressure monitoring in labour, although it forms part of routine practice in some countries. This has its advantages as discontinuation of uterine contraction recording much earlier than the time of delivery leads to failure to recognize that the uterus is contracting more than

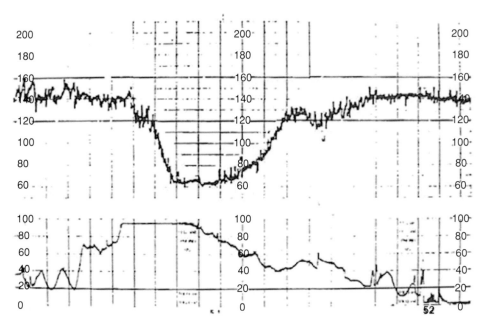

Figure 5.8 Tetanic contractions caused by accidental bolus infusion of oxytocin when the infusion was run fast to check whether the intravenous line was patent.

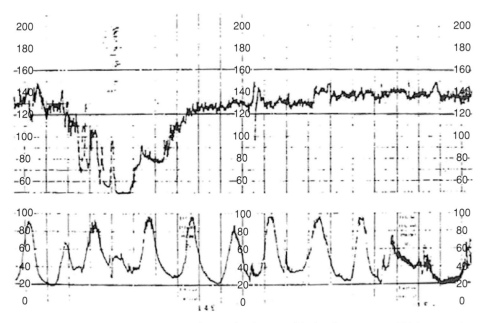

Figure 5.9 Hypertonic uterine contractions showing the elevation of the baseline pressure, which has caused a transient bradycardia.

five times in 10 min, and pathological FHR patterns that are caused by uterine hyper-stimulation (Figure 5.1). Uterine contraction monitoring is a must with the use of oxytocin infusion to help regulate the dose of oxytocin infusion to achieve optimal uterine activity. The FIGO guidelines provide information on methods of uterine activity monitoring [68]. Computer-assisted automated analysis of uterine activity along with FHR interpretation may aid the improvement of reporting criteria and clinical management of cases [69]. The results of a large RCT – the INFANT study with 45 000 women recruited – will be published soon and are likely to provide us with the direction on the future of FHR and uterine contraction monitoring.

References

1. Selin L, Wallin G, Berg M. Dystocia in labour: risk factors, management and outcome – a retrospective observational study in a Swedish setting. *Acta Obstet Gynecol Scand.* 2008; 87: 216–21.

2. Arulkumaran S, Koh CH, Ingemarsson I, Ratnam SS. Augmentation of labour: mode of delivery related to cervimetric progress. *Aust & NZ J Obstet Gynaecol.* 1987; 27: 304–8.

3. Zhang J, Troendle J, Mikolajczyk R, *et al.* The natural history of the normal first stage of labor. *Obstet Gynecol.* 2010; 115(4): 705–10.

4. Thomas J, Callwood A, Paranjothy S. National Sentinel Caesarean Section Audit: update. *Pract Midwife.* 2000; 3(11): 20.

5. Arulkumaran S. Uterine activity in labour. In Grudzinskas JG, Yovich JL, Simpson JL, Chard T (eds), *Uterine Physiology* (pp. 356–77). Cambridge: Cambridge University Press; 1995.

6. Sanborn BM. Cell and molecular biology of myometrial smooth muscle function. *Semin Cell Dev Biol.* 2007; 18: 287–8.

7. Garfield RE, Maner WL. Physiology and electrical activity of uterine contractions. *Semin Cell Dev Biol.* 2007; 18: 289–95.

8. Marshall JM. Regulation of activity in uterine smooth muscle. *Physiol Rev Suppl.* 1962; 5: 213–27.

9. Cottrill HM, Barton JR, O'Brien JM, Rhea DL, Milligan DA. Factors influencing maternal perception of uterine contractions. *Am J Obstet Gynecol.* 2004; 190: 1455–7.

10. Gibb D. *Uterine Activity in Labour.* Tunbridge Wells: Castle House Publications; 1989.

11. Steer PJ. Standards in fetal monitoring: practical requirements for uterine activity measurement and recording. *Br J Obstet Gynaecol.* 1993; 100(suppl. 9): 32–6.

12. Miles AM, Monga M, Richeson KS. Correlation of external and internal monitoring of uterine activity in a cohort of term patients. *Am J Perinatol.* 2001; 18(3): 137–40.

13. LaCroix GE. Monitoring labor by an external tokodynamometer. *Am J Obstet Gynecol.* 1968; 101: 111–19.

14. Nageotte M. *Uterine Contraction Monitoring,* 3rd edition, Philadelphia, PA: Lippincott Williams and Wilkins; 2003.

15. Chua S, Arulkumaran S, Yang M, Steer PJ, Ratnam SS. Intrauterine pressure: comparison of extra vs. intra amniotic methods using a transducer tipped catheter. *Asia Oceania J Obstet Gynaecol.* 1994; 20: 35–8.

16. Chan WH, Paul RH, Toews J. Intrapartum fetal monitoring: maternal and fetal morbidity and perinatal mortality. *Obstet Gynecol.* 1973; 41: 7–13.

17. Nuttall ID. Perforation of a placental fetal vessel by an intrauterine pressure catheter. *Br J Obstet Gynaecol.* 1978; 85: 573–4.

18. Devoe LD, Gardner P, Dear C, Searle N. Monitoring intrauterine pressure during active labor: a prospective comparison of two methods. *J Reprod Med.* 1989; 34: 811–14.

19. Svenningsen L, Jensen O. Application of fiberoptics to the clinical measurement of intra-uterine pressure in labor. *Acta Obstet Gynecol Scand.* 1986; 65: 551–5.

20. Vanner T, Gardosi J. Intrapartum assessment of uterine activity. *Baillieres Clin Obstet Gynaecol.* 1996; 10: 243–57.

21. Arulkumaran S, Yang M, Tien CY, Ratnam SS. Reliability of intrauterine pressure measurements. *Obstet Gynecol.* 1991; 78: 800–2.

22. Chua S, Arulkumaran S, Yang M, Ratnam SS, Steer PJ. The accuracy of catheter-tip pressure transducers for the measurement of intrauterine pressure in labour. *Br J Obstet Gynaecol.* 1992; 99: 186–9.

23. Chua S, Kurup A, Arulkumaran S, Ratnam SS. Augmentation of labor: does internal tocography result in better obstetric outcome than external tocography? *Obstet Gynecol.* 1990; 76: 164–7.

24. Bakker JHJ, Janssen PF, van Halem K *et al.* Internal versus external tocodynamometry during induced or augmented labour. *Cochrane Database Syst Rev.* 2013; 8. CD006947. doi: 10.1002/14651858.CD006947

25. Chia YT, Arulkumaran S, Soon SB, Norshida S, Ratnam SS. Induction of labour: does internal tocography result in better obstetric outcome than external tocography. *Aust NZ J Obstet Gynaecol.* 1993; 33: 159–61.

26. Haran G, Elbaz M, Fejgin MD, Biron-Shental T. A comparison of surface acquired uterine electromyography and intrauterine pressure catheter to assess uterine activity. *Am J Obstet Gynecol.* 2012; 206(5): e1–e5.

27. Maul H, Maner WL, Olson G, Saade GR, Garfield RE. Non-invasive transabdominal uterine electromyography correlates with the strength of intrauterine pressure and is predictive of labor and

delivery. *J Matern Fetal Neonatal Med.* 2004; 15: 297–301.

28. Marque CK, Terrien J, Rihana S, Germain G. Preterm labour detection by use of a biophysical marker: the uterine electrical activity. *BMC Pregnancy Childbirth.* 2007; 7: S5.

29. Jiang W, Li G, Lin L. Uterine electromyogram topography to represent synchronization of uterine contractions. *Int J Gynaecol Obstet.* 2007; 97: 120–4.

30. Odendaal HJ, Brink S, Steytler JG. Clinical and haematological problems associated with severe abruptio placentae. *S Afr Med J.* 1978; 54: 476–80.

31. Woolfson J, Steer PJ, Bashford CC, Randall NJ. The measurement of uterine activity in induced labour. *Br J Obstet Gynaecol.* 1976; 83: 934–7.

32. Bakker PC, van Geijn HP. Uterine activity: implications for the condition of the fetus. *J Perinat Med.* 2008; 36: 30–7.

33. Althaus JE, Petersen S, Driggers R, *et al.* Cephalopelvic disproportion is associated with an altered uterine contraction shape in the active phase of labor. *Am J Obstet Gynecol.* 2006; 195: 739–42.

34. Caldeyro-Barcia R, Sica-Blanco Y, Poseiro JJ, *et al.* A quantitative study of the action of synthetic oxytocin on the pregnant human uterus. *J Pharmacol Exp Ther.* 1957; 121: 18–31.

35. El-Sahwi S, Gaafar AA, Toppozada HK. A new unit for evaluation of uterine activity. *Am J Obstet Gynecol.* 1967; 98: 900–3.

36. Miller FC, Yeh SY, Schifrin BS, Paul RH, Hon EH. Quantitation of uterine activity in 100 primiparous patients. *Am J Obstet Gynecol.* 1976; 124: 398–405.

37. Steer PJ, Carter MC, Beard RW. Normal levels of active contraction area in spontaneous labour. *Br J Obstet Gynaecol.* 1984; 91: 211–19.

38. Phillips GF, Calder AA. Units for the evaluation of uterine contractility. *Br J Obstet Gynaecol.* 1987; 94: 236–41.

39. Arulkumaran S, Yang M, Ingemarsson I, Singh P, Ratnam SS. Augmentation of labour: does oxytocin titration to achieve preset active contraction area values produce better obstetric outcome? *Asia Oceania J Obstet Gynaecol.* 1989; 15: 333–7.

40. Gibb DM, Arulkumaran S, Ratnam SS. A comparative study of methods of oxytocin administration for induction of labour. *Br J Obstet Gynaecol.* 1985; 92: 688–92.

41. Arulkumaran S, Chua S, Chua TM, *et al.* Uterine activity in dysfunctional labour and target uterine activity to be aimed with oxytocin titration. *Asia Oceania J Obstet Gynaecol.* 1991; 17: 101–6.

42. Bakker PC, Kurver PH, Kuik DJ, Van Geijn HP. Elevated uterine activity increases the risk of fetal acidosis at birth. *Am J Obstet Gynecol.* 2007; 196: e311–16.

43. Peebles DM, Spencer JA, Edwards AD, *et al.* Relation between frequency of uterine contractions and human fetal cerebral oxygen saturation studied during labour by near infrared spectroscopy. *Br J Obstet Gynaecol.* 1994; 101: 44–8.

44. Arulkumaran S, Gibb DMF, Ratnam SS, Heng SH, Lun KC. Total uterine activity in induced labour: an index of cervical and pelvic tissue resistance. *Br J Obstet Gynaecol.* 1985; 92: 693–7.

45. Cowan DB, van Middelkoop A, Philpott RH. Intrauterine-pressure studies in African nulliparae: normal labour progress. *Br J Obstet Gynaecol.* 1982; 89: 364–9.

46. Fairlie FM, Phillips GF, Andrews BJ, Calder AA. An analysis of uterine activity in spontaneous labour using a microcomputer. *Br J Obstet Gynaecol.* 1988; 95: 57–64.

47. Arulkumaran S, Gibb DM, Lun KC, Heng SH, Ratnam SS. The effect of parity on uterine activity in labour. *Br J Obstet Gynaecol.* 1984; 91: 843–8.

48. Zhang J, Bricker L, Wray S, Quenby S. Poor uterine contractility in obese women. *Br J Obstet Gynaecol.* 2007; 114: 343–8.

49. Wray S. Insights into the uterus. *Exp Physiol.* 2007; 92: 621–31.

50. Parratt JR, Taggart MJ, Wray S. Changes in intracellular pH close to term and their possible significance to labour. *Pflugers Arch.* 1995; 430: 1012–14.

51. Quenby S, Pierce SJ, Brigham S, Wray S. Dysfunctional labor and myometrial lactic acidosis. *Obstet Gynecol.* 2004; 103: 718–23.

52. Arulkumaran S, Gibb DM, Ingemarsson I, Kitchener HC, Ratnam SS. Uterine activity during spontaneous labour after previous lower-segment caesarean section. *Br J Obstet Gynaecol.* 1989; 96: 933–8.

53. Chua S, Arulkumaran S, Singh P, Ratnam SS. Trial of labour after previous caesarean section: obstetric outcome. *Aust NZ J Obstet Gynaecol.* 1989; 29: 12–17.

54. Arulkumaran S, Ingemarsson I, Ratnam SS. Oxytocin augmentation in dysfunctional labour after previous caesarean section. *Br J Obstet Gynaecol.* 1989; 96: 939–41.

55. Arulkumaran S, Chua S, Ratnam SS. Symptoms and signs with scar rupture: value of uterine activity measurements. *Aust NZ J Obstet Gynaecol.* 1992; 32: 208–12.

56. Beckley S, Gee H, Newton JR. Scar rupture in labour after previous lower uterine segment caesarean section: the role of uterine activity measurement. *Br J Obstet Gynaecol*. 1991; 98: 265–9.

57. Gee H, Taylor EW, Hancox R. A model for the generation of intrauterine pressure in the human parturient uterus which demonstrates the critical role of the cervix. *J Theor Biol*. 1988; 133: 281–91.

58. Paul RH, Phelan JP, Yeh SY. Trial of labor in the patient with a prior cesarean birth. *Am J Obstet Gynecol*. 1985; 151: 297–304.

59. Arulkumaran S, Gibb DM, Ratnam SS, Heng SH, Lun KC. Uterine activity in oxytocin induced labour. *Asia Oceania J Obstet Gynaecol*. 1986; 12: 533–40.

60. Oppenheimer LW, Bland ES, Dabrowski A, *et al.* Uterine contraction pattern as a predictor of the mode of delivery. *J Perinatol*. 2002; 22: 149–53.

61. Steer PJ, Carter MC, Beard RW. The effect of oxytocin infusion on uterine activity levels in slow labour. *Br J Obstet Gynaecol*. 1985; 92: 1120–6.

62. Arulkumaran S, Ingemarsson I, Ratnam SS. Oxytocin titration to achieve preset active contraction area values does not improve the outcome of induced labour. *Br J Obstet Gynaecol*. 1987; 94: 242–8.

63. Hauth JC, Hankins GD, Gilstrap LC III. Uterine contraction pressures achieved in parturients with active phase arrest. *Obstet Gynecol*. 1991; 78: 344–7.

64. Crane JM, Young DC, Butt KD, Bennett KA, Hutchens D. Excessive uterine activity accompanying induced labor. *Obstet Gynecol*. 2001; 97: 926–31.

65. Pacheco LD, Rosen MP, Gei AF, Saade GR, Hankins GD. Management of uterine hyperstimulation with concomitant use of oxytocin and terbutaline. *Am J Perinatol*. 2006; 23: 377–80.

66. Chandraharan E, Arulkumaran S. Acute tocolysis. *Curr Opin Obstet Gynecol*. 2005; 17(2): 151–6.

67. Gibb DM, Arulkumaran S, Lun KC, Ratnam SS. Characteristics of uterine activity in nulliparous labour. *Br J Obstet Gynaecol*. 1984; 91: 220–7.

68. FIGO Study Group on the Assessment of New Technology. International Federation of Gynecology and Obstetrics. Intrapartum surveillance: recommendations on current practice and overview of new developments. *Int J Gynaecol Obstet*. 1995; 49: 213–21.

69. Ayres-de Campos D, Bernardes J, Garrido A, Marquesde-Sa J, Pereira-Leite L. SisPorto 2.0: a program for automated analysis of cardiotocograms. *J Matern Fetal Med*. 2000; 9: 311–18.

The Management of Intrapartum 'Fetal Distress'

Laura Coleman and Bryony Strachan

Introduction

Each Baby Counts is the Royal College of Obstetricians' quality improvement programme to reduce the unnecessary suffering and loss of life from brain injury or death in labour by 50% by 2020. This is an ambitious target, and will take reflection and learning across units by all professionals. Fetal asphyxia in labour causes brain injury and stillbirth. The aim of good obstetric care is to reduce the number of infants that die or are damaged due to birth asphyxia. Permanent brain damage or death resulting from asphyxia around the time of birth is a major tragedy for any family. The challenge is to find the baby at risk of asphyxia without causing harm from unnecessary intervention for the mother or fetus.

Fetal Asphyxia and 'Fetal Distress' in Labour: Definitions

The term 'asphyxia' is derived from the Greek and means 'without pulse'. Its current usage in obstetrics is to describe fetal distress before or during labour. Fetal distress or fetal asphyxia are poorly defined terms, but have been widely used for a number of different meanings to describe a range of pathological conditions. Asphyxia is defined experimentally as impaired respiratory gas exchange accompanied by the development of metabolic acidosis. It is usually reserved for experimental situations in which these changes can be accurately established. In the clinical context, fetal asphyxia is progressive hypoxaemia and hypercapnia with a significant metabolic acidaemia. Fetal distress is a commonly used, but poorly defined, term. Its common usage is to describe concern about a fetal condition that pre-empts a caesarean section (CS) or instrumental delivery. It is not a diagnosis as such, but a concern or indication for delivery. Presumed fetal distress was the indication for 22% of caesarean births in the UK [1]. The underlying cause (for example, hyperstimulation, placental insufficiency, cord compression or abruption) is often not known, even after delivery. Therefore obstetricians need to think about the cause for the fetal distress and not take 'fetal distress' as a diagnosis.

Perinatal Mortality and Morbidity

Labour has been described as the most dangerous journey of our lives, and remains so in many parts of the world. Perinatal mortality has declined considerably over the last 50 years in developed countries as a result of greatly improved antenatal and intrapartum care. In 1960, the perinatal mortality rate in England and Wales was 33 per 1000 births, with one-third of these deaths caused by intrapartum asphyxia [2]. In 2013, the combined stillbirth and neonatal mortality rate had fallen to 6.7 per 1000 births, with less than one-tenth of these deaths caused by intrapartum events. In the UK, each year around 500 babies die or are left with severe brain injury during labour [3].

In the developing countries of the world, the perinatal mortality rate is over six times greater than that of the UK, at rates of 47 and 60 per 1000 births, respectively. Intrapartum deaths still account for one-third of these deaths. The World Health Organization argues that intrapartum deaths are largely avoidable with skilled care. In developing countries, just over 40% of births will occur in a healthcare facility, and little more than one in two will have the assistance of a doctor, nurse or midwife [4].

Therefore there are challenges for healthcare professionals on a worldwide and UK basis to reduce the

Best Practice in Labour and Delivery, Second Edition, ed. Sir Sabaratnam Arulkumaran. Published by Cambridge University Press. © Cambridge University Press 2016.

risk of dying for babies, so that the day of your birth is no longer the most dangerous day of your life.

The Consequences of Intervention for Fetal Distress

Interventions for presumed fetal distress are common. Although CS is becoming safer, it still has 2–4 times the mortality and 5–10 times the morbidity of a spontaneous vaginal birth for the mother. Similarly, operative intervention for presumed fetal distress in the form of forceps delivery or vacuum extraction is not without risk to mother and to fetus. The risks of haemorrhage, urinary and bowel symptoms, perineal trauma and pain, and post-traumatic syndrome to the mother are greater with an instrumental delivery. Operative delivery for the fetus is also not without risk. Delivering a fetus by a forceps or vacuum delivery increases the chance of a cephalhaematoma, facial nerve injury, retinal haemorrhage, life-threatening intracranial haemorrhage or skull fracture [1,5].

The movements for 'normal birth' have highlighted concerns of 'over-intervention' because our current tests for predicting fetal asphyxia in labour lack specificity.

A Cochrane review in 2012 compared operative delivery with conservative management for fetal distress in labour and found no significant difference in perinatal mortality in the two groups. Unfortunately there was only one contributing study, which was outdated, and there were no data available on maternal or neonatal morbidity. Contemporary practice often involves expedition of delivery; however, it is important to note that this practice has evolved in the absence of any randomized evidence [6].

Ideally, fetal monitoring should identify the fetus at risk without causing undue harm to the mother or fetus from unnecessary intervention. The challenge is to accurately identify those babies that are coping well with the 'stress' of labour from those which are getting 'distressed' with enough time to expedite delivery before asphyxia occurs.

During labour the baby's physiology changes from transplacental oxygenation through the mother to a new circulation and having to take in oxygen through newly expanded lungs. During this transition the baby is subjected to increasing contractions during which the placental circulation is repeatedly interrupted while the baby negotiates its way through the birth canal. Babies are 'designed' to withstand this

Table 6.1 Antenatal factors affecting fetal reserve

Presumed fetal growth restriction
Pre-eclampsia
Intrapartum bleeding
Infection, e.g. chorioamnionitis
Postmaturity
Prematurity
Antepartum haemorrhage

journey with an ability to preferentially deliver oxygen at low tension to the tissue, utilize glycogen reserves and undergo anaerobic metabolism when required.

Management of 'Fetal Distress': Decision Making

We have described a pragmatic approach to the management of 'fetal distress' in labour based on three key decision-making criteria:

1. *The fetal reserve*, i.e. how well grown and developed the fetus is to cope with the stresses of labour.
2. *The likely cause* of the fetal distress, i.e. is it the type and frequency of contractions or a sudden event such as an abruption or cord prolapse.
3. *The potential response to resuscitation*, i.e. is there a reversible interruption to oxygen supply such as uterine hyper-stimulation.

The Fetal Reserve

Assess the reserve of the fetus to cope with the stress of labour by reviewing the antenatal history (Table 6.1). The effect of antenatal factors on the development of fetal hypoxia in labour is complex. In the Western Australia series, antenatal factors were common findings in the infants that developed neonatal encephalopathy [7]. These included intrauterine growth restriction, postmaturity and pre-eclampsia. These conditions affect placental function and transfer, making hypoxia in labour more likely. If fetal growth is impaired, glycogen stores in the fetal liver are depleted, which reduces the ability of the fetus to cope with a hypoxic insult. Growth restriction or placental insufficiency make the fetus more likely to be delivered for presumed fetal distress. However, routine antenatal care including abdominal palpation and symphyseal fundal height will only detect one-third of

Table 6.2 Comparison of grading systems for anaesthesia and fetal reserve for labour

ASA grading before anaesthesia [9]	Fetal reserve before labour
P1 Normal healthy patient	F1 Normal healthy term infant
P2 Mild systemic disease	F2 Mild systemic disease, e.g. mild to moderate pre-eclampsia, minor antepartum haemorrhage, postmaturity, mild IUGR, 34–36 weeks' gestation
P3 Severe systemic disease	F3 Severe systemic disease, e.g. severe IUGR or 27–33 weeks' gestation
P4 Severe systemic disease that is a constant threat to life	F4 Severe systemic disease that is an imminent threat to life, e.g. severe IUGR with abnormal CTG
	Suspected severe chorioamnionitis with abnormal CTG in preterm infant
P5 Moribund patient	F5 Fetus with lethal congenital malformations or unlikely to survive because of extreme prematurity
P6 Brain-dead patient	F6 Stillbirth

'small for gestational age' babies before birth. Using a customized growth centile chart where maternal characteristics such as height, weight, ethnicity and parity are considered, the sensitivity increases to 48% [8]. Half of growth-restricted babies will not be recognized before labour.

In the presence of infection, the fetus will increase its metabolic and oxygen requirement, making the fetus more likely to become hypoxic. Inflammatory cytokines compound the effects of hypoxia on cell damage.

Assessment of Fetal Reserve: Preparation Before Labour

An anaesthetist will assess the risk of a patient before an anaesthetic according to a standardized grading. In a similar way, an obstetrician could assess the fetus before labour (Table 6.2). For example, a normal healthy fetus will have a low risk for developing fetal distress in labour and with the aim of reducing unnecessary intervention, intermittent auscultation is appropriate. For a fetus known to be growth-restricted or postmature, the risk of developing fetal distress is higher, warranting a careful plan for the type and frequency of monitoring and the intervention required.

Some babies are at such a high perceived risk of developing fetal distress and asphyxia that a prelabour CS may be recommended. Other babies will have a very poor outcome after birth because of severe congenital problems or extreme prematurity. A careful and sensitive discussion is needed to make a plan for appropriate monitoring in labour, taking into account parental wishes and the neonatal plan for assessment and resuscitation at birth. For a stillbirth, although there is no need for fetal monitoring, a plan for monitoring maternal vital signs should be made, particularly in the presence of a uterine scar.

The Cause of Fetal Distress in Labour

The second key 'decision maker' for the obstetrician is to consider the underlying cause of the fetal distress. This will determine the likely response to intrauterine resuscitation and the likelihood of continuing with the labour or expediting delivery.

Contractions and Placental Blood Flow

The fetus is at risk during labour because the supply of oxygen from the mother may be interrupted by contractions of the uterus affecting placental exchange, and compressing the cord. The exchange of oxygen and carbon dioxide with the maternal circulation is compromised by uterine contractions. This was demonstrated by Borell *et al.* in 1965 [10]. Using arteriographic techniques on three women in labour, who were carrying congenitally lethal fetuses, they demonstrated that maternal blood entering the villous spaces was considerably delayed at the height of a contraction, reducing placental perfusion and thus the gaseous exchange during normal labour. At full dilatation of the cervix the Ferguson reflex releases further oxytocin, increasing the strength of contractions, and may cause further compromise to gaseous exchange during the second stage. The start of maternal pushing (the active phase of the second stage) increases the risk of acidaemia with higher levels of lactic acid and carbon dioxide and increasing acidosis. No changes were seen with the passive second stage [11]. Thus the two parts of the second stage of labour actually differ in their potential to stimulate fetal acidosis. The Valsalva manoeuvre does not have an additive effect to this.

Therefore hyper-stimulation and/or tachysystole will increase the risk of fetal hypoxia by reducing the time the uterus spends at rest with optimum placental perfusion. A diseased placenta will be more susceptible to the effects of uterine activity on the reduction of gaseous exchange.

Cord Compression

The delivery of oxygenated blood to the fetus is via the umbilical cord. This is prone to compression against the fetal part during contractions. The presence of Wharton's jelly in the cord is usually protective of severe compression. Infants with intrauterine growth restriction (IUGR) have a reduction of Wharton's jelly, and both the total and lumen vein areas are reduced [12]. Thus a growth-restricted infant is more susceptible to cord compression. A normally grown fetus is protected from the effects of cord compression except in the extremes of cord prolapse or severe entanglement.

Failure to Progress or Dystocia

In study and audit data, reasons for performing an emergency caesarean are categorized as fetal distress or failure to progress in labour to aid audit data. In reality these definitions overlap. A prolonged or obstructed labour will eventually exhaust the fetus. Therefore an accurate assessment of the progress of labour is important in considering the causes of fetal distress.

Maternal Positioning

As early as the eighteenth century, obstetricians favoured mothers delivering in the left lateral position. Most historical pictures of birth are in the upright position. Aorto-caval compression by the term gravid uterus can exacerbate any fetal compromise by reducing the preload to the mother's heart, reducing cardiac output and uterine artery flow. Aorto-caval compression can be measured using toe phlesmography, where changes in blood pressure in the toe can reflect poor perfusion to the lower limbs associated with aorto-caval compression. Using this technique, aorto-caval compression was seen in about half of women in labour, which disappeared using the left or right lateral position. Aorto-caval compression was seen most commonly in the supine position, and less frequently in the standing and semi-recumbent positions. An occipito-posterior position in labour increased the likelihood. Ten per cent of women will have a 'revealed' aorto-caval compression syndrome with hypotension in the supine position. However, in about one-third of women, this aortocaval compression is concealed with no apparent drop in blood pressure as measured in the upper arm. Fetal heart decelerations were not seen in all cases of aortocaval compression, presumably because of the collaterals from the ovarian arteries and placental reserve. Pelvic tilt alone was not good enough to relieve aortocaval compression. A lateral tilt of 15° is recommended; however, angle of tilt is often overestimated, and even at 15°, both left and right pelvic tilt failed to reverse the decreased blood flow in the leg associated with the supine position [13].

Sudden Dramatic Events

Most 'fetal distress' is of an insidious onset as the strength of the contractions increase and the head descends in the pelvis. However, sudden events such as a cord prolapse, abruption or vasa praevia can cause profound dramatic distress.

Vasa Praevia

Vasa praevia is rare and must be considered to be diagnosed. The blood loss is from the fetal side and this carries high mortality. The diagnosis should be considered with any bleed after a spontaneous or artificial rupture of membranes accompanied by acute fetal distress. Alerting the attending neonatologist to the possibility of vasa praevia is vital to ensure the immediate provision of blood for transfusion of the fetus. The characteristic sinusoidal pattern of the cardiotocograph (CTG) with anaemia can be present (Figure 6.1). Prolonged decelerations of the fetal heart rate (FHR) coinciding with membrane rupture can be another pattern.

Cord Prolapse

The diagnosis of cord prolapse is made on vaginal examination. The management is to deliver the fetus promptly. Elevation of the presenting part above the pelvic brim will relieve cord compression. This can be achieved by digital displacement, keeping the hand in the vagina until delivery. Alternatively, a knee–elbow position or an exaggerated Sims' position can be used. Bladder filling with 500 ml of saline using a Foley catheter can also be useful. Tocolysis will help reduce compression of the cord from contractions. If the FHR recovers with these measures then a rapid sequence spinal block can be used in favour of a general anaesthetic.

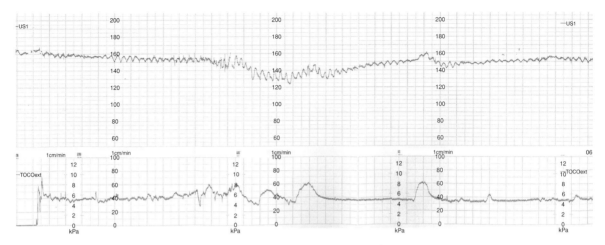

Figure 6.1 Sinusoidal pattern seen after ruptured membranes associated with anaemia from vasa praevia.

Abruption

The presence of continued pain between contractions with or without bleeding may suggest an intrapartum abruption as a cause of the fetal distress. This is unlikely to respond to resuscitation.

Uterine Rupture

Fetal distress may be the first sign of impending uterine rupture. The presence of pain between contractions, vaginal bleeding, sudden cessation of contractions or a rise of the presenting part should alert the obstetrician to the possibility of uterine rupture, particularly in a woman at risk. Again, this will not respond to resuscitation.

Fetal distress caused by sudden dramatic labour events will not be reversed with intrauterine resuscitation. However, intrauterine resuscitation is rarely contraindicated, even when immediate delivery is planned, as it will optimize fetal oxygenation during preparation for delivery. Table 6.3 summarizes the potential response to intrauterine resuscitation.

Table 6.3 Potential response to intrauterine resuscitation

Yes	Maybe	No
Hyper-stimulation	Cord compression	Placental abruption
Supine hypotension	Placental insufficiency	Uterine rupture
Dehydration	Infection	Vasa praevia
Hypotension, e.g. following regional anaesthetic	Cord prolapse	

Intrauterine Resuscitation

Maternal Positioning in Left Lateral

An upright or left lateral position reduces the risk of fetal heart decelerations. It makes sense to prevent the effects of aorto-caval compression by discouraging the use of supine or tilt positions in favour of the lateral or upright position. If fetal distress is suspected, then using the lateral position is good practice to correct any revealed or concealed aorto-caval compression.

Stopping the Contractions

Maternal blood flow to the placental villous space is reduced or altered during a contraction. Increasing the frequency of contractions above four in 10 min will reduce gaseous exchange across the placenta.

Recognizing hyper-stimulation is the first step in preventing this. Commonly, this is missed. In the Swedish survey of malpractice claims, 71% had injudicious use of oxytocin, with greater than six contractions observed in 10 min [14]. With hyper-stimulation, the oxytocin infusion must be stopped for a short period of time before recommencing at a lower rate once the fetus has recovered. Oxytocin has a half-life of 15 min; therefore, reducing the rate of the infusion will reduce the serum levels quickly. An infusion should be stopped for at least 15 min before recommencing. Tocolytics should be considered in addition to stopping oxytocin.

Tocolysis

Acute tocolysis or uterine relaxation can be a valuable tool in the management of fetal distress. By correcting

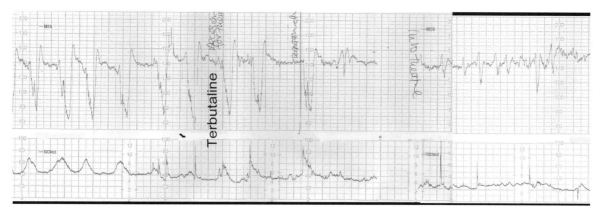

Figure 6.2 Cardiotocograph showing the effect of terbutaline on contraction frequency and fetal heart rate.

the hyper-stimulation causing the fetal distress, it may be possible to continue with the labour or convert an immediate category 1 caesarean to a less-urgent category 2.

Terbutaline, a betasympathomimetic, is the tocolytic with most published data. The NICE guidance recommends a dose of 250 mcg given subcutaneously [15]. The effect of abolishing contractions can be seen in Figure 6.2. Fears regarding risk of postpartum haemorrhage are largely unfounded in practice. If this does occur, the action can be reversed with 1 mg of propranolol given intravenously.

Atosiban, an oxytocin antagonist developed for the treatment of preterm labour, has the potential for use as an acute tocolytic as it has a favourable side-effect profile and is currently being evaluated. Nitroglycerin as a sublingual preparation (400 mg) has been shown to be useful for acute tocolysis. Its very short duration of action (2–3 min) makes it ideal for use at caesarean section to aid delivery – for example in a transverse lie with no liquor – but not so good for tocolysis in labour, as the dose has to be repeated every 2 min. Side-effects such as hypotension, nausea and headache are common.

Intravenous Fluids

Maternal hypovolaemia and hypotension can decrease the uteroplacental blood supply. For this reason, the NICE guidance recommends assessing the mother for signs of dehydration and/or hypotension when assessing a suspicious CTG in labour, and treatment with a bolus of 500 ml crystalloid is recommended [15]. There are no randomized trials looking at the use

of an intravenous fluid bolus for the management of fetal distress, and caution must be used in the presence of pre-eclampsia because of the risk of pulmonary oedema. However, it does seem sensible to correct dehydration and hypotension if present. Intravenous fluid boluses of glucose-containing solutions should be avoided because of potentially detrimental effects on fetal status, including increased fetal lactate and decreased fetal pH.

Amnioinfusion

Amnioinfusion has been used as a treatment for fetal distress with some promising results in trials in resource-poor areas. One potential use is in the case of meconium staining of the liquor to dilute the meconium and therefore make the incidence of meconium aspiration less likely. Unfortunately, trials have not shown the benefit of this [15]. It is likely that the meconium has already been inhaled in utero down to the alveoli levels. Therefore adding more fluid once thick meconium has been seen is unlikely to be of significant benefit.

The other potential use is in the presence of variable decelerations thought to be due to cord compression. The addition of fluid would cushion the cord compression occurring during a contraction. A meta-analysis did show a modest reduction in FHR abnormalities and a reduction in low Apgars and low arterial pH at birth. However, the trials included were too small to address rare but serious maternal side-effects of amnioinfusion [16].

Trials based in centres with standard peripartum surveillance have not demonstrated benefit in either scenario and therefore amnioinfusion is not recommended for management of fetal distress.

Oxygen

Oxygen administration has been shown to increase fetal oxygenation as measured by pulse oximetry, and some studies have shown improvements in FHR patterns. However, oxygen administration may be potentially harmful. Studies have demonstrated that routine oxygenation in the second stage caused deterioration in cord blood gas values. Other studies in animals have shown raised harmful free radicals as a result of maternal oxygen administration, and neonatal resuscitation uses air initially to avoid high concentrations of oxygen, again because of free radical formation.

There is increasing evidence that maternal facial oxygen administration can be a frightening experience for mothers and partners at a particularly stressful time and may distract attention from other preparations for emergency delivery. Based on current evidence, maternal oxygen administration cannot be recommended for intrauterine resuscitation for the fetus [15]. However, pre-oxygenation for the mother is useful if a general anaesthetic is being considered.

Delivering the Fetus

Having considered the fetal reserve, the nature of the insult and the potential or actual response to resuscitation, the decision is whether to expedite delivery.

There is only one randomized trial comparing delivery for fetal distress to a conservative approach which was published in 1959 from South Africa. Women were randomized to intervention (delivery by caesarean, symphysiotomy or forceps), or a conservative approach to fetal distress as picked up by FHR abnormalities on intermittent auscultation or the presence of meconium staining of the liquor. There was a high perinatal mortality rate in both arms of the study, with a significant number of deaths in the intervention group due to trauma. The study was underpowered for differences in perinatal mortality. The Cochrane reviewers concluded that there was too little evidence to show whether operative management is more beneficial than treating factors which may be causing the baby's distress, and that further contemporary research is needed. Such a trial will be difficult to perform [7].

Caesarean Section or Operative Delivery

Having decided to deliver a distressed baby, the next decision is how to do so. During preparation for delivery, resuscitation methods can continue. In the first stage of labour the option is CS, except in rare circumstances (for example, rapid progress in a multiparous patient or a second twin) where a vaginal birth can be considered.

The classification of urgency is useful in determining good communication with the anaesthetist. The choice of anaesthesia has to be made between the anaesthetist and the mother. Increasingly, regional analgesia is favoured in preference to general anaesthesia. With the use of a 'rapid sequence' spinal anaesthetic, a decision interval can be less than the gold standard of 30 min [1]. The use of an urgency classification helps communication between the whole team in preparing for delivery, balancing the need for urgency and adequate careful preparation for the mother.

Poor fetal outcome with instrumental vaginal births relate to inappropriate application and/or excessive traction, particularly at mid-cavity and rotational deliveries in the presence of fetal distress.

A prospective cohort study of 393 women experiencing operative delivery in the second stage of labour reported an increased risk of neonatal trauma and admission to the special care baby unit (SCBU) following excessive pulls (more than three pulls) and sequential use of instruments. The risk was further increased where delivery was completed by CS following a protracted attempt at operative vaginal delivery [17].

The bulk of malpractice litigation results from failure to abandon the procedure at the appropriate time, particularly the failure to eschew prolonged, repeated or excessive traction efforts in the presence of poor progress. The choice of instrument will depend on the skill and expertise of the operator and the assessment of the ease and difficulty of the planned delivery. Mid-cavity and rotational deliveries will have a higher complexity (and thus higher morbidity) than low-cavity and non-rotational deliveries. Opting for CS is not always the safest way for mother or baby, and considerable morbidity can occur to either.

The wise obstetrician in the presence of fetal distress will choose the instrument that will have the best chance of delivering the baby the safest and quickest way with the least risk of failure or use of multiple instruments.

Forceps or Vacuum Delivery

Forceps and vacuum extraction are associated with different benefits and risks. The options available for rotational delivery include Kielland forceps, manual rotation followed by direct traction forceps or rotational vacuum extraction. There is an increasing trend for opting for a manual rotation, despite this being the least assessed by research. Rotational deliveries should be performed by experienced operators, the choice depending upon the expertise of the individual operator.

Average decision-to-delivery time for CS in the presence of fetal distress is 30–40 min. In instrumental birth this time is 20–30 min [15]. There appears to be no advantage of forceps over a vacuum delivery in the presence of fetal distress, and the decision-to-delivery intervals are similar between these instruments. Delivery in theatre compared to the room will result in a longer decision-to-delivery interval, but this must be balanced against the risk of failure in the room causing increased morbidity [18].

Managing Fetal Distress: Non-technical Skills

In a recent survey of malpractice cases in Sweden, the most common events were neglecting to supervise fetal well-being in 173 cases (98%), neglecting signs of fetal asphyxia in 126 cases (71%), including incautious use of oxytocin in 126 cases (71%), and choosing a non-optimal mode of delivery in 92 cases (52%). The authors conclude that there is a great need and a challenge to improve cooperation and to create security barriers within our labour units. Similar findings are seen in the UK Confidential Enquiries, which found substandard care in 75% of intrapartum-related deaths, related to failure to recognize a problem to act appropriately or to communicate. A long delay has been highlighted as a major contribution to intrapartum deaths. This suggests that there is often a window of opportunity where intervention could make a difference.

Brian Goldman, in a Ted X talk on why doctors make mistakes, talks about how we are trained to believe that if we work hard enough and learn hard enough, we will not make mistakes. Great baseball players are described as '300 hitters', i.e. they hit the ball, don't get caught and make it to first base three out of ten times. We expect to be '1000 hitters' and manage 1000 out of 1000 women in complex labour perfectly each time. We are all human and we will all make mistakes [14,19]. The *Each Baby Counts* campaign will help us to investigate the human factors involved when things go wrong, allowing the profession to design better systems to reduce the number of mistakes we make [20].

The complexity of patient care in modern obstetrics demands a wide range of skills and attributes. Conventional training has placed great emphasis on acquisition of the necessary knowledge and practical skills to ensure competent practice. However, good outcomes will only be realized if appropriate plans can be put in place effectively. This requires both technical and non-technical skills, such as communication, team working, planning, resource management and decision making. Such skills are not new in obstetrics; good practitioners have always demonstrated these competencies, but they have not featured explicitly in formal training programmes. These skills are sometimes referred to under the general heading of 'human factors'. There are several teamwork dimensions, based on commercial and military aviation models, which have been applied in medical settings [21]. There are barriers to teamwork, particularly in labour wards with complex hierarchy, communication and decision-making structures.

How Do We Make the 'Right' Decisions?

Most work on medical decision making is 'low-velocity'; i.e. time constraints are modest, and there is a cooling-off period for adjustment and reconsideration. 'High-velocity' decision making in the busy labour ward is different.

The Nature of High-Velocity Decision Making

In the heat of an emergency situation, a decision needs to be made within huge time pressure, and the impact of the decision (delivery or not) may have major implications.

In this situation, the human mind works in a different way. Understanding this enables the clinician to improve their decision making. In simple terms,

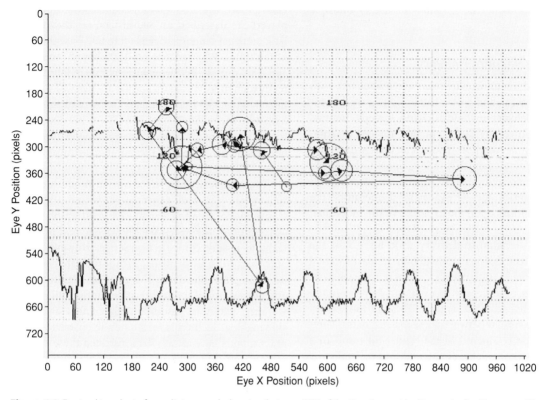

Figure 6.3 Eye-tracking chart of a cardiotocograph showing that over 90% of the time is spent looking at the fetal heart rate. The circles represent the fixation point, with the larger circles indicating a longer fixation time. The arrows indicate the saccadic movements of the eye.

the human brain filters visual and auditory information under stressful conditions. This prevents 'information overload'. Visually, data are concentrated on the focal field with reduced input from the periphery. When reading the two lines of data such as on a CTG, the focal field cannot take in both the heart rate and the contractions, and only a small part of the time looking at the CTG is spent looking at contractions (Figure 6.3).

Auditory information is also filtered by the task concerned. For example, when an obstetrician is concentrating on an examination or the start of a difficult delivery, a fetal bradycardia may not be heard by them although clearly audible to all others in the room. Understanding this allows the clinician to make concerted efforts to gain the vital information and to rely on their 'wing men', the fellow members of the team, to alert them to danger.

Filtering of Information is Crucial

A good decision maker is able to filter the correct information and compute the information correctly. Not being able to filter the information leads to information overload and an inability to make a timely decision. Filtering the wrong information and concentration of the minutia leads to the wrong decision.

Conclusions

Fetal distress is an imprecise term for a fetus at risk of intrapartum asphyxia.

Losing a baby from intrapartum asphyxia is now uncommon in the developed world. We are still dealing with an imperfect tool to monitor the baby, namely CTG. An obstetrician needs to balance the risk of unnecessary intervention with the need to correctly identify babies that are distressed. Normal labour involves challenges to the normal gaseous exchange of the fetus for which a normal healthy baby will almost certainly cope. Good decision making involves assessing the fetal reserve to identify the fetus at risk of distress in labour, the likely cause of the fetal distress and the likely response to resuscitation. Starting intrauterine resuscitation is rarely contraindicated

Table 6.4 Summary of management options

1. Make a decision – assess:
   - the fetal reserve;
   - the likely cause of distress;
   - the likely response to resuscitation.
2. Resuscitate the fetus:
   - place mother in left lateral;
   - stop the contractions by stopping oxytocin and give tocolysis;
   - give intravenous fluids.
3. Communicate clearly with the team.

and should be started even when immediate delivery is planned. Intrauterine resuscitation includes positioning in left lateral, stopping the contractions and giving intravenous fluids. Understanding how we make decisions in the acute setting will help develop our decision-making skills. Good communication and team working on the labour ward is vital (Table 6.4).

References

1. National Collaborating Centre for Women's and Children's Health. *Caesarean Section: Clinical Guideline*. London: RCOG Press; 2004.

2. Fryer JG, Ashford JR. Trends in perinatal and neonatal mortality in England and Wales 1960–69. *Br J Prev Soc Med*. 1972; 26: 1–9.

3. Office for National Statistics. Child mortality statistics: childhood, infant and perinatal, 2013; 2013. www.web. ons.gov.uk/ons/rel/vsob1/child-mortality-statistics–childhood–infant-and-perinatal/index.html (accessed 16 May 2016).

4. World Health Organization. *Neonatal and Perinatal Mortality: Country, Regional and Global Estimates in 2004*. Geneva: WHO Maternal Health and Safe Motherhood Programme; 2007.

5. Towner D, Castro MA, Eby-Wilkens E, Gilbert WM. Effect of mode of delivery in nulliparous women on neonatal intracranial injury. *New Engl J Med*. 1999; 341: 1709–14.

6. Hofmeyr GJ, Kulier R. Operative versus conservative management for 'fetal distress' in labour. *Cochrane Database of Syst Rev*. 2012; 6. CD001065. doi: 10.1002/14651858.CD001065.pub2.

7. Badawi N, Kurinczuk JJ, Keogh JM, *et al.* Antepartum risk factors for newborn encephalopathy: the Western Australian case-control study. *Br Med J*. 1998; 317: 1549–53.

8. RCOG. *The Investigation of the Small-for-Gestational-Age Fetus*. London: RCOG Press; 2002.

9. American Society of Anesthesiologists. ASA physical status classification system. www.asahq.org/clinical/physicalstatus.htm (accessed 22 November 2005).

10. Borell U, Fernstrom I, Ohlsen L, Wiqvist N. Influence of uterine contractions on the uteroplacental blood flow at term. *Am J Obstet Gynecol*. 1965; 93: 44–57.

11. Piquard F, Schaefer A, Hsiung R, Dellenbach P, Haberey P. Are there two biological parts in the second stage of labor? *Acta Obstet Gynecol Scand*. 1989; 69: 713–18.

12. Gill P, Jarjoura D. Wharton's jelly in the umbilical cord: a study of its quantitative variations and clinical correlates. *J Reprod Med*. 1993; 38: 611–14.

13. Kinsella SM, Lee A, Spencer JA. Maternal and fetal effects of the supine and pelvic tilt positions in late pregnancy. *Eur J Obstet Gynecol Reprod Biol*. 1990; 36: 11–17.

14. Berglund S, Grunewald C, Pettersson H, Cnattingius S. Severe asphyxia due to delivery-related malpractice in Sweden 1990–2005. *Br J Obstet Gynaecol*. 2008; 115: 316–23.

15. National Collaborating Centre for Women's and Children's Health. *Intrapartum Care of Healthy Women and their Babies during Childbirth*. London: RCOG Press; 2014.

16. Hofmeyr GJ. Amnioinfusion for potential or suspected umbilical cord compression in labour. *Cochrane Database Syst Rev*. 1996; 2. CD000013. doi: 10.1002/14651858.CD000013.

17. Murphy DJ, Liebling RE, Patel R, Verity L, Swingler R. Cohort study of operative delivery in the second stage of labour and standard of obstetric care. *Br J Obstet Gynaecol*. 2003; 110: 610–15.

18. Murphy DJ, Koh DK. Cohort study of the decision to delivery interval and neonatal outcome for emergency operative vaginal delivery. *Am J Obstet Gynecol*. 2007; 196: e1–7.

19. Confidential Enquiry into Stillbirths and Deaths in Infancy. *4th Annual Report*. London: Maternal and Child Health Research Consortium; 1997.

20. Goldman B. Doctors make mistakes: Can we talk about that? [Video file]; 2011. www.ted.com/talks/brian_goldman_doctors_make_mistakes_can_we_talk_about_that#t-1150935 (accessed 16 May 2016).

21. Fletcher G, Flin R, McGeorge P, *et al.* Anaesthetists' non-technical skills (ANTS): evaluation of a behavioural marker system. *Br J Anaesth*. 2003; 90: 580–8.

Nutrition and Hydration in Labour

David Fraser and Jonathon Francis

Given the increasing interest in many aspects of peri-natal physiology, it is regrettable that there remains a lack of reliable evidence to guide clinical practice in the vexed interest of what – if any – oral intake – would be safe for low-risk labouring women. As a result, views appear to have become somewhat polarized across the Atlantic. The background to the issues and the evidence from the limited number of studies conducted in this area is the subject of this chapter.

Introduction

At a meeting of the New York Obstetrical Society in December 1945, Curtis Mendelson first described his studies on aspiration of stomach contents associated with general anaesthesia (GA) in pregnant women – these findings were published the following year [1]. Mendelson had noted 66 cases of aspiration of stomach contents into the lungs in over 44 000 pregnancies at the New York Lying-In Hospital from 1932 to 1945, an incidence of 1.5 per 1000 deliveries. In 45 of these cases, the aspirated material was recorded; 40 mothers had aspirated liquid and 5 had aspirated solid food. Only two of the mothers actually died, both dying on the delivery table as a result of suffocation after ingesting solid material. The surviving women went on to develop an aspiration pneumonitis, thought to be due to the aspiration of gastric acid. So the risks of gastric aspiration were noted to be two-fold: the aspiration of solid particles sufficiently large to obstruct the airway, and the pneumonitis secondary to acidic gastric contents.

The significance of this seminal paper lies not only in the description of this eponymous condition for the first time, but also on the profound effect it had on the subsequent management of labouring women. Nil-by-mouth (NBM) policies were introduced into many Western labour wards in the 1940s and 1950s in the belief that this would reduce the incidence of pulmonary aspiration of acidic gastric contents should GA be required.

Pulmonary aspiration is increasingly rare, and in the years 1994–2012 only one maternal death from the aspiration of gastric contents under general anaesthesia has been recorded in the UK, an 18-year period when approximately 12 million women delivered [2–7].

The fact that maternal death from pulmonary aspiration of gastric contents has virtually disappeared has led to relaxations in the 'NBM rule', in Europe, at least. In a postal survey of 351 maternity units in England and Wales, almost 33% allowed labouring women to both eat and drink [8]. In a smaller study of clinical practice in the Netherlands, only 14% of the obstetricians surveyed had a restrictive policy during normal labour [9]. This non-restrictive policy was not associated with a higher mortality due to Mendelson's syndrome.

By contrast, the practice of restricted oral intake in normal labour appears to persist in the United States. In an anonymous survey of obstetricians and anaesthetists, approximately 90% restricted patients to clear fluids throughout labour – although this view represented a response rate of only 33% of those surveyed [10]. In April 2007, the American Society of Anesthesiologists, in a practice guideline for obstetric anaesthesia, recommended that 'solid foods should be avoided in labouring patients' [11]. This advice was echoed two years later in an American College of Obstetricians and Gynecologists (ACOG) Committee Opinion published in September 2009 [12].

Best Practice in Labour and Delivery, Second Edition, ed. Sir Sabaratnam Arulkumaran. Published by Cambridge University Press. © Cambridge University Press 2016.

Practical Obstetric Considerations

A number of anatomical and physiological changes occur in pregnancy and labour which increase the risk of pulmonary aspiration, if GA is required. Many of these have been exacerbated by the rising rates of maternal obesity witnessed in the last decade.

The anatomical changes that can increase the difficulty of tracheal intubation in obstetric patients include raised body mass index (BMI) and enlarged breasts.

National data published for the UK in 2010 identified the growing numbers of obese pregnant women [13]. The study found that almost 5% of the UK maternity population were severely obese (BMI ≥35), while just over 2% were morbidly obese (BMI ≥40). An increased risk of obstetric complications, including operative delivery, was also noted in obese women.

This obesity and enlarged breasts can make laryngoscopy more difficult, particularly if the situation is exacerbated by the laryngeal oedema that may complicate common obstetric conditions, such as pre-eclampsia.

These considerations may also jeopardize effective airway protection by making it more difficult to apply cricoid pressure correctly.

In pregnancy, symptomatic gastro-oesophageal reflux is much more likely to occur. This occurs due to a combination of rising intra-abdominal pressure caused by the gravid uterus, and the steady decline in lower oesophageal sphincter tone as a result of high progesterone levels. The tone of the sphincter is also reduced by GA – increasing the likelihood of reflux of gastric contents into the oropharynx, and their subsequent pulmonary aspiration.

Labour also causes significant depression of gastric motility and delays in gastric emptying in proportion to its duration [14]. Following a standard 'meal' of 750 ml of water containing a dye, the volume of fluid remaining in the stomach after 30 min was compared in three groups of women: non-pregnant, late pregnancy (pregnancy of at least 34 weeks' gestation) and labouring. The mean volume remaining during labour was significantly higher than in non-pregnant women and pregnant women before labour. The authors proposed that these results might be attributed to the pain and emotional disturbances that accompany labour.

Finally, narcotic analgesics exacerbate the problem of delayed gastric emptying in labour, and women who have received intramuscular narcotic analgesics such as pethidine or diamorphine in labour are more likely to vomit or to have increased volumes of gastric residuals at delivery [15].

A postal survey of UK obstetric practice published in 2008 found that the use of such intramuscular opioids is still widespread, at least in consultant-led maternity units. A total of 234 consultant-led obstetric units in the UK were questioned about their use of intramuscular opioids, and of units responding to the survey questionnaire over 84% were using pethidine and 34% used diamorphine [16].

Changes in Obstetric Anaesthetic Practice

In the 68 years since the publication of Mendelson's seminal paper, anaesthetic practice in obstetrics has changed profoundly. This has contributed to the extremely low rates of maternal mortality and morbidity witnessed today.

General Anaesthesia

Until the 1970s, when commercially produced epidural catheters and needles became more widely available, GA was used almost universally to provide anaesthesia for operative obstetrics [17]. The inherent dangers of aspiration highlighted by Mendelson in the 1940s were widely appreciated, and measures taken to avoid these. In the 1950s this included restriction of oral intake during labour, inducing anaesthesia in a steep head-up position and sometimes emptying the stomach before induction of anaesthesia either by inserting a gastric tube or by administering an emetic drug such as apomorphine. It was also at this time that the use of thiopentone and suxamethonium was shown to be an excellent combination for inducing anaesthesia and muscle relaxation to facilitate tracheal intubation [18].

In the 1960s Sellick first described the use of cricoid pressure as an additional measure to prevent regurgitation of stomach contents during induction of anaesthesia prior to intubation of the trachea [19]. This manoeuvre was widely adopted in modern practice and is still considered best practice when inducing GA in any patient who is at high risk of aspiration.

The techniques mentioned above of inducing anaesthesia using thiopentone and suxamethonium while applying cricoid pressure prior to intubation of the trachea have remained the standard general anaesthetic technique used in obstetrics. More recently other agents have been developed and discussion is ongoing in the anaesthetic community about whether this standard practice should be modified [20].

Diminishing Rates of General Anaesthesia

The major change that has taken place with regards to general anaesthesia in obstetrics is the frequency with which it is used. Although the rates of obstetric intervention – including caesarean section (CS) – are increasing, the proportion of women receiving GA in obstetrics is now low.

A UK-wide survey of obstetric anaesthetic departments estimated that in 1982 over three-quarters (77%) of CSs were carried out under GA, with some units having a 100% rate [21]. The same survey estimated that the GA rate had fallen to 44% in 1992.

The UK National Obstetric Anaesthesia Data (NOAD) online report of 2011, produced by the Obstetric Anaesthetists' Association, found the national rate of GA for caesarean delivery was only 8.2% [22]. In 2011 there were a total of 6495 de novo GAs for CS and 4783 cases when a regional technique was converted to a GA – the vast majority being for emergency CS. NOAD also reports that the overall number of CSs performed under GA in 2011 appeared to have reduced when compared to previous years.

These figures show that in modern obstetric practice the substantial majority of labouring women will *not* require a GA. Unfortunately, it is often difficult to predict those women for which GA will ultimately be required.

One approach to this problem is to assume that *all* women in normal labour are at equal risk of requiring a GA (with the associated risks of pulmonary aspiration of gastric contents) and offer everyone routine prophylactic antacid medication. However, a Cochrane review of the limited number of randomized controlled trials of this approach found no evidence that either H_2-receptor antagonists or antacids in labour reduced the incidence of gastric aspiration, and recommended that they should not be routinely given to low-risk women in normal labour [23].

Regional Anaesthesia and Analgesia

The risks associated with GA can largely be avoided if a GA is not administered at all and an alternative technique used instead. The increased availability of, and expertise in, regional anaesthesia and analgesia over

the past 40 years has contributed to reducing the number of GAs required for women in labour.

Epidural analgesia for labour has evolved over the past three decades. A common technique used nowadays is the 'low-dose' or 'mobile' epidural. This uses a mixture of relatively weak local anaesthetic combined with a low concentration of the short-acting opiate fentanyl. A typical solution would be 0.1% levobupivacaine and 2 mcg/ml fentanyl. This combination usually gives sufficient analgesia without the dense motor block and leg weakness that can occur when higher concentrations of local anaesthetic are used.

Data from the NOAD 2011 report referred to above [22] showed a national regional analgesia rate in the UK of 22.7% (range 4.1–37.6%).

There are several advantages of epidural analgesia for labour with regards to aspiration risk to the mother. It should reduce (or abolish) the requirement for systemic opioid analgesic medication. A Cochrane review from 2011 reports that, on average, 34% of women in labour in the UK receive systemic opioid analgesia, 10% of whom also receive epidural analgesia (almost certainly after they had received systemic opioid). The same review found that systemic opiates are associated with increased rates of maternal nausea and vomiting [24].

Fentanyl administered via an epidural catheter has also been shown to decrease gastric emptying but only after it had been infused for more than 4.5 hours, after which time the women had received a total dose of fentanyl of more than 100 mcg [25]. It seems likely, therefore, that any delay in gastric emptying in women with an epidural will be directly related to the duration of their labour and the dose of epidural fentanyl.

Another advantage of an effective labour epidural is that it can be 'topped up' with much stronger local anaesthetic to give a more profound anaesthetic block should operative delivery of the fetus be required. This helps reduce the chance of GA being required, avoiding the risks associated with it.

Women who are considered at high risk of complications from a GA, including aspiration (such as morbidly obese parturients), are often advised to have an epidural in labour in an attempt to minimize the chances of a GA being needed if an operative obstetric intervention is necessary.

The overall emphasis on the anaesthetic management of women in labour for the past few decades has been a drive to decrease the number of GAs and utilize regional anaesthetic techniques. This has been achieved to a large extent and it is likely that GA rates will continue to decline, although they will almost certainly never reach zero! This change has been brought about by increased awareness of the benefits of regional anaesthesia, and better training of anaesthetists, obstetricians and midwives. The sub-specialization of obstetric anaesthetists and the early identification of 'at-risk' patients who are administered H_2-receptor antagonists during labour have also helped reduce the risk of pulmonary aspiration of gastric contents.

Oral Intake in Labour

Labour is a metabolically challenging time for mother and fetus. Non-diabetic women in late pregnancy have been shown to exhibit a state of 'accelerated starvation' if denied food and drink [26]. This results in the increased production of ketones – in particular β-hydroxybutyrate and aceto-acetic acid – and the non-esterified fatty acids from which they are derived, and significant reductions in plasma glucose and insulin levels. The changes seem to occur equally in lean and obese women. These physiological changes are exacerbated by the metabolic changes of labour, and the authors caution against the common practice of skipping breakfast in pregnant women.

The production of ketones is a normal physiological adaptation to generate an alternative energy supply when glucose supply is limited. Despite this, concerns about the detrimental effects of maternal starvation and subsequent ketosis in labour in the 1960s and 1970s led to the intrapartum administration of high-dose intravenous dextrose solutions as a preventative measure. However, it is now clear that ketones are not so detrimental to the mother and fetus as once thought. In addition, it quickly became apparent that while strategies employing high-dose intravenous dextrose throughout labour could swiftly correct maternal ketosis, the practice was associated with adverse consequences for the mother and fetus, so the practice was abandoned [27].

Attention subsequently switched to intrapartum measures that might attenuate the metabolic consequences of eating and drinking in labour. These have been evaluated in a limited number of randomized controlled studies of labouring women considered as at low risk of needing a GA (there are no studies looking at high-risk women in labour).

Unrestricted Diet in Labour

Only one randomized study has assessed the effect of unrestricted oral intake in labour compared with complete restriction [28]. In 2005, Tranmer et al. reported on the effect of oral intake in 328 low-risk nulliparous women in Canada. Women randomized to the 'usual care' arm of the study ($N = 165$) were permitted only ice chips, popsicles or sips of fluid during the active phase of labour. Those in the intervention group ($N = 163$) were allowed unrestricted access to their choice of foods and fluid during labour, although encouraged to eat 'easily digestible' foods or fluids. The primary outcome of this study was the incidence of labour dystocia and there were no significant differences in this, or any other labour and delivery outcomes, between the two groups. The reported rates of thirst, hunger and nausea were also comparable. Interestingly, only 56% of those allocated to the unrestricted diet group reported that they actually ate or drank some form of carbohydrate in labour.

Restricted Diet in Labour

Two studies have assessed the comparison of low-residue food in labour with restriction to water only.

In 1999, Scrutton et al. published the results of a prospective study examining the effect of light diet on the metabolic profile, outcome of labour and the risk of aspiration in a group of 94 women delivering in a university teaching hospital [29]. Women presenting in early labour (cervical dilatation less than 5 cm) were randomly allocated to one of two groups; those in the eating group ($N = 48$) were permitted to select from a low-residue diet throughout their labour, whereas those in the starved group ($N = 46$) were permitted water only. The two groups were similar with respect to age, parity, induction status and cervical dilatation at the time of randomization. By the end of labour, plasma β-hydroxybutyrate and non-esterified fatty acids were significantly lower in the eating group. Conversely, the plasma glucose and insulin levels were higher in the eating group. However, those women who ate had significantly higher gastric volumes within an hour of delivery, and were twice as likely to vomit at or around delivery. The volumes vomited by women in the eating group were also significantly larger than volumes vomited by women in the starved group (309 ml vs. 104 ml). The vomit contained a considerable amount of solid and semi-solid residue.

There were no significant differences between groups with respect to duration of labour, mode of delivery or neonatal outcome. The rates of assisted delivery in this relatively small study were only 25% in each group, implying that those studied were genuinely representative of a low-risk population.

The restricted diet was generally well tolerated by those in the intervention group, though there was a progressive decrease in food consumption as labour advanced.

These results suggest that those women allowed a light diet in labour are at reduced risk of developing ketosis without any discernible benefit to the labour progress or outcome for mother or fetus. However, the residual gastric volume around the time of birth is significantly higher in the eating group, who are almost certainly at greater risk of pulmonary aspiration should they require an emergency GA.

A far larger prospective, randomized study from the same unit was published in 2009 [30]. A total of 2426 nulliparous, low-risk women were randomized on admission to either the 'eating' group ($N = 1219$) or to the 'water-only' group ($N = 1207$). The two groups were comparable with respect to their age, ethnic origin, prelabour food intake, need for intravenous fluids and use of prostaglandin and oxytocin.

Both groups of women had free access to water, but the women in the 'water-only' group received water or ice chips only and were encouraged not to eat if they requested to do so. Those randomized to the 'eating' group were encouraged to consume a low-fat, low-residue diet at will during their labour, and the foods they consumed included fruit juice, soup, cereal, biscuits, fruits, chocolate, toast, vegetable stew, sandwiches, burgers, chicken and rice.

Over 5% of all women recruited to this study consumed nothing during labour. Of the women allocated to the 'water-only' group, 20% failed to adhere to the study protocol and consumed food in their labour. Conversely, 29% of those who had been actively encouraged to eat during their labour chose not to do so.

There were no significant differences between the two groups in any of the following outcome measures:

- rate of normal vaginal delivery;
- duration of labour;
- rate of instrumental vaginal delivery;
- rate of CS;
- use of epidural analgesia;
- use of oxytocin for labour augmentation;

- incidence of maternal vomiting;
- neonatal Apgar scores; and
- neonatal admission to NICU/SCBU.

This study found that eating in low-risk labour did not influence obstetric outcomes, including mode of delivery and the duration of labour. The study was not powered to show any difference in rates of gastric aspiration, since the prevalence of this condition is now so low that any such study would need to recruit vast numbers of women.

Although the women recruited to the study were all 'low risk', the intervention rates were quite high, with CS rates of 30% in both groups – implying quite a highly medicalized birthing environment. Notwithstanding this, the findings from this large study dominate the findings in subsequent meta-analysis of the benefits and harms of restricting oral intake during labour [31].

Low-Carbohydrate 'Sport Drinks'

Sport drinks have become very popular in the last decade. Most contain mixtures of carbohydrates (such as glucose and dextrose), sodium, potassium and calcium, together with flavouring to make them more palatable.

Three studies have compared the effects of restricting women to water only compared with allowing them access to carbohydrate drinks.

The results of the first of the studies of the effect of a sport drink on the outcome of labour were published by Kubli *et al.* in 2002 [32]. Sixty women in early labour (cervical dilatation less than 5 cm) were randomly allocated to either an 'isotonic sport drink' group ($N = 30$) or to a 'water-only (control)' group ($N = 30$). In this case, the oral sport drink used was Lucozade Sport™. Women in the sport drink group were permitted to consume up to 500 ml in the first hour and then a further 500 ml every 3–4 h. By the end of labour, plasma β-hydroxybutyrate and non-esterified fatty acids were significantly increased and the plasma glucose significantly decreased in the water-only group.

There was no difference between the two groups in duration of labour, mode of delivery or neonatal outcome.

There were no significant differences between the groups in gastric volume measured within 45 min of delivery, or in the volume vomited or number of vomiting episodes within 1 h of birth or throughout labour. The mean volume of liquid consumed in the sport drink group (925 ml) was significantly greater than in the water-only group (478 ml), implying active engagement with the study protocol. The mean calorific intake in the sport drink group was 47 kcal/h – it was zero in the water-only group.

Thus, isotonic sport drinks appear to prevent the ketosis of labour without the increase in gastric volumes and tendency to vomit sometimes seen in women who eat during labour. Despite these metabolic improvements, though, there were no significant differences in maternal or neonatal outcomes.

The second of the randomized controlled trials evaluating the effects of carbohydrate versus placebo were published by an active group of researchers on this subject in the Netherlands [33].

In the first of a number of studies published by this group, 201 consecutive nulliparous women in early labour (cervical dilatation 2–4 cm at entry) were randomized into one of two treatment groups. One group of women ($N = 99$) were randomized to the placebo arm of the study and received flavoured water. The other group ($N = 102$) received an isotonic carbohydrate solution containing 12.6 g carbohydrate per 100 ml. Both solutions had an identical taste and colour. All patients were permitted to drink at will, and no additional food or drinks were offered.

In contrast to studies cited above, a high proportion of women recruited to this study had high-risk pregnancies (80% of the carbohydrate and 82% for the placebo – not statistically significant), presumably because in the Netherlands women considered at low risk are delivered by independent midwives.

The median total intake of the study solution was 300 ml in the placebo group and 400 ml in the carbohydrate group (p value 0.04). The median total calorific intake during the study was 0 kJ in the placebo group and 802 kJ in the carbohydrate group (p value <0.001). There was no statistically significant difference in the percentage of those women who required augmentation or pain relief.

Although there was no significant difference between the carbohydrate and placebo groups for spontaneous births or for instrumental vaginal delivery, the CS rate for the carbohydrate group (21%) was significantly higher than that noted in the placebo group (7%). The reasons for the use of CS are listed in Table 7.1.

The low rate of CS in the placebo arm of the study is particularly surprising given that 82% of the women allocated to this treatment arm were regarded as 'high-

Table 7.1 Reasons for performing caesarean section

	Carbohydrate group	Placebo group [33]
Non-progressing labour	12	3
Fetal distress	4	2
Combination of factors	5	2

risk'. The authors postulated that the increase in CS for non-progress in the carbohydrate group was due to a redistribution of blood in favour of the gastrointestinal tract at the expense of the myometrium. This, in turn, might lead to less energy for uterine contractions.

There were no significant differences in neonatal outcome between the carbohydrate and placebo groups.

The apparent reduction in CS rates for women confined to water only is an unusual finding in the context of the other studies published and referred to above. The difference may have arisen from the small numbers of women recruited, and prompted the authors to recommend further studies before drawing any firm conclusions about the maternal and neonatal effects of carbohydrate administration to labouring women.

In the third randomized study, the effects of oral carbohydrate intake on fetal acid–base status were assessed in 100 nulliparous women who were randomized at 8–10 cm of dilatation [34]. All women were asked to drink 200 ml of either a carbohydrate solution (containing 25 g carbohydrate) or placebo. Subsequent analysis of the fetal arterial umbilical cord blood revealed identical pH and base excess in both groups.

The combined number of women recruited to these five studies is only approximately 3100, the majority of which were recruited to the O'Sullivan *et al.* study [30]. In summary, the pooled data identify no benefits or harms of restricting foods and fluids in women at low risk of needing a GA. The pooled data are underpowered to assess the incidence of Mendelson's syndrome, since this is such a rare outcome.

One study did report an increase in CS rates in women taking carbohydrate drinks in labour [33]. However, in a later publication assessing the metabolic consequences of carbohydrate supplements to 202 nulliparous women at 8–10 cm cervical dilatation, this same group of workers found a *lower* rate of CS in women allocated to the carbohydrate arm of a similar study [35].

In the absence of any compelling evidence of benefit or harm associated with restriction of fluids and food in women at low risk of complications, the most recent Cochrane review of this subject concluded that there is no justification for continuing to do so [31].

Finally, the evidence relating to the benefits (or otherwise) of eating and drinking in labour has recently been summarized by the authors of recently published national guidance on intrapartum care, published in December 2014 [36].

This guideline emphasizes the importance of attempting to promote normality in intrapartum care whenever appropriate. Low-risk multiparous women are advised that birth at home or in a midwifery-led unit is particularly suitable for them because obstetric intervention rates are lower and the outcome for the baby is comparable with birth in a consultant obstetric unit. Low-risk nulliparous women are advised that birth in a midwifery-led unit (freestanding or alongside a consultant obstetric unit) is particularly suitable for them for similar reasons.

This emphasis on maintaining normality includes a more liberal approach to eating and drinking in labour. For example, with particular reference to controlling gastric acidity, the NICE summary guidance makes the following recommendations:

- Do not offer either H_2-receptor antagonists or antacids routinely to low-risk women.
- Either H_2-receptor antagonists or antacids should be considered for women who receive opioids or who have or develop risk factors that make a GA more likely.
- Inform women that they may drink during established labour and that isotonic drinks may be more beneficial than water.
- Inform women that they may eat a light meal in established labour unless they have received opioids or develop risk factors that make a GA more likely.

None of these studies assessed women's views of feeding regimens in labour.

Patient Choice

There is a paucity of high-quality data exploring women's preferences with respect to eating and drinking in labour.

Even when oral intake is unrestricted, labouring patients do not always avail themselves of the opportunity to eat and drink. In the Tranmer *et al.* study [28], only 56% of those women in the intervention group

actually reported that they ate or drank in labour. Similarly, in the largest study of its kind published to date, O'Sullivan *et al.* note that 29% of women allocated to the eating group chose not to eat in labour [30].

In a study published in 1997, a multidisciplinary team comprising a research midwife, a consultant anaesthetist and a consultant obstetrician formulated a written policy in favour of oral intake in labour with an uncomplicated pregnancy [37]. A subsequent audit of 250 low-risk primiparous women reported that 40% said they felt hungry at some point in labour, and 92% felt thirsty. Approximately 68% of women questioned drank water only while in labour in hospital and many stated this was all they wanted, although the actual number was not reported. The main reason why oral intake was restricted from eating and drinking to fluids only was the use of regional analgesia or Entonox – as per the departmental protocol. The study also reported that a 'considerable number' of women questioned did not eat while they were in labour in hospital, usually because they did not feel like eating. However, many appreciated the option of eating and drinking, even if few chose to do so.

In a Scottish study published in 2000, 149 postnatal women were invited to complete an audit questionnaire within 36 hours of delivery that incorporated questions on their oral intake in labour [38]. Only a minority of women questioned (30%) said that they would wish to eat during their labour, generally in the early stages. When the 'food' and 'no food' groups were compared, there were no statistical differences in the duration of labour, choice of analgesia or mode of delivery.

So while a desire to eat in early labour may be common, on the basis of what little information is currently available, it would appear that many women do not usually wish to eat – or even drink – once they are in the active phase of labour, and it may be inappropriate to encourage them do so.

Conclusion

The NBM policy of starvation in labour was introduced over 50 years ago in order to prevent maternal morbidity and mortality from pulmonary aspiration of gastric contents (Mendelson's syndrome) in those labouring women who required a GA.

The maternal mortality and morbidity due to the pulmonary aspiration of gastric contents is now so rare in Western obstetric practice as to make the NBM policy questionable for low-risk women in normal labour.

The randomized controlled studies that have been published have recruited relatively few patients, but based on these data there seems little justification for restricting food and fluids to labouring women considered at low risk of complications.

Carbohydrate-based isotonic sport drinks containing calories consumed in labour also appear to reduce markers of 'starvation' in labour, while preventing the significant fall in plasma glucose levels seen in the water-only group. Gastric volumes, incidence and volume of vomiting were comparable to the water-only group, and there were no significant differences between the groups in maternal or neonatal outcomes.

The use of carbohydrate solutions in labour appears to have little effect on neonatal outcome when compared to placebo-treated women. Similarly, there appears to be no difference in rates of spontaneous birth and instrumental vaginal delivery rates. There appears to be conflicting evidence about the effect of drinking carbohydrate solutions in labour on the risk of subsequently requiring a CS.

It is reasonable to inform low-risk women that they may drink during established labour and that isotonic drinks may be more beneficial than water. Furthermore, women can be advised that they may eat a light meal in established labour unless they have received opioids or develop risk factors that make a GA more likely.

There are no studies of women at increased risk of potentially needing a GA. Nonetheless, for those women at high risk of obstetric intervention, it would seem prudent to avoid solids and semi-solids and patients should probably be advised to restrict their intake to isotonic drinks.

Finally, there is some evidence that even when given the choice, only a minority of labouring women actually wish to eat in labour, particularly near to delivery. Ultimately, the matter of what to drink and eat in labour must be a matter of patient choice. Information should be made widely available to allow women to make an informed choice.

References

1. Mendelson CL. The aspiration of stomach contents into the lungs during obstetric anesthesia. *Am J Obstet Gynecol*. 1946; 52: 191–205.

2. Department of Health, Welsh Office, Scottish Office Department of Health and Department of Health and Social Services, Northern Ireland. *Why Mothers Die: Report on Confidential Enquiries into Maternal Deaths in the United Kingdom, 1994–1996*. London: The Stationary Office; 1998.

3. Department of Health, Welsh Office, Scottish Office Department of Health and Department of Health and Social Services, Northern Ireland. *Why Mothers Die: Report on Confidential Enquiries into Maternal Deaths in the United Kingdom, 1997–1999*. London: RCOG Press; 2001.

4. Lewis G (ed.). *The Confidential Enquiry into Maternal and Child Health (CEMACH): Why Mothers Die 2000–2002. The Sixth Report on Confidential Enquiries into Maternal Deaths in the United Kingdom*. London: RCOG Press; 2004.

5. Lewis G (ed.). *The Confidential Enquiry into Maternal and Child Health (CEMACH). Saving Mothers' Lives: Reviewing Maternal Deaths to Make Motherhood Safer – 2003–2005. The Seventh Report on Confidential Enquiries into Maternal Deaths in the United Kingdom*. London: CEMACH; 2007.

6. Lewis G (ed.). *The Confidential Enquiry into Maternal and Child Health (CEMACH). Saving Mothers' Lives: Reviewing Maternal Deaths to Make Motherhood Safer – 2006–2008. The Eighth Report on Confidential Enquiries into Maternal Deaths in the United Kingdom*. London: CEMACH; 2011.

7. Knight M, Kenyon S, Brocklehurst P, *et al.* (eds). *Saving Lives, Improving Mothers' Care: Lessons Learned to Inform Future Maternity Care from the UK and Ireland Confidential Enquiries into Maternal Deaths and Morbidity 2009–12*. Oxford: National Perinatal Epidemiology Unit, University of Oxford; 2014.

8. Michael S, Reilly CS, Caunt JA. Policies for oral intake during labour: a survey of maternity units in England and Wales. *Anaesthesia*. 1991; 46: 1071–3.

9. Scheepers HCJ, Essed GGM, Brouns F. Aspects of food and fluid intake during labour: policies of midwives and obstetricians in the Netherlands. *Eur J Obstet Gynecol Reprod Biol*. 1998; 78: 37–40.

10. Hawkins J, Gibbs CP, Martin-Salvaj G, *et al.* Oral intake policies on labor and delivery: a national survey. *J Clin Anesthesia*. 1998; 10: 449–51.

11. American Society of Anesthesiologists. Practice guidelines for obstetric anesthesia. *Anesthesiology*. 2007; 106(4): 843–63.

12. American College of Obstetricians and Gynecologists. Committee opinion no. 441. *Obstet Gynecol*. 2009; 114: 714.

13. Centre for Maternal and Child Enquiries (CMACE). *Maternal Obesity in the UK: Findings from a National Project*. London: CMACE; 2010.

14. Davison JS, Davison MC, Hay DM. Gastric emptying time in late pregnancy and labour. *J Obstet Gynaecol Br Commonw*. 1970; 77: 37–41.

15. Nimmo WS, Wilson J, Prescott LF. Narcotic analgesics and delayed gastric emptying during labour. *Lancet*. 1975; I: 890–3.

16. Tuckey JP, Prout RE, Wee MY. Prescribing intramuscular opioids for labour analgesia in consultant-led maternity units: a survey of UK practice. *Int J Obstet Anesth*. 2007; 17: 3–8.

17. Chadwick HS. Obstetric anesthesia: then and now. *Minerva Anestiol*. 2005; 71(9): 517–20.

18. Hodges RJ, Bennett JR, Tunstall ME, Knight RF. General anaesthesia for operative obstetrics: with special reference to the use of thiopentone and suxamethonium. *Br J Anaesth*. 1959; 31: 152–63.

19. Sellick BA. Cricoid pressure to control regurgitation of stomach contents during induction of anaesthesia. *Lancet*. 1961; 2(7199): 404–6.

20. Levy DM. Traditional rapid sequence induction is an outmoded technique for caesarean section and should be modified: proposed. *Int J Obstet Anesth*. 2006; 15(3): 227–9.

21. Brown GW, Russell IF. A survey of anesthesia for caesarean section. *Int J Obstet Anesth*. 1995; 4(4): 214–18.

22. Obstetric Anaesthetists' Association. National obstetric anaesthesia data 2011; 2011. www.oaa-anaes. ac.uk/assets/_managed/editor/File/NOAD/NOAD %202011%20final.pdf (accessed 12 May 2016).

23. Gyte GML, Richens Y. Routine prophylactic drugs in normal labour for reducing gastric acid aspiration and its effects. *Cochrane Database Syst Rev*. 2006; 3. CD005298. doi: 10.1002/146551858.CD005298.pub2.

24. Ullmann R, Smith LA, Burns E, Mori R, Dowswell T. Parenteral opioids for maternal pain management in labour. *Cochrane Database Syst Rev*. 2010; 9. CD007396. doi: 10.1002/146551858.CD007396.pub2.

25. Porter JS, Bonello E, Reynolds F. The influence of epidural administration of fentanyl infusion on gastric emptying in labour. *Anesthesia*. 1997; 52: 1151–6.

26. Metzger BE, Ravnikar V, Vileisis RA, Freinkel N. 'Accelerated starvation' and the skipped breakfast in late normal pregnancy. *Lancet*. 1982; I: 588–92.

27. Lawrence GF, Brown VA, Parsons RJ, Cooke ID. Feto-maternal consequences of high-dose glucose infusion during labour. *Br J Obstet Gynaecol*. 1982; 89: 27–32.

28. Tranmer JE, Hodnett ED, Hannah ME, Stevens BJ. The effect of unrestricted oral carbohydrate intake on labor progress. *J Obstet Gynecol Neonatal Nurs*. 2005; 34: 319–28.

29. Scrutton MJ, Metcalfe GA, Lowy C, Seed PT, O'Sullivan G. Eating in labour: a randomised controlled trial assessing risks and benefits. *Anaesthesia*. 1999; 54: 329–34.

30. O'Sullivan G, Liu B, Hart D, Seed P, Shennan A. Effect of food intake during labour on obstetric outcome: randomised controlled trial. *BMJ*. 2009; 338: b784.

31. Singata M, Tranmer J, Gyte GML. Restricting oral fluid and food intake during labour. *Cochrane Database Syst Rev*. 2013; 8. CD003930. doi: 10.1002/146551858. CD003930.pub3.

32. Kubli M, Scrutton MJ, Seed PT. An evaluation of isotonic 'sport drinks' during labour. *Anesth Analg*. 2002; 94: 404–8.

33. Scheepers HCJ, Thans MCJ, de Jong PA, *et al*. A double-blind, randomised, placebo controlled study on the influence of carbohydrate solution intake during labour. *Br J Obstet Gynaecol*. 2002; 109: 178–81.

34. Scheepers HC, Thans MC, de Jong PA, Essed GG, Kanhai HH. The effects of oral carbohydrate administration on fetal acid base balance. *J Perinat Med*. 2002; 30(5): 400–4.

35. Scheepers HCJ, de Jong PA, Essed GGM, Kanhai HHH. Carbohydrate solution intake during labour just before the start of the second stage: a double-blind study on metabolic effects and clinical outcome. *Br J Obstet Gynaecol*. 2004; 111: 1382–7.

36. National Institute for Health and Care Excellence. *Intrapartum Care: Care of Healthy Women and their Babies during Childbirth*: NICE Clinical Guideline 190. London: NICE; 2014.

37. Newton C, Champion P. Oral intake in labour: Nottingham's policy formulated and audited. *Br J Midwif*. 1997; 5: 418–22.

38. Armstrong TS, Johnston IG. Which women want food during labour? Results of an audit in a Scottish DGH. *Health Bulletin*. 2000; 58: 141–4.

Chapter

8

Prolonged Second Stage of Labour Including Difficult Decision Making on Operative Vaginal Delivery and Caesarean Section

Deirdre J. Murphy

Introduction

The second stage of labour is an important element of the natural process of childbirth. From the perspective of the mother, her partner and the midwife it is often seen as the climax of the birth process, and from the perspective of the obstetrician it is the period of increased risk. The second stage begins with full dilatation of the cervix and ends with birth of the baby. It is difficult to ascertain exactly when full dilatation of the cervix has occurred, as it is an event in the continuum of the labour process. It is diagnosed by either routine vaginal examination during labour or when the patient reports experiencing the sensation to bear down, or when the presenting part is visible. The definition of prolonged second stage of labour is controversial and has changed over time with use of regional analgesia.

The second stage of labour has two phases:

1. A passive phase that begins with full dilatation of the cervix and ends when bearing down efforts begin.
2. An active phase when the mother feels the sensation of bearing down due to pressure of the presenting part on the rectum and pelvic floor musculature, and active maternal pushing occurs.

The desired outcome following effective management of the second stage of labour is safe delivery of a healthy infant to a mother who has had a rewarding experience retaining both physical and psychological well-being. The ideal management of the second stage of labour is where spontaneous vaginal birth is facilitated without use of instruments or additional procedures. This should be possible in most cases. There are,

however, difficult decisions to be made in cases that deviate from normal. The optimal approach in these circumstances is one where the midwife and obstetrician work together (with the anaesthetist and neonatal specialist if required) in supporting a woman through appropriate intervention including episiotomy, operative vaginal delivery or caesarean section (CS).

Duration of the Second Stage of Labour

It is perhaps surprising that there is no single accepted definition of an appropriate duration for the second stage of labour. The approach in recent years has been to manage the second stage of labour expectantly for as long as possible so that the woman can achieve a spontaneous vaginal birth, particularly with epidural anaesthesia. Guidelines differentiate between nulliparous and parous low-risk women but limited guidance is available for high-risk women, including women with a prior CS, or medical or obstetrical complications. The American College of Obstetricians and Gynecologists (ACOG) define the normal limits for the second stage of labour without regional anaesthesia as 2 h for nulliparous women and 1 h for multiparous women [1]. When a woman is given regional anaesthesia, an extra hour is added in both cases. The 'green-top' guideline of the Royal College of Obstetricians and Gynaecologists (RCOG) [2] describe a prolonged second stage as lack of continuous progress for three hours with regional anaesthesia or two hours without regional anaesthesia in nulliparous women. In multiparous women, prolonged second stage is no progress for two hours with, or one hour without, regional anaesthesia. The RCOG guideline emphasizes that the durations stated are a combined total of both active

Best Practice in Labour and Delivery, Second Edition, ed. Sir Sabaratnam Arulkumaran. Published by Cambridge University Press. © Cambridge University Press 2016.

and passive phases of the second stage. The National Institute for Health and Care Excellence (NICE) guideline on intrapartum care allows longer intervals of active second stage to achieve spontaneous vaginal birth as follows [3]:

- Nulliparous women:
  - birth would be expected to take place within three hours of the start of the active second stage in most women;
  - a diagnosis of delay in the active second stage should be made when it has lasted two hours and women should be referred to a healthcare professional trained to undertake an operative vaginal birth if birth is not imminent.

- Parous women:
  - birth would be expected to take place within two hours of the start of the active second stage in most women;
  - a diagnosis of delay in the active second stage should be made when it has lasted one hour and women should be referred to a healthcare professional trained to undertake an operative vaginal birth if birth is not imminent.

With the original NICE criteria (2007) it would be considered acceptable for the second stage of labour to last a total of five hours for a nulliparous woman with an epidural, where up to two hours are allowed for passive descent and three hours for the active phase. The risks of intervention in the second stage of labour because an arbitrary time limit has been exceeded must be balanced with the risks of an adverse outcome for the mother or her baby as a result of a prolonged second stage of labour. The updated guideline (2014) reflects this with a suggested upper limit of four hours for women of all parities [3]:

- After diagnosis of full dilatation in a woman with regional analgesia, agree a plan with the woman in order to ensure that birth will have occurred within four hours regardless of parity.

Outcomes of Prolonged Second Stage of Labour

Undue prolongation of the second stage of labour can result potentially in maternal and/or fetal compromise, although the published data are far from consistent. A large US cross-sectional study ($n = 15\,759$)

investigated the relationship between prolonged duration of the second stage (defined as more than four hours) and morbidity outcomes in nulliparous women [4]. Logistic regression analyses, controlling for various confounders, showed that there was evidence of an association between a prolonged second stage of labour and an increased incidence of chorioamnionitis (OR 1.79 [95% CI 1.44–2.22]), third- or fourth-degree lacerations (OR 1.33 [95% CI 1.07–1.67]), caesarean section (OR 5.65 [95% CI 4.46–7.16] and operative vaginal birth (OR 2.83 [95% CI 2.38–3.36]). There was no evidence of an association between prolonged second stage of labour and endomyometritis (OR 0.79 [95% CI 0.49–1.26]), postpartum haemorrhage (PPH) (OR 1.05 [95% CI 0.84–1.31]), meconium-stained liquor (OR 1.11 [95% CI 0.93–1.33]) or admission to the neonatal unit (OR 0.59 [95% CI 0.35–1.03]). In a study of 5158 women, the same authors concluded that multiparous women with a second stage of three hours or greater have an increased risk of operative delivery, peripartum morbidity, five minute Apgar score less than 7, fetal acidosis (umbilical artery pH <7.0, base excess (BE) <−12) and admission to neonatal intensive care unit [5].

Similarly, a population-based cohort study of 121 517 women in Canada reported an increase in risk of maternal obstetric trauma, PPH, puerperal febrile morbidity, low five minute Apgar score, birth depression and admission to the neonatal intensive care unit among both nulliparous and multiparous women, with increasing duration of the second stage of labour. Risks of both maternal and perinatal adverse outcomes rose with increased duration of the second stage, particularly for durations longer than three hours in nulliparous women and longer than two hours in multiparous women [6]. A large UK cross-sectional study ($n = 25\,069$) investigated prolonged second stage of labour and perinatal outcomes [7]. Logistic regression analysis showed that there was evidence of a dose-response association between a longer duration and a higher rate of PPH (durations: 120–179 min OR 1.6 [95% CI 1.3–1.9]; 180–239 min OR 1.7 [95% CI 1.3–2.3]; 240+ min OR 1.9 [95% CI 1.2–2.8]. A UK prospective cohort study of complex operative deliveries conducted at full dilatation in an operating theatre ($n = 393$) reported that a prolonged second stage of greater than three hours was associated with an increased risk of extended uterine incision at failed instrumental delivery (adjusted OR 4.1 [95% CI 1.1–16.5]) [8].

There is no clear consensus on the optimal duration of the second stage of labour, and the research addressing this question is currently limited. The well-recognized association between operative vaginal delivery and pelvic floor trauma confounds the relationship between prolonged second stage of labour and pelvic floor morbidity. The question of 'how long is too long' needs to be addressed, ideally by prospective randomized studies with both short- and long-term outcomes. Against this is the need to individualize care in the context of the needs and wishes of the woman, with appropriate attention given to the fetal status and its ability to tolerate the stress of prolonged pushing. The ACOG practice bulletin and the RCOG guideline both emphasize the need to individualize care for the specific circumstances, stating that 'the length of the second stage of labour is not in itself an absolute or even strong indication for operative termination of labour' [1], and that 'the question of when to intervene should involve balancing the risks and benefits of continuing pushing as against operative delivery' [2]. However, the potential for maternal or perinatal adverse outcomes is reflected in the NICE guideline recommendation that 'following initial obstetric assessment for women with delay in the second stage of labour, ongoing obstetric review should be maintained every 15–30 minutes' [3]. The practical implications for an obstetrician of being available for regular reviews at close intervals needs to be considered in the context of busy maternity units and competing demands on their time.

Causes of Prolonged Second Stage of Labour

At a physiological level, prolonged second stage of labour can be considered in terms of deviations from normal of the powers, passages or passenger (the 3 Ps), or a combination of these factors. The powers reflect maternal uterine activity and maternal effort when actively pushing. Various factors influence the powers, including support and encouragement, rate, rhythm, duration and strength of contractions, maternal position when pushing and degree of motor and sensory blockage with analgesia or anaesthesia. The bony pelvis (passages) is pre-determined in terms of maximum dimensions; however, repositioning of the mother may optimize the available diameters at the pelvic outlet. Occasionally, a cervical fibroid, ovarian cyst or placental tissue may obstruct the passages, although this is usually apparent long before the second stage of labour. More commonly there may be resistance in the pelvic floor musculature and perineal tissues of a nulliparous woman, or a multiparous woman may have extensive perineal scarring.

The passenger (the baby) may be too large for the woman (cephalo-pelvic disproportion, CPD) or may descend into the pelvis with an abnormal presentation (brow or face), abnormal position (occipito-posterior or occipito-transverse), or may fail to rotate and flex fully, resulting in asynclitism and deflexion. Most fetuses orientate with a cephalic vertex presentation because of the pelvic shape. In labour, 80–90% of vertex presentations become occipito-anterior (OA) position. Of the remaining 10–20%, almost 90% will become occipito-anterior with progress of labour. Persistent occipito-posterior position (POP) can occur in 2–5% of cases. This results in a larger head diameter being presented, resulting in poor progress in both first and second stages of labour. Any presentation other than vertex is defined as a malpresentation. The various types are breech, face, brow, shoulder and cord presentation. Vaginal breech delivery is addressed separately. Shoulder presentation could result in prolapse of the arm and obstructed labour, and therefore requires delivery by CS. If the umbilical cord presents at the cervix and the membranes are intact, it is a cord presentation. This should be delivered by CS, otherwise cord prolapse will occur after rupture of the membranes. Face presentation is diagnosed by palpation of the orbital ridges, nose, mouth and chin. A mento-anterior position can deliver vaginally due to presenting diameters similar to vertex OA. If the face is in a mento-posterior position, the presenting diameter will be larger than the pelvis and vaginal delivery is not possible. The safe option in this case is CS. A deflexed head causes a brow presentation. If the head becomes flexed due to the mechanics of labour, a brow presentation can become vertex. On the other hand, if further deflexion occurs, brow presentation becomes a face presentation. Persistent brow needs to be delivered by CS.

In general terms, assessment of progress should include observation by the midwife of maternal behaviour, effectiveness of pushing and fetal well-being, taking into account the fetal position and station at the onset of the second stage. These factors will assist in deciding the timing of further vaginal examinations and the need for obstetric review.

Epidural Anaesthesia and Prolonged Second Stage of Labour

Epidural anaesthesia may contribute to the likelihood of a prolonged second stage of labour and subsequent intervention, but equally it may have a role to play in the successful management of prolonged second stage of labour.

An updated Cochrane systematic review of epidural anaesthesia in labour concluded that epidural anaesthesia provides significantly better, safer and effective pain relief than non-epidural techniques [9]. It is the method of choice for many women, particularly nulliparous women. A systematic review of the effects of epidural analgesia on labour, maternal and neonatal outcomes was performed with a meta-analysis of 38 randomized controlled trials (RCTs) involving 9658 women. The following observations were made:

- Epidural analgesia was found to offer better pain relief (mean difference (MD) −3.36, [95% CI −5.41 to −1.31], three trials, 1166 women) and a reduction in the need for additional pain relief (risk ratio (RR) 0.05 [95% CI 0.02–0.17], 15 trials, 6019 women).
- Epidural was associated with prolongation of the second stage and more frequent oxytocin augmentation. The duration of the second stage was increased by an average of 14 min in the epidural group.
- The total operative vaginal delivery rate was higher for epidural (23 trials, $n = 7935$, OR 1.42 [95% CI 1.28–1.57]).
- There was an increased risk of CS for fetal distress (RR 1.43 [95% CI 1.03–1.97], 11 trials, 4816 women) but no evidence of a significant difference in the risk of CS overall (RR 1.10 [95% CI 0.97–1.25], 27 trials, 8417 women).

Certain side-effects are specifically associated with epidural anaesthesia, including itching, shivering, maternal pyrexia >38 °C and urinary retention, hypotension (affecting fetal heart rate (FHR)), headache due to accidental dural puncture and, rarely, respiratory arrest. Some interventions can be avoided if the woman does not have an epidural – these include intravenous lines, intravenous fluids, bladder catheterization and continuous electronic fetal monitoring.

However, the corollary is that epidural anaesthesia provides safe and effective anaesthesia in the second stage of labour for interventions such as labour augmentation, episiotomy, operative vaginal delivery and emergency CS. The NICE intrapartum care guideline specifically recommends effective anaesthesia in these circumstances [3]:

- Consideration should be given to the use of oxytocin, with the offer of regional analgesia, for nulliparous women if contractions are inadequate at the onset of the second stage.
- Tested effective analgesia should be provided prior to carrying out an episiotomy, except in an emergency due to acute fetal compromise.
- Instrumental birth is an operative procedure that should be undertaken with tested effective anaesthesia.

When effective epidural analgesia has been achieved it should not be discontinued. There is insufficient evidence to support the hypothesis that discontinuing epidural analgesia reduces the incidence of operative vaginal delivery (23% vs. 28%; RR 0.84 [95% CI 0.61–1.15]), but there is evidence that it increases women's pain (22% vs. 6%; RR 3.68 [95% CI 1.99–6.80]) [9].

How to Avoid Prolonged Second Stage of Labour

There are several approaches that may help a woman achieve a spontaneous vaginal birth within the limits set for a normal duration for the second stage of labour and thereby avoid operative vaginal delivery (OVD) or CS. First line measures include support, change of position, emptying of the bladder and encouragement.

Support in Labour

There is evidence to show that continuous support for women during childbirth can reduce the incidence of OVD, particularly when the carer is not a member of staff (22 trials; $n = 15\ 288$) [10]. Women allocated to continuous support had shorter labours (MD −0.58 hours [95% CI −0.85 to −0.31]) and were less likely to have a CS (RR 0.78 [95% CI 0.67–0.91]) or instrumental vaginal birth (fixed-effect, RR 0.90 [95% CI 0.85–0.96]). All women should be encouraged to have continuous support during labour.

Women's Position in the Second Stage of Labour

The position or positions a woman adopts in the second stage of labour may have an important impact on the duration of the second stage and the need for operative intervention. The NICE intrapartum care guideline and the RCOG guideline reflect this in the following recommendation:

> Women should be discouraged from lying supine or semi-supine in the second stage of labour and should be encouraged to adopt any other position that they find most comfortable.

A systematic review has assessed the benefits and risks of the use of different positions during the second stage of labour [11]. The review included 19 trials involving 5764 women. The use of any upright or lateral position compared with supine or lithotomy was associated with reduced duration of the second stage of labour: weighted mean reduction duration 16.9 min [95% CI 14.3–19.5 min]; a reduction in assisted births: RR 0.84 [95% CI 0.73–0.98]; and a reduction in episiotomies RR 0.84 [95% CI 0.79–0.91]. A large RCT is in progress evaluating alternative positions in the second stage of labour for women with epidural analgesia.

Pushing in the Second Stage of Labour

When and how a woman is encouraged to push requires consideration and is summarized in the following NICE recommendations:

- Women should be informed that in the second stage they should be guided by their own urge to push.
- Upon confirmation of full cervical dilatation in a woman with regional analgesia, unless the woman has an urge to push or the baby's head is visible, pushing should be delayed for at least one hour and longer if the woman wishes, after which actively encourage her to push during contractions.

A meta-analysis demonstrated that nulliparous women with epidurals were likely to have fewer rotational or mid-cavity operative interventions when pushing was delayed for 1–2 hours or until they had a strong urge to push [12]. Allowing passive descent and rotation is recommended where the fetal status is satisfactory.

Two US RCTs of good quality have compared coached with uncoached pushing in the second stage of labour [13,14]. The mean duration of the second stage of labour was significantly shorter for women in the coached group compared with the uncoached group (46 min vs. 59 min, $p = 0.014$) [13]. There were no differences noted in any other maternal or neonatal outcomes in either trial. There is therefore no high-level evidence that directed pushing affects outcomes other than the duration of the second stage of labour.

Oxytocin Augmentation

Consideration should be given to the use of oxytocin, with the offer of regional analgesia, for nulliparous women if contractions are inadequate at the onset of the second stage [3]. However, caution is required, particularly for multiparous women. While it may be desirable to augment the uterine contractions with the use of oxytocin, clearly this should not be contemplated where uterine activity is already optimal and if CPD or obstructed labour is suspected.

Role of Episiotomy in Prolonged Second Stage of Labour

Episiotomy can be used to facilitate delivery if there is a clinical need, such as for OVD or suspected fetal compromise (e.g. fetal bradycardia), or where the perineum is very tight and impeding delivery despite good maternal effort. However, it should be limited to specific clinical indications and not employed routinely. This is reflected in guideline recommendations [3]:

- A routine episiotomy should not be carried out during spontaneous vaginal birth.
- An episiotomy should be performed if there is a clinical need, such as instrumental birth or suspected fetal compromise.
- Where an episiotomy is performed, the recommended technique is a mediolateral episiotomy originating at the vaginal fourchette and usually directed to the right side. The angle to the vertical axis should be between 45 and 60 degrees at the time of the episiotomy.
- Tested effective analgesia should be provided prior to carrying out an episiotomy, except in an emergency due to acute fetal compromise.

A Cochrane review of eight randomized trials involving 5541 women found that as compared to routine use (75%), restrictive episiotomy use (28%) was more beneficial as it was associated with less posterior perineal trauma, less need for suturing and fewer healing complications [15]. On the other hand, it was associated with more anterior perineal trauma and there was no difference in severe vaginal or perineal trauma, dyspareunia, urinary incontinence or severe pain. The evidence overall was in favour of a restrictive approach to episiotomy.

Operative Delivery in the Second Stage of Labour

Episiotomy is only likely to be effective when the presenting part is distending the perineum and close to crowning. When delay occurs in the second stage of labour prior to this, the choice is between OVD and CS.

Assessment Prior to Operative Delivery

The vast majority of avoidable maternal and neonatal morbidity at OVD relates to inappropriate application of the instrument and operator inexperience [2]. Therefore an essential prerequisite for OVD is a skilled operator. The obstetrician must be able to assess the bony pelvis and unequivocally determine the fetal position and station, as well as any degree of flexion, caput, moulding and asynclitism [16,17]. The instrument must then be correctly placed and an appropriate amount of traction applied in the right direction. In such circumstances, successful operative vaginal delivery rates are high and morbidity low. However, these skills are not easy to acquire, and certainly cannot be self-taught. In addition, the trainee obstetrician must know when to ask for help. Predictors of failed operative vaginal delivery include occipito-posterior position, high presenting part (station spines +0), inadequate analgesia and birth weight >4000 g, and these criteria should alert the obstetrician to be cautious and seek senior support [18–20].

In a survey conducted in the UK and Ireland, obstetricians of all grades reported occasional difficulty in assessing the station and position of the presenting part [21]. Errors in defining the position were reported by both trainees and experts in up to 10% of deliveries. An ultrasound assessment in order to confirm the fetal head position prior to OVD has been shown to be feasible and acceptable to women and the health professionals caring for them [22]. A subsequent RCT ($n = 514$) was conducted to evaluate whether an ultrasound scan prior to OVD could improve the accuracy of diagnosis of the fetal head position in a routine clinical setting [23]. The ultrasound assessment reduced the incidence of incorrect diagnosis of the fetal head position (4/257, 1.6% versus 52/257, 20.2%, odds ratio 0.06 [95% CI 0.02–0.19], p value <0.001) without delaying delivery but did not reduce morbidity. This suggests that while ultrasound is very accurate in defining the fetal head position, a more integrated clinical skills-based approach is likely to be required to prevent adverse outcomes at instrumental delivery.

The RCOG has recommended that obstetricians be confident and competent in the use of both vacuum and forceps, and that operators should choose the instrument most appropriate to the clinical circumstances and their level of skill [2]. This reflects the need in up to 20% of vacuum extractions to complete the delivery by forceps, and the absolute and relative contraindications of the different instruments. Clear and detailed guidelines are available and should be adapted within local practice-based protocols and followed up with regular audit and multidisciplinary review of adverse incidents. A UK study demonstrated substantial differences between consultant assessment regarding fetal position and station compared with specialist registrars, and that the consultant was more likely to reverse a decision for CS and safely conduct an OVD [24]. Clearly, appropriate supervision and the availability of skilled obstetricians on the labour ward at all times will be an essential component of training initiatives. Simulation-based training has a role to play, as do training courses specifically dedicated to acquiring the skill of OVD [16].

The following minimum prerequisites must be fulfilled when assessing a woman before attempting an OVD:

- no more than one-fifth of the head should be palpable on abdominal palpation;
- cervix fully dilated and membranes ruptured;
- station at the level of ischial spines or below;
- exact position of the fetal head should be determined;
- excessive caput or moulding should not be present;

Table 8.1 Choice of instrument for OVD [17]

Non rotational low-cavity delivery	Mid-cavity delivery +/− rotation
Favour vacuum if: No working epidural Good expulsive efforts Good contractions No marked caput/moulding Birth canal is roomy	Having judged that attempting OVD is suitable, the following factors influence the selection of a particular method
	Select manual rotation and traction forceps if: Good analgesia Rotational movement is possible Descent of fetal head with maternal effort Birth canal is roomy Absence of signs of true CPD
Favour forceps if: Dense epidural block No good expulsive efforts Contractions not good Marked caput/moulding Birth canal is not roomy	
	Select Kielland's if: Dense regional block Descent of fetal head with maternal effort Birth canal is roomy Absence of signs of true CPD
	Select vacuum (with metal cup or Kiwi Omnicup) if: No dense regional block Good maternal effort Descent of fetal head with maternal effort No significant caput/moulding No signs of true CPD

Notes

1. A method should only be used if the operator is adequately trained. The operator should use the instrument he or she prefers.
2. The mother's preferences should be taken into account where appropriate.
3. Vacuum delivery is contraindicated at gestational age <34 weeks and face presentation.
4. Fetal status in itself should not determine the choice of instrument. There is no evidence that one instrument leads to quicker delivery than another.

- there should be noticeable descent of head with uterine contraction and bearing down efforts; and
- pelvis is deemed adequate.

Vacuum vs. Forceps

The choice between forceps or vacuum delivery will depend on the clinical circumstances and on the operator's competence and preference [2]. Forceps delivery may be preferred in instances where there is diminished maternal effort (e.g. maternal exhaustion, dense epidural block, general anaesthesia), for preterm deliveries (<34 weeks' gestation), after a failed vacuum extraction and for low-cavity deliveries with suspected fetal thrombocytopenia. A vacuum delivery may be preferred for outlet deliveries and for rotational deliveries with limited analgesia. A qualitative study explored the decision making of expert obstetricians and the criteria they use when choosing between instruments (see Table 8.1) [17].

There have been no recent RCTs comparing vacuum and forceps, but a systematic review of existing RCTs reported that use of the vacuum extractor was associated with significantly less maternal trauma (OR 0.41 [95% CI 0.33–0.50]), and this is one of its main advantages. It also reported that vacuum was associated with more completed deliveries (OR 1.69 [95% CI 1.31–2.19]) than forceps delivery [25]. However, this is potentially misleading, as attempted vacuum delivery has a higher failure rate than forceps as a first line instrument, with failed vacuum deliveries frequently completed by forceps. Vacuum failure rates of between 20% and 30% have been reported in two RCTs comparing different vacuum devices, with higher failure rates for the handheld disposable vacuum device [26,27]. Failure of vacuum delivery is three to four times more likely with a fetal malposition. An updated Cochrane review places a greater emphasis on choosing an appropriate instrument based on differing risks and benefits [28]. In a prospective cohort study of women with complex deliveries transferred to theatre for arrested progress in the second stage of labour, attempted forceps was more likely to result in completed vaginal delivery than attempted vacuum (63% vs. 48%, $p < 0.01$) [18].

Operative vaginal delivery is associated with increased pelvic floor morbidity. Forceps delivery incurred a higher risk of third-degree laceration than vacuum in two population-based studies (OR 1.94 [95% CI 1.30–2.89] and OR 3.33 [95% CI 2.97–3.74], respectively) [29,30]. In a randomized trial assessing anal sphincter function, symptoms of altered faecal continence were significantly more common following forceps delivery than vacuum [31]. More reassuringly, there was no difference in rates of urinary and bowel dysfunction at five-year follow-up of a previous randomized controlled study comparing forceps and vacuum delivery [32].

The neonatal outcome is critical to the debate on the role of OVD in modern obstetric practice and on the choice of instrument. The operator's expertise may ultimately determine the preferred mode of delivery, but each obstetrician should have the necessary skills to deliver the baby by the safest means according to the degree of fetal urgency. The neonatal morbidity related to operative delivery needs to be evaluated where OVD is successfully achieved, where a failed attempt at OVD results in CS, and where delivery is by immediate CS. In a systematic review of trials comparing vacuum extraction with forceps delivery, the use of the vacuum extractor was associated with an increase in neonatal cephalhaematoma and retinal haemorrhages, whereas forceps delivery was associated with an increase in facial palsy [25]. If speed is of the essence, particularly in the presence of suspected fetal hypoxia, then there is a higher chance of completed OVD with forceps as a single instrument than vacuum, thereby avoiding the risks of sequential use of instruments [33]. However, a population-based cohort study in Scotland ($n = 1021$) reported no difference between the decision-to-delivery intervals (DDIs) for forceps and vacuum deliveries but a 15 min difference between the DDIs for deliveries completed in a labour room compared to those requiring transfer to an operating theatre [34]. Different types of morbidity occur with vacuum and forceps and in all cases a backup plan needs to be in place in the event of abandoning or failing an attempted OVD [2].

In situations where the baby is born in poor condition, fears about early morbidity are quickly replaced by concerns about survival and long-term neurological disability. A large Australian population-based study reported an increased risk of neonatal encephalopathy following both OVD and emergency CS (OR 2.3 [95% CI 1.2–4.7] and OR 2.2 [95% CI 1.0–4.6], respectively) [35]. Moderate and severe neonatal encephalopathy are strongly associated with cerebral palsy and death. The use of sequential instruments, particularly vac-

Table 8.2 Vacuum extraction compared to forceps assisted delivery [2,25]

Vacuum compared to forceps is:	
More likely to fail at achieving vaginal delivery	OR 1.7; 95% CI 1.3–2.2
More likely to be associated with cephalhaematoma	OR 2.4; 95% CI 1.7–3.4
More likely to be associated with retinal haemorrhage	OR 2.0; 95% CI 1.3–3.0
More likely to be associated with maternal worries about baby	OR 2.2; 95% CI 1.2–3.9
Less likely to be associated with significant maternal perineal and vaginal trauma	OR 0.4; 95% CI 0.3–0.5
No more likely to be associated with delivery by caesarean section	OR 0.6; 95% CI 0.3–1.0
No more likely to be associated with low five minute Apgar scores	OR 1.7; 95% CI 1.0–2.8
No more likely to be associated with the need for phototherapy	OR 1.1; 95% CI 0.7–1.8

uum and forceps, has been associated with scalp trauma, intracranial haemorrhage and neonatal death [33]. Reassuringly, a five-year follow-up of the UK second stage prospective cohort study reported low overall rates of neurodevelopmental morbidity with comparable outcomes for each mode of delivery [36].

The relative merits of vacuum extraction and forceps are summarized in Table 8.2 [2,25].

Manual rotation either with or without traction forceps has been explored as a strategy to correct fetal malpositions and is recommended in the guideline of the Society of Obstetricians and Gynaecologists of Canada [37]. A large, retrospective cohort study reported a reduction in caesarean delivery associated with the use of manual rotation (9% versus 41%, $p < 0.001$) [38]. Of the 731 women in this study who underwent manual rotation, none experienced an umbilical cord prolapse and there was no difference in either birth trauma or neonatal acidaemia between neonates who had experienced an attempt at manual rotation versus those who had not. Given these data, manual rotation of the fetal occiput in the setting of fetal malposition in the second stage of labour warrants further evaluation as a potential strategy to consider before moving to OVD or caesarean delivery.

Kielland's rotational forceps has decreased in popularity, reflecting concerns about morbidity but perhaps more realistically as a result of the need for greater obstetric skill. Two recent studies compared rotational vacuum, manual rotation with forceps and Kielland's rotational forceps and reported similar maternal and neonatal morbidity rates but a higher failure rate with attempted rotational vacuum delivery [39,40].

Deciding Between Operative Vaginal Delivery and Caesarean Section

Rotational delivery and mid-cavity arrest in the second stage of labour present the obstetrician with a choice between a potentially difficult operative vaginal delivery and CS at full dilatation, each with inherent risks. In a prospective cohort study of women transferred to theatre for second stage arrest, CS was associated with an increased risk of major haemorrhage (adjusted OR 2.8 [95% CI 1.1–7.6]) and prolonged hospital stay (OR 3.5 [95% CI 1.6–7.6]) [18]. However, caesarean delivery (OR 0.63 [95% CI 0.38–1.00]) and major haemorrhage were less likely with delivery by an experienced obstetrician (OR 0.5 [95% CI 0.3–0.9]). High rates of third- and fourth-degree tears are reported following OVD and there was a three-fold increased risk of urinary incontinence at three years following OVD compared to second stage CS [41]. The comparable morbidity at CS relates to extension of the uterine incision into the cervix, vagina or broad ligaments. Long-term follow-up studies will determine whether this results in subsequent difficult deliveries or an increased risk of uterine rupture.

To date, there has been inconsistency in the reported early neonatal morbidity when comparing OVD with CS in the second stage of labour. In a prospective cohort study of women transferred to theatre in the second stage of labour, delivery by CS was associated with an increased risk of admission to the special care baby unit (SCBU) compared to OVD (OR 2.6 [95% CI 1.2–6.0]) [18]. Of note, there were equal rates of pathological FHR tracings in the two groups. However, neonatal trauma was significantly less common following caesarean delivery compared to operative vaginal delivery (OR 0.4 [95% CI 0.2–0.7]). A low umbilical artery pH was more frequently recorded following failed operative vaginal delivery, but there was no increase in admissions to SCBU. Similarly, a recent US study found no increase in neonatal morbidity among women who had a failed OVD when non-reassuring fetal heart rate tracings were accounted for [42]. In a further large North American population-based study, the sequential use of vacuum and forceps was associated with an increased need for mechanical ventilation in the infant [43]. These findings suggest that neonatal complications could be reduced, with careful selection of cases for attempted operative vaginal delivery and a judicious choice of instrument.

A previous delivery experience can have important implications for future pregnancies, not least whether a woman would contemplate another pregnancy. In the UK second stage prospective cohort study, women were far more likely to aim for a future vaginal delivery (79% vs. 39%) and to achieve a subsequent vaginal delivery (78% vs. 31%) following OVD than CS, although fear of childbirth was a frequently reported reason for avoiding a further pregnancy in both groups [44,45]. Women who have experienced a previous CS at full dilatation generate anxiety in subsequent labours relating to the risk of further emergency CS and potential uterine rupture. Mid-cavity and rotational OVD have become unpopular in the United States and are increasingly abandoned in favour of CS. This may be a short-sighted view, however, if one fails to consider the outcome of future deliveries in the assessment of overall morbidity.

Clearly, choice of operative delivery in the second stage of labour presents a difficult risk–benefit dilemma in terms of short- and long-term maternal and infant outcomes. Caesarean section at full dilatation with anhydramnios and a deeply engaged fetal head is a difficult procedure. This is reflected in high rates of major obstetric haemorrhage, extension of the uterine incision and prolonged hospital admission. These risks must be balanced with the potential for pelvic floor trauma and neonatal injury with OVD. Although there is a published protocol for a Cochrane systematic review comparing OVD with CS for difficult deliveries in the second stage of labour, as yet there have been no RCTs addressing this important question. At present, the decision relies on experience, judgement and clinical skill.

Conclusion

Decisions regarding the most appropriate management of prolonged second stage of labour continue to be challenging. Individual clinical circumstances, maternal preferences and the skill of the obstetric team will influence the approach taken. A balance needs to be achieved between avoiding unnecessary intervention and preventing avoidable morbidity. Every woman has a right to expect high-quality care in labour, and in the event of a prolonged second stage she should be assessed carefully and advised on a course of action that will result in a safe and timely delivery. Most women who have reached the second stage of labour will prefer an OVD to a CS if this can be achieved safely with a minimum of morbidity. In such circumstances women should be encouraged that the probability of a spontaneous vaginal birth in a subsequent pregnancy is very high. Some women will express a preference for a CS and should be counselled on the differences between lift-out, low-cavity, mid-cavity and rotational OVDs, and on the implications of a second stage CS for subsequent births. Good decision making is founded on mutual respect and trust between the labouring woman and her care givers. The skilled obstetrician will demonstrate competency in both the technical and non-technical aspects of care in the second stage of labour.

References

1. American College of Obstetricians and Gynecologists. Operative vaginal delivery: use of forceps and vacuum extractors for operative vaginal delivery. *ACOG Prac Bull.* 2000; 17: 1–6.

2. Royal College of Obstetricians and Gynaecologists. *Operative Vaginal Delivery.* London: RCOG Press; 2011.

3. NICE. *Intrapartum Care: Care of Healthy Women and their Babies during Childbirth*: NICE Clinical Guideline 190. London: NICE; 2014.

4. Cheng YW, Hopkins LM, Caughey AB. How long is too long: does a prolonged second stage of labor in nulliparous women affect maternal and neonatal outcomes? *Am J Obstet Gynecol.* 2004; 194: 933–8.

5. Cheng YW, Hopkins LM, Laros RK Jr, Caughey AB. Duration of the second stage of labour in multiparous women: maternal and neonatal outcomes. *Am J Obstet Gynecol.* 2007; 196: e1–e6.

6. Allen VM, Baskett TF, O'Connell CM, McKeen D, Allen AC. Maternal and perinatal outcomes with increasing duration of the second stage of labor. *Obstet Gynecol.* 2009; 113(6): 1248.

7. Saunders NS, Pearson CM, Wadsworth J. Neonatal and maternal morbidity in relation to the length of the second stage of labour. *Br J Obstet Gynaecol.* 1992; 99: 381–5.

8. Murphy DJ, Liebling RE, Patel R, Verity L, Swingler R. Cohort study of operative delivery in the second stage of labour and standard of obstetric care. *Br J Obstet Gynaecol.* 2003; 110: 610–15.

9. AnimSomuah M, Smyth RM, Jones L. Epidural versus non-epidural or no analgesia in labour *Cochrane Database Syst Rev.* 2011; 12: CD000331.

10. Hodnett ED, Gates S, Hofmeyr GJ, Sakala C. Continuous support for women during childbirth. *Cochrane Database Syst Rev.* 2013; 7: CD003766.

11. Gupta JK, Hofmeyr GJ. Position for women during second stage of labour. *Cochrane Database Syst Rev.* 2003; 3: CD002006.

12. Roberts CL, Torvaldsen S, Cameron CA, Olive E. Delayed versus early pushing in women with epidural analgesia: a systematic review and meta-analysis. *Br J Obstet Gynaecol.* 2004; 111: 1333–40.

13. Bloom SL, Casey BM, Schaffer JI, *et al.* A randomized trial of coached versus uncoached maternal pushing during the second stage of labor. *Am J Obstet Gynecol.* 2006; 194: 10–13.

14. Schaffer JI, Bloom SL, Casey BM, *et al.* A randomized trial of coached versus uncoached maternal pushing during the second stage of labor on postpartum pelvic floor structure and function. *Am J Obstet Gynecol.* 2005; 192: 1692–6.

15. Carroli G, Mignini L. Episiotomy for vaginal birth. *Cochrane Database Syst Rev.* 2009; 1: CD000081.

16. Murphy DJ, Ramphul M. Indications and assessment for operative vaginal birth. In Attilakos G, Draycott T, Gale A, Siassakos D, Winter C (eds), *ROBuST Course Manual.* Cambridge: Cambridge University Press; 2014.

17. Bahl R, Murphy DJ, Strachan B. Decision making in operative vaginal delivery: when to intervene, where to deliver and which instrument to use? Qualitative analysis of expert practice. *Eur J Obstet Gynecol Reprod Biol.* 2013; 170(2): 333–40.

18. Murphy DJ, Liebling RE, Verity L, Swingler R, Patel R. Cohort study of the early maternal and neonatal morbidity associated with operative delivery in the second stage of labour. *Lancet.* 2001; 358: 1203–7.

19. Ben-Haroush A, Melamed N, Kaplan B, Yogev Y. Predictors of failed operative vaginal delivery: a single-center experience. *Am J Obstet Gynecol.* 2007; 197: e5–47.

20. Aiken CE, Aiken AR, Brockelsby JC, Scott JG. Factors influencing the likelihood of instrumental delivery success. *Obstet Gynecol.* 2014; 123(4): 796–803.

21. Ramphul M, O'Brien Y, Murphy DJ. Strategies to enhance assessment of the fetal head position before instrumental delivery: a survey of obstetric practice in the United Kingdom and Ireland. *Eur J Obstet Gynecol Reprod Biol.* 2012; 165(2): 181–8.

22. Ramphul M, Kennelly M, Murphy DJ. Establishing the accuracy and acceptability of abdominal ultrasound to

identify the foetal head position in the second stage of labour: a validation study. *Eur J Obstet Gynecol Reprod Biol*. 2012; 164(1): 35–9.

23. Ramphul M, Ooi PV, Burke G, *et al*. Instrumental delivery and ultrasound: a multicentre randomised controlled trial of ultrasound assessment of the fetal head position versus standard care as an approach to prevent morbidity at instrumental delivery. *BJOG*. 2014; 121(8): 1029–38.

24. Olah KS. Reversal of the decision for caesarean section in the second stage of labour on the basis of consultant vaginal assessment. *J Obstet Gynecol*. 2005; 25: 115–16.

25. Johanson RB, Menon BK. Vacuum extraction versus forceps for assisted vaginal delivery. *Cochrane Database Syst Rev*. 2000; 2: CD000224.

26. Attilakos G, Sibanda T, Winter C, Johnson N, Draycott T. A randomised controlled trial of a new handheld vacuum extraction device. *Br J Obstet Gynaecol*. 2005; 112: 1510–15.

27. Groom KM, Jones BA, Miller N, Paterson-Brown S. A prospective randomised controlled trial of the Kiwi Omnicup versus conventional ventouse cups for vacuum-assisted vaginal delivery. *Br J Obstet Gynaecol*. 2006; 113: 183–9.

28. O'Mahony F, Hofmeyr GJ, Menon V. Choice of instruments for assisted vaginal delivery. *Cochrane Database Syst Rev*; 2010, 11: CD005455.

29. Damron DP, Capeless EL. Operative vaginal delivery: a comparison of forceps and vacuum for success rate and risk of rectal sphincter injury. *Am J Obstet Gynecol*. 2004; 191: 907–10.

30. De Leeuw JW, Struijk PC, Vierhout ME, Wallenburg HC. Risk factors for third degree perineal ruptures during delivery. *Br J Obstet Gynaecol*. 2001; 108: 383–7.

31. Fitzpatrick M, Behan M, O'Connell PR, O'Herlihy C. Randomised clinical trial to assess anal sphincter function following forceps or vacuum assisted vaginal delivery. *Br J Obstet Gynaecol*. 2003; 110: 424–9.

32. Johanson RB, Heycock E, Carter J, *et al*. Maternal and child health after assisted vaginal delivery: five-year follow up of a randomised controlled study comparing forceps and ventouse. *Br J Obstet Gynaecol*. 1999; 106: 544–9.

33. Towner D, Castro MA, Eby-Wilkens E, Gilbert WM. Effect of mode of delivery in nulliparaous women on neonatal intracranial injury. *N Engl J Med*. 1999; 341: 1709–14.

34. Murphy DJ, Koh DM. Cohort study of the decision to delivery interval and neonatal outcome for 'emergency' operative vaginal delivery. *Am J Obstet Gynecol*. 2007; 196: e1–7.

35. Badawi N, Kurinczuk JJ, Keogh JM, *et al*. Intrapartum risk factors for newborn encephalopathy: the Western Australian case-control study. *Br Med J*. 1998; 317: 1554–8.

36. Bahl R, Patel RR, Swingler R, Ellis N, Murphy DJ. Neurodevelopmental outcome at 5 years after operative delivery in the second stage of labor: a cohort study. *Am J Obstet Gynecol*. 2007; 197: e1–6.

37. Cargill YM, MacKinnon CJ, Arsenault MY, *et al*. Guidelines for operative vaginal birth: Clinical Practice Obstetrics Committee. *J Obstet Gynaecol Can*. 2004; 26: 747–61.

38. Shaffer BL, Cheng YW, Vargas JE, Caughey AB. Manual rotation to reduce caesarean delivery in persistent occiput posterior or transverse position. *J Matern Fetal Neonatal Med*. 2011; 24: 65–72.

39. Tempest N, Hart A, Walkinshaw S, Hapangama DK. A re-evaluation of the role of rotational forceps: retrospective comparison of maternal and perinatal outcomes following different methods of birth for malposition in the second stage of labour. *BJOG*. 2013; 120(10): 1277–84.

40. Bahl R, Van de Venne M, Macleod M, Strachan B, Murphy DJ. Maternal and neonatal morbidity in relation to the instrument used for midcavity rotational operative vaginal delivery: a prospective cohort study. *BJOG*. 2013; 120(12): 1526–32.

41. Bahl R, Strachan B, Murphy DJ. Pelvic floor morbidity at three years after instrumental delivery and caesarean section in the second stage of labor and the impact of a subsequent delivery. *Am J Obstet Gynecol*. 2005; 192: 789–94.

42. Alexander JM, Leveno KJ, Hauth JC, *et al*. Eunice Kennedy Shriver National Institute of Child Health and Human Development (NICHD) Maternal-Fetal Medicine Units Network (MFMU): failed operative vaginal delivery. *Obstet Gynecol*. 2009; 114(5): 1017–22.

43. Demissie K, Rhoads GG, Smulian JC, *et al*. Operative vaginal delivery and neonatal and infant adverse outcomes: population based retrospective analysis. *Br Med J*. 2004; 329: 24–9.

44. Murphy DJ, Liebling R. Cohort study of maternal views on future mode of delivery following operative delivery in the second stage of labour. *Am J Obstet Gynecol*. 2003; 188: 542–8.

45. Bahl R, Strachan B, Murphy DJ. Outcome of subsequent pregnancy three years after previous operative delivery in the second stage of labour: cohort study. *Br Med J*. 2004; 328: 311–14.

Instrumental Vaginal Deliveries
Indications, Techniques and Complications

Gabriel Kalakoutis, Stergios Doumouchtsis and Sabaratnam Arulkumaran

Introduction

Instrumental vaginal delivery (IVD) is one of the commonest surgical operations performed in obstetric practice. This chapter will deal with forceps and ventouse delivery. Manipulative delivery such as breech, twins and shoulder dystocia are dealt with in different chapters. Difficult decision making regarding whether to proceed with IVD or caesarean section (CS) is discussed in detail in Chapter 8. The two instruments that have been used for IVDs are different forms of forceps and ventouse that help in the rotation and traction of the head along the pelvis to assist delivery. A new instrument, the 'Odon' device, is undergoing evaluation by clinical trials. If found to be effective and safe for mother and newborn, it will become another instrument to help with assisted vaginal delivery. The principle with all the instruments is based on traction of a flexed head in the antero-posterior diameter along the axis of the pelvis with the flexion point of the head as the leading part. The flexion point is 3 cm anterior to the occiput along the sagittal suture. Achieving the antero-posterior direction of the head may be by digital or manual rotation with the hand, assistance with forceps specially designed for rotation or auto-rotation with vacuum. Ventouse delivery is performed by traction of the fetal scalp with a suction cup. Forceps cradle the parietal and malar bones of the fetal skull to allow application of traction. During this process it also laterally displaces maternal tissues.

The incidence of IVD in different countries varies between 10% and 15% [1,2]. The use in many countries is on the decline, with ventouse becoming more popular than forceps. There is also an increase in second stage CS. Over the past two decades, in the UK, the use of forceps has decreased by 50% in favour of vacuum extraction or CS [3]. In the United States,

the rate of vacuum delivery exceeded the rate of forceps delivery in 1992 [2,4]. In Canada, forceps delivery has decreased in the last decade from 11.2% in 1991 to 6.8% in 2001 [5]. Ventouse delivery is associated with less maternal morbidity compared to forceps [6]. However, failure rates with vacuum are higher (RR 1.7) [7,8] and in some instances the delivery is completed with forceps with the consequence of risk of higher neonatal morbidity with sequential instrumentation [9].

It is best to classify IVD based on the station of the leading bony point of the fetal head and the degree of rotation of the sagittal suture from the midline. When the fetal scalp is visible on separation of the labia it is an *outlet* delivery and invariably the sagittal suture is in an antero-posterior diameter or right or left occipito-anterior or posterior position (rotation does not exceed 45°). The fetal head is virtually on the perineum. When the leading point of the skull is at station $\geq \pm 2$ cm and not on the pelvic floor it is a low-cavity IVD. Low-cavity IVD is subdivided into cases that need $\leq 45°$ or $>45°$ of rotation. *Mid-cavity* deliveries are those with an engaged fetal head but in which the leading point of the skull is above +2 cm station [10]. Abdominal examination before vaginal examination is of paramount importance to make sure the head is zero-fifths or one-fifth palpable. If more than one-fifth of the head is palpable, IVD is contraindicated.

Indications

The recently published NICE guidelines (2014) suggest that IVD should be offered if there is concern about fetal health or there is a prolonged second stage [11]. Occasionally the indication may be when supportive care has not effected spontaneous vaginal delivery.

Best Practice in Labour and Delivery, Second Edition, ed. Sir Sabaratnam Arulkumaran. Published by Cambridge University Press. © Cambridge University Press 2016.

Prolonged second stage in nulliparas is longer than two hours in the active second stage and one hour of active phase in multiparous women. In nulliparas, consideration should be given to oxytocin if contractions are inadequate at the onset of the second stage. Inadequate uterine contractions, poor expulsive maternal efforts and minor disproportion or malposition of the fetal head may be the cause and these should be identified and recorded.

The natural tone of pelvic musculature is reduced with an epidural. This alters the shape of the forward and medially sloping pelvic floor and reduces the chances for the fetal head to rotate for the occiput to become anterior. This predisposes to less flexion of the head and more occipito-posterior or lateral positions. Epidural also abolishes the 'Ferguson reflex', which is a surge of oxytocin and increase in uterine activity produced by distension of the cervix and vagina in the late first and second stage of labour. The increased incidence of use of oxytocin in the second stage and IVDs with epidural may be attributed to these two factors [12]. The possibility of fetal compromise is greater in the second stage due to possible compression of the uterine vessels with contractions and the head exerting pressure on the uterine vessels that traverse the pelvic floor, or occult cord compression or the prolonged nature of the contractions. Prolonged deceleration or rising baseline rate with increase in the depth and width of the decelerations and much less time at the baseline rate compared to the duration of the decelerations are indications for IVD.

Maternal indications are most commonly maternal distress or maternal exhaustion. Medically significant conditions are less common indications. These include cardiac disease, cerebral vascular disease and pre-eclampsia. Vaginal birth after previous CS may be a relative indication to minimize the risk of scar rupture if the second stage is likely to be prolonged. There is no evidence that the use of ventouse after dural tap will benefit the parturient unless her headache deteriorates [13].

Contraindications

IVD is contraindicated in fetal malpresentation (e.g. brow, face mento-posterior), unengaged fetal head (fetal head is above the ischial spines or more than one-fifth of the head is palpable abdominally), cephalo-pelvic disproportion (signified by severe caput, +++ of moulding, high station and non-descent of the head

during contractions and bearing down effort), fetal coagulopathy or bone demineralization disorder. IVD is best avoided when the cervix is not fully dilated. Vacuum delivery (not forceps) is exceptionally performed for cord prolapse at 9 cm in a multiparous woman or a second twin [1] and situations where the benefits significantly outweigh the risks and there is no viable alternative [5].

The most common relative contraindications are high presenting part and fetal prematurity. Among premature newborns delivered by vacuum extraction, 14.29% exhibit scalp oedema, 21.43% bone fracture and 21.43% cephalhaematoma [14]. The Royal College of Obstetricians and Gynaecologists (RCOG) recommends avoiding the use of ventouse below 34 weeks because of the susceptibility of the preterm fetus to trauma [1]. Subsequent guidelines also suggested its limited use between 30 and 34 weeks' gestation as its safety is not known [15].

Forceps may only be applied in vertex presentation, face presentation if the fetal position is mento-anterior and in breech presentation for the delivery of the after-coming head. Unknown position of the fetal head is a contraindication for both vacuum and forceps delivery due to the increased risks of failure and fetal trauma [16,17]. Vaginal examination during operative delivery fails to identify the correct fetal head position in 25% [18] to 65% [19] of cases. Intrapartum ultrasound may provide objective information on the fetal head station, position and progress of labour [20], and hence some authors recommend routine performance of abdominal and translabial ultrasound scanning in the labour room [21]. The use of ultrasound in the second stage to assist IVD is discussed in the previous chapter.

Prerequisites for Safe IVD

There should be a clear maternal or fetal indication to perform an IVD. The maternal and fetal condition should be evaluated by the person who is planning to perform the IVD. Examination and communication should be in the presence of a chaperone. The mother and her partner should be able to understand the reason for IVD, possible benefits and complications, and also the consequence of not performing the IVD and the alternatives. Consent should be obtained, either verbal or written following discussion, based on the unit's policy.

Consideration should be given for good analgesia. If the mother is on regional analgesia the sensation at the perineum should be tested and the dose adequately increased. If not on regional blockade, pudendal block and local perineal infiltration with 1% lignocaine may be adequate for low forceps or ventouse deliveries. Epidural or spinal anaesthesia are more suitable for optimal pain relief in cases of mid-cavity IVD and trial of IVD. In cases of cord prolapse, antepartum bleeding or prolonged deceleration, delivery should be expedited and actions should be undertaken without delay.

Prior to proceeding with an IVD, an abdominal examination should be performed to assess the size of the fetus, the uterine contractions and the descent of the fetal head in 'fifths' above the pelvic brim. Oxytocin infusion should be considered if contractions are inadequate (less than four in 10 min, each lasting <40 s) in the absence of signs of fetal compromise and if there are no signs of severe disproportion such as significant caput or +++ moulding. Descent of the head with contractions and bearing down effort is a good indicator that the use of oxytocin may be of benefit. The bladder should be empty and therefore not abdominally palpable. The mother can be asked to void urine and if there is difficulty in voiding due to the head being impacted in the pelvis, the bladder should be emptied by catheterization. A big fetus, especially known asymmetrical macrosomic fetus (e.g. abdominal circumference well over 90th centile and head circumference along the 50th centile), prolonged second stage, obese mother, postterm pregnancy and rotational IVD are associated with shoulder dystocia. A plan to tackle this eventuality should be in place, including additional assistants and a paediatrician in attendance.

On vaginal examination the cervix should be fully dilated with vertex presentation. The presence of liquor, its colour, station, position, the degree of caput and moulding should be noted in addition to the descent of the vertex with contraction and bearing down efforts. For a safe IVD the leading bony part of the fetal head should be below spines; but this should be correlated to the abdominal findings. It is stated that in some women the severe caput and moulding may give an impression that the head is low but abdominally the head is more than one-fifth palpable. The accurate assessment of the true descent of the fetal head requires both abdominal and vaginal examination. The degree of asynclitism is critical for the correct application of forceps or vacuum. When there is synclitism, the parietal eminences are at the same level

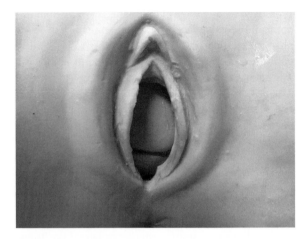

Figure 9.1 Anterior asynclitism: more parietal bone and the sagittal suture in the anterior half of the pelvis.

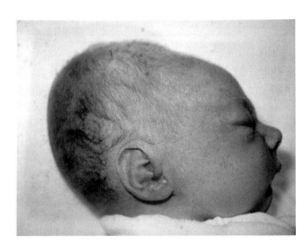

Figure 9.2 The newborn's head showing the larger suboccipito-bregmatic diameter well above the position of the ear. See the colour plate section for a colour version of this figure.

and indicated by the sagittal suture placed centrally in the pelvis and equal portions of the skull are felt on either side. Figure 9.1 shows a case with anterior asynclitism. If the large diamond-shaped anterior fontanelle is felt in the centre of the pelvis, there is likely to be some degree of extension as in the well-flexed head the anterior fontanelle will be more towards the side facing the pelvic wall. In cases with extension it is useful to feel for the ear of the fetus if possible, which will give some idea of the position (based on the direction of the pinna of the ear) and station, i.e. that the maximal suboccipito and biparietal diameter is low as the ear is well below the parietal eminences (Figure 9.2).

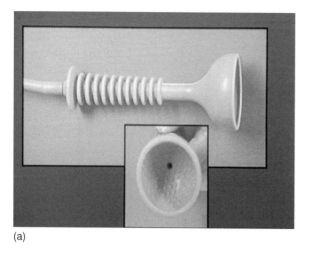

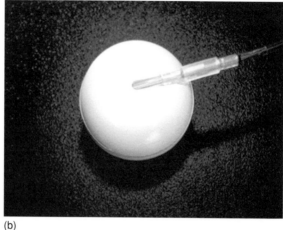

(a)   (b)

Figure 9.3 (a) Silk cup; (b) Kiwi™ posterior cup (Omnicup) showing the tubing used for creating suction and also used for traction, going through a groove to the centre of the cup. See the colour plate section for a colour version of this figure.

The IVD should be carried out in a room with adequate facilities and personnel. The procedure should be carried out under adequate antiseptic and aseptic conditions. There is inadequate evidence to recommend antibiotic prophylaxis [22]. The clinician should have the competence to perform the procedure, be capable of managing any complications and be prepared to abandon the procedure and carry out a CS. The CS in such situations is fraught with difficulties and complications and hence the help of an experienced clinician may become necessary. Compressive and traction forces on the head due to the application of an instrument may give rise to prolonged decelerations, and should there be difficulties in delivery with a prolonged period of traction it may be best to abandon the procedure and carry out a CS. To identify the fetal condition, intermittent or continuous fetal heart rate (FHR) monitoring is recommended. Difficulty or failure are likely to arise when the head is one-fifth or more palpable on abdominal examination, the presenting part is at or above the level of spines, there is occipito-posterior position, excessive moulding of the fetal head, fetal macrosomia, dysfunctional or prolonged labour and body mass index >30 kg/m^2 [23]. In such cases, a trial of IVD should be performed in the operating theatre under effective epidural or spinal anaesthesia, with facilities and personnel available for CS. Such an eventuality should have been mentioned to the mother and her partner and appropriate consent taken.

Vacuum-assisted Deliveries

The vacuum extractor is a device with a suction cup attached with tubing to a vacuum source and a handle, which is used to apply traction to the cup. Traction is applied to the fetal head along the axis of the birth canal. Malmström devised the stainless steel vacuum cup in the 1950s. It has rounded edges and a diameter of 60 mm, with the vacuum tubing and the traction chain attached to the centre of the upper surface of the cup. Bird modified the Malmström vacuum extractor by attaching the vacuum tubing and the traction chain on the side of the cup. This allows the placement of the cup close and anterior to the occiput in occipito-posterior and lateral positions. Kobayashi introduced a single unit silastic cup with a diameter of 65 mm and a stainless steel valve that allows the release of suction between contractions without loss of application of the cup to the head (Figure 9.3a). Kiwi Omnicup (Clinical Innovations Inc., Murray, Utah) is a disposable vacuum extractor with a rigid flat plastic cup and a hand-pump traction system directly applied to the vacuum cup (Figure 9.3b). The accurate development of negative pressure can be monitored via an indication gauge on the traction handle. Randomized studies [24] suggest that rigid cups are more likely to result in vaginal birth than soft cups, but they are more likely to cause scalp trauma.

The parturient should be in lithotomy position with adequate analgesia. Prior to cup placement, the fetal presentation, the amount of fetal head in 'fifths'

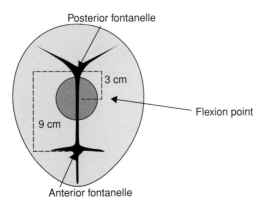

Figure 9.4 The flexion point about 3 cm anterior to the posterior fontanelle along the sagittal suture.

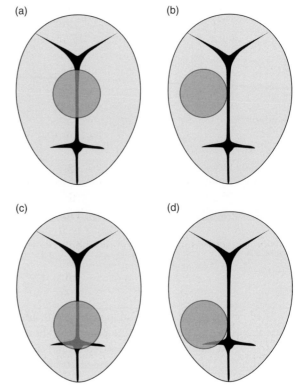

Figure 9.5 (a) Flexing median application of the vacuum cup (correct application). (b–d) Various malapplications of the vacuum cup: (b) flexing paramedian; (c) deflexing median; (d) deflexing paramedian.

palpable abdominally above the symphysis pubis, the position of the fetal head and the station should be confirmed. Correct placement of the cup is a major determinant of the outcome. The 'flexion point' is the site on the fetal scalp over which the centre of the vacuum cup should be placed to achieve a flexing median application. Flexion point is on the sagittal suture 3 cm anterior to the posterior fontanelle (Figure 9.4). Application of the vacuum cup on this point promotes synclitism and flexion of the fetal head, presenting the optimal diameter of the fetal head (suboccipito-bregmatic, 9.5 cm) to the maternal pelvis. By incorrect application of the vacuum cup (deflexing and para-median, Figure 9.5), the fetal head will present with a larger diameter that will increase the difficulty and risk of failure or fetal injury [25,26]. In occipito-lateral or posterior positions, a vacuum cup with the tubing emerging from the lateral aspect (posterior metal cup) or through a groove in the cup (posterior rigid plastic cup – Omnicup) (Figure 9.3b) should be used, as it can be inserted between the vaginal wall and the head to reach the flexion point. Soft silk, plastic or anterior metal cups, where the tubing is attached in the centre of the cup, are not suitable for occipito-posterior or lateral positions as the lateral vaginal wall would not permit a cup with the central stem or suction tubing on the dorsum to be shifted to the flexion point. These cups are suitable for occipito-anterior positions as the flexion point is directly accessible.

After the application of the cup to the fetal head and before inducing negative pressure, any maternal tissue entrapment between the cup and the fetal head should be excluded. Apart from causing significant vaginal or cervical trauma and maternal haemorrhage,

entrapment of maternal tissue may cause detachment of the cup and failure of the procedure. Detachment of the cup is associated with increased incidence of cranial fractures (9.58%; RR 2.11) cephalhaematoma (18.56%; RR 1.86) and scalp oedema (26.34%; RR 1.41) [14].

The vacuum is created by mechanical, electrical or a hand pump and the cup is held in place by atmospheric pressure acting on the dorsum of the cup. Hence the maximum pressure that can be created is less than 760 mmHg. In the past it was thought that the formation of chignon, i.e. the soft tissue sucked into the cup, was important for traction and suction was created in a gradual stepwise manner. Based on studies it is known that quick development of negative pressure is as effective as the gradual stepwise process [27]. Effective traction usually requires a negative pressure of at least 0.6 kg/cm^2 (440 mmHg) and usually 0.8 kg/cm^2 (588 mmHg). Higher pressures are associated with increased risk of fetal head injury. The traction force indicators of the vacuum devices should be checked throughout the delivery as attention to the force and duration may help to reduce the incidence of fetal injuries [28]. Traction should be in line with the axis of the pelvis, and ideally it should be perpendicular to the plane of the vacuum cup. Each effort at traction should be with uterine contractions and coordinated with maternal expulsive efforts. Descent must be observed with the initial and subsequent traction efforts. The initial lengthening of the traction tube in an occiptio-posterior and lateral position signifies that the first traction has resulted in flexion of the head, resulting in the flexion point coming as the leading part of the presentation. This should result in progressive descent with successive traction efforts. If the cup is dislodged, the reason for the 'pop-off' should be evaluated, and if there are no contraindications it can be reapplied after careful inspection of the fetal scalp for injury. There is no consensus on the maximum number of traction attempts, the duration of a vacuum application or the number of 'pop-offs' that should be allowed. Vacca suggests that the traction force should not exceed 11.5 kg, the duration of the procedure should be restricted to 15 min and the number of pulls limited to three for the descent phase and three for the perineal phase [29]. A traction force exceeding 13.5 kg is associated with an increased risk of fetal scalp injury [29]. Higher levels of traction force and a greater number of pulls may, however, be required during the outlet phase of the vacuum delivery as resistance is greatest at this stage. For this reason, additional time and pulls should be allowed for the perineum to stretch over the head, especially if the birth is managed without episiotomy [29]. The 'pop-offs' are due to change in direction of the pull to upwards before the maximum biparietal diameter emerges from underneath the sub-pubic arch, large caput underneath the pubic arch acting as a 'door stopper' or sudden excess force due to the belief that the head is just going to come out on seeing the portion of the head that may be the scalp and not the bony skull.

The traction force is less when the head descends with the cup during traction compared with a situation when the head does not descend with traction. Hence additional pulls with descent are less likely to be harmful compared with traction on a head that does not descend with three pulls. The RCOG guidelines recommend that 'operative vaginal delivery should be abandoned where there is no evidence of progressive descent with each pull or where delivery is not imminent following three pulls of a correctly applied instrument by an experienced operator' [1]. The SOGC guidelines advise that if delivery has not occurred after four contractions the intended method of delivery should be reassessed [5]. With efficient uterine contractions and good maternal expulsive efforts, almost all vacuum-assisted deliveries should be completed within 15 min. If a 20 min limit is exceeded, the procedure should be abandoned unless delivery is imminent [16]. The procedure should also be abandoned if there is evidence of fetal scalp trauma.

Forceps Deliveries

Forceps are a paired instrument with a handle, shank, lock and blade. The blades have a cephalic and a pelvic curve between the heel and toes (at the distal end) and are attached to each other by a lock on the shank. Forceps are used for traction of the fetal head. Specially made forceps that allow sliding of one shank over the other and with minimal pelvic curve, i.e. Kielland's forceps, can be used for correction of asynclitism and rotation of the head followed by traction. The Barton's forceps are used for transverse arrest in a flat pelvis and the Piper's forceps with long shanks for the delivery of the after-coming head in breech presentations.

The mechanism of action of forceps includes correction of deflexion, asynclitism or positional abnormalities of the fetal head, extraction by working in synchrony with the maternal expulsive forces and transient reduction of the resistance of the outlet by enlargement of the soft tissue of the birth canal. The cephalic curve grasps the fetal head over the maxilla or malar eminences, while the length of the blade grasps the sides of the head from the malar area along the side of the head in front of the ear and the parietal bones in front of the occiput (Figure 9.6). This bimalar–biparietal application exerts uniform pressure on the head. In this position the shank is over the flexion point, allowing the correct direction of traction.

The choice of forceps depends on the indication, clinical situation and preferences of the obstetrician, as well as the availability of instruments. For occipito-anterior positions in the mid- or low-cavity or low-direct occipito-posterior positions, the Neville–Barnes with or without axis traction handle or the Simpson's forceps can be used. Wrigley's forceps are ideal for outlet deliveries. If the position is occipito-lateral or posterior, Kielland's forceps can achieve rotation without inflicting trauma to the fetus or the maternal passages.

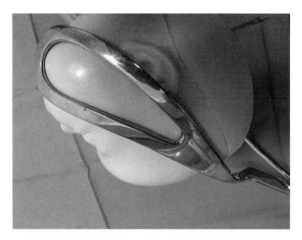

Figure 9.6 Bimalar–biparietal application of the forceps which when checked before traction will allow one finger between the head and heel of the blade on either side, the sagittal suture would be perpendicular to the shank and the occiput would be 3 cm above the shank, allowing the traction on a flexed head with the line of pull along the flexion point. See the colour plate section for a colour version of this figure.

Non-fenestrated blades are indicated in cases with oedematous soft maternal tissues to minimize risk of tearing. Face presentation with mento-anterior position can be delivered using Kielland's or Simpson's forceps.

Proper application of the forceps to the fetal head is extremely important for a safe procedure with a successful outcome. The exact location of the sagittal suture and posterior fontanelle should be ascertained. The arrangement of the blades should be rehearsed prior to insertion. The forceps blades should be applied gently between contractions. The left blade is applied first to the left side of the maternal pelvis using the left hand, while the right hand guides and protects the head and the vagina. The right blade is applied to the right side of the maternal pelvis using the right hand. No force should be required. If there is resistance the blade should be removed and reapplied. The blades are correctly placed when they are situated in the spaces between the fetal orbits and ears and this will be reflected by the shanks and handles being horizontal and there being easy locking of the blades. When the blades are locked and prior to applying traction, the obstetrician should confirm correct application by ensuring that the sagittal suture is symmetrically and perpendicularly in the midline between the two shanks, the occiput is 3–4 cm above the shanks (so that the traction line is along the flexion point, thus

promoting flexion and exposing the minimal diameter) and the space between the heel of the blade and the head does not admit more than a finger breadth (ensures synclitism).

Analgesia before forceps delivery includes pudendal nerve block, spinal analgesia, diazepam, and ketamine or vinydan ether. The available evidence shows that none of these agents or methods is superior to the others [30].

Once the forceps have been applied and the position of the blades checked, traction should be coordinated with uterine contractions and maternal bearing down efforts. The axis of the traction forces should follow the pelvic curve (curve of Carus). The traction is initially downward and as the head descends in the birth canal, the angle moves forward and upward at the outlet. The Pajot manoeuvre involves the combined exertion of outward and downward forces, which produce a vector that follows the pelvic curve. Traction should be released between contractions in order to reduce the intracranial pressure and the associated vagally induced bradycardia. An episiotomy is usually indicated when the head is crowning at the perineum.

Delivery in Malposition of the Fetal Head

Malpositions of occipito-transverse or -posterior position may be associated with some degree of extension of the head and asynclitism. One needs to carefully consider whether to use digital or manual rotation or rotational forceps delivery, ventouse delivery or CS. If the head is rotating and descending with uterine contractions and bearing down efforts, it may be possible to keep a finger on the suture line and assist, i.e. digital rotation. Alternatively the whole hand can be used to assist with manual rotation. In a digital rotation the index and middle fingers are placed onto the part of the anterior parietal bone that overlaps the occipital bone in the area of the posterior fontanelle and gentle pressure is applied with the tips of the fingers to rotate the posterior fontanelle upward and toward the symphysis pubis. In a manual rotation, the hand under the posterior parietal bone and the thumb on the anterior parietal bone applies rotational pressure (Figure 9.7) [31].

For mid-cavity or rotational assisted vaginal birth it is recommended that a skilled operator be present for all attempts [15]. Insufficient training is likely to result in poor outcomes [32]. Correction of asynclitism and

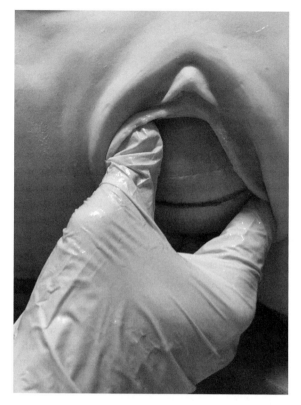

Figure 9.7 Manual rotation of the fetal head from left occipito-transverse to occipito-anterior position. See the colour plate section for a colour version of this figure.

of the fetus will lie equidistant from the two blades of the forceps. If the blades cannot be locked easily, their position should be checked and they should be removed and reinserted.

An abnormal position (e.g. occipito-transverse) is corrected by rotating the handles of the forceps blades and directing the fetal occiput to the anterior position to emerge underneath the symphysis pubis. The risk of injury can be minimized by avoiding excessive torsion during rotation, rotation in the wrong direction, forceful rotation or combined rotation with traction. In a rotational delivery the movements of traction and rotation should always be separate unless rotation occurs spontaneously with traction. Rotation should be avoided during a uterine contraction [33].

Complications

Maternal Injuries

Vaginal, cervical, labial, periurethral lacerations, pelvic haematomas, perineal injuries, episiotomy extension and the associated haemorrhage are the most common complications. Severe maternal morbidity is increased after operative vaginal deliveries [34] and maternal deaths from traumatic operative delivery have been reported [17].

Maternal injury is less frequent and less extensive with the use of vacuum compared to forceps [8,35,36]. Maternal complications of vacuum delivery include cervical lacerations, severe vaginal lacerations, periurethral lacerations, vaginal haematomas, and third- and fourth-degree tears [8]. The use of forceps has been associated with a higher rate of episiotomies and third- and fourth-degree perineal and vaginal tears [37].

The most common vaginal lacerations are the posterior midline tears or the anterior periurethral tears. Inadvertent entrapment of the cervix or the vaginal wall with consequent lacerations can occur during an operative delivery. Posterior tears should be repaired if they involve more than the vaginal mucosa. Anterior labial and periurethral tears do not usually require repair unless they are bleeding. Injury to the bladder or the urethra may cause urinary retention secondary to oedema or haematoma and late fistula formation. The first volume of urine passed should be checked and the residual urine measured if the bladder is palpable or there was difficulty in voiding. Insertion of a Foley catheter is advisable if the tear is close to the urethra.

auto-rotation is expected with traction and descent of the head with a ventouse delivery if the cup was placed over the flexion point. Twisting or rotational motions of the vacuum cup may result in injury. The auto-rotation occurs as the head descends by virtue of the anatomy of the pelvis. Rotation of the fetal head can be attempted using special rotational forceps (Kielland's). Before Kielland's forceps are used, it is essential to identify abdominally the side of the baby's back and the occiput on vaginal examination. The forceps are applied with the 'knobs' facing towards the baby's occiput. The anterior or posterior blade may be applied first directly depending on the preference of the obstetrician. The anterior blade can be positioned by direct, reverse or classical and wandering method. In the wandering method the anterior blade is placed over the face and then moved to lie on the side of the fetal head. The posterior blade can be applied directly. The blades are locked and asynclitism corrected by sliding the shanks on each other until the sliding locks come to the same level. If there is no asynclitism the sagittal suture

Vaginal lacerations may extend into the ischiorectal fossae.

A third- or fourth-degree perineal tear with anal sphincter injury is a potentially severe complication of vaginal delivery, which may result in anal incontinence and rectovaginal fistula formation. A third-degree perineal tear and altered faecal continence occurs more frequently after forceps than vacuum deliveries [38] and in occipito-posterior positions [39,40]. The incidence of third- or fourth-degree perineal tears with forceps-assisted delivery can be as high as 31% and 17% with the use of vacuum, respectively. This rate is significantly higher than at an unassisted delivery [36]. However, normal vaginal delivery without evidence of sphincter injury is also associated with significant effect on anal sphincter function [41]. Anal incontinence can occur regardless of the mode of delivery [42].

Trauma to the pelvic floor musculature and its innervation as a result of forceps and vacuum delivery may contribute to the occurrence of urinary incontinence [43]. Arya *et al.* found that in primiparous women, urinary incontinence after forceps delivery is more likely to persist compared with spontaneous vaginal or vacuum delivery [44]. Liebling *et al.* studied the symptoms of pelvic floor morbidity after difficult operative vaginal deliveries and CSs during the second stage of labour, and concluded that although a CS does not completely protect women from pelvic floor morbidity, operative vaginal delivery was associated with a greater prevalence of urinary symptoms and dyspareunia for up to a year after delivery [45].

Psychological morbidity following IVD is also of concern. Instrumental vaginal delivery can be associated with fear of subsequent childbirth, which may present as a post-traumatic stress type syndrome termed 'tokophobia'. Midwife-led debriefing after assisted vaginal birth did not reduce maternal depression [46]. After delivery the obstetrician that conducted the birth should discuss the indications and complications of operative delivery with the woman if anxieties and fear of the next childbirth are to be alleviated [47].

Fetal Injuries

Scalp Bruises and Lacerations

Fetal scalp injuries occur in most operative vaginal deliveries. They are usually transient and of no clinical significance. The more significant injuries are related to incorrect application of the instrument, excessive or incorrectly directed traction or cephalo-pelvic disproportion.

During application of the vacuum cup to the fetal head a collection of interstitial fluid and microhaemorrhages (chignon) fill the internal diameter of the vacuum cup. This is less pronounced when using soft cups, and resolves within 12–18 hours. The incidence of scalp abrasions and lacerations after vacuum extraction is 10%. The incidence of scalp abrasions is higher in infants delivered by Kiwi Omnicup vacuum or metal cup devices compared to those delivered by silastic cup [48]. Correct cup placement and traction, and avoidance of cup detachments ('pop-offs') reduce the risk of scalp injuries [16].

Cephalhaematoma

Cephalhaematoma is secondary to rupture of blood vessels between the skull and the periosteum. It is delineated by the suture lines and thus can be differentiated from subgaleal haemorrhage. As the capacity of the subperiosteal space is limited, these haematomas are small. Cephalhaematoma occurs in 1–2% of spontaneous vaginal deliveries, in 6–10% of vacuum extractions (range 1–26%) [8,14,24,25] and in 4% of forceps deliveries [8]. Vacuum extraction therefore has a stronger association with cephalhaematoma compared with forceps (odds ratio: 2.38) [8]. Metal cups are more likely to cause cephalhaematoma than silastic cups or the Omnicup [49]. Vacuum extractions at mid or low station are associated with a higher incidence of cephalhaematoma (13.11% and 13.56% respectively) when compared with vacuum applied at the outlet (6.81%; RR 1.92; RR 1.99) [14].

Subgaleal Haemorrhage and Cranial Trauma

Subgaleal, also known as subaponeurotic haemorrhage develops between the skull periosteum and the galea aponeurotica. This space has a capacity of up to 260 ml in term infants. The pathogenesis includes avulsion of the aponeurosis from the cranium and haemorrhage caused by traction forces during operative delivery, skull fracture or rupture of an interosseous synchondrosis. Subgaleal haemorrhage with a loss of 20–40% of the circulating blood volume will result in hypovolaemic shock, disseminated intravascular coagulation, multi-organ failure and neonatal death in up to 25% of cases.

Vacuum extraction (OR = 7.17 [95% CI: 5.43–10.25]) and forceps delivery (OR = 2.66 [95% CI:

1.78–5.18]) are risk factors for subgaleal haemorrhage [50]. The incidence after spontaneous vaginal deliveries is 4 per 10 000 [51] and ranges between 0% and 21% following vacuum extractions [14,26,51]. Maternal nulliparity, placement of vacuum cup over the sagittal suture close to the infant's anterior fontanelle and failed vacuum extraction predispose to subgaleal haemorrhage [26].

Skull fractures can be caused by compression from forceps blades or from the skull pushing against the maternal bony pelvis and are usually linear, affecting the parietal bones, or depressed, forming the so-called 'ping-pong ball-type' fracture. A skull fracture must be suspected in any cephalhaematoma or subarachnoid haemorrhage. A registry of neonatal deaths attributable to intrapartum trauma revealed that cranial injury was almost always associated with physical difficulty at delivery, the use of instruments, poor judgement and persistence in continuing with the operative vaginal delivery in the presence of failure to progress or signs of fetal compromise [52].

Intracranial Trauma

Intracranial haemorrhage occurs in approximately 5–6 per 10 000 live births and can be potentially fatal or cause lifelong disability. Forceps and vacuum delivery, precipitous delivery, prolonged second stage of labour and macrosomia are recognized risk factors. Caesarean section after a failed attempt at IVD and the sequential use of vacuum and forceps are additional risk factors.

Epidural haemorrhage is a blood collection between a calvarial bone and its inner periosteum or between the periosteal membrane and the underlying outer dura fibrous stratum [53]. It is usually a result of injury to the middle meningeal artery, and is frequently associated with a cephalhaematoma or skull fracture. In neonates, the meningeal arteries are not embedded in the cranial bones and they are therefore less susceptible to injury. This probably explains the rarity of epidural haemorrhage in neonates, which accounts for approximately 2% of all cases of intracranial haemorrhage [54]. It is associated with difficult parturition and operative delivery in nulliparous women. It typically results from the mechanical forces exerted on the fetal head with or without the use of instruments. During labour an increased degree of moulding leading to excessive displacement of the skull bones may cause considerable injury to the dura matter.

Subdural haemorrhage is associated with mechanical compression and distortion of the fetal cranium, tearing of veins and venous sinuses and bleeding into the subdural space. The incidence is 2.9 per 10 000 after spontaneous delivery, 4.1 per 10 000 after CS without labour, 8.0 per 10 000 after vacuum delivery, 9.8 per 10 000 after forceps delivery, 25.7 per 10 000 after CS following failed IVD and 21.3 per 10 000 after combined vacuum and forceps delivery [9]. Subdural haematomas can also occur antenatally in utero and after uncomplicated vaginal deliveries.

Subarachnoid haemorrhage is most frequently caused by rupture of the small bridging vessels of the leptomeninges. The incidence of subarachnoid haemorrhage after spontaneous vaginal delivery is 0.1–1.3 per 10 000, after vacuum extraction 0.6–2.2 per 10 000, after forceps delivery 0.1–3.3 per 10 000 and after combined vacuum and forceps delivery 10.7 per 10 000 [9,36].

Nerve Injury

The incidence of brachial plexus injury ranges from 0.13 to 3.6 per 1000 births. Risk factors include macrosomia, shoulder dystocia, operative deliveries and malpresentation. Studies have shown that the risk of brachial plexus injury is higher in forceps deliveries than vacuum extractions [9,55], although other studies have shown that the risk between the two modes of delivery is similar [36]. There are three types of brachial plexus injury: injury to the upper plexus (C5–C7, Erb's palsy) accounts for approximately 90% of cases, injury to C8–T1 (Klumpke's palsy) accounts for less than 1% of brachial plexus injury, and injury to the entire plexus (approximately 10% of cases) results in a flaccid extremity with absent reflexes. The pathogenesis of injury often involves stretch injury when shoulder dystocia requires extreme lateral flexion and traction of the head. However, there are reports of injury that occurs when lateral flexion and traction of the head has not been applied, such as during precipitous deliveries or when there is injury to the posterior shoulder.

Facial nerve palsy is a rare complication of forceps deliveries with an incidence rate of 2.9–5 per 1000 forceps deliveries. However, one-third of facial nerve injuries occur in spontaneous delivery.

Forceful pushing of the blades to achieve locking may cause the 'toes' of the blades to apply pressure on the side of the neck, causing laryngeal nerve injury and rarely, phrenic nerve palsy if the pressure reaches the root of the neck. In such cases the abrasion marks made by the blades of the forceps would usually be seen and will remain for a few days. Laryngeal nerve compression can cause vocal fold paralysis. It is noted that 5–26% of congenital vocal fold paralysis may be due to birth trauma. The paralysis of that side of the diaphragm can be diagnosed by radiological studies, which will not show any movements of the dome on that side.

Upper cervical spinal cord injury is extremely rare and may occur in one baby in every 80 000 deliveries [56]. Misjudged high or upper mid-cavity rotational forceps deliveries that are associated with greater traction and rotation may give rise to high cervical injuries. Higher incidence of 0.7 per 1000 deliveries also have been reported and are considered to be due to excess force and 'unphysiological torsional forces' [25].

Vacuum deliveries are associated with retinal haemorrhage in the newborn and the incidence is higher compared with normal or forceps-assisted deliveries [57,58]. These haemorrhages are innocuous and get absorbed with no long-term ophthalmological consequences.

Choice of Instrument

In current obstetrics the choice of forceps or vacuum seems to depend on how the operator was trained in using the forceps or vacuum devices. The size of mother, baby, parity, progress of labour, station, position, synclitism, caput, moulding, the descent of the fetal head with contractions and maternal bearing down efforts, and operator experience will influence the outcome. It is wise to check the instruments before they are applied. It is not uncommon to find a vacuum set with leaks or a pair of blades that does not form a matching pair. If force is needed to apply or lock the blades, it is suggestive of malposition or asynclitism. Proceeding with such an application and traction may lead to a difficult delivery and maternal and fetal injury. Once properly applied, the traction should be synchronized with contractions and bearing down effort. Failure of progressive descent with each pull indicates that there may be some disproportion. If traction over three contractions does not result in significant descent or if the duration of traction exceeds 20 min, the process needs to be re-evaluated and the

operative delivery abandoned unless vaginal delivery is imminent [17].

Forceps are more successful in achieving a vaginal delivery than ventouse (RR 0.65 [95% CI: 0.45–0.94]) but with the risk of more use of general anaesthetic, more CSs, more vaginal trauma, more third- and fourth-degree tears, more flatus incontinence, more facial injuries and fewer cephalhaematomas. The ventouse type with the greatest success in vaginal deliveries is the metal cup over the soft cup or the disposable rigid vacuum extractor, but with more scalp injuries and cephalhaematomas [59].

When one instrument has failed to effect delivery, sequential use of instruments offers the advantage of avoiding the complications of CS at full dilatation with a low head, but increases the risks of fetal trauma [60,61]. If the head has descended to the introitus, a sequential operative delivery is less likely to cause harm compared with the use of a second instrument when there is no or minimal descent. Request should be made for a neonatologist to be present at delivery in case the baby needs resuscitation.

Conclusion

Increasing success of safe IVD is of paramount importance to reduce maternal and fetal trauma and to reduce unnecessary CS. Training and assessment on the theoretical and technical aspects of IVD should improve successful and safe IVDs. The initial training can be on specially designed mannequins by an experienced trainer. The next step is to perform the IVD, with the trainer assisting in normal occipito-anterior deliveries. In doing so the essential steps should be followed – communication with the woman and partner; consent for the procedure; positioning and draping; checking whether the bladder is empty; checking the abdominal and vaginal findings; checking the instruments; adequate analgesia; proper non-forceful application; checking correctness of the application, etc. – before the traction is synchronized with uterine contractions and bearing down efforts. The formulation of objective structured assessment of technical skills (OSATS) that describes these steps and helps assessment as to whether the individual can do this independently or whether they need assistance has been a forward step in training and is discussed in Chapter 32.

Operation details
Ventouse Delivery

Name ....

MRN ....

NHS No. ....

Ward ....

Consultant ....

Date _____ Obstetrician _____ Assistant _____ Midwife _____

Indication _____

Location ☐ Delivery room ☐ Theatre I ☐ Theatre II

Anaesthetic ☐ GA ☐ Pudendal ☐ Regional ☐ Perineal

Consent ☐ Verbal ☐ Written ☐ Decision made by _____

Bladder emptied ☐ Yes ☐ No   **Indwelling catheter** ☐ Yes ☐ No   **Balloon deflated** ☐ Yes ☐ No

Abdo examination ☐ Cephalic 0/5 ☐ 1/5

Vaginal examination Dilation_____ Position_____ Station_____ Caput_____ Moulding_____ Liquor_____

Type ☐ Silastic ☐ Metal ☐ Omnicup (Kiwi)

Fontanelles and sutures

Please indicate cup placement

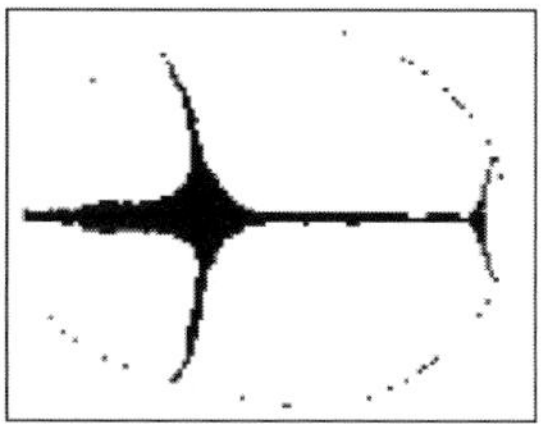

Cup applied ☐ Easily ☐ With difficulty

Negative pressure _____ kg/cm² over _____ mins

Vaginal wall and cervix checked to exclude entrapment ☐ Yes ☐ No

Checked cup application

☐ Flexing Median ☐ Deflexing Median

☐ Flexing Paramedian ☐ Deflexing Paramedian ☐ Not sure

Cup dislodged ☐ Yes (how many times?)_____ ☐ No

Station when cup dislodged_____ Reason why _____

How many pulls _____ Contractions _____

Episiotomy performed ☐ Yes ☐ No ☐ Median ☐ Right mediolateral

Delivery of head in ☐ OA ☐ OP ☐ OL in _____ mins

Time started _____ Time of delivery _____

Indications and outcome discussed with patients ☐ Yes ☐ No

Instruments correct ☐   **Swabs correct** ☐   **Estimated blood loss** _____

Examination of baby's head Application ☐ Injury ☐

Action taken if failed/comments

Figure 9.8 Proforma used for recording a ventouse delivery.

Operation details

Forceps Delivery

Name	
MRN	
NHS No...	

Ward ....

Consultant ....

Date _____ Obstetrician _____ Assistant _____ Midwife _____

Indication _____

Location ☐ Delivery room ☐ Theatre I ☐ Theatre II

Anaesthetic ☐ GA ☐ Pudendal ☐ Regional ☐ Perineal

Consent ☐ Verbal ☐ Written ☐ Decision made by _____

Bladder emptied ☐ Yes ☐ No   Indwelling catheter ☐ Yes ☐ No   Balloon deflated ☐ Yes ☐ No

Abdo examination ☐ Cephalic 0/5 ☐ 1/5

Vaginal examination Dilation_____ Position _____ Station _____ Caput _____ Moulding _____ Liquor _____

Type ☐ Andersons ☐ Wrigleys ☐ Other ☐ Keillands

Easy application of blades ☐ Yes ☐ No   Number of pulls?_____   Number of Contractions _____

Episiotomy performed ☐ Yes ☐ No ☐ Median ☐ Right mediolateral

Delivery of head in ☐ OA ☐ OP ☐ OL   in_____mins

Time started _____ Time of delivery _____

Indications and outcome discussed with patients ☐ Yes ☐ No

Instruments Correct ☐   Swabs correct ☐   Estimated blood loss_____

Action taken if failed / comments

_____

Figure 9.9 Proforma used for forceps delivery.

It is also important to document the procedure carefully for the purpose of debriefing staff, explaining the procedure and outcome to the couple and for writing a report in the unexpected event of medical litigation. Many hospitals use their own format; those used for vacuum and forceps delivery at St George's Hospital, London are given in Figures 9.8 and 9.9. Regular audit of the individual and the unit's performance on IVDs should be carried out to reduce unnecessary interventions and also to reduce morbidity to the mother and baby.

References

1. Royal College of Obstetricians and Gynaecologists. *Operative Vaginal Delivery: Guideline No. 26*. London: RCOG Press; 2005.

2. Kozak LJ, Weeks JD. US trends in obstetric procedures, 1990–2000. *Birth*. 2002; 29: 157–61.

3. Patel RR, Murphy DJ. Forceps delivery in modern obstetric practice. *Br Med J*. 2004; 328: 1302–5.

4. Miksovsky P, Watson WJ. Obstetric vacuum extraction: state of the art in the new millennium. *Obstet Gynecol Surv*. 2001; 56: 736–51.

5. Society of Obstetricians and Gynaecologists of Canada. Guidelines for operative vaginal birth. *J Obstet Gynaecol Can*. 2004; 26: 747–53.

6. Chalmers JA, Chalmers I. The obstetric vacuum extractor is the instrument of first choice for operative vaginal delivery. *Br J Obstet Gynaecol*. 1989; 96: 505–6.

7. Ben-Haroush A, Melamed N, Kaplan B, Yogev Y. Predictors of failed operative vaginal delivery: a single-center experience. *Am J Obstet Gynecol*. 2007; 197: e301–5.

8. Johanson RB, Menon BK. Vacuum extraction versus forceps for assisted vaginal delivery. *Cochrane Database Syst Rev*. 2000; 2. CD000224.

9. Towner D, Castro MA, Eby-Wilkens E, Gilbert WM. Effect of mode of delivery in nulliparous women on neonatal intracranial injury. *N Engl J Med*. 1999; 341: 1709–14.

10. American College of Obstetricians and Gynecologists. *Operative Vaginal Delivery*. Washington, DC: ACOG; 2000.

11. NICE. Intrapartum care: care of healthy women and their babies during childbirth: clinical guideline 190; 2014. www.nice.org.uk.

12. NICE. *Intrapartum Care: Care of Healthy Women and their Babies during Childbirth*: Clinical Guideline 190. London: National Institute for Health and Clinical Excellence; 2007.

13. Stride PC, Cooper GM. Dural tap revisited: a 20 year survey from Birmingham Maternity hospital. *Anaesthesia*. 1993; 48: 247–55.

14. Simonson C, Barlow P, Dehennin N, *et al*. Neonatal complications of vacuum-assisted delivery. *Obstet Gynecol*. 2007; 109: 626–33.

15. RCOG. Operative vaginal delivery: Green-top Guideline No. 26; 2011. www.rcog.org.uk/en/guidelines-research-services/guidelines/gtg26/.

16. McQuivey RW. Vacuum-assisted delivery: a review. *J Matern Fetal Neonatal Med*. 2004; 16: 171–80.

17. Edozien LC. Towards safe practice in instrumental vaginal delivery. *Best Pract Res Clin Obstet Gynaecol*. 2007; 21: 639–55.

18. Akmal S, Kametas N, Tsoi E, Hargreaves C, Nicolaides KH. Comparison of transvaginal digital examination with intrapartum sonography to determine fetal head position before instrumental delivery. *Ultrasound Obstet Gynecol*. 2003; 21: 437–40.

19. Sherer DM, Miodovnik M, Bradley KS, Langer O. Intrapartum fetal head position II: comparison between transvaginal digital examination and transabdominal ultrasound assessment during the second stage of labor. *Ultrasound Obstet Gynecol*. 2002; 19: 264–8.

20. Henrich W, Dudenhausen J, Fuchs I, Kamena A, Tutschek B. Intrapartum translabial ultrasound (ITU): sonographic landmarks and correlation with successful vacuum extraction. *Ultrasound Obstet Gynecol*. 2006; 28: 753–60.

21. Zahalka N, Sadan O, Malinger G, *et al*. Comparison of transvaginal sonography with digital examination and transabdominal sonography for the determination of fetal head position in the second stage of labor. *Am J Obstet Gynecol*. 2005; 193: 381–6.

22. Liabsuetrakul T, Choobun T, Peeyananjarassri K, Islam Q. Antibiotic prpophylaxis for operative vaginal delivery. *Cochrane Database Syst Rev*. 2014; 10. CD004455. doi: 10.1002/14651858.CD004455.pub3.

23. Murphy DJ, Liebling RE, Verity L, Swingler R, Patel R. Early maternal and neonatal morbidity associated with operative delivery in second stage of labour: a cohort study. *Lancet*. 2001; 358: 1203–7.

24. Johanson R, Menon V. Soft versus rigid vacuum extractor cups for assisted vaginal delivery. *Cochrane Database Syst Rev*. 2000; 11. CD000446. doi: 10.1002/14651858.CD000446.pub2.

25. Vacca A. Vacuum-assisted delivery. *Best Pract Res Clin Obstet Gynaecol*. 2002; 16: 17–30.

26. Boo NY, Foong KW, Mahdy ZA, Yong SC, Jaafar R. Risk factors associated with subaponeurotic haemorrhage in full-term infants exposed to vacuum extraction. *Br J Obstet Gynaecol*. 2005; 112: 1516–21.

27. Suwannachat B, Lumbiganon P, Laopaiboon M. Applying negative pressure rapidly or in steps for vacuum extraction assisted vaginal delivery. *Cochrane Database Syst Rev*. 2012; 8. CD006636. doi: 10.1002/14651858.CD006636.pub3.

28. Whitlow BJ, Tamizian O, Ashworth J, *et al*. Validation of traction force indicator in ventouse devices. *Int J Gynecol Obstet*. 2005; 90: 35–8.

29. Vacca A. Vacuum-assisted delivery: an analysis of traction force and maternal and neonatal outcomes. *Aust NZ J Obstet Gynaecol*. 2006; 46: 124–7.

30. Nikpoor P, Bain E. Analgesia for forceps delivery. *Cochrane Database Syst Rev*. 2013; 9. CD008878.

31. Barth WH. Persistent occiput posterior. *Obstet Gynecol*. 2015; 125: 695–709.

32. Johnstone T. Minimising risk: obstetric skills training. *Clin Risk*. 2003; 9; 99–102.

33. Menticoglou SM, Perlman M, Manning FA. High cervical spinal cord injury in neonates delivered with forceps: report of 15 cases. *Obstet Gynecol*. 1995; 86: 589–94.

34. Pallasmaa N, Ekblad U, Gissler M. Severe maternal morbidity and the mode of delivery. *Acta Obstet Gynecol Scand*. 2008; 87: 662–8.

35. Johanson RB, Rice C, Doyle M, *et al*. A randomised prospective study comparing the new vacuum extractor policy with forceps delivery. *Br J Obstet Gynaecol*. 1993; 100: 524–30.

36. Wen SW, Liu S, Kramer MS, *et al*. Comparison of maternal and infant outcomes between vacuum extraction and forceps deliveries. *Am J Epidemiol*. 2001; 153: 103–7.

37. Johnson JH, Figueroa R, Garry D, Elimian A, Maulik D. Immediate maternal and neonatal effects of forceps and vacuum-assisted deliveries. *Obstet Gynecol*. 2004; 103: 513–18.

38. Harkin R, Fitzpatrick M, O'Connell PR, O'Herlihy C. Anal sphincter disruption at vaginal delivery: is recurrence predictable? *Eur J Obstet Gynecol Reprod Biol*. 2003; 109: 149–52.

39. Damron DP, Capeless EL. Operative vaginal delivery: a comparison of forceps and vacuum for success rate and risk of rectal sphincter injury. *Am J Obstet Gynecol*. 2004; 191: 907–10.

40. Wu JM, Williams KS, Hundley AF, Connolly A, Visco AG. Occiput posterior fetal head position increases the risk of anal sphincter injury in vacuum-assisted deliveries. *Am J Obstet Gynecol*. 2005; 193: 525–8; discussion 528–9.

41. Rieger N, Schloithe A, Saccone G, Wattchow D. The effect of a normal vaginal delivery on anal function. *Acta Obstet Gynecol Scand*. 1997; 76: 769–72.

42. Nygaard IE, Rao SS, Dawson JD. Anal incontinence after anal sphincter disruption: a 30-year retrospective cohort study. *Obstet Gynecol*. 1997; 89: 896–901.

43. Dimpfl T, Hesse U, Schussler B. Incidence and cause of postpartum urinary stress incontinence. *Eur J Obstet Gynecol Reprod Biol*. 1992; 43: 29–33.

44. Arya LA, Jackson ND, Myers DL, Verma A. Risk of new-onset urinary incontinence after forceps and vacuum delivery in primiparous women. *Am J Obstet Gynecol*. 2001; 185: 1318–23; discussion 1323–4.

45. Liebling RE, Swingler R, Patel RR, *et al*. Pelvic floor morbidity up to one year after difficult instrumental delivery and cesarean section in the second stage of labor: a cohort study. *Am J Obstet Gynecol*. 2004; 191: 4–10.

46. Lavender T, Walkinshaw SA. Can midwives reduce postpartum psychological morbidity? A randomized trial. *Birth*. 1998; 25: 215–19.

47. Murphy DI, Pope C, Frost J, Liebling RE. Women's views on the impact of operative delivery in the second stage of labour: quality interview study. *BMJ*. 2003; 327: 1132.

48. Hayman R, Gilby J, Arulkumaran S. Clinical evaluation of a 'hand pump' vacuum delivery device. *Obstet Gynecol*. 2002; 100: 1190–5.

49. Attilakos G, Sibanda T, Winter C, Johnson N, Draycott T. A randomised controlled trial of a new handheld vacuum extraction device. *Br J Obstet Gynaecol*. 2005; 112: 1510–15.

50. Gebremariam A. Subgaleal haemorrhage: risk factors and neurological and developmental outcome in survivors. *Ann Trop Paediatr*. 1999; 19: 45–50.

51. Uchil D, Arulkumaran S. Neonatal subgaleal hemorrhage and its relationship to delivery by vacuum extraction. *Obstet Gynecol Surv*. 2003; 58: 687–93.

52. O'Mahony F, Settatree R, Platt C, Johanson R. Review of singleton fetal and neonatal deaths associated with cranial trauma and cephalic delivery during a national intrapartum-related confidential enquiry. *Br J Obstet Gynaecol*. 2005; 112: 619–26.

53. Doumouchtsis SK, Arulkumaran S. Head injuries after instrumental vaginal deliveries. *Curr Opin Obstet Gynecol*. 2006; 18: 129–34.

54. Perlman JM. Brain injury in the term infant. *Semin Perinatol*. 2004; 28: 415–24.

55. Gilbert WM, Nesbitt TS, Danielsen B. Associated factors in 1611 cases of brachial plexus injury. *Obstet Gynecol*. 1999; 93: 536–40.

56. Mills JF, Dargaville PA, Coleman LT, Rosenfeld JV, Ekert PG. Upper cervical spinal cord injury in neonates: the use of magnetic resonance imaging. *J Pediatr*. 2001; 138: 105–8.

57. Berkus MD, Ramamurthy RS, O'Connor PS, Brown K, Hayashi RH. Cohort study of silastic obstetric vacuum cup deliveries: I. Safety of the instrument. *Obstet Gynecol*. 1985; 66: 503–9.

58. Williams MC, Knuppel RA, O'Brien WF, *et al*. Obstetric correlates of neonatal retinal hemorrhage. *Obstet Gynecol*. 1993; 81: 688–94.

59. O'Mahoney F, Hofmeyr G, Menon V. Choice of instruments for assisted vaginal delivery. *Cochrane*

Database Sys Rev. 2010; 11. CD005455. doi: 10.1002/14651858.CD005455.pub2.

60. Sadan O, Ginath S, Gomel A, *et al.* What to do after a failed attempt of vacuum delivery? *Eur J Obstet Gynecol Reprod Biol.* 2003; 107: 151–5.

61. Gardella C, Taylor M, Benedetti T, Hitti J, Critchlow C. The effect of sequential use of vacuum and forceps for assisted vaginal delivery on neonatal and maternal outcomes. *Am J Obstet Gynecol.* 2001; 185: 896–902.

Chapter 10

Caesarean Deliveries
Indications, Techniques and Complications

Gerard H. A. Visser

Introduction

Caesarean sections (CSs) are nowadays one of the most frequently performed operative procedures. Although relatively safe, they are associated with both short- and long-term complications. Moreover, incidences of up to 50% and even higher have nothing to do with evidence-based medicine and may result in an impaired long-term outcome of the offspring, rather than in a better outcome. In this chapter, classification, indications, techniques and complications of CSs are reviewed. The rising CS rates are discussed critically. This chapter is an updated and thoroughly revised version of the one published in 2009 [1].

Classification of CS

The traditional classification of CS as elective or emergency is too simplistic, making detailed comparison impossible. Distinguishing between prelabour CS (which varies from elective to emergency) and intrapartum CS (which are, by definition, more or less emergency) is preferable (Table 10.1, part A). With such a classification the urgency of the procedure is indicated, which is important for the anaesthesiology team. In case of emergency the time between indication and first incision should preferably be less than 30 min. In the other cases the timing may (should) be decided together with the anaesthesiologist. In the UK, NICE has recommended a system of classification based on the urgency of the situation, irrespective of a prelabour or intrapartum indication, and is given in Table 10.1, part B [2].

For quality assessment and (inter)national comparison, one may also use the so-called ten-group classification (Table 10.2) [3]. In a comparison between nine institutional cohorts it was found that overall CS rates correlate strongly with CS rates in singleton cephalic nullipara ($r = 0.99$). So, if you consider your CS rate too high, then review the indications in this subgroup. CS rates in induced labour were found to be similar to spontaneous labours and greatest institutional variation was found in spontaneously labouring multipara (6.7-fold difference) and nulliparas (3.7-fold difference). The World Health Organization (WHO) proposes this classification system as a global standard for assessing, monitoring and comparing CS rates within healthcare facilities over time, and between facilities [4].

Indications for CS

A CS is performed when it is perceived to be a safer method of delivery for the mother and/or baby than delivery by the vaginal route. However, when considering a CS the future reproductive career of the woman should also be taken into account. For instance, a CS in case of breech presentation is likely to reduce perinatal mortality [5,6], but the risk of uterine rupture and/or placenta accreta/increta in a subsequent pregnancy may hamper some of this advantage. This is illustrated by case reports of maternal death due to and following a pregnancy ending in a CS because of breech presentation [7]. Caesarean section for twins has become standard in many countries, but in a recent large randomized controlled trial no improved outcome was found in women randomized to CS [8].

There are numerous indications for CS. A not-exhaustive list is shown in Box 10.1.

Best Practice in Labour and Delivery, Second Edition, ed. Sir Sabaratnam Arulkumaran. Published by Cambridge University Press. © Cambridge University Press 2016.

Table 10.1 Classification of urgency of caesarean section. (A) Differentiation between prelabour and intrapartum; (B) the system used in the UK based on the NICE Guidelines

A. Differentiation between prelabour and intrapartum

1. Prelabour	Emergency because of immediate threat to the life of the woman or fetus (e.g. abruption)
	Maternal or fetal compromise, not immediately life threatening (e.g. pre-eclampsia, severe fetal growth restriction)
	Timed delivery (e.g. previous CS with fibroids; breech presentation at term)
	Elective (e.g. maternal request)
2. Intrapartum	Emergency because of immediate threat to the life of the woman or fetus (e.g. abruption, uterine rupture, cord prolapse, fetal bradycardia)
	Sub-acute (e.g. failure to progress)
B. UK system based on the NICE Guidelines [2]	The urgency of CS should be documented using the following standardized scheme in order to aid clear communication between healthcare professionals about the urgency of a CS:
	1. Immediate threat to the life of the woman or fetus (*immediate*)
	2. Maternal or fetal compromise which is not immediately life threatening (*urgent*)
	3. No maternal or fetal compromise but needs early delivery (*scheduled*)
	4. Delivery to suit the woman or staff (*elective*)

Table 10.2 Ten-group CS classification as a global standard for assessing, monitoring and comparing CS rates within healthcare facilities over time, and between facilities [3, with permission]

Group	Classification
1	Nulliparous, single cephalic, ≥37 weeks, in spontaneous labour
2	Nulliparous, single cephalic, ≥37 weeks induced (including prelabour CS)
3	Multiparous (excluding previous CS), single cephalic, ≥37 weeks, in spontaneous labour
4	Multiparous (excluding previous CS), single cephalic, ≥37 weeks, induced (including prelabour CS)
5	Previous CS, single cephalic, ≥37 weeks
6	All nulliparous breeches
7	All multiparous breeches (including previous CS)
8	All multiple pregnancies (including previous CS)
9	All transverse/oblique lies (including previous CS)
10	All preterm single cephalic, <37 weeks, including previous CS

The Incidence of CS

CS rates have dramatically increased during the last few decades, without evidence of substantial improvements in outcome [11]. Factors related to this increase are summarized in Figure 10.1, starting with electronic fetal monitoring introduced in the early 1970s, to medico-legal issues, financial incentives to attending physicians and traffic jams preventing the doctor arriving in time from a private office to the hospital (see [11]).

Nowadays, CS rates vary considerably, from less than 20% in the north of Europe to 50% in the south of Europe and China and to even higher rates in South America [11]. This large range indicates that CS rates have nothing to do with evidence-based medicine. It is more likely due to a loss of practical skills, erroneous interpretation of fetal electronic monitoring tracings, an increase in inductions of labour (without giving it a proper try), the loss of care during labour, financial incentives, outpatient clinics far away from the birthing centre and – last but not least – medico-legal issues. In 2015, the WHO issued a revised statement on CS rates [3]. They conducted two studies: a systematic review of available studies that had sought to find the ideal CS rate within a given country or population, and a worldwide country-level analysis using the latest available data. Based on these available data, and using internationally accepted methods to assess the evidence with the most appropriate analytical techniques, the WHO concluded: '1) That CSs are effective in saving maternal and infant lives, but only when they are required for medically indicated reasons, and 2) That at population level, CS rates higher than 10% are not associated with reductions in maternal and newborn mortality rates' [4].

Attempts to reduce CS rates have not been effective thus far, maybe with the exception of the north of Portugal. In 2011 a project started that included: (a) a uniform classification of CS; (b) dissemination of knowledge; (c) publication of CS rates per hospital; (d) equal doctor's fee for CS and vaginal delivery; (e) financing of hospitals based on CS rate (a lower amount in cases of high rates); and (f) implementation of STAN technology for fetal surveillance. Since then the CS rate not only was reduced in the north of

Box 10.1 Indications for Caesarean Section

1. Prelabour – maternal

Surgical Scarred uterus following previous myomectomy. Previous classical CS, more than two previous lower segment CSs. In case of one previous lower segment incision there is an estimated 0.5% risk of scar rupture and maternal preference should influence the mode of delivery. Previous anal sphincter damage with symptoms, or abnormal endoanal ultrasound or manometry may worsen during a subsequent vaginal delivery and these women should be given the option of an elective CS.

Ovarian cyst/myoma Allows surgical removal of the cyst, and in cases in which they obstruct the pelvis.

Medical Certain maternal diseases may necessitate a CS, such as Marfan syndrome with a dilated aortic root.

Psychological The reasons why a woman wishes to have a CS 'on maternal request' should be explored. Counselling, starting preferably early in pregnancy, might be indicated should they describe fear of childbirth. The risks and benefits of the procedure should be explained in order to ensure the woman has made a fully informed decision. A clinician has the right to refuse to perform a CS on the grounds of maternal request alone [8] but all efforts should be directed towards a consensus between patient and doctor.

2. Prelabour – fetal

Mechanical Transverse lie, certain congenital malformations, breech presentation. In case of breech presentation, external cephalic version should be offered. The benefits of a CS for the current pregnancy outcome should be discussed in relation to future reproductive wishes and associated complications (placenta accreta, uterine rupture, etc.).

Fetal compromise/severe IUGR In case of antenatal fetal heart rate (FHR) abnormalities indicative of hypoxaemia or anaemia, a CS should be performed. The same holds for early IUGR with severe fetal Doppler abnormalities. At present there are no data to suggest that a term small-for-gestational-age fetus is better off by being delivered by CS.

Vasa praevia This may be detected antenatally by ultrasound and Doppler. Elective CS is indicated to avoid rapid exsanguination that is associated with tearing of the fetal vessels.

3. Prelabour–feto-maternal

Placental abruption, placenta praevia and eclampsia may be put in this category. In case of maternal eclampsia, (blood pressure) stabilization is indicated before CS.

4. Intrapartum fetal distress

Emergency CS is indicated in acute causes of fetal distress, like cord prolapse, uterine rupture, abruptio placentae or ruptured vasa praevia. In other cases of abnormal CTG patterns adjunct technologies like fetal scalp blood sampling or scalp stimulation may prevent unnecessary CSs and the same holds for therapeutic measures such as amnioinfusion and reduction of excessive (induced) contractions. Acute tocolysis with either beta-mimetic drugs or oxytocin receptor blockers may also improve the fetal condition while awaiting a CS [9,10].

5. Intrapartum feto-maternal

Failure to progress and cephalo-pelvic disproportion/malpresentation are the most frequent reasons for intrapartum CS. In case of failure to progress in the absence of obvious disproportion or malpresentation, rupture of the membranes and oxytocin administration should be considered.

Portugal, but in the whole country, from about 36% to 33% [12].

Techniques

Discussions concerning the technique of CS mostly concentrate on the more classical approach, cutting all layers, as compared to a more digital approach, the so-called Joel-Cohen method, and to the closure of the uterus in one or two layers.

The modified Joel-Cohen method is associated with a lower duration of the operation, less blood loss, lower rate of need for postoperative analgesia and lower febrile morbidity as compared to the

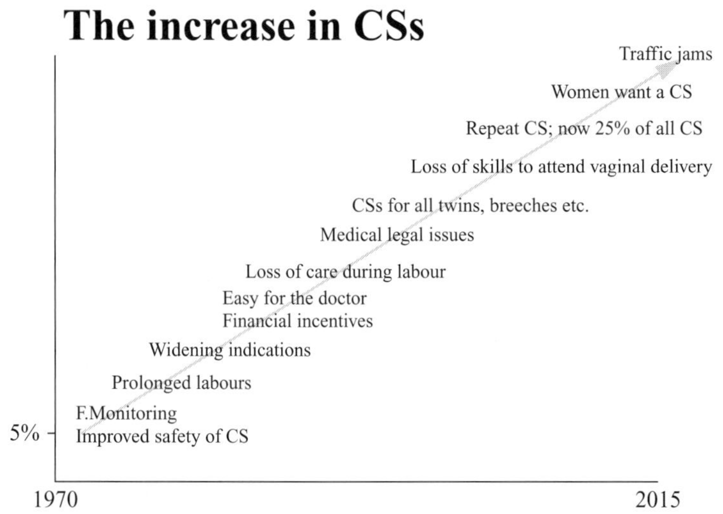

The increase in CSs

Figure 10.1 Schematic representation of factors that (may) have contributed to an increase in CS rate with time [11].

Traffic jams

Women want a CS

Repeat CS; now 25% of all CS

Loss of skills to attend vaginal delivery

CSs for all twins, breeches etc.

Medical legal issues

Loss of care during labour

Easy for the doctor

Financial incentives

Widening indications

Prolonged labours

F.Monitoring

5% — Improved safety of CS

1970   2015

Pfannenstiel method [13,14,15] and is, therefore, the current method of first choice, despite the fact it initially looks a more barbaric method used by doctors who do not seem to know the correct surgical procedures. The procedure is summarized – and recommended and referenced – in the latest NICE guidelines [2], and is shown in Box 10.2.

Some comments that can be made regarding the NICE guidelines relate to the use of oxytocin or carbetocin after the baby has been delivered, to exteriorization of the uterus, to single- or double-layer closure of the uterus and closure of the skin.

The long-acting oxytocin derivate carbetocin has been developed to reduce postpartum haemorrhage following a CS. A recent Cochrane review has indicated that this agent significantly reduced the need for therapeutic uterotonics as compared to oxytocin (RR 0.62 [95% CI 0.44–0.88]), without reducing the overall incidence of postpartum haemorrhage [16].

Exteriorization of the uterus after the baby has been delivered is generally not necessary and should not be performed routinely. However, it may be useful in case inspection and suturing of the wound is found to be difficult, for instance in case of lateral tears and/or substantial blood loss.

Earlier studies have shown that single-layer closure using locked stitches was associated with a higher risk of uterine rupture in subsequent pregnancies, as compared to double-layer closure (RR 4.96, significant) [17]. This was not found when unlocked stitches were used (RR 0.49, ns (not significant)). A review

published in 2014 did not find an increased risk for uterine scar rupture (RR 0.86, ns) in those with single-layer closure when compared with double-layer closure [18]. The thickness of the lower uterine segment, however, was found to be slightly but significantly thinner in the subsequent pregnancy (15 as compared to 17.6 mm). Operation time was significantly shorter in the former group. Finally, in a recent large Swedish cohort study it was found that factors from the first delivery by CS that were associated with uterine rupture in a subsequent pregnancy were maternal age ≥35 years (adjusted odds ratio (OR) 2.1), maternal height <160 cm (OR 1.7), large-for-gestational-age infant (OR 2.4) and infection (OR 2.1), but not one-layer closure of the uterus [19]. So, for the time being it may be concluded that one-layer closure of the uterus is sufficient. Stitches should not be locked, since this may affect the local circulation, resulting in necrosis.

Suturing the skin is likely to be associated with a lower incidence of wound complications than closure using staples (adjusted OR 0.4; [20]). Subcuticular suture is definitely the preference of the patient and also an objective overall cosmetic assessment favours sutures as compared to staples [20,21].

Finally, in cases of difficulties delivering the fetal head, a (disposable) ventouse may be used instead of forceps. Delivery of the placenta by controlled traction instead of by manual removal is not only associated with a lower incidence of endometritis, but also with a lower amount of blood loss [22].

Box 10.2 Procedure for CS according to the 2011 NICE guidelines [2]

Abdominal wall incision CS should be performed using a transverse abdominal incision because this is associated with less postoperative pain and an improved cosmetic effect compared with a midline incision. The transverse incision of choice should be the Joel-Cohen incision (a straight skin incision, 3 cm above the symphysis pubis; subsequent tissue layers are opened bluntly and, if necessary, extended with scissors and not a knife), because it is associated with shorter operating times and reduced postoperative febrile morbidity.

Instruments for skin incision The use of separate surgical knives to incise the skin and the deeper tissues at CS is not recommended because it does not decrease wound infection.

Extension of the uterine incision When there is a well-formed lower uterine segment, blunt rather than sharp extension of the uterine incision should be used because it reduces blood loss, incidence of postpartum haemorrhage and the need for transfusion at CS.

Fetal laceration Women who are having a CS should be informed that the risk of fetal laceration is about 2%.

Use of forceps Forceps should only be used at CS if there is difficulty delivering the baby's head. The effect on neonatal morbidity of the routine use of forceps at CS remains uncertain.

Use of uterotonics Oxytocin 5 IU by slow intravenous injection should be used at CS to encourage contraction of the uterus and to decrease blood loss.

Method of placental removal At CS, the placenta should be removed using controlled cord traction and not manual removal as this reduces the risk of endometritis.

Exteriorization of the uterus Intraperitoneal repair of the uterus at CS should be undertaken. Exteriorization of the uterus is not recommended because it is associated with more pain and does not improve operative outcomes such as haemorrhage and infection.

Closure of the uterus The effectiveness and safety of single-layer closure of the uterine incision is uncertain. Except within a research context, the uterine incision should be sutured with two layers.

Closure of the peritoneum Neither the visceral nor the parietal peritoneum should be sutured at CS because this reduces operating time and the need for postoperative analgesia, and improves maternal satisfaction.

Closure of the abdominal wall In the rare circumstances that a midline abdominal incision is used at CS, mass closure with slowly absorbable continuous sutures should be used because this results in fewer incisional hernias and less dehiscence than layered closure.

Closure of subcutaneous tissue Routine closure of the subcutaneous tissue space should not be used, unless the woman has more than 2 cm subcutaneous fat, because it does not reduce the incidence of wound infection.

Use of superficial wound drains Superficial wound drains should not be used at CS because they do not decrease the incidence of wound infection or wound haematoma.

Closure of the skin Obstetricians should be aware that the effects of different suture materials or methods of skin closure at CS are not certain.

Complications

Complications of CS may be directly related to the operation itself (direct complications) or to consequences for future pregnancies. Complications for the infant concern an iatrogenic early delivery, which may result in direct neonatal morbidity, or to long-term consequences of being born by CS.

Early Maternal Complications

Direct maternal morbidity due to a CS is infrequent. Still, a publication from Asia on maternal complications following elective CS showed a 2.7-fold increased risk of composite morbidity/mortality (maternal mortality, ICU admission, blood transfusion, hysterectomy and internal iliac artery ligation) for an elective antepartum CS and a relative risk of 14.2 for an elective intrapartum CS [23]. Rather frequent complications are bladder injury while opening the peritoneum and haemorrhage from the uterus or incision site, usually the edges. Tachycardia, oliguria or pallor should alert the care giver of a postoperative haemorrhage, either intrauterine, intraperitoneal or in the abdominal wound. Normal blood pressure should not reassure, as hypotension is a late sign. Early return to the theatre may be indicated.

Women having a CS are at increased risk of venous thromboembolic disease (VTE) due to their pregnancy and surgery. Other risk factors include obesity, immobility, thrombophilia, family history and previous history of VTE. It is one of the leading causes of maternal death in the UK [24], and substandard care is

Table 10.3 Placenta praevia and accreta associated with prelabour CS [28]

Prior CS	Number of women	Placenta accreta	Hysterectomy	Percentage of cases of accreta in women with placenta praevia
0	6201	15 (0.24%)	40 (0.65%)	3
1	15 808	49 (0.31%)	67 (0.42%)	11
2	6324	36 (0.57%)	57 (0.9%)	40
3	1452	31 (2.13%)	35 (2.4%)	61
4	258	6 (2.33%)	9 (3.49%)	67
≥5	89	6 (6.74%)	8 (8.99%)	

most commonly due to a failure to recognize the signs and symptoms or failure to implement appropriate thrombo-prophylaxis.

Late maternal complications include a lesser desire for future children, as well as a decreased ability to conceive [25]. The risk of stillbirth in a subsequent pregnancy has been found to be double in women who had a CS compared to women who had a vaginal delivery; however, this population of women form a higher-risk group, which introduces bias [26]. Recently it was found that the risk for spontaneous preterm birth might be increased following a previous CS [27].

The largest risks of a previous CS are uterine rupture, placenta praevia and placenta accreta/increta in a subsequent pregnancy. The risk of uterine rupture is approximately 0.5–1% in subsequent labours. In about 10% of cases of rupture the fetus will die. Counselling of women as to these risks is important and most obstetricians will do a CS if the patient requests one. However, a vaginal birth after caesarean (VBAC) is a good alternative, provided that an experienced team and operating room facilities are readily available 24 hours per day, seven days per week. The more CS a woman has had, the greater the chance of placenta praevia in a future pregnancy, and the higher the risk of a placenta praevia/accreta [28]; Table 10.3). The risk of a hysterectomy due to a placenta increta is about 1 in 25 000 in women without a CS scar and 1 in 500 after one CS [29].

The most important *direct fetal complications* are related to iatrogenic early prelabour CS. In some countries, 30–40% of CSs for breech presentation or repeat CS are performed before 39 weeks of gestation, putting the infant at a four-fold increased risk of pulmonary problems at 37–38 weeks and a two-fold increased risk at 38–39 weeks, with additional risks related to treated hypoglycaemia, admission to the NICU, neonatal sepsis and hyper bilirubin-

aemia [30,31]. Elective prelabour CSs should not be performed before 39 weeks of gestation, unless there is evidence of fetal lung maturity [32]. However, many doctors ignore this advice and give antenatal corticosteroids to enhance fetal lung maturation. This medication works, also close to term [33,34], but corticosteroids are powerful drugs with significant side-effects. Elective prelabour CS should not be performed before 39 weeks of gestation!

Large observational studies have shown associations between CSs and *immunological and weight problems in the offspring*. The incidence of both type 1 diabetes and childhood asthma is increased by 20–30%, and the same holds for overweight and obesity. These relations are most likely causal and may – among others – be induced by an altered colonization of the gastrointestinal tract [11,35]. These data emphasize the consequences of the current exaggerated interference with the normal birth process.

Conclusions

The rate of CS is increasing; however, the procedure has become safer due to the use of antibiotics, awareness of the need for thrombo-prophylaxis and coherent delivery suite guidelines for the management of postpartum haemorrhage. There is, however, no place for complacency; the decision to perform each CS should be taken critically, balancing the pros and cons for that particular individual. Meticulous planning and surgical attention to detail should help to minimize the risks of the procedure, and good analgesia and early mobilization should help limit postoperative morbidity. Local procedures should be in place to monitor CS practice in terms of indications for the procedure, standards of clinical care provided and complications encountered. Active critical review should help to inform practice and capitalize on safety.

It should not be forgotten that women are designed to deliver vaginally and not by CS [11].

References

1. Story L, Paterson-Brown S. Cesarean deliveries: indications, techniques and complications. In Warren R, Arulkumaran S (eds), *Best Practice in Labour and Delivery* (pp. 104–15). Cambridge: Cambridge University Press; 2009.

2. RCOG, RCM, NICE. *Caesarean Section*. London: RCOG Press; 2011.

3. Brennan DJ, Robson MC, Murphy M, O'Herlihy C. Comparative analysis of international cesarean delivery rates using 10-group classification identifies significant variation in spontaneous labor. *Am J Obstet Gynecol*. 2009;201: 308.e1–8.

4. WHO. WHO statement on caesarean section rates. WHO/RHR/15.02. 2015. www.who.int/reproductive health/publications/maternal_perinatal_health/cs-statement/en.

5. Hannah ME, Hannah WJ, Hewson SA, *et al.* Planned caesarean section versus planned vaginal birth for breech presentation at term: a randomized multicenter trial. *Lancet*. 2000;356: 1375–83.

6. Rietberg CCT, Elferink-Stinkens PM, Visser GHA. The effect of the Term Breech Trial on medical intervention behaviour and neonatal outcome in the Netherlands: an analysis of 35,453 term breech infants. *Brit J Obstet Gynaecol*. 2005;112: 205–9.

7. Schutte JM, de Boer K, Briët JW, *et al.* Moedersterfte in Nederland: het topje van de ijsberg. *Ned Tijdschr Obstet Gynaecol*. 2005;118: 89–91. (In Dutch)

8. Barrett JF, Hannah ME, Hutton EK, *et al.* A randomized trial of planned cesarean or vaginal delivery for twin pregnancy. *N Engl J Med*. 2013;369: 1295–305.

9. Briozzo L, Martinez A, Nozar M, *et al.* Tocolysis and delayed delivery versus emergency delivery in cases of non-reassuring fetal status during labor. *J Obstet Gynaecol Res*. 2007;33: 266–73.

10. De Heus R, Mulder EJ, Derks JB, *et al.* A prospective randomized trial of acute tocolysis in term labour with atosiban or ritodrine. *Eur J Obstet Gynecol Reprod Biol*. 2008;139(2): 139–45.

11. Visser GHA. Women are designed to deliver vaginally and not by Cesarean Section; an obstetrician's view. *Neonatology*. 2015;107: 8–13.

12. Ayres-De-Campos D, Cruz J, Medeiros-Borges C, Costa-Santos C, Vicente L. Lowered national cesarean section rates after a concerted action. *Acta Obstet Gynecol Scand*. 2015;94: 391–8.

13. Darj E, Nordström ML. The Misgav Ladach method for cesarean section compared to the Pfannenstiel method. *Acta Obstet Gynecol Scand*. 1999;78: 37–41.

14. Mathai M, Hofmeyr GJ, Mathai NE. Abdominal surgical incisions for caesarean section. *Cochrane Database Syst Rev*. 2013;5: CD004453.

15. Gizzo S, Andrisani A, Noventa M, *et al.* Caesarean section: could different transverse abdominal incision techniques influence postpartum pain and subsequent quality of life? A systematic review. *PLoS One*. 2015;10(2): e0114190.

16. Su LL, Chong YS, Samuel M. Carbetocin for preventing post-partum haemorrhage. *Cochrane Database Syst Rev*. 2012;2: CD005457.

17. Roberge S, Chaillet N, Boutin A, *et al.* Single- versus double-layer closure of the hysterotomy incision during cesarean delivery and risk of uterine rupture. *Int J Gynaecol Obstet*. 2011;115: 5–10.

18. Roberge S, Demers S, Berghella V, *et al.* Impact of single- vs double-layer closure on adverse outcomes and uterine scar defect: a systematic review and metaanalysis. *Am J Obstet Gynecol*. 2014;211: 453–60.

19. Hesselman S, Hogberg U, Ekholm-Selling K, Råssjö EB, Jonsson M. The risk of uterine rupture is not increased with single- compared with double-layer closure: a Swedish cohort study. *Brit J Obstet Gynaecol*. 2014; 122(11): 1535–41. doi: 10.1111/1471-0528.13015.

20. Mackeen AD, Schuster M, Berghella V. Suture versus staples for skin closure after cesarean: a metaanalysis. *Am J Obstet Gynecol*. 2015;212: e1–621.

21. Aabakke AJ, Krebs L, Pipper CB, Secher NJ. Subcuticular suture compared with staples for skin closure after cesarean delivery: a randomized controlled trial. *Obstet Gynecol*. 2013;122(4): 878–84.

22. Anorlu RI, Maholwana B, Hofmeyr GJ. Methods of delivering the placenta at caesarean section. *Cochrane Database Syst Rev*. 2008;16(3): CD004737.

23. Lumbiganon P, Laopaiboon M, Gülmezoglu AM, *et al.* Method of delivery and pregnancy outcomes in Asia: the WHO global survey on maternal and perinatal health. *Lancet*. 2010;375: 490–9.

24. CEMACH. *Saving Mothers' Lives*. London: CEMACH; 2007.

25. Jolly J, Walker J, Bhara K. Subsequent obstetric performance related to primary mode of delivery. *Br J Obstet Gynaecol*. 1999;106: 227–32.

26. Smith GC, Pell JP, Dobbie R. Caesarean section and risk of unexplained stillbirth in subsequent pregnancy. *Lancet*. 2003;362: 1779–84.

27. Di Renzo GC, Giardina I, Rosati A, *et al*. GC maternal risk factors for preterm birth: a country-based population analysis. *Eur J Obstet Gynecol Reprod Biol*. 2011;159: 342–6.

28. Silver RM, Landon MB, Rouse DJ, *et al*. Maternal morbidity associated with multiple repeat cesarean deliveries. *Obstet Gynecol*. 2006;107: 1226–32.

29. Kwee A, Bots ML, Visser GH, Bruinse HW. Emergency peripartum hysterectomy: a prospective study in the Netherlands. *Eur J Obstet Gynecol Reprod Biol*. 2006;124(2): 187–92.

30. Tita AT, Landon MB, Spong CY, *et al*. Timing of elective repeat cesarean delivery at term and neonatal outcomes. *N Engl J Med*. 2009;360: 111–20.

31. Wilmink FA, Hukkelhoven CW, Lunshof S, *et al*. Neonatal outcome following elective cesarean section beyond 37 weeks of gestation: a 7-year retrospective study of a national registry. *Am J Obstet Gynecol*. 2010;202: e1–8.

32. ACOG. Committee opinion no. 394: cesarean delivery on maternal request. *Obstet Gynecol*. 2007;110: 1501.

33. Stutchfield P, Whitaker R, Russell I. Antenatal betamethasone and incidence of neonatal respiratory distress after elective caesarean section: pragmatic randomised trial. *BMJ*. 2005;331(7518): 662.

34. Ahmed MR, Sayed Ahmed WA, Mohammed TY. Antenatal steroids at 37 weeks, does it reduce neonatal respiratory morbidity? A randomized trial. *J Matern Fetal Neonatal Med*. 2014;22: 1486–90.

35. Cho CE, Norman M. Cesarean section and development of the immune system in offspring. *Am J Obstet Gynecol*. 2013;208(4): 249–54. doi: 10.1016/j.ajog.2012.08.009.

Breech and Twin Delivery

Stephen Walkinshaw

Approximately 3–4% of singleton births involve a breech presentation. Experience with vaginal breech birth is reducing in 'Westernized' healthcare settings. Twins account for an increasing proportion of births, usually around 1%, but in some populations it is 2–3%, with contributions from both reproductive technology and increasing age. Like breech birth, there has been a move towards caesarean section (CS) as the mode of twin birth and a consequent reduction in exposure to the range of manoeuvres needed to manage the second twin.

Despite these trends, vaginal breech births and vaginal twin births occur regularly on the labour ward, and all practitioners will need both an understanding of the mechanisms of birth and skills in safe conduct of such births.

Breech Birth

Breech Birth at Term

Whatever the criticisms of the Term Breech Trial [1], in most healthcare settings its publication accelerated the trend to elective caesarean birth for breech presentation at term. Overall the trial showed benefit in serious short-term outcomes, but no increased long-term morbidity in survivors. Although many have downplayed the importance of some of the transient short-term morbidity, common sense would dictate that most women would prefer their newborn infants not to suffer potentially avoidable trauma or admission to a neonatal unit. Population data from Holland, Sweden and Denmark [2,3,4], among others, have shown the predicted improvement in perinatal mortality following a move to elective caesarean birth, although French data did not support increased perinatal risk [5].

Other data from France [6] confirmed a lack of increased risk, particularly where very strict consensus guidelines were in place, that was subtly different from the Term Breech vaginal birth guidance. Subsequent Norwegian data [7] and the French data argue that where vaginal breech labour rates are traditionally high and clear guidance is in place, there is no reason to advocate planned CS. The Lille Group, using such an approach, increased the vaginal breech birth rate in an eight-year period without change in neonatal outcome measures [8].

Others have debated the number needed to prevent harm. Hannah and Hofmeyr suggest 29 elective CSs to avoid an adverse outcome, although for perinatal death it is nearer 200. A Dutch study [9] proposed a number needed to treat (NNT) of 175, and the Swedish study [3] proposed 400 for avoidance of perinatal mortality.

Maternal morbidity, either short or medium term, was not different in the Term Breech Trial, although elective CS clearly carries an increased risk for the mother. Villar *et al.* [10] showed risks of death of 4 in 10 000, risk of ICU admission of 2.7% and risk of hysterectomy of 3.5 per 1000 for women undergoing planned CS compared with planned vaginal birth, results not dissimilar to a large US cohort. Risks in subsequent pregnancies include late stillbirth, placenta praevia accreta and uterine rupture and its consequences. Dutch data [9] put this last risk as equivalent to that of the increase in perinatal mortality associated with vaginal breech birth. Risk to the baby from elective caesarean birth is not zero, as seen in the Term Breech data, and at all gestations up to 39–40 weeks there is an increased risk of neonatal respiratory distress.

This suggests that directive advising of elective caesarean birth for the term breech is not necessarily

---

Best Practice in Labour and Delivery, Second Edition, ed. Sir Sabaratnam Arulkumaran. Published by Cambridge University Press. © Cambridge University Press 2016.

appropriate and that the more measured approach advised by RCOG [11], ACOG [12], RANZOG [13] and most recent Canadian [14] guidelines is more useful.

External Cephalic Version (ECV)

Efficacy

Given the controversies, the logical first step would seem to be to remove the problem by ECV. It has been an RCOG audit standard for some time to offer ECV to women with a diagnosed breech presentation at term.

There is significant reduction in the risk of CS in women where there is an intention to undertake ECV (OR 0.55 [95% CI 0.33–0.91]) with no increased risk to the baby [15]. Although high success rates were achieved in the trials, studies of practice show success rates nearer 50–60% (reviewed by Impey and Hofmeyr [16]). Parity is the main factor that affects success, with nulliparous success rates around one in three and multiparous success rates around two in three or greater. Amniotic fluid volume may affect success, although there is no consensus on whether there should be an absolute cut-off for attempting the procedure. Maternal weight and height affect success and fetal weight (both macrosomia and small for gestation) may be a factor. Operator experience may play a role.

Reversion to breech occurs after successful ECV, with 3–7% being reported for term ECV. Reversion rates of over 20% have been reported for preterm ECV.

Techniques to Improve Success

Tocolysis and anaesthesia have been advocated to improve success rates. The most recent Cochrane review [17] shows a reduction in ECV failures with beta-agonist tocolysis (RR 0.75 [95% CI 0.60–0.82]) and a reduction in CS rate (RR 0.77 [95% CI 0.67–0.88]). No other tocolytic drugs or interventions reviewed show evidence of efficacy and the review concluded that no further trials of nitric oxide donors are required.

There has been consideration of moving the traditional timing of ECV to earlier in gestation, arguing that the breech is less likely to be engaged and that amniotic fluid volumes are more favourable. A large multinational trial [18] showing a reduction in breech presentations in labour did not demonstrate a reduction in CS rates. In addition, preterm birth rates were

Table 11.1 Setting and preparation

Regular service
Immediate access to operative birth
Ultrasound facilities
Fetal monitoring facilities
Comfortable bed with wedge
Establish fetal health (CTG)
Ultrasound examination – size, liquor, position, head
Flexion

slightly higher in the early (34–36 week) arm of the trial. The authors recommend discussion and choice with regard to gestation of ECV, and this seems sensible advice given the results (Table 11.1).

Safety

Systematic reviews of the randomized trials showed no increase in perinatal mortality or morbidity and other reviews of safety have been reassuring [19]. Transient fetal heart rate (FHR) abnormalities occur in 5.7%, with persisting abnormal CTG in approximately 1 in 300. Placental abruption was very rare, occurring in 1 in 1000 cases. A detailed examination of perinatal deaths in series of ECV suggests a perinatal mortality of 1.6 per 1000. This is not different from the perinatal mortality of pregnancies between 37 and 40 weeks. This older safety profile has been replicated in the early ECV trial [18].

Overall the need for emergency birth occurs around 1 in every 200 attempts [16].

Contraindication should be rare, being only 4% in one series. They would include recent antepartum haemorrhage, some uterine anomalies, abnormal cardiotocography (CTG), rupture of the membranes and multiple pregnancies in the antenatal period. Other factors such as suspected growth restriction or oligohydramnios might be relative contraindications.

Uptake

Most women would choose ECV to allow vaginal delivery. However, more recent surveys have suggested a substantial minority of eligible women would decline ECV, opting for CS. In part this may be a failure of education, and uptake can be increased by well-constructed information packages.

Table 11.2 Conduct of ECV

Ensure comfortable position (wedge or tilt, partial Trendelenburg)
Consider tocolysis
Disengage breech (palmar surface fingers pulling or modified Paulik's grip pushing) (Figure 11.1)
Manipulate breech laterally to encourage fetal flexion (forward somersault)
Consider use of other hand on fetal occiput to encourage flexion (Figure 11.2)
Continuous feedback on discomfort
If successful, place woman sitting upright
Auscultate or visualize fetal heart rate
If that fails, ask woman if she wishes a further attempt
Consider tocolysis if not used initially
Repeat procedure
When completed, repeat CTG
Check Rh (D) status and give appropriate dose of Rh immunoglobin

Conduct of ECV

There are no studies comparing different methods of performing ECV. Training is largely 'hands-on', although Burr and colleagues developed a model that has some promise [20].

A variety of healthcare professionals carry out ECV, including midwives. There are no studies comparing techniques, and practitioners should be able to vary their technique if necessary (Table 11.2).

Vaginal Breech Birth

Selection for Vaginal Breech Birth

Practitioners need to be aware when considering vaginal breech birth that published studies usually work within guidance and exclusions. The Term Breech Trial had clear guidance for conduct of the vaginal birth arm of the trial [1] that was agreed by a consensus group. Other published studies have other exclusions [5] and have argued that selection and guidance for conduct can influence outcomes (see Table 11.3).

Success is more likely if both the mother's pelvis and the baby are of average proportions, and the Term Breech Trial excluded fetuses known to be over 4 kg, as do other groups [5]. The presentation should be either frank (hips flexed, knees extended) or complete (hips

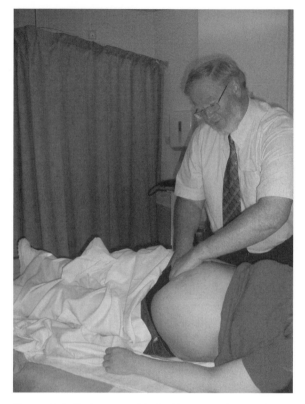

Figure 11.1 Displacement of the fetal breech at ECV using the 'one pole' method.

Table 11.3 Contraindications (relative and absolute) to vaginal breech birth

Other indication for caesarean birth
Footling breech or kneeling (feet below the buttocks) breech presentation
Known hyperextension of neck (ultrasound or clinical impression)
Large fetus (more than 4 kg)
Suspected fetal growth restriction
Previous caesarean section
Clinically inadequate pelvis
Lack of availability of experienced obstetrician
Insufficient throughput to maintain safety

flexed, knees flexed but feet not below the fetal buttocks). Where presentation was not so, the risk of cord prolapse was 5.6% [11].

Hyperextension of the fetal head increases the risk of nuchal arms and head entrapment. Assessment of pelvic size is rarely carried out in modern practice, but should be considered if contemplating vaginal

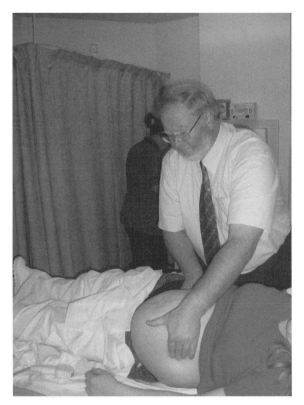

Figure 11.2 Flexing the fetal head after displacement of the breech.

breech birth; there appears no advantage to formal pelvimetry.

Neither presentation for the first time in labour nor previous caesarean birth are absolute contraindications to vaginal breech birth, although the French groups have this as part of their consensus guideline.

There has been much debate about facilities and personnel. Subanalysis of the Term Breech Trial showed the absence of an experienced practitioner (variously defined) increased the risk of poor outcomes [11]. Analysis of the French multi-centre study showed that a senior obstetrician was present at 95% of births [6].

The birth setting is more contentious. There are midwifery practitioners who conduct vaginal breech births and a number of case reports and individual stories, but no published series that allow a systematic assessment of either safety or success. At present any recommendation to women would need to be giving birth in a hospital setting. As contentious is whether size and throughput should matter. There is some evidence that adverse neonatal outcome at

caesarean birth for breech is higher (three-fold) in units with fewer than 1000 births in a US setting. The PREMODA group analysed factors that were associated with adverse outcomes and one was birth in a unit delivering fewer than 1500 women [21]. Logically, teams working in smaller centres will have less exposure to vaginal breech birth, and need to consider whether they can safely support such requests. The RCOG [11] recommended consideration of referral in some circumstances.

Conduct of Labour

The 7th Report of the Confidential Enquiry into Stillbirth and Deaths in Infancy [22] highlighted the need for senior involvement in supervising labour in intended or unexpected breech births. The Term Breech Trial and others have confirmed the importance of such involvement early.

Although there are few data to guide labour conduct in breech presentation, few experienced practitioners believe that labour progress should be allowed to be the same as for cephalic presentation. Groups who have demonstrated comparable outcomes with planned CS and who achieve higher vaginal breech birth rates rarely regard a rate of progression of the first stage of less than 0.5 cm/h as normal [5,7] and these data provide strong evidence for intrapartum guidance to differ [14]. The mean length of the active second stage in these studies is an hour, and given the good outcomes reported advice on shortening the duration of active pushing before resorting to CS may be wise.

There is no robust evidence that epidural analgesia is an advantage for breech birth. Similarly, the evidence supporting the use of continuous electronic FHR monitoring is no more robust for breech presentation than it is for general use, but most authorities advise its use. The CESDI report [22] was critical of the management of fetal monitoring. Again, groups with good vaginal breech rates and safety advocate continuous electronic FHR monitoring as part of their guidance. The data on fetal blood sampling from the buttock are too few to justify its use outside a research setting.

Induction of labour can be considered for a planned breech birth, as the evidence against is not substantial, but augmentation in current practice should be avoided unless there is careful review of uterine activity and labour progress at consultant/specialist level. Subgroup analysis of the Term Breech Trial

Table 11.4 First stage of labour

Admission assessment (most senior staff available)
Fetal size, pelvic size, breech type, attitude fetal head
If ultrasound equipment or the skills to assess the above are not available, recommend caesarean section Inform consultant/specialist staff of admission
Advise continuous electronic fetal heart rate monitoring
Discuss analgesia requirements; consider epidural analgesia
Careful review of first stage progress Careful review of descent as well as cervical progress Oxytocin augmentation only after senior review and where clinically poor uterine activity (not simply for failure of cervical dilatation)
Where electronic fetal heart rate monitoring changes, senior review; fetal blood sampling not indicated

Table 11.5 Assisted breech birth

Place in lithotomy when breech distending perineum
Consider episiotomy
Hands off the baby until the umbilicus appears (unless sacro-posterior)
Avoid handling the umbilical cord unless clearly under tension
If extended legs and do not deliver, flex the leg outwards using two or three fingers; no traction is needed
Allow spontaneous birth of the arms, then support the body if necessary
Encourage an assistant to carry out suprapubic pressure on the head to keep it flexed
If arms do not deliver and are flexed, then you can use pelvic grip (Figure 11.3) to rotate baby to bring the elbow into view and sweep the arms out
Once arms are delivered, support the baby; do not let it 'hang'
Use forceps or Mauriceau–Smellie–Viet manoeuvre to deliver the head (Figures 11.4–11.6)

suggested poorer outcomes if augmentation occurred [11], confirming the advice of the CESDI report [22] (see Table 11.4).

Conduct of Breech Birth

There are no compelling data comparing safety or efficacy of the various techniques utilized in breech birth. Therefore debates on whether classical techniques are superior to Bracht manoeuvres, or whether forceps are superior to Mauriceau–Smellie–Viet techniques are simply personal opinions. Comparison of Bracht techniques versus classical techniques in 1953 recommended the Bracht technique. A study in 1991 showed some subtle neurodevelopmental differences in neonatal outcomes comparing classical and Bracht techniques. In the most recent study [23], Bracht and similar manoeuvres appeared associated with less neonatal morbidity. The techniques used by midwifery practitioners are essentially derived from Bracht.

The Mauriceau technique was compared with other techniques by one French group and showed no differences in neonatal outcomes. Older studies suggested improved neonatal outcomes where forceps were used for the after-coming head. Manoeuvres for difficulty with the arms, such as the classical method described by Kunzel and Kirschbaum [24], the method of Muller [25] or Lovset's manoeuvre [26], have rarely been compared.

Therefore there are only four general rules for birth of the breech:

1. learn and become comfortable with one set of techniques;

2. keep your hands to yourself until the umbilicus is delivered;

3. use rotation, not traction, if in trouble; and

4. make sure an experienced practitioner is present, as well as anaesthetic and paediatric help.

Assisted Breech Delivery

Current advice is to use the dorsal lithotomy position until such time as convincing evidence appears for alternatives. One recent study audited outcomes for a small cohort of births using the all-fours position compared with the classical position [26]. Although perineal trauma was reduced and there were no serious neonatal complications, cord artery pH was significantly lower in the all-fours group (see Table 11.5).

Much of assisted breech birth is common sense and allowing normal birth to occur. Although episiotomy may not always be strictly necessary, particularly in a parous woman, it is advised in case more complex manoeuvres become necessary.

The manoeuvres to deliver the normal positions of the arms and legs require simple flexion and it should not be necessary to pull on the trunk to gain access.

There is debate on whether the baby should 'hang' near-vertically, as traditional teaching has it. Unsupported 'hanging' can result in uncontrolled birth of the head, and increases extension of the neck. It is best to support at an angle, resting the baby on the forearm.

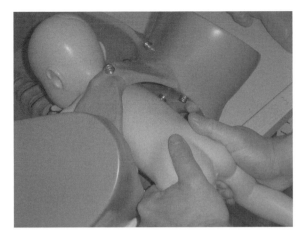

Figure 11.3 Pelvic grip for manipulation at vaginal breech birth.

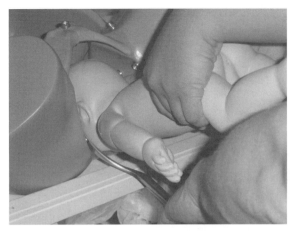

Figure 11.4 Forceps to the after-coming head.

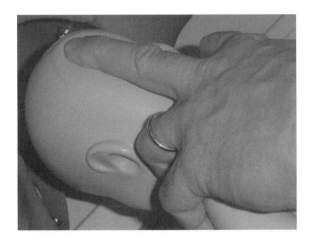

Figure 11.5 Upper hand position at Mauriceau–Smellie–Viet procedure.

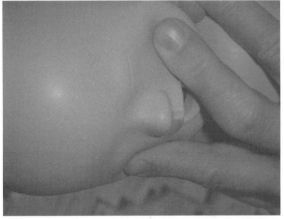

Figure 11.6 Lower hand position at Mauriceau–Smellie–Viet manoeuvre.

Before attempting any of the manoeuvres to deliver the head, allow some time for the nape of the neck to become visible. Where using forceps, an assistant will be needed to support the body and keep the arms out of the way. Wrigley's forceps are adequate for this task, unless Piper's forceps are available; these were designed for this task, having a longer shank (Figure 11.4).

The Mauriceau–Smellie–Viet manoeuvre requires draping of the baby over the forearm with the legs on either side. The classic description by Smellie, and before him, Gifford [25], involved placing a finger in the mouth, but current advice is that this is not necessary. The manoeuvre involves placing the index and middle fingers of one hand on either side of the fetal maxilla to allow some flexion, and the other hand is placed on the back with the middle finger up the occiput. Birth is by flexion (Figures 11.5 and 11.6).

Bracht Technique

This technique has been utilized for many years in mainland Europe [24]. It follows and exaggerates the planes of a spontaneous breech birth. The French studies showing better outcomes predominately use this technique. The key is the particular grasp of the baby, keeping the thighs flexed against the abdomen and then rotating the baby, using gentle pressure around the maternal symphysis (see Table 11.6 and Figure 11.7).

Table 11.6 Bracht technique

Place in lithotomy when breech distending perineum

Consider episiotomy

Hands off the baby until the umbilicus appears (unless sacro-posterior)

Avoid handling the umbilical cord unless clearly under tension

Abdominal then suprapubic pressure to maintain head flexion

Grasp the baby with the thumbs pressing the baby's thigh against its stomach and the rest of the hands over the sacral and loin area (pelvic grip)

While the woman is pushing, gently rotate or lift the baby around the maternal symphysis, maintaining upwards movement but without traction (Figure 11.7).

Spontaneous birth of the legs and arms.

Mauriceau–Smellie–Viet or forceps for the head

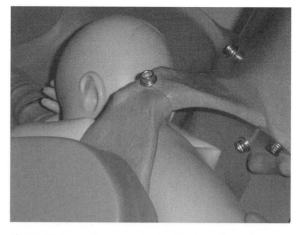

Figure 11.8 Lovset's manoeuvre showing entry of posterior shoulder into pelvis.

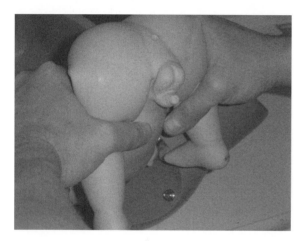

Figure 11.7 Initial rotation during Bracht technique.

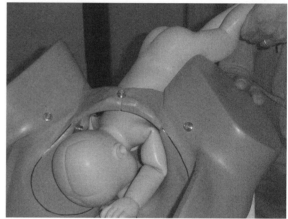

Figure 11.9 Classical arm manoeuvre showing entry of posterior shoulder into pelvis.

Manoeuvres for Delay in Delivery of the Arms

This can present as either extended arms or where one or both arms are flexed behind the head. Careful observation of the shoulder blade should forewarn.

Lovset's Manoeuvre

This manoeuvre was described in 1937. It involves using the fact that the posterior shoulder will be lower in the pelvis. Using the pelvic grip, the baby is rotated to an oblique position and gentle traction applied. The baby is then lifted in that plane to fur-

ther encourage descent of the posterior shoulder and arm (Figure 11.8). The baby is then rotated through 180°, presenting the arm under the symphysis, where it can be hooked out. The baby is then rotated through 180° again to present the other shoulder and arm.

Classical Arm Development

This uses similar principles to Lovset's approach by making the posterior shoulder available. The baby is grasped by the feet and swung outwards and upwards in an oblique plane away from the shoulder of interest (Figure 11.9). The other hand is then inserted into the posterior vagina and along the arm. When sufficiently confident the arm is then swept across the chest and out. To deliver the other arm the baby is held along its sides and rotated through 180° to bring the other shoulder into the posterior vagina. The 'swinging' manoeuvre is repeated to effect delivery of the other arm.

An alternative method has been suggested in which the anterior arm is delivered first by swinging the baby in the opposite direction.

Nuchal Arms

This should not happen and is usually a consequence of inappropriate traction. Where only one arm is involved, Lovset's manoeuvre should be enough to free the arm.

An alternative method is simply to rotate, using the pelvic grip, in the direction the arm is pointing. This will usually bring the elbow under the symphysis.

When both arms are involved, management is difficult and one may have to try both rotations to see which is the most likely arm to be deliverable. Even in very skilled hands trauma is common.

Alternatively the classical technique described before can be successful for this. Rotate (swing) the fetus towards the hand of the posterior nuchal arm and above the level of the maternal symphysis. This may result in delivery of the posterior arm, but if not it allows room for the occiput to slip below the elbow. A hand can be placed over the shoulder and behind the humerus to allow pressure on the humerus with delivery in front of the face.

If these manoeuvres fail, it is legitimate, in the author's opinion, to force the arm across the face to deliver. Humeral or clavicular fractures are very likely, but will not cause long-term harm; perinatal hypoxia does.

Head Entrapment

Other than advice on incising the cervix at 4 and 7 o'clock where entrapment is secondary to incomplete dilatation, there is little in the literature to guide clinicians on this rare but feared complication.

William Smellie's original description of the manoeuvre that bears his name was for its use for a head trapped high in the pelvis.

Symphysiotomy is the classic technique that is suggested, although its morbidity in unskilled hands

Table 11.7 Head entrapment drill

Call for anaesthetic support; prepare for caesarean birth
Check cervix is fully dilated; if not, consider incision of cervix (4 and 7 o'clock)
Try combination of Mauriceau–Smellie–Viet and suprapubic pressure
Repeat with McRoberts' position
Mid-cavity forceps
Rotate and lift the body into a lateral position, apply suprapubic pressure to flex the head into the pelvis, then rotate back and continue with previous techniques
Symphysiotomy if adequate training
Caesarean section; use ventouse to aid extraction if necessary

is formidable. More recently, case reports using McRoberts' position have appeared, and there is logic in consideration of this position, where obstruction is above the symphysis. Smellie's manoeuvre or forceps should be able to deliver where the head is trapped in the mid-pelvis (see Table 11.7).

Multiple Birth

Multiple Birth at Term

There has been a steady increase in the proportion of multiple pregnancies delivered by elective caesarean birth. The most marked impetus came from Keily's review [27] of over 16 000 multiple births in New York, where he demonstrated increased overall neonatal mortality rates for infants weighing between 2501 g and 3000 g and over 3001 g, and demonstrated intrapartum mortality rates that, although low (1.22 per 1000), were 3.5 times those of similar birth weight singleton infants. There remained debate over mode of birth, and particularly whether guidance could be tailored to presentation, birth weight or gestation.

In contrast, a systematic review carried out by the group planning the Twin Birth Study did not demonstrate differences in mortality in the literature from 1980 to 2001. This group showed an increased rate of low five minute Apgar scores, but increased overall neonatal morbidity associated with CS [28].

A series of papers using UK national data from Smith and colleagues consistently demonstrated increased risk for the second twin, culminating in a large study of twins in England, Wales and Northern Ireland using the perinatal death reporting system [29].

There were no differences linked to mode of birth for births less than 36 weeks' gestation, but a relative risk of perinatal death secondary to anoxia of 3.4 for second twins where birth was planned vaginally. The absolute risk to the second twin was 3.2 per 1000 compared with planned caesarean birth. He consistently identified twin birth weight discrepancy as the variable associated with the highest risk.

US data were conflicting. The analyses by Wen and colleagues [30] in term pregnancies showed an increased risk of overall mortality and asphyxial mortality only in those infants born by CS after vaginal birth of the first twin, with low rates overall (1 per 10 000 for caesarean birth and 2.4 per 1000 for vaginal then caesarean birth). There were no differences where both delivered vaginally. The rate of second twin CS was 9.45%. In contrast, the massive study by Sheay et al. [31] of over 290 000 twin pregnancies from national data sets showed no difference in neonatal mortality between twins 1 and 2, even when broken down into birth weight groups. Looking at their data by mode of birth, there was a significant increase in neonatal deaths at vaginal birth, but odds ratios were only 1.08. These data were not controlled for gestation or birth weight. Examination of cause of death (through ICD coding) showed no differences in deaths coded as intrauterine hypoxia or birth asphyxia. Nova Scotian data, from a well-validated data set, followed [32], although looking at composite outcomes. This data set showed a three-fold increase in composite perinatal morbidity for the second twin in planned vaginal births, with no differences in outcomes by birth order when planned caesarean birth. The relative presentation of twins did not seem to influence outcomes, but once again inter-twin size difference did. The odds of poor outcome were 3.75 times greater where twin 2 was more than 20% larger than twin 1.

More recent non-randomized data that have examined planned mode of birth rather than actual mode have shown no substantial clinical differences in outcomes by planned mode of birth [33,34]. The WHO study [35] of twins in low- and middle-income countries did not find differences in maternal or neonatal morbidity by presentation of the second twin. This was reassuring data, given the overall higher rates of morbidity and the more variable access to skills and facilities. Systematic review of planned birth data [36] shows no difference in maternal or neonatal outcomes. This review was also unable to demonstrate any difference when analysis was performed on actual birth mode.

To some extent the debate was on hold until the Twin Birth Study was reported [37]. This was a large multinational trial of planned vaginal birth versus planned CS for twin pregnancies between 32 and 37 + 6 weeks' gestation. It involved 2800 twin pairs where the first twin was a cephalic presentation. Ultimately 90.7% of the planned CS group had CS and 39.6% of the planned vaginal birth group had CS for both twins. No differences in composite neonatal morbidity or maternal outcomes were seen and there was no difference in neonatal mortality.

Although, like the Term Breech Study, this trial is unlikely to be the last word on the topic, its findings combined with recent analyses of planned mode of birth provide strong evidence that planned CS for uncomplicated twin pregnancies should not be recommended practice. Where there are no other contraindications to vaginal birth, vaginal birth should be the default position.

Vaginal Twin Birth

Selection

Approximately 40% of twins will present at birth as vertex–vertex, 40% as vertex–non-vertex and 20% with the first twin non-vertex. Given the data on singleton breech births, it would seem logical to recommend elective CS where the presenting twin is breech or transverse. Published data do not show large differences in outcomes where labour occurs, and a recent systematic review [38] was unable to find support for a view that CS should be recommended practice where the first twin is non-cephalic. National guidance may need to be more considered and current French guidance [39] states that a non-cephalic presentation is not an indication to prefer one mode of birth over the other. Interlocking of twins is extraordinarily rare (1/600–800) and should not be used to influence choice of mode of birth.

There is general agreement that mono-amniotic twins should be delivered by elective CS. Timing remains controversial. UK guidance [40] is for birth by 36 weeks' gestation, but others challenge the need for early birth where there is no evidence of twin complications.

The only other group where CS might be considered with a vertex first twin is where the second twin is significantly larger than the first. In a number of studies, morbidity and mortality appears greater if the second twin is 20–25% larger or where the absolute difference is more than 250 g [29,41].

Available evidence suggests that vaginal birth of twins after CS does not carry additional risk compared with vaginal birth after CS in singleton pregnancies [28], and although most practitioners would suggest caesarean birth, women should have a choice.

Conduct of Labour

Birth in a hospital setting is recommended for twin birth, and the key areas are preparation and the presence of skilled practitioners [8,37,42]. The Twin Birth Study achieved 95% compliance with the presence of an experienced practitioner skilled in twin birth, and this may have contributed to the good outcomes in both groups. Australian data [42] demonstrated higher risks for twins less than 36 weeks' gestation in smaller units and, as for singleton breech birth, smaller services or services where there is less exposure or experience in complex twin births may need to consider an offer of transfer to another unit where feasible.

The conduct of labour and the support provided during labour should conform to usual standards.

There is evidence that the length of the first stage of labour is prolonged by about one hour [43], with differences more marked for multiparous women. There is interesting evidence of differences in myometrial contraction behaviour in twin births in laboratory studies [44], which could account for this. This may need to be factored into guidance on progress and augmentation.

Fetal Monitoring

Most texts recommend continuous electronic FHR monitoring, although there is no specific evidence to support this. There needs to be certainty that two separate heart rates are being monitored, and this may involve the use of ultrasound to pick out both fetal heart positions. Where external monitoring has been used for both twins, very high signal loss rates have been reported (up to 33% in the first stage and 60% in the second stage), and there is a strong case for early

Table 11.8 First stage of labour

Assess presentation and relative size of twins
   Non-cephalic presentation: consider caesarean birth
   Twin 2 larger by 20–25%: recommend caesarean birth

Care coordinated by senior staff
Intravenous access
Continuous one-to-one midwifery care

Continuous electronic fetal heart rate monitoring
   More frequent maternal pulse estimate
   Twin 1 by direct ECG as soon as feasible

Consider early offer of epidural analgesia
Use oxytocin under senior supervision for usual indications

Prepare for the second stage and birth
   Ultrasound equipment
   Access to obstetric theatre
   Prepare oxytocin infusion
   Have tocolytic agent available

amniotomy and direct fetal scalp electrode monitoring of the first twin. More regular monitoring of the maternal heart rate is wise to ensure no confusion.

Analgesia

All options should be available, although most authorities recommend earlier or elective use of epidural analgesia [14,39]. The logic of this argument is that vaginal operative birth rates are high (8% in one study where the first twin delivered spontaneously), internal manipulation may be needed and that CS for the second twin may occur (between 4% and 10%).

As in singleton labour, maternal informed choice should be paramount.

Oxytocin Augmentation

There is no evidence that the use of oxytocin to augment poor progress in the first stage of labour is contraindicated for twin labour and it should be considered for similar indications to singleton labour. Data showing that twin labour may not progress at the same rate as singleton labour [43] should be factored into decisions for augmentation. The laboratory data [44] that the response of twin myometrium to exogenous oxytocin is greater than that of singletons should lead to caution in both the timing of intervention with oxytocin and dosages used (see Table 11.8).

Birth of Twin 1

Where the first twin is cephalic, then birth should follow the usual guidance for the length of the second stage and the indications for operative birth.

If labour with a breech first twin occurs, this should follow national or local guidance for singleton breech birth.

Birth of Twin 2

Once the first twin is born, the presentation of the second twin should be sought by abdominal palpation followed by digital vaginal examination. Ultrasound is more widely available and should be used in addition where practicable, and its use should be mandatory where there is any doubt.

Twin 2 Cephalic

Where the head is not fully engaged in the pelvis it should be stabilized by an assistant.

Many recommend the immediate use of oxytocin following the birth of the first twin, to ensure that the second enters the pelvis and to shorten the birth interval [14,37]. There is little concrete evidence for this outside its logical use where uterine contractions cease. It is important that an infusion has been prepared in advance.

There is increasing literature that 'active management' of the second twin results in better outcomes [41,45]. French guidance [39] where the head is engaged is for pushing to immediately restart with amniotomy and oxytocin infusion.

Where the head is not engaged the decision is more complex. There are advocates of conservative management with stabilization of the head abdominally and oxytocin if there are no abnormal CTG features. Others advocate, if skills allow, internal version and breech extraction [39].

Twin 2 Non-cephalic

Where the lie of the second twin is not longitudinal or where the presentation is high, then internal manipulation or ECV may be needed. As in vaginal operative birth for malposition, failed vaginal birth carries the highest morbidity [36] and therefore the choice of procedure should be that with the best success rate provided this is not at the expense of increased morbidity for either the woman or the baby.

Reviews of non-randomized studies are consistent [46], showing higher vaginal birth rates without any excess of injury or perinatal hypoxia when IPV with breech extraction is used. Failure rates with IPV are consistently around 5%, as in the Twin Birth Study [37]. Breech extraction success rates are high, in excess of 90% in second twins.

ECV is the alternative and the average practitioner is likely to be more familiar with this technique. However success rates are generally less than 50%; it was 42% in the Twin Birth Study.

All the evidence is that IPV and/or breech extraction does not increase either maternal or neonatal morbidity.

Logically there appears little doubt that breech extraction with or without internal version should be the first-choice procedure for the non-cephalic second twin.

Skills and preparation are the key elements for these procedures. There is concern that skills in internal procedures are being lost [47] despite the evidence that this should be best practice. This is not dissimilar to the loss of skills required for vaginal operative birth requiring rotation. Both were fuelled by the erroneous belief that second stage CS was the safer option.

For ECV and IPV to be successful and safe, the uterus needs to be relaxed. This may be achieved by switching off any oxytocin infusion in progress, or by giving tocolysis [48]. The most frequently used acute tocolytic is terbutaline, either as 250 mcg subcutaneously, or given intravenously over 5 min.

The approach where the membranes are left intact is now favoured since the studies of Rabinovici *et al.* in the 1980s [49]. Skills and drills can be useful, but best preparation is to practise the initial techniques (see below) during CS for transverse lie or for twins.

Where the membranes are already ruptured and the lie is transverse or oblique, ECV is unlikely to succeed. An experienced practitioner using good uterine relaxation techniques may be able to achieve birth with IPV, but if uterine relaxation cannot be readily achieved or if the practitioner does not feel sufficiently competent under these circumstances, then CS should be undertaken. Where the membranes rupture early in the process of attempted IPV, it may be possible to continue provided the operator still has hold of the foot and there is good uterine relaxation,

Table 11.9 Internal podalic version and breech extraction

Requirements

    Continuous fetal heart rate monitoring

    Uterine relaxation (including tocolysis)

    Adequate analgesia

    Immediate access to obstetric theatre

    Ultrasound equipment

Technique

    Grasp the anterior or both feet through the membranes

    Use other hand to guide fetal head to longitudinal lie

    Gentle continuous traction towards introitus

    Continuous pressure on abdomen to flex the fetal head (as in vaginal breech birth by Bracht technique; some may find it easier to use an assistant)

    Leave membranes intact until feet either below the level of the ischial spines or at introitus

    Once the umbilicus is delivered, proceed using either Bracht manoeuvre or Lovset's manoeuvre to deliver the arms

    Birth of the head using conventional techniques

but attempts should not be prolonged or vigorous (Table 11.9).

Inter-Twin Delivery Interval

There is continuing debate on whether arbitrary time constraints need to be applied to the interval between the birth of the twins where FHR monitoring is reassuring. Traditional teaching was that the birth of the second twin should be achieved within 30 min of the first. Data following the introduction of electronic FHR monitoring showed no differences in measures of short-term morbidity [46]. There is a linear decrease in cord artery pH with an increasing interval that reaches statistical but not clinical significance by 30 min. Others have shown increasingly frequent neonatal acidosis (cord artery pH less than 7.0 or base deficit greater than 12 mmol/l) with longer time intervals [50]. In one study the rate was 27% after 30 min, and in another the difference in severe acidosis reached statistical significance at 60 min. Stein and colleagues [41], in a population cohort, found inter-twin delivery interval to be an independent risk factor for short-term neonatal adverse outcomes.

It is of note that the mean interval in the planned vaginal birth arm of the Twin Birth Study was 10 min and the range was 1–33 min. Most recent authors demonstrating good outcomes for second twins with a

low risk of CS, including French guidance [39], advocate 'active management'.

Overall the data suggest that sooner is better and that a relaxed approach to the interval may be unwise.

Preterm Breech and Twin Birth

There is a separate debate on whether or not CS should be recommended for preterm breech presentation and for preterm twins. The conduct of labour or birth is not different to that described above (Figure 11.10).

Detailed audit in the UK of births between 27 and 28 weeks' gestation suggested increased mortality for breech presentations at these gestations born vaginally (22.6% compared with 13.5% for births by CS) [51]. US data examining neonatal outcomes by planned route of birth [52] in a cohort of pregnancies less than 32 weeks' gestation showed no differences in neonatal outcomes by planned mode of birth where the presentation was cephalic, but increased neonatal mortality in planned vaginal birth where the presentation was breech. The relative risks were three for birth below 28 weeks' gestation and over five for between 28 and 32 weeks' gestation. Systematic review of the non-trial literature [53] on mode of delivery also shows increased mortality in pregnancies between 25 and 36 + 6 weeks' gestation where the presentation was breech.

It appears the pendulum is swinging towards CS for the preterm breech in the absence of adequate randomized trials.

For multiple pregnancies, a number of studies, including one with long-term follow-up [54], have shown no advantage to caesarean preterm birth based on gestation or birth weight cut-offs [28] for multiple births. Others [55] suggested advantages to caesarean birth in terms of mortality and morbidity where the birth weights were less than 1000 g, but not above this limit. The Twin Birth Study trial [37] appears to confirm that planned vaginal birth above 32 weeks' gestation is safe. They were not able to demonstrate in subgroup analysis any gestation effect between 32 and 36 weeks' gestation.

Therefore, for twins over 32 weeks' gestation there is strong evidence to advise vaginal birth.

The situation for twin births before 32 weeks' gestation is uncertain, with singleton data [52] strongly suggesting no advantage to CS if cephalic. In these circumstances individualized care is best.

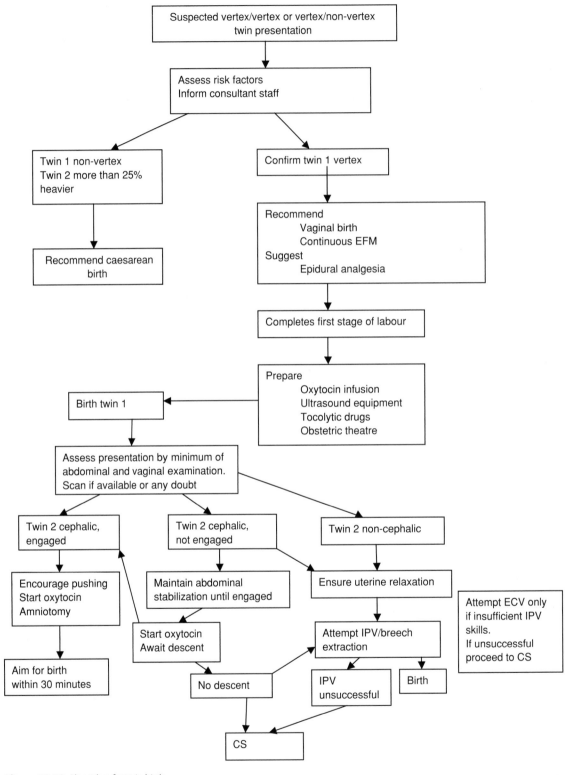

Figure 11.10 Algorithm for twin birth.

References

1. Hannah ME, Hannah WJ, Hewson SA, *et al.* Planned caesarean section versus planned vaginal birth for breech presentation at term: a randomised multicentre trial. *Lancet.* 2000; 356: 1375–83.

2. Viemmix F, Bergenhenegouwen L, Schaaf JM, *et al.* Term breech deliveries in the Netherlands: did the increased caesarean section rate affect neonatal outcome? A population-based cohort study. *Acta Obstet Gynaecol Scand.* 2014; 93: 888–96.

3. Swedish Collaborative Breech Study Group. Term breech delivery in Sweden: mortality relative to fetal presentation and planned mode of delivery. *Acta Obstet Gynecol Scand.* 2005; 84: 593–601.

4. Hartnack Tharin JE, Rasmussen S, Krebs L. Consequences of the Term Breech Trial in Denmark. *Acta Obstet Gynaecol Scand.* 2011; 90: 767–71.

5. Goffinet F, Carayol M, Foidart JM, *et al.* Is planned vaginal delivery for breech presentation at term still an option? Results of an observational prospective survey in France and Belgium. *Am J Obstet Gynecol.* 2006; 194: 1002–11.

6. Vendittelli F, Pons JC, Lennery D, Mamelle N. The term breech presentation: neonatal results and obstetric practices in France. *Eur J Obstet Gynecol Reprod Biol.* 2006; 125: 176–84.

7. Vistad I, Cvancarova M, Hustad BL, Henriksen T. Vaginal breech delivery: results of a prospective registration study. *BMC Pregnancy Childbirth.* 2013; 13, 153.

8. Michel S, Drain A, Closset E, *et al.* Evaluation of a decision protocol for type of delivery of infants in breech presentation at term. *Eur J Obstet Gynecol Reprod Biol.* 2011; 158, 194–8.

9. Rietberg CC, Elferink-Stenkens PM, Visser GHA. The effect of the Term Breech Trial on medical intervention behaviour and neonatal outcome in The Netherlands: an analysis of 35,453 term breech infants. *Br J Obstet Gynaecol.* 2005; 112: 205–9.

10. Villar J, Carroli G, Zavaleta N, *et al.* Maternal and neonatal individual risks and benefits associated with caesarean delivery: multicentre prospective study. *Br Med J.* 2007; 335: 1025–7.

11. Hofmeyr GJ, Impey L. *The Management of Breech Presentation.* London: RCOG Press; 2006.

12. ACOG. Committee opinion no. 340: mode of term singleton breech delivery. *Obstet Gynecol.* 2006; 108: 235–7.

13. Royal Australian and New Zealand College of Obstetricians and Gynaecologists. Breech deliveries at term: College Statement No. C-Obs 11; 2005. www.ranzcog.edu.au/component/docman/doc_view/945-c-obs-11-management-of-term-breech-presentation-.html (accessed 16 May 2016).

14. SOGC. Vaginal delivery of breech presentation: Clinical Practice Guideline No. 226; 2009. www.sogc.org/guidelines/vaginal-delivery-of-breech-presentation (accessed 16 May 2016).

15. Hofmeyr GJ, Kulier R. External cephalic version for breech presentation at term. *Cochrane Database Syst Rev.* 1996; 2: CD000083. doi: 10.1002/14651858.CD000083.

16. Impey L, Hofmeyr GJ. *External Cephalic Version and Reducing the Incidence of Breech Presentation.* London: RCOG Press; 2006.

17. Cluver C, Gyte GM, Sinclair M, Dowswell T, Hofmeyr GJ. Interventions for helping to turn term breech babies to head first presentation when using external cephalic version. *Cochrane Database Syst Rev.* 2015; 9: CD000184.

18. Hutton EK, Hannah ME, Ross SJ, *et al.* The Early External Cephalic Version (ECV) 2 Trial: an international multicentre randomised controlled trial of timing of ECV for breech pregnancies. *BJOG.* 2011; 118: 564–77.

19. Collaris RJ, Guid Oei S. External cephalic version: a safe procedure? A systematic review of version-related risks. *Acta Obstet Gynecol Scand.* 2004; 83: 511–18.

20. Burr R, Helyer P, Robson SC. A training model for external cephalic version. *Eur J Obstet Gynecol Reprod Biol.* 2001; 99: 199–200.

21. Azria E, Le Meaux JP, Khoshnood B, *et al.* Factors associated with advserse perinatal outcomes for term breech fetuses with planned vaginal delivery. *Am J Obstet Gynecol.* 2012; 207: e1–9.

22. Confidential Enquiry into Stillbirths and Deaths in Infancy. *Breech Presentation at the Onset of Labour: 7th Annual Report.* London: Maternal and Child Health Consortium; 2000.

23. Vranjes M, Habek D. Perinatal outcome in breech presentation depending on the mode of vaginal delivery. *Fetal Diagn Ther.* 2008; 23: 54–9.

24. Kunzel W, Kirschbaum M. Management of vaginal delivery in breech presentation at term. In: *European Practice in Gynaecology and Obstetrics: Breech Delivery* (pp. 99–126). Paris: Elsevier; 2002.

25. Baskett TF, Calder A, Arulkumaran S. Breech delivery In: *Munro Kerr's Operative Obstetrics* (pp. 181–94). London: Saunders Elsevier; 2007.

26. Bogner G, Strobl M, Schausberger C, *et al.* Breech delivery in the all fours position: a prospective observational comparative study with classic assistance. *J Perinat Med.* 2014; 43: 707–13.

27. Keily JL. The epidemiology of perinatal mortality in multiple births. *Bull NY Acad Med.* 1990; 66: 618–37.

28. Hogle KL, Hutton EK, McBrien KA, Barrett JFR, Hannah ME. Cesarean delivery for twins: a systematic review and meta-analysis. *Am J Obstet Gynecol.* 2003; 188: 220–7.

29. Smith GC, Fleming KM, White IR. Birth order of twins and risk of perinatal death related to delivery in England, Northern Ireland, and Wales, 1994–2003: retrospective cohort study. *Br Med J.* 2007; 334: 576–8.

30. Wen SW, Fung KFF, Oppenheimer L, *et al.* Neonatal mortality in second twin according to cause of death, gestational age, and mode of delivery. *Am J Obstet Gynecol.* 2004; 191: 778–83.

31. Sheay W, Ananth CV, Kinzler WL. Perinatal mortality in first- and second-born twins in the United States. *Obstet Gynecol.* 2004; 103: 63–70.

32. Armson BA, O'Connell C, Persad V, *et al.* Determinants of perinatal mortality and serious neonatal morbidity in the second twin. *Obstet Gynecol.* 2006; 108: 556–64.

33. Wenckus DJ, Gao W, Kominiarek MA, Wilkins I. The effects of labor and delivery on maternal and neonatal outcomes in term twins: a retrospective cohort study. *BJOG.* 2014; 121: 1137–44.

34. Herbst A, Källén K. Influence of mode of delivery on neonatal mortality in the second twin, at and before term. *BJOG.* 2008 115: 1512–17.

35. Vogel JP, Holloway E, Cuesta C, *et al.* Outcomes of non-vertex second twins, following vertex vaginal delivery of first twin: a secondary analysis of the WHO Global Survey on maternal and perinatal health. *BMC Pregnancy Childbirth.* 2014; 14: 55.

36. Rossi AC, Mullin PM, Chmait RH. Neonatal outcomes of twins according to birth order, presentation and mode of delivery: a systematic review and meta-analysis. *BJOG.* 2011; 118: 523–32.

37. Barrett JF, Hannah ME, Hutton EK, *et al.* A randomized trial of planned cesarean or vaginal delivery for twin pregnancy. *N Engl J Med.* 2013; 369: 1295–305.

38. Steins Bisschop CN, Vogelvang TE, May AM, Schuitemaker NW. Mode of delivery in non-cephalic presenting twins: a systematic review. *Arch Gynecol Obstet.* 2012; 286: 237–47.

39. Vayssière C, Benoist G, Blondel B, *et al.* Twin pregnancies: guidelines for clinical practice from the French College of Gynecologists and Obstetricians (CNGOF). *Eur J Obstet Gynecol Reprod Biol.* 2011; 156: 12–17.

40. Visintin C, Mugglestone MA, James D, Kilby MD. Antenatal care for twin and triplet pregnancies: summary of NICE guidance. *BMJ.* 2011; 343: d5714.

41. Stein W, Misselwitz B, Schmidt S. Twin-to-twin delivery time interval: influencing factors and effect on short-term outcome of the second twin. *Acta Obstet Gynecol Scand.* 2008; 87: 346–53.

42. Algert CS, Morris JM, Bowen JR, Giles W, Roberts CL Twin deliveries and place of birth in NSW 2001–2005. *Aust N Z J Obstet Gynaecol.* 2009; 49: 461–6.

43. Leftwich HK, Zaki MN, Wilkins I, Hibbard JU. Labor patterns in twin gestations. *Am J Obstet Gynecol.* 2013; 209: e1–5.

44. Turton P, Arrowsmith S, Prescott J, *et al.* A comparison of the contractile properties of myometrium from singleton and twin pregnancies. *PLoS One.* 2013; 8: e63800.

45. Fox NS, Silverstein M, Bender S, *et al.* Active second-stage management in twin pregnancies undergoing planned vaginal delivery in a U.S. population. *Obstet Gynecol.* 2010; 115: 229–33.

46. Cruikshank DP. Intrapartum management of twin gestations. *Obstet Gynecol.* 2007; 109: 1167–76.

47. Jonsdottir F, Henriksen L, Secher NJ, Maaløe N. Does internal podalic version of the non-vertex second twin still have a place in obstetrics? A Danish national retrospective cohort study. *Acta Obstet Gynecol Scand.* 2015; 94: 59–64.

48. Baskett TF, Calder A, Arulkumaran S. Procedures and techniques: acute tocolysis. In: *Munro Kerr's Operative Obstetrics* (pp. 285–8). London: Saunders Elsevier; 2007.

49. Rabinovici J, Barkai G, Reichman B, Serr DM, Mashiach S. Internal podalic version with unruptured membranes for the second twin in transverse lie. *Obstet Gynecol.* 1988; 71: 428–30.

50. Leung TY, Tam WH, Leung TN, Lok IH, Lau TK. Effect of twin-to-twin delivery interval on umbilical cord blood gas in the second twins. *Br J Obstet Gynaecol.* 2002; 109: 63–7.

51. Confidential Enquiry into Stillbirths and Deaths in Infancy. *Survival Rates of Babies Born Between 27 and 28 Weeks' Gestation in England, Wales and Northern Ireland 1998–2000: 8th Annual Report.* London: Maternal and Child Health Consortium; 2002.

52. Reddy UM, Zhang J, Sun L, *et al.* Neonatal mortality by attempted route of delivery in early preterm birth. *Am J Obstet Gynecol.* 2012; 207: e1–8.

53. Bergenhenegouwen LA, Meertens LJ, Schaaf J, *et al.* Vaginal delivery versus caesarean section in preterm breech delivery: a systematic review. *Eur J Obstet Gynaecol Reprod Biol.* 2014; 172: 1–6.

54. Rydhstrom H. Prognosis for twins with birth weight less than 1500 g: the impact of caesarean section in relation to fetal presentation. *Am J Obstet Gynecol.* 1999; 163: 528–33.

55. Zhang J, Bowes WA, Grey TW, McMahon MJ. Twin delivery and neonatal and infant mortality: a population-based study. *Obstet Gynecol.* 1996; 88: 593–8.

Chapter 12

Cord Prolapse and Shoulder Dystocia

Joanna F. Crofts

Umbilical Cord Prolapse

Definition

Umbilical cord prolapse is the descent of the umbilical cord through the cervix alongside, or past, the fetal presenting part in the presence of ruptured membranes. Umbilical cord prolapse is an acute obstetrical emergency requiring rapid identification and intervention [1].

Pathophysiology of Cord Prolapse

Cord prolapse most commonly occurs after the amniotic membranes rupture (spontaneously or artificially) where the fetal presenting part is poorly applied to the maternal cervix. The umbilical cord may subsequently be compressed, compromising the fetal blood supply.

Neonatal Morbidity and Mortality Associated With Cord Prolapse

The perinatal mortality rate associated with cord prolapse has declined over the last century. At the National Maternity Hospital in Dublin, Ireland perinatal survival following cord prolapse has increased from 46% in the 1940s to 94% in the last decade [2]. Undoubtedly some of this improvement will be due to improved obstetric management, but the parallel improvements in neonatal care cannot be underestimated. However, the mortality rate over recent decades has remained static: 36–162 per 1000 [1], with cases of cord prolapse appearing consistently in perinatal mortality enquiries.

Birth asphyxia (due to cord compression preventing venous return to the fetus and arterial vasospasm secondary to exposure to vaginal fluids and/or air) may result in hypoxic-ischaemic encephalopathy, cerebral palsy or neonatal death. Prematurity and congenital malformation account for the majority of adverse outcomes associated with cord prolapse in hospital [3], but birth asphyxia and perinatal death does occur in normally formed term babies following cord prolapse, especially if the cord prolapse occurs outside the hospital setting (e.g. during home births or in a standalone midwifery-led unit) [4]. The inevitable delay from diagnosis of cord prolapse to delivery because transfer to hospital is required appears to be a contributing factor.

Incidence and Risk Factors

The incidence of cord prolapse is 0.1–0.6% in all presentations, increasing to 1% in breech presentation [1]. The National Maternity Hospital, Dublin, Ireland has reported a significant reduction in the incidence of cord prolapse over a 69-year period from 6.4 per 1000 live births in the 1940s to 1.7 per 1000 live births in the last decade [2]. Of note, the rate of grand multiparity has also fallen over this time period, which may, in part, account for the reduction in the incidence of umbilical cord prolapse.

Most risks factors for cord prolapse are associated with a poorly applied fetal presenting part. A stepwise multivariate logistic regression model study [5] of 456 cases of cord prolapse in a population of 121 227 women identified the following risk factors for cord prolapse (odds ratio [95% confidence interval]):

- malpresentation (5.1 [4.1–6.3]);
- polyhydramnios (3.0 [2.3–3.9]);
- true knot of the umbilical cord (3.0 [1.8–5.1]);
- preterm delivery (2.1 [1.6–2.8]);
- induction of labour (2.2 [1.7–2.8]);

Best Practice in Labour and Delivery, Second Edition, ed. Sir Sabaratnam Arulkumaran. Published by Cambridge University Press. © Cambridge University Press 2016.

Table 12.1 Risk factors for cord prolapse

Antenatal	Intrapartum
Breech presentation	Aminiotomy (especially with a high presenting part)
Unstable lie	Prematurity
Oblique or transverse lie	Breech presentation
External cephalic version	Second twin
Amnio-reduction	Amnioinfusion
Expectant management of premature rupture of membranes	Fetal scalp electrode application
Male fetus	Disimpaction of the fetal head during rotational assisted delivery
Previous cord prolapse	

- grand multiparity (1.9 [1.5–2.3]);
- lack of prenatal care (1.4 [1.02–1.8]); and
- male gender (1.3 [1.1–1.6]).

A case control study of 709 cases of cord prolapse and 2407 randomly selected controls found that infants affected by cord prolapse were more likely to weigh less than 2500 g (4.8 [3.7–6.2]) and to be born prematurely (2.9 [2.2–3.7]). Other risk factors included second twin (5.0 [3.3–11.7]) and breech presentation (birth weight-adjusted 2.5 [1.7–3.9]) [4]. Expectant management of preterm ruptured membranes is also associated with cord prolapse [1].

Obstetric interventions (amniotomy, fetal scalp electrode application, external cephalic version and amnio-reduction) are associated with an increased risk of umbilical cord prolapse, especially in the presence of a high presenting part (Table 12.1).

Prediction

Ultrasound has been proposed as a method of detecting cord presentation and therefore predicting pregnancies at greatest risk of cord prolapse. However, there is currently insufficient evidence to support such practice, and it is therefore not recommended except in a research setting [1]. Selective ultrasound screening may be considered for women with breech presentation at term who are considering vaginal birth [1].

Prevention

The RCOG recommends that women with transverse, oblique or unstable lie should be offered elective admission to hospital at 37 + 0 weeks (or sooner if there are signs of labour or suspicion of ruptured membranes). Women who choose to remain in the com-munity should be advised to present urgently if there are signs of labour or suspicion of membrane rupture [1]. Women with preterm prelabour rupture of membranes and a non-cephalic presentation should be managed as an inpatient due to the higher risk of umbilical cord prolapse in this group.

Elective admission does not prevent cord prolapse; however, if cord prolapse does occur in hospital, immediate diagnosis and emergency treatment is possible, thereby improving neonatal outcome. Women with a transverse, oblique or unstable lie should be offered stabilizing induction after correcting the lie or an elective caesarean section (CS) at term. An emergency CS is indicated if labour or ruptured membranes are associated with an abnormal lie, or if the cord is palpated below the presenting part on vaginal examination during labour; in this situation artificial rupture of membranes should be avoided [1].

Any obstetric intervention after the membranes have ruptured (application of fetal scalp electrode, manual rotation of vertex, internal podalic version) carries a risk of cord prolapse, and upwards displacement of the presenting part after membrane rupture should therefore be minimized. Fundal pressure or stabilization of a longitudinal lie may reduce the risk of cord prolapse during artificial rupture of the membranes if the vertex is high. Artificial rupture of membranes should be avoided whenever possible if the presenting part is unengaged and mobile; if it becomes necessary, it should be performed in, or near, the operating theatre with facilities to perform an immediate emergency CS if required [1].

Management

See Figure 12.1 for an algorithm for the management of cord prolapse.

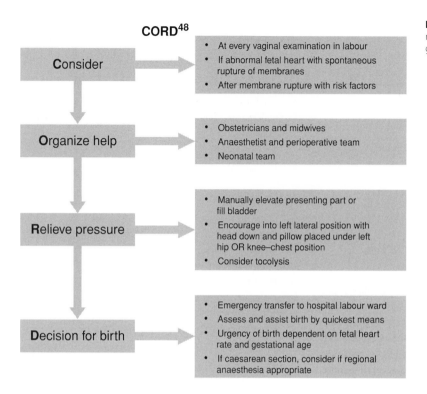

CORD[48]

Consider
- At every vaginal examination in labour
- If abnormal fetal heart with spontaneous rupture of membranes
- After membrane rupture with risk factors

Organize help
- Obstetricians and midwives
- Anaesthetist and perioperative team
- Neonatal team

Relieve pressure
- Manually elevate presenting part or fill bladder
- Encourage into left lateral position with head down and pillow placed under left hip OR knee–chest position
- Consider tocolysis

Decision for birth
- Emergency transfer to hospital labour ward
- Assess and assist birth by quickest means
- Urgency of birth dependent on fetal heart rate and gestational age
- If caesarean section, consider if regional anaesthesia appropriate

Figure 12.1 Algorithm for the management of cord prolapse (RCOG guideline).

Recognition of Cord Prolapse

Cord prolapse should be suspected when there is an abnormal fetal heart rate (FHR) pattern (e.g. bradycardia, decelerations) in the presence of ruptured membranes, particularly if such changes commence soon after membrane rupture. A speculum and/or a digital vaginal examination should be performed when cord prolapse is suspected, regardless of gestation. Mismanagement of abnormal FHR patterns is one of the commonest aspects of substandard care identified in cord prolapse associated with perinatal death [1].

Call for Help

When cord prolapse is diagnosed, urgent help should immediately be called, including (if possible) a senior midwife, additional midwifery staff, the most experienced obstetrician available, an anaesthetist, the theatre team and neonatologist.

If cord prolapse occurs outside hospital an emergency ambulance should be called immediately to transfer the patient to an appropriate obstetric unit. Even if delivery appears imminent a paramedic ambulance should still be called in case of neonatal compromise at birth.

When help arrives, 'cord prolapse' should be clearly stated so that all in attendance immediately understand the problem. Staff outside the obstetric unit (midwives, ambulance staff, general practitioners) should liaise directly with the obstetric unit, clearly stating they are transferring in a patient with a cord prolapse, giving an estimated time of arrival at hospital, so that the appropriate hospital staff are aware, and preparations can be made to ensure timely delivery on arrival at hospital.

Prepare for Immediate Delivery and Minimize Cord Compression

As soon as cord prolapse has been recognized, cord compression should be minimized and preparations should be made for immediate, emergency delivery. Unless the patient is fully dilated delivery should be by emergency CS [1].

Reducing Cord Compression

There are several methods described to minimize compression of the cord between the cervix and presenting part.

Digital Elevation

When cord prolapse is diagnosed the presenting part should be digitally elevated away from the cord by maintaining the examination hand within the vagina and applying upwards pressure on the presenting part. Handling of the cord should be kept to a minimum to reduce the risk of cord vasospasm.

Maternal Positioning

The presenting part may be displaced away from the prolapsed cord using different maternal positions: knee–chest position (woman kneeling on bed with her head down and pelvis in the air), or tilting the bed so that the foot of the bed is steeply raised with the mother lying in the left lateral position.

Bladder Filling

If the decision-to-delivery interval is likely to be prolonged, particularly if it involves ambulance transfer, elevation of the presenting part through bladder filling may be helpful [1]. The bladder should be catheterized with an indwelling urinary catheter and filled with 500–700 ml of fluid by connecting a bag of intravenous fluid to the catheter. The catheter should be clamped once 500–750 ml of fluid have been instilled. It is essential to empty the bladder just before attempted delivery, whether this is to be a vaginal delivery or a CS.

When bladder filling was first described there was one neonatal death in 28 cases, with a decision-to-delivery interval of 25–115 min [6]. Two subsequent studies of a total of 112 cases of cord prolapse managed with bladder filling reported no fetal deaths despite an average decision-to-delivery interval of over 30 min [1].

Assess Fetal Well-being

The fetus should be continuously monitored once cord prolapse has been diagnosed, if possible. If there is no audible fetal heart an ultrasound scan should be performed as soon as possible to confirm fetal viability.

Prepare for Immediate Delivery

Wide-bore intravenous access should be established and blood taken for full blood count and group and save. While preparing for immediate delivery, the fetal condition should be optimized. If an oxytocin infusion is running, this should be stopped and a 500 ml bolus of intraveneous fluid given. Tocolysis to inhibit uterine contractions can be considered (e.g. terbutaline

sulphate 0.25 mg subcutaneously). However, although terbutaline has been demonstrated to reduce contractions and abolish bradycardia in the absence of cord prolapse, there is no direct evidence that terbutaline is of benefit during cord prolapse [1]. Manipulation of the cord or exposure to air may cause reactive vasoconstriction and fetal hypoxia/acidosis, therefore some authorities advise that swabs soaked in warm saline wrapped around the cord may be beneficial, but there are no data to support or refute this [1].

Although the measures described above may be useful during preparation for delivery, delivery must never be delayed.

Delivery

Emergency CS is the recommended mode of delivery when vaginal delivery is not imminent. Caesarean section is associated with lower perinatal mortality and low Apgar score at five minutes compared to spontaneous vaginal birth. However, when vaginal delivery is imminent, outcomes appear to be similar or better with vaginal delivery.

There is poor correlation between the decision-to-delivery interval and umbilical cord pH [1]. Neonatal outcomes after emergency CS occurring up to 60 minutes from decision appear to be no worse than those following immediate delivery, in cases without a non-resolving bradycardia. However, a CS should be performed within 30 minutes (category 1) if there are fetal heart rate abnormalities associated with cord prolapse. A CS of urgency category 2 is appropriate in cases where the fetal heart rate is reassuring.

In the majority of cases regional, rather than general, anaesthesia may be used; however, prolonged and repeated attempts at regional anaesthesia must be avoided. The presenting part should be kept elevated while the anaesthesia is undertaken. Clear communication about the urgency and timing of delivery is required between the obstetric and anaesthetic team to ensure the safest method of anaesthesia for both mother and fetus.

Vaginal birth can be attempted at full dilatation when it can be rapidly accomplished, ideally within 10 min of the diagnosis. Ventouse or forceps delivery should only be considered if the prerequisites for operative delivery are met. In general, poor fetal outcomes are associated with more difficult attempts at achieving vaginal birth. In multiparas, or for second twins, a ventouse extraction may be attempted by experienced operators at 9 cm dilatation when there is cord prolapse with severe CTG abnormalities and delivery is considered easily achievable. Breech extraction may be performed under some circumstances (e.g. after internal podalic version for the second twin or when delivery is imminent in singleton breech presentation).

Neonatal Resuscitation

An experienced neonatal team must be present at delivery to ensure full cardiorespiratory support is given, if required, to the neonate.

Documentation

Documentation should include the time cord prolapse occurred, the time help was called and arrived, methods used to alleviate cord compression, the time the decision to deliver was made, as well as the time and mode of birth. The neonatal condition at birth should also be documented. This should include the Apgar score at 1, 5 and 10 min of age and arterial and venous cord pH levels.

Shoulder Dystocia

Definition and Incidence

Shoulder dystocia is a vaginal cephalic delivery that requires additional obstetric manoeuvres to deliver the fetus after gentle downward traction has failed [7]. Shoulder dystocia occurs when either the anterior, or less commonly the posterior, fetal shoulder impact on the maternal symphysis or the sacral promontory respectively, preventing delivery of the body after delivery of the fetal head. The incidence of shoulder dystocia in the largest case series (34 800–267 228 births) ranges between 0.58% and 0.70% [7].

Shoulder dystocia remains a largely unpredictable event that can result in serious long-term morbidity for both mother and baby. Brachial plexus injury (BPI) is the most frequent serious neonatal morbidity associated with shoulder dystocia. The incidence varies substantially between studies [7,8] (2–16% of births complicated by shoulder dystocia), suggesting that at least some of these injuries may be preventable. Aside from any personal harm and health costs, poor outcomes can result in very significant litigation costs. In England, the NHS Litigation Authority paid more than £100 million in legal compensation over a decade for preventable harm associated with shoulder dystocia [9], and in the United States shoulder dystocia is the second most commonly litigated complication of childbirth [10].

Pathophysiology of Shoulder Dystocia

In the majority of women the antero-posterior diameter of the pelvic inlet is narrower than the oblique or transverse diameter. Shoulder dystocia occurs when the diameter of the maternal pelvis through which the fetal shoulders attempt to pass is less than the bisacromial diameter of the fetus, usually when the fetal shoulders do not rotate to the wider oblique pelvic diameter.

Antenatal Risk Factors for Shoulder Dystocia

Macrosomia

The greater the fetal birth weight, the higher the risk of shoulder dystocia [11]. A review of vaginal births of infants born to non-diabetic mothers reported rates of shoulder dystocia of 5.2%, 9.1%, 14.3% and 29.0% in infants weighing 4000–4250 g, 4250–4500 g, 4500–4750 g and 4750–5000 g respectively [12]. Infants weighing over 4000 g are significantly more likely to suffer shoulder dystocia compared to those weighing less than 4000 g (11.1% and 0.6% respectively) [13].

Previous Shoulder Dystocia

Previous shoulder dystocia is a risk factor for recurrent shoulder dystocia. The recurrence rate is reported to be approximately 15% [7]. However, rates may be underestimated due to selection bias; elective CS may be performed in some pregnancies following shoulder dystocia.

Maternal Diabetes Mellitus

Maternal diabetes mellitus increases the risk of shoulder dystocia [8]. Infants of diabetic mothers have a three- to four-fold increased risk of shoulder dystocia compared to infants of non-diabetic mothers for the same birth weight.

Instrumental Delivery

Compared to a spontaneous delivery, shoulder dystocia is approximately twice as likely to occur with instrumental delivery [12].

Maternal Obesity

Shoulder dystocia is associated with obesity; however, obese women tend to have larger babies and the association may be due to fetal macrosomia rather than maternal obesity per se. In a study that controlled for potential confounding effects of other variables associated with obesity, there was no significant increase in the risk of shoulder dystocia associated with maternal obesity (OR 0.9 [95% CI 0.5–1.6]) [14].

Parity

There appears to be no relationship between parity and shoulder dystocia.

Gestational Age

Studies investigating births between 37 and 43 weeks' gestation suggest there is no significant difference in the gestational age at delivery of births complicated by a shoulder dystocia and births without shoulder dystocia.

Intrapartum Risks

The risk of shoulder dystocia is increased in any labour in which progress is slow (prolonged first stage, prolonged second stage, use of Syntocinon® for augmentation of labour).

Prediction

Macrosomia alone is a weak predictor of shoulder dystocia. The majority of infants with a birth weight of ≥4500 g do not develop shoulder dystocia [15] and, equally importantly, 30–48% of shoulder dystocia occurs in infants with a birth weight of less than 4000 g. Furthermore, antenatal detection of macrosomia is poor. Clinical fetal weight estimation is unreliable; third trimester ultrasound scans have at least a 10% margin for error for actual birth weight and sensitivity of just 60% for macrosomia (>4.5 kg).

A retrospective review of 267 228 vaginal births reported that even the most powerful predictors for shoulder dystocia have a sensitivity of just 12% and positive predictive value of under 5% [16]. The majority of cases of shoulder dystocia occur with women with no risk factors. Shoulder dystocia is, therefore, an unpredictable and largely unpreventable event. Clinicians should be aware of existing risk factors but must always be alert to the possibility of shoulder dystocia with any delivery [7].

Prevention

Shoulder dystocia can only be prevented by CS. However, a decision-analysis model estimated that an additional 2345 caesarean deliveries would be required to prevent one permanent injury from shoulder dystocia [17]. Estimation of fetal weight is unreliable, and the large majority of macrosomic infants do not experience shoulder dystocia; therefore elective CS is not recommended in cases of suspected fetal macrosomia [7]. However, elective CS should be considered for a woman with diabetes and suspected fetal macrosomia (estimated fetal weight >4500 g), reflecting the higher incidence of BPI in this subgroup, and may be considered if the estimated fetal weight is over 5000 g in non-diabetic pregnancies.

Management

There are numerous techniques described that can be used to relieve shoulder dystocia. The Royal College of Obstetricians and Gynaecology have published an evidence-based algorithm for the management of shoulder dystocia (Figure 12.2) [7].

There is no evidence that one manoeuvre is superior to another. The algorithm begins with simple measures, which are often effective, and leads progressively to more invasive manoeuvres.

Recognition of Shoulder Dystocia

There may be difficulty with delivery of the face and chin. When the head delivers it remains tightly applied to the vulva, retracts and depresses the perineum – the 'turtle-neck' sign. There may be a failure of restitution and the anterior shoulder then fails to deliver with routine traction.

Call for Help

As soon as shoulder dystocia is suspected, help must be summoned immediately. Help should include (if possible) a senior midwife and additional midwifery staff, the most experienced obstetrician available and a neonatologist. If shoulder dystocia is not resolved quickly then the obstetric consultant and anaesthetist should be urgently called.

Clearly State the Problem

'Shoulder dystocia' should be clearly stated as help arrives so that attendants immediately understand the

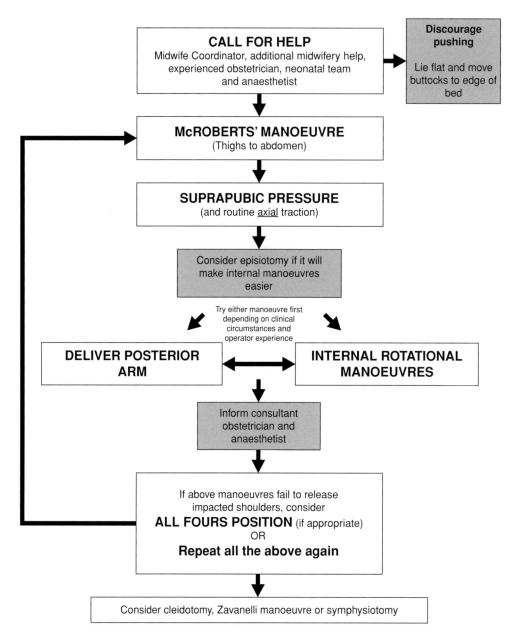

Baby to be reviewed by neonatologist after birth and referred for Consultant Neonatal review if any concerns

DOCUMENT ALL ACTIONS ON PROFORMA AND COMPLETE CLINICAL INCIDENT REPORTING FORM.

Figure 12.2 Algorithm for the management of shoulder dystocia (RCOG guideline).

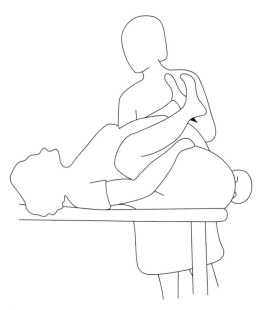

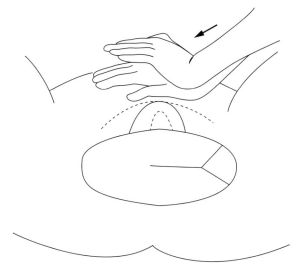

Figure 12.4 Suprapubic pressure (from the SaFE study).

Figure 12.3 The McRoberts' manoeuvre (from the SaFE study).

problem. Maternal pushing should be discouraged as it may increase the impaction of the shoulders, and will not resolve the dystocia.

McRoberts' Position

McRoberts' position (hyperflexion of the maternal legs) is the most widely advocated first line manoeuvre and was first described in 1983 [18]. McRoberts' position increases the relative antero-posterior diameter of the pelvic inlet by rotating the maternal pelvis cephaloid and straightening the sacrum relative to the lumbar spine. The reported success rate is between 40% and 90% [8]. McRoberts' position is associated with less neonatal trauma than other resolution manoeuvres; however, this may be because more severe cases of shoulder dystocia, which are more likely to result in injury, often require more than one resolution manoeuvre.

There is no evidence that using McRoberts' position in anticipation of shoulder dystocia is helpful; therefore prophylactic McRoberts' positioning is not recommended [7].

To perform McRoberts' position, the mother should be laid flat and her legs hyperflexed against her abdomen by an assistant on each side (Figure 12.3). Routine traction (the same degree of traction applied during a normal delivery) should be applied to the fetal

head. If the shoulders are not released an additional resolution manoeuvre should be attempted.

Suprapubic Pressure

Suprapubic pressure was first described by Rubin in 1964 [19]. The aim of suprapubic pressure is to reduce the diameter of the fetal shoulders (the bisacromial diameter) by adduction and rotate the shoulders into the wider oblique angle of the maternal pelvis.

Suprapubic pressure should be applied superior to the maternal symphysis pubis in a downward and lateral direction by an assistant from the side of the fetal back (if this is known) to adduct the shoulders (Figure 12.4). Again, if the anterior shoulder is not released with suprapubic pressure and routine traction, a different manoeuvre should be attempted.

Evaluate the Need for an Episiotomy

An episiotomy will not relieve the bony obstruction that causes shoulder dystocia and therefore an episiotomy will not resolve the dystocia. However, an episiotomy may be required to improve access to the pelvis, facilitating internal vaginal manoeuvres.

Internal Manoeuvres

There are two types of internal manoeuvre that can be performed – delivery of the posterior arm or internal rotation. There is no evidence that one is superior to the other [7]. All internal manoeuvres start with the

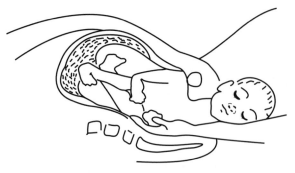 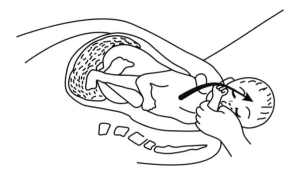

Figure 12.5 Delivery of the posterior arm (from the SaFE study).

same action – gaining access to the pelvis; this is best achieved posteriorly, as the sacral hollow is the most spacious part of the pelvis. The whole hand is inserted into the vagina posteriorly (sacral hollow) and, if the fetal arms are flexed across the fetal chest, delivery of the posterior arm should be attempted first. If the posterior fetal arm is extended behind the fetal back, internal rotation is likely to be the better option.

Delivery of the Posterior Arm

Delivery of the shoulder may be facilitated by delivery of the posterior arm, first described by Barnum in 1945 [20]. The rationale is that by delivering the posterior arm the diameter of the fetal shoulders is narrowed by the width of the arm, providing enough room to resolve the shoulder dystocia.

If the fetal arms flexed, the posterior fetal hand and forearm will be encountered on entry into the sacral hollow. The fetal wrist can be grasped by the accoucheur and the posterior arm can then be removed from the maternal pelvis with the application of gentle traction in a straight line (Figure 12.5). Once the posterior arm has been delivered, gentle traction can be applied to the fetal head; if the shoulder dystocia has resolved the fetus should be easily delivered. However, if despite delivering the posterior arm the shoulder dystocia has not resolved, the fetus can be rotated through 180°. As the posterior shoulder rotates to an anterior position it will move down the pelvis below the symphysis pubis, thus the shoulder dystocia will be resolved.

The posterior arm is much more difficult to deliver if it is extended, and in this situation it is best to attempt internal rotation first. An extended posterior arm needs to be flexed before it can be delivered. Flexion can be achieved by the application of backward pressure to the upper arm, followed by pressure in the

antecubital fossa when this can be reached. Once the posterior arm has been flexed, the wrist can be grasped and delivered as previously described. Direct traction on the upper arm should be avoided as it may result in humeral fracture.

Internal Rotational Manoeuvres

The aims of internal rotation are to:

1. move the fetal shoulders out of the narrowest diameter of the pelvis (the antero-posterior) and into a wider diameter (the oblique or transverse);
2. reduce the fetal bisacromial diameter by adducting the shoulders; and
3. utilize the pelvic anatomy: as the shoulders rotate they descend through the pelvis due to the pelvic bony architecture.

Rotation can be most easily achieved by pressing on the anterior or posterior aspect of the posterior shoulder. Pressure on the posterior aspect of the posterior shoulder has the additional benefit of adducting the shoulders and reducing the shoulder diameter. Rotation should move the shoulders into the wider oblique diameter, resolving the shoulder dystocia, so delivery becomes possible with routine traction. If delivery does not occur with the shoulders in the oblique, pressure can be continued to rotate the shoulders through 180°.

If pressure in one direction is not effective, efforts should be made to rotate the shoulders in the opposite direction by pressure on the opposite aspect of the fetal posterior shoulder. If pressure on the posterior shoulder is unsuccessful, pressure can be applied to the more difficult to reach anterior fetal shoulder.

An assistant providing suprapubic pressure while internal rotation is being attempted may also help. The person performing internal rotation needs to ensure suprapubic pressure is applied in the correct direction and rotation is with, not against, each other.

Internal rotational manoeuvres were described by Woods [21] and Rubin [19] in 1943 and 1964, respectively. However, both Woods and Rubin included the application of fundal pressure in their descriptions. Fundal pressure is no longer recommended as it can be associated with uterine rupture and BPI [22]. Therefore, internal rotational manoeuvres should no longer be described as a 'Woods' screw' or 'Rubin'. A simple description of what was done is sufficient; for example: 'Rotation and subsequent delivery of the fetal shoulders was achieved by applying pressure on the anterior aspect of the fetal posterior shoulder in a clockwise direction.'

All-fours Position

The all-fours manoeuvre may dislodge the anterior shoulder and facilitate access to the posterior shoulder to enable internal manoeuvres to be performed. In 82 reported cases the success rate was 83% without the need for additional manoeuvres and with few injuries to mother and babies [23]. The mother should be asked to transfer onto her hands and knees and gentle traction should be applied to the fetal head to determine if the shoulders have been released. It may be difficult for some mothers to assume this position, particularly with an epidural block.

Additional Manoeuvres

Surgical manoeuvres such as cephalic replacement followed by CS and symphysiotomy are uncommon and have serious potential maternal morbidity. They are considered to be last resort measures and should only be performed if the fetal heartbeat is still present [7].

Cephalic Replacement Followed by Caesarean Section

Cephalic replacement of the head and subsequent delivery by CS was first performed by Zavanelli. In a case series of 59, cephalic replacement was unsuccessful in six cases (10%), and two mothers (3%) suffered a ruptured uterus. Furthermore, two (3%) babies died and of the survivors, two (4%) babies had permanent neurological injury and five (9%) experienced a permanent BPI. It is important to note that the uterus retracts after delivery of the fetal head, so tocolysis is required prior to un-restituting, flexing and replacing the fetal head into the uterine cavity.

Symphysiotomy

Symphysiotomy is the surgical division of the symphyseal ligament to increase pelvic dimensions. It is associated with high incidence of serious maternal morbidity, including urethral and bladder injury, infection, pain and long-term walking difficulty, and poor neonatal outcome.

What Not To Do

Do Not Pull Hard, Do Not Pull Quickly, Do Not Pull Down

It is instinctive to apply traction to the fetal head in an attempt to deliver the baby. However, strong downward traction on the fetal head is associated with neonatal trauma, including permanent BPI. Traction will not resolve the dystocia and traction above that used during a normal delivery should be avoided. Evidence suggests that traction applied quickly with a 'jerk' rather than applied slowly may be more damaging to the nerves of the brachial plexus; therefore traction should be applied slowly, carefully and in an axial direction.

Do Not Apply Fundal Pressure

Fundal pressure has been described as a manoeuvre in the management of shoulder dystocia; indeed, fundal pressure is described by both Woods and Rubin in their original description of internal rotational manoeuvres. However, a study in 1987 reported fundal pressure, in the absence of other manoeuvres, was associated with a 77% complication rate, including uterine rupture [21] and BPI in the neonate [22]. Therefore, fundal pressure is no longer a recommended manoeuvre in the management of shoulder dystocia and should not be used.

Documentation

A review of fatal cases of shoulder dystocia in the United Kingdom reported that the sequence of events during delivery was often inadequately recorded and stressed the need for a clear, complete, contemporaneous record of the sequence of events. The RCOG shoulder dystocia guideline suggests that a pro forma may be helpful in documenting key events after delivery [7]. Documentation should include time of delivery of the head and body, manoeuvres performed (with timings and sequence), anterior fetal shoulder at the time of the dystocia, degree of traction applied, staff in attendance and the time they arrived, fetal condition at birth (including any evidence of arm weakness, cord pH measurements and resuscitation required) and an explanation to the parents.

After the Birth

Shoulder dystocia is a frightening and potentially traumatic experience for the mother and her attending family. It is important to inform the parents what is happening and give the mother clear instructions during the emergency. The birth and the reason for the use of manoeuvres should be discussed after delivery.

A neonatologist should immediately review any baby with a suspected injury following shoulder dystocia. For those babies suspected of having a BPI, early intervention is key to a good outcome. Babies should commence physiotherapy at about five days of age and progress should be reviewed regularly. If arm function remains unequal by eight weeks of age a referral should be made to a specialist centre for assessment regarding future treatments. In the UK the Erb's Palsy Group is an excellent source of information and supports families and healthcare practitioners caring for children with brachial plexus injuries (www.erbspalsygroup.co.uk).

A woman who has had a previous shoulder dystocia should be referred to a consultant-led antenatal clinic in subsequent pregnancies to discuss antenatal care and mode of delivery.

Maternal Morbidity Associated With Shoulder Dystocia

There is significant maternal morbidity associated with shoulder dystocia; particularly postpartum haemorrhage (11%) and fourth-degree perineal tears (3.8%). Many women also experience psychological trauma and guilt following shoulder dystocia, especially if their child has suffered a birth injury.

Neonatal Morbidity and Mortality Associated With Shoulder Dystocia

Brachial Plexus Injury

The brachial plexus is the most complex structure in the peripheral nervous system conveying motor, sensory and sympathetic nerve fibres to the arm and shoulder. The brachial plexus contains five roots (C5–C8, T1) that terminate in five main peripheral nerves. Sympathetic nerve fibres from the first thoracic root

provide the autonomic nerve supply to the head, neck and upper limbs, and control sweat glands, pupil dilatation and eyelid movement.

The brachial plexus is vulnerable to trauma due to its large size, superficial location and position between two highly mobile structures: the neck and arm. The incidence of BPI in the UK and Republic of Ireland in 1998–99 was 1 in 2300 live births [24]. The proportion of BPIs reported to be permanent, an injury lasting more than 12 months, ranges between 8% and 12% – a rate of approximately one permanent injury per 10 000 births.

Risk of Brachial Plexus Injury

Brachial plexus injuries are associated with shoulder dystocia with a wide incidence range: 8.5–32% of shoulder dystocias. BPI in association with shoulder dystocia has been repeatedly found to occur regardless of the procedure used to disimpact the shoulder and appears to be independent of the experience of the accoucheur conducting the delivery. BPIs, however, have been reported to arise without concomitant shoulder dystocia in up to 47% of cases, indicating that injury can occur without recognized shoulder dystocia.

Brachial plexus injury is nearly 20 times more common in infants of diabetic mothers compared to those of non-diabetics. Assisted vaginal delivery and increased birth weight are also associated with a significantly increased risk compared to spontaneous vaginal delivery. Conversely, delivery by CS appears protective. As with shoulder dystocia, the risk factors for BPI are not independent and accurate prediction of pregnancies at risk is currently not possible.

Classification of Brachial Plexus Injury
Erb's Palsy

Erb's palsy, or upper BPI, is the most common form of BPI, with a frequency of 73–86% [22]. The affected cervical nerve roots are the fifth (C5) and sixth (C6), with the seventh cervical root (C7) sometimes also involved. The classic Erb's palsy posture is a result of paralysis or weakness in the shoulder muscles, the elbow flexors and the forearm supinators. The affected arm hangs down and is internally rotated, extended and pronated. If C7 is involved, the wrist and finger extensors are also paralysed. The loss of extension causes the wrist to flex and the fingers to curl up in the 'waiter's tip position'. Full functional recovery is reported to occur in 65–90% of cases; the prognosis is worse with C7 involvement.

Klumpke's Palsy

Klumpke's palsy, an isolated lower BPI, is rare, accounting for 0.6–2% of obstetric BPIs. The affected cervical nerve roots are the eighth cervical (C8) and first thoracic (T1), with occasional C7 involvement. Klumpke's palsy is characterized by weakness of the triceps, forearm pronators and wrist flexors. The classic physical findings are a 'claw-like' paralysed hand with good elbow and shoulder function. Full functional recovery is reported to occur in less than 50% of cases.

Total Brachial Plexus Injury

Complete involvement of the brachial plexus occurs in approximately 20% of BPIs. The entire plexus from C5 to T1 is involved, with total sensory and motor deficits of the entire arm, resulting in a paralysed arm with no sensation. Horner's syndrome, caused by sympathetic nerve injury, resulting in contraction of the pupil and ptosis on the affected side may also be present with a total BPI and is associated with a worse prognosis. Functional recovery is not possible without surgical intervention.

Other Fetal Injuries

Other reported fetal injuries include fractures of the humerus and clavicle, pneumothoraxes and hypoxic brain damage.

Lessons for Training

There is a need for shoulder dystocia training. Poor outcomes following shoulder dystocia are commonly a result of inappropriate clinical management. Between 1995 and 2010 the NHS Litigation Authority (NHSLA) received around 555 claims related to shoulder dystocia and paid out over £189 million [9]. The fifth Confidential Enquiries into Stillbirths and Deaths in Infancy in England and Wales found grade three suboptimal care in 66% of neonatal deaths following shoulder dystocia. In a large simulation study involving over 140 staff conducted in the south-west of England, only 43% of midwives and doctors were able to successfully manage severe shoulder dystocia prior to training [25].

Simulation has been used to identify common errors made by staff when managing shoulder dystocia. The most common error was the inability to gain vaginal access to enable internal manoeuvres to be performed; access should be gained posteriorly into the sacral hollow with the whole hand [26]. The use of acronyms and eponyms, both in training and in clinical practice, appears to be counterproductive. Acronyms such as HELPERR (Call for Help, Evaluate for Episiotomy, elevate Legs, apply Pressure, Enter, Remove, Rotate) can be confusing and should no longer be used. Staff that have been taught the eponyms such as 'Woods' screw' or 'Rubin manoeuvre' often remember the name of the manoeuvre but are unsure of the actual intervention. The purpose and technical description of the manoeuvre should be taught rather than the eponymous name.

Not all shoulder dystocia training is equal. Some shoulder dystocia training programmes have been associated with improvements in outcomes, while others have seen no improvement or even worsening outcomes. Those training programmes that have been associated with improvements have all had the following in common: (1) annual training has been conducted in the clinical area; (2) midwives and obstetricians have been trained together; and (3) high-fidelity training mannequins have been used. A recent paper reported no permanent BPIs in 562 cases of shoulder dystocia over a four-year period in a single healthcare institution [27]. That no baby suffered permanent BPI challenges the commonly held view that permanent BPI is largely unavoidable.

Poor neonatal outcome following shoulder dystocia has been associated with a lack of staff confidence and competence in managing this unpredictable and largely unpreventable condition. Therefore, training for the management of shoulder dystocia might be the most effective means of reducing the associated morbidity and mortality. The fifth CESDI report recommended a 'high level of awareness and training for all birth attendants' as 'professionals will be exposed to it (shoulder dystocia) relatively infrequently, but urgent action is needed when it does occur'. If performed properly, training will reduce both the severity of shoulder dystocia complications and the number of children suffering a debilitating BPI.

References

1. Royal College of Obstetricians and Gynaecologists. *Umbilical Cord Prolapse*. London: RCOG Press; 2014.

2. Gibbons C, O'Herlihy C, Murphy JF. Umbilical cord prolapse: changing patterns and improved outcomes –

a retrospective cohort study. *BJOG*. 2014;121(13): 1705–8.

3. Murphy DJ, MacKenzie IZ. The mortality and morbidity associated with umbilical cord prolapse. *BJOG*. 1995;102(10): 826–30.

4. Critchlow CW, Leet TL, Benedetti TJ, Daling JR. Risk factors and infant outcomes associated with umbilical cord prolapse: a population-based case-control study among births in Washington state. *Am J Obstet Gynecol*. 1994;170(2): 613–18.

5. Kahana B, Sheiner E, Levy A, Lazer S, Mazor M. Umbilical cord prolapse and perinatal outcomes. *Int J Gynecol Obstet*. 2004;84(2): 127–32.

6. Katz Z, Shoham Z, Lancet M, *et al.* Management of labor with umbilical cord prolapse: a 5-year study. *Obstet Gynecol*. 1988;72: 278–81.

7. Royal College Obstetricians and Gynaecologists. *Shoulder Dystocia*, 2nd edition, London: RCOG Press; 2012.

8. Gherman RB. Shoulder dystocia: an evidence-based evaluation of the obstetric nightmare. *Clin Obstet Gynecol*. 2002;45(2): 345–62.

9. NHS Litigation Authority. *Ten Years of Maternity Claims: An Analysis of NHS Litigation Authority Data*. London: NHSLA; 2012.

10. Angelini DJ, Greenwald L. Closed claims analysis of 65 medical malpractice cases involving nurse-midwives. *J Midwifery Womens Health*. 2005;50(6): 454–60.

11. Acker DB, Sachs BP, Friedman EA. Risk factors for shoulder dystocia. *Obstet Gynecol*. 1985;66(6): 762–8.

12. Nesbitt TS, Gilbert WM, Herrchen B. Shoulder dystocia and associated risk factors with macrosomic infants born in California. *Am J Obstet Gynecol*. 1998;179(2): 476–80.

13. Nocon JJ, McKenzie DK, Thomas LJ, Hansell RS. Shoulder dystocia: an analysis of risks and obstetric maneuvers. *Am J Obstet Gynecol*. 1993;168(6 Pt 1): 1732–7; discussion 37–9.

14. Robinson H, Tkatch S, Mayes DC, Bott N, Okun N. Is maternal obesity a predictor of shoulder dystocia? *Obstet Gynecol*. 2003;101(1): 24–7.

15. Gross SJ, Shime J, Farine D. Shoulder dystocia: predictors and outcome – a five-year review. *Am J Obstet Gynecol*. 1987;156(2): 334–6.

16. Ouzounian JG, Gherman RB. Shoulder dystocia: are historic risk factors reliable predictors? *Am J Obstet Gynecol*. 2005;192(6): 1933–5.

17. Rouse DJ, Owen J, Goldenberg RL, Cliver SP. The effectiveness and costs of elective cesarean delivery for fetal macrosomia diagnosed by ultrasound. *JAMA*. 1996;276(18): 1480–6.

18. Gonik B, Allen R, Sorab J. Objective evaluation of the shoulder dystocia phenomenon: effect of maternal pelvic orientation on force reduction. *Obstet Gynecol*. 1989;74(1): 44–8.

19. Rubin A. Management of shoulder dystocia. *JAMA*. 1964;189: 835–7.

20. Barnum CG. Dystocia due to the shoulders. *Am J Obstet Gynecol*. 1945;50: 439–42.

21. Woods CE, Westbury NY. A principle of physics as applicable to shoulder delivery. *Am J Obstet Gynecol*. 1943;45: 796–804.

22. Gross TL, Sokol RJ, Williams T, Thompson K. Shoulder dystocia: a fetal-physician risk. *Am J Obstet Gynecol*. 1987;156(6): 1408–18.

23. Bruner JP, Drummond SB, Meenan AL, Gaskin IM. All-fours maneuver for reducing shoulder dystocia during labor. *J Reprod Med*. 1998;43(5): 439–43.

24. Evans-Jones G, Kay SP, Weindling AM, *et al.* Congenital brachial palsy: incidence, causes, and outcome in the United Kingdom and Republic of Ireland. *Arch Dis Child Fetal Neonatal Ed*. 2003;88(3): F185–9.

25. Crofts JF, Bartlett C, Ellis D, *et al.* Training for shoulder dystocia: a trial of simulation using low-fidelity and high-fidelity mannequins. *Obstet Gynecol*. 2006;108(6): 1477–85.

26. Crofts JF, Fox R, Ellis D, *et al.* Observations from 450 shoulder dystocia simulations: lessons for skills training. *Obstet Gynecol*. 2008;112(4): 906–12.

27. Crofts JF, Bentham G, Tawfik S, Claireaux H, Draycott T. Can accurate training and management for shoulder dystocia prevent all permanent brachial plexus injuries? *BJOG*. 2013;120: 412.

Chapter 13

Antepartum Haemorrhage

Neelam Potdar, Osric Navti and Justin C. Konje

Introduction

Antepartum haemorrhage (APH) is defined as any bleeding from the genital tract between the 24th week of pregnancy and the onset of labour. This definition of gestational age is based on the UK professional guidance for viability cut-off point of 24 weeks [1]. APH complicates 2–5% of all pregnancies [2] and is associated with significant maternal and perinatal morbidity and mortality. Globally, obstetric haemorrhage remains one of the most important causes of maternal mortality, accounting for 11% of maternal deaths. In the last *UK Confidential Enquiries into Maternal Mortality and Morbidity report (2009–12)*, mortality rate due to obstetric haemorrhage was 0.49 per 100 000 maternities [3]. The WHO estimates a 1% case fatality rate for the 14 million annual cases of obstetric haemorrhage [4].

Aetiology

Table 13.1 shows the various causes for APH; however, these are identifiable only in approximately half of cases. Bleeding from the placental bed is the commonest cause and in some cases a local cause in the genital tract can be ascertained.

Diagnosis and Management

Antepartum haemorrhage by nature is unpredictable, and the bleeding at presentation can be significant or non-substantial. The management of any patient with significant APH should ideally be in a hospital with adequate facilities for transfusion, delivery by caesarean section (CS) and neonatal intensive care. Initial management includes history-taking, evaluation of the general condition, initiation of appropriate investigations and treatment including delivery.

Table 13.1 Causes of antepartum haemorrhage

	Causes	Incidence (%)
Placental	Placenta praevia	31
	Placental abruption	22
	Vasa praevia	0.5
Unclassified	Marginal	34
Genital tract	Cervicitis	8.0
	Trauma	5.0
	Vulvovaginal varicosities	2.0
	Genital infections	0.5
	Genital tumours	0.5
	Others	0.5

History

This must include the amount, character and duration of bleeding. It is also important to ascertain whether there are any associated abdominal pains or regular uterine contractions. Initiating or contributory factors such as trauma or coitus should be excluded. The gestational age as confirmed by either a booking ultrasound scan or the last menstrual period and information regarding placental site should be obtained. Additional useful information includes the number of past bleeding episodes, history of ruptured membranes, past obstetric and cervical smear history.

Physical Examination

This is aimed at assessing both maternal and fetal conditions and includes a general examination for evidence of shock (pallor, restlessness, cold-clammy extremities and poor skin perfusion), assessing maternal pulse, respiratory rate and blood pressure. Abdominal examination includes fundal height measurement, consistency of uterus (soft or firm), presence of tenderness, palpable uterine contractions, fetal lie, presentation and viability. Vulval inspection should include an

Best Practice in Labour and Delivery, Second Edition, ed. Sir Sabaratnam Arulkumaran. Published by Cambridge University Press. © Cambridge University Press 2016.

assessment of the amount of bleeding and determination of whether the bleeding is continuing or not. A speculum examination is essential but should only be done after placenta praevia has been excluded.

Initial Management and Investigations

The initial assessment/resuscitation and investigations is generic for all types of APH, with further treatment tailored according to the severity of bleeding, gestational age of the pregnancy and the cause of bleeding. These should include:

1. Access to intravenous line with one or two wide-bore cannulae (preferably size 14–16 French gauge).
2. Obtaining blood for a full blood count, urea and electrolytes, group and save, and holding of serum for potential cross-matching depending upon the severity of bleeding. In the presence of heavy bleeding, at least four units of blood should be cross-matched. If placental abruption is suspected a coagulation profile should also be checked. Other tests include a Kleihauer Betke test on maternal blood and urine dipstick for protein.
3. Administration of intravenous fluids if bleeding continues or the woman is haemodynamically compromised, while awaiting cross-matched blood. Colloids are the preferred intravenous fluids in such circumstances. Consideration should be given to transfusing O Rhesus (D) negative blood where cross-matching is delayed.
4. An ultrasound scan assessment to confirm placental site once the feto-maternal status is satisfactory. This may not always be necessary.

Subsequent management (conservative or immediate) will depend on the feto-maternal condition and the gestational age of the fetus. These will be discussed under the various types of APH.

Placenta Praevia

Placenta praevia is defined as a placenta sited partially or wholly in the lower uterine segment. If the placenta lies over the cervical os, it is considered as major praevia. Traditionally, different grades have been defined based on the relationship of the placenta to the internal cervical os (Table 13 2). In clinical practice, ultrasound definitions with relation to the cervical os are

Table 13.2 Grading of placenta praevia

Grade	Description
I	Placenta is in the lower segment, but the lower edge does not reach the internal os
II	Lower edge of the placenta reaches but does not cover the internal os
III	Placenta covers the internal os partially
IV	Placenta covers the internal os completely

more commonly used. A placenta that overlaps the cervical os or has its edges less than 20 mm from the os is considered praevia on ultrasound scan.

The prevalence of clinically identified placenta praevia is approximately 4–5/1000 pregnancies [5]. The exact aetiology of placenta praevia is unknown, but it has been shown to be associated with increasing maternal age, parity, smoking, in-vitro fertilization, multiple pregnancies and previous CS. A single CS increases the risk of placenta praevia by 0.65%, three by 2.2% and four or more by 10% [6]. Furthermore, Hershkowitz *et al.* [7] showed a recurrent risk of 4–8% after one pregnancy was affected by placenta praevia.

Clinical Implication

Placenta praevia can lead to varying degrees of maternal haemorrhage at different gestations, with a significant impact on materno-fetal well-being.

Maternal Risks

These include:

1. Maternal mortality: primarily due to haemorrhage, has reduced from 5% to less than 0.1% since the use of conservative management [8]. In the *2009–12 Confidential Enquiry into Maternal Deaths and Morbidity* report, two maternal deaths were reported secondary to placenta praevia [3].
2. Postpartum haemorrhage: this occurs due to inadequate occlusion of the sinuses in the lower uterine segment at the site of the placental bed.
3. Placenta accreta: occurring in approximately 15% of cases with placenta praevia.
4. Air embolism: this is possible if the sinuses in the placental bed are torn.
5. Postpartum sepsis: often secondary to ascending infection.

6. Recurrence: after one previous placenta praevia the recurrence rate is approximately 4–8%.

Fetal Risks

These include:

1. Perinatal mortality, primarily due to prematurity. Previously, the perinatal mortality for cases presenting between 27 and 32 weeks was approximately 20%; however, with conservative management and improved neonatal care this has dropped to 42–81/1000 [9]. In women with placenta praevia the odds ratios for having a preterm delivery, need for neonatal intensive care and low birth weight are 27.7, 3.4 and 7.4 respectively [10].
2. Fetal growth restriction: may occur in approximately 16% of cases and is more likely in women with recurrent bleeding episodes.
3. Major congenital malformations: reports indicate a doubling in women with placenta praevia. The most common are those of the central nervous, cardiovascular, respiratory and gastrointestinal systems.
4. Unexpected fetal death secondary to vasa praevia or severe maternal haemorrhage can occur.
5. Other associated risks are fetal malpresentation, fetal anaemia, umbilical cord prolapse and compression.

Diagnosis

Clinical

Placenta praevia characteristically presents with painless vaginal bleeding. The initial bleed usually occurs in most cases at about 34 weeks and before 36 weeks in more than 50% of cases [11]. In some cases, threatened miscarriage in the second trimester of pregnancy precedes the bleeding due to placenta praevia. The bleeding episodes are not uncommonly recurrent, with the severity of subsequent episodes usually being greater than the previous one.

The absence of abdominal pain is regarded as a significant differentiating feature between placenta praevia and abruption, although 10% of women with placenta praevia will have a co-existing abruption. Since most women undergo a second trimester ultrasound scan and placental localization, low-lying placentae should have been diagnosed. Other findings

on abdominal examination include malpresentation of the fetus, which occurs in about 35% of cases [12]. Vaginal examination is avoided in known cases of placenta praevia as speculum or digital examination may further aggravate bleeding. Historically, in cases of suspected placenta praevia with mild to moderate bleeding, where delivery was being considered, a digital vaginal examination was performed in theatre with or without anaesthesia. This so called 'double set-up examination' allowed immediate access to CS if the placental edge was felt on examination [13]. With the advent of better imaging modalities this approach is rarely undertaken; however, in the parts of the world where ultrasound is not routinely available this can be useful.

Screening for Low-Lying Placenta

Various radiological methods have been used in the past to localize the placenta, including soft tissue placentography, radioisotope radiography, pelvic angiography and thermography. Currently the gold standard for localizing low-lying placenta is ultrasound scan, with an emerging role for magnetic resonance imaging (MRI). Transabdominal ultrasound scan has a high false-positive rate for detection of low-lying placentae, whereas transvaginal scanning is safe in the presence of placenta praevia and is more accurate. In most obstetric units in the UK, fetal anomaly screening is undertaken between 20 and 24 weeks of pregnancy and includes documentation on placental localization. This examination is used to predict the likelihood of placenta praevia at term. Women with low-lying placentae at 20–24 weeks are offered a repeat scan between 34–36 weeks of gestation to confirm the diagnosis. In cases with asymptomatic suspected major placenta praevia, a transvaginal scan is performed at 32 weeks to confirm the diagnosis (Figure 13.1) and allow planning for third trimester management. A few studies have shown that before 24 weeks' gestation the placenta can be low-lying in 28% of the scans, but by term only 3% of placentae are low-lying [9]. This is because the placenta 'migrates' to the upper uterine segment as the pregnancy advances. The mean rate of placental migration is about 5.4 mm per week. In recent years, ultrasound has been used to predict the likelihood and extent of placental migration and the occurrence of placenta praevia at term. Studies using transvaginal ultrasound have shown that unless the placental edge is reaching the internal cervical os at mid-pregnancy,

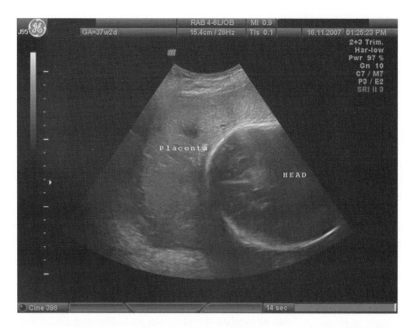

Figure 13.1 A transvaginal ultrasound image showing a low-lying anterior placenta (placenta praevia) below the fetal head.

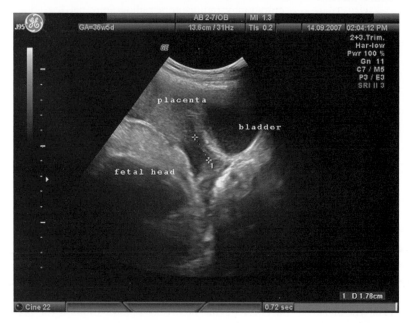

Figure 13.2 Placenta praevia approximately 18 mm from the cervical os. See the colour plate section for a colour version of this figure.

placenta praevia is unlikely to be present at term [14,15]. Oppenheimer *et al.* showed that at mid-trimester, if the placental edge overlapped the internal cervical os by >2 cm, placental migration did not occur [16]. When the placental edge was >2 cm away from the internal os, migration always occurred, whereas if the edge was <2 cm from the os (Figure 13.2), placental migration occurred in 88.5% of cases. The significance of the shape of the placental edge

to predict placental migration has also been studied. A thick placental edge, defined as thickness of 1 cm or less, within 1 cm from the edge and/or an angle between the basal and chorionic plate of >45° is associated with a higher rate of APH and a lesser chance of placental migration [16,17].

A false-negative scan for a low-lying placenta has been reported in 7% of cases. This is primarily seen when the placenta is posterior, the bladder is full, the fetal head obscures the placental margin or the operator fails to scan the lateral uterine wall [18].

Management Options

These are either (a) immediate delivery or (b) expectant management. Both of these are influenced by the severity of haemorrhage, fetal well-being and gestational age.

Immediate Delivery

Where there is severe life-threatening haemorrhage, irrespective of the gestational age, CS is the only delivery option. With mild to moderate bleeding occurring after 34 weeks' gestation, delivery should be planned after stabilizing the maternal condition.

Expectant Management

In cases where the bleeding is small and self-limiting, expectant management has a role. This provides time to achieve fetal maturity, thereby reducing perinatal morbidity and mortality. Another advantage is that in some cases with advancing gestation, the placenta migrates and vaginal delivery might be considered reasonable. There has been a controversy regarding the expectant management as inpatient or outpatient. Cotton et al. reported no difference in the perinatal or maternal mortality rates in cases managed either at home or in the hospital, whereas others have reported an increase in the neonatal morbidity with those managed at home [9]. For women with asymptomatic placenta praevia, conservative management at home is becoming increasingly acceptable [19]. The RCOG in the UK has recommended that women with major placenta praevia who have previously bled should be admitted and managed as inpatients from 34 weeks of gestation [20]. Those with major praevia who have never bled and are asymptomatic require careful counselling before offering outpatient care. These cases require close proximity with the hospital and constant presence of a companion. During expectant management preterm delivery is a major problem, with approximately 40% occurring before 37 weeks [21]. Papinniemi et al. showed that 88.2% of women with placenta praevia underwent CS before term [10]. Furthermore, the use of tocolysis for uterine contractions with vaginal bleeding is controversial. There is a 10% association of abruption in cases of praevia, and in

these the use of tocolysis can mask the features of hypovolaemia. Others have shown reduced perinatal morbidity and mortality with use of tocolysis in preterm labour and placenta praevia [22]. Similarly, the use of cervical cerclage to reduce bleeding and prolong pregnancy is not recommended as sufficient evidence is lacking [23].

Liberal use of blood transfusion has been advocated in cases where there is excessive bleeding. The aim is to optimize oxygen supply to the fetus and restore maternal blood volume, aiming for a haemoglobin of at least 10 g/dl and a haematocrit of 30%. If the bleeding settles, conservative management can be continued on an inpatient basis. Once a significant bleeding episode has occurred, four units of cross-matched blood should be made readily available. Maternal steroids should be administered for fetal lung maturity where indicated. With prolonged inpatient care, mobility and thrombo-prophylaxis should be encouraged and delivery planned around 38 weeks' gestation.

Mode of Delivery

This is determined by the clinical state of the patient, fetus and the ultrasound findings. Caesarean section is the recommended method for major placenta praevia, whereas vaginal delivery may be possible with minor degrees. Currently, as the diagnosis of praevia is based on ultrasound findings, the distance of the placental edge from the internal os can guide decision making. The RCOG have recommended that the placenta needs to be at least 2 cm from the cervical os for an attempted vaginal delivery [20]. Bhide et al. have suggested that if the placental edge is further than 2 cm from the cervical internal os but within 3.5 cm, vaginal delivery can be attempted [24]. In the UK, the RCOG recommends that for a planned CS for placenta praevia, a consultant obstetrician and anaesthetist should be present within the delivery suite. In the case of an emergency, consultant staff should be alerted and attend as soon as possible. Specialized multidisciplinary personnel like the haematologist and interventional radiologist should be informed and their help sought promptly if required. The American College of Obstetricians and Gynecologists and the Royal Australian and New Zealand College of Obstetricians and Gynaecologists are of the consensus that, when hysterectomy is anticipated, consent should include the same [25,26]. The anaesthetist, in consultation with the obstetrician and the mother, must make the choice of anaesthetic technique for CS. If the patient is not actively bleeding and is in a stable condition, an experienced anaesthetist may consider regional anaesthesia, otherwise general anaesthesia is used. For all cases, whether elective or emergency, cross-matched blood is kept available and the amount depends upon the clinical features of the individual case and availability of the local blood bank services. If the woman has atypical antibodies, specific arrangements for appropriately typed blood should be made with the blood bank. There is no evidence to support the use of autologous blood transfusion in the management of placenta praevia, although cell salvage should be considered where available. The uterine incision in placenta praevia is usually made in the lower segment; however, in difficult cases it may be converted to a T-, J- or U-shaped incision. In the presence of an anterior placenta, the approach can be of either going through the placenta to deliver the baby or identifying the placental edge and going through the membranes above or below the placenta. Some authors advise against cutting or tearing through the placenta as the fetal vessels are torn [27]. Inevitably, the placental bed sinuses bleed as the lower segment is less muscular, with reduced ability for retraction. Where uterotonics are not effective, figure-of-eight haemostatic sutures can be applied to the placental bed. Other modalities shown to be effective include intramyometrial prostaglandins, intrauterine hydrostatic balloon and uterine brace sutures. In uncontrolled bleeding, an early decision may be required for uterine or internal iliac artery ligation or even hysterectomy. Embolization of the uterine arteries has been shown to be extremely useful in selective cases. Where the placenta is morbidly adherent it may be left *in situ* with prophylactic or therapeutic uterine artery embolization and internal iliac artery ligation. The value of methotrexate is debatable. Successful pregnancies have been reported thereafter with a risk of subsequent haemorrhage and need for hysterectomy [28].

Vasa Praevia

Vasa praevia is a rare condition in which the fetal blood vessels traverse the fetal membranes in the lower part of the uterus, unsupported by placental tissue or the umbilical cord. It occurs in 1 per 6000 deliveries [29] and is associated with high perinatal mortality. As the fetal vessels precede the presenting part, they may rupture before or during labour, leading to

fetal blood loss. Before the widespread use of ultrasound, vasa praevia was diagnosed retrospectively and the perinatal mortality was high. Characteristic ultrasound features for the diagnosis of vasa praevia include echogenic parallel or circular lines near the cervix representing the umbilical cord, which can be further confirmed by Doppler and transvaginal scan [30,31]. Three-dimensional ultrasound has been shown to be useful in diagnosing vasa praevia [32]. It is important to diagnose these cases antenatally and offer elective CS at term.

Placenta Percreta/Accreta

Placenta accreta or the morbidly adherent placenta occurs due to abnormalities in implantation. It is associated with high maternal morbidity and mortality. In the UK Obstetric Surveillance Study (UKOSS) of women requiring peripartum hysterectomy, 38% had a morbidly adherent placenta, placenta accreta or increta [33]. The prevalence is higher if the placenta is low-lying or there is a prior scar on the uterus. An anterior low-lying placenta with a history of prelabour CS is more likely to be morbidly adherent and for such cases the index of suspicion should be high. Recent reports suggest antenatal diagnosis on ultrasound scan with a high positive predictive value for placenta accreta [34] (Figure 13.3). Three-dimensional colour power Doppler has also been used for diagnosis [35]. One of the specific recommendations of the 2007 CEMACH report is that all women who have had a previous CS should have their placental site determined by ultrasound scan [36]. Magnetic resonance imaging has a poor sensitivity of about 38% and is still considered as a research tool [37]. Management of a morbidly adherent placenta requires multidisciplinary care and planning in the antenatal and intrapartum period.

Placental Abruption

Placental abruption is the most common cause of bleeding in the second and third trimester of pregnancy. It is defined as the partial or complete premature separation of a normally situated placenta. It complicates approximately 0.3–1% of births [38,39], although temporal trends in some countries have shown an increase in the rates of abruption [40,41]. The wide variation in the reported incidence reflects discrepancy in the clinical and histological diagnosis. In one study, histologic evidence of abruption was seen

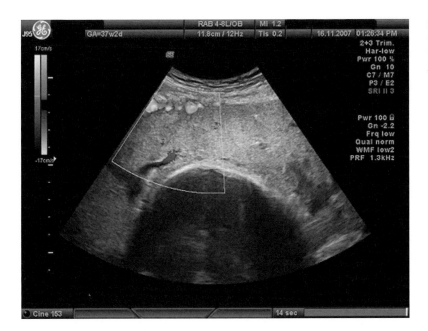

Figure 13.3 Placenta accreta: note the increased vascularity at the poorly defined placenta–uterine interface. See the colour plate section for a colour version of this figure.

in 4.5% of routinely examined placentae, suggesting that small episodes are more common than the clinical diagnosis [42]. In addition, the incidence of abruption is highest at 24–26 weeks' gestation, and decreases with advancing gestational age [43].

Placental abruption in 65–80% of cases is 'revealed' where the blood tracks between the membranes and the decidua, and escapes into the vagina. In the other 20–35% of cases, abruption is 'concealed', and the blood accumulates behind the placenta with no obvious external bleeding. Traditionally, four grades of placental abruption have been described (Table 13.3); the most severe grade is reported in 0.2% of pregnancies.

Table 13.3 Grading of abruption

Grade	Description
0	Asymptomatic-small retro-placental clot
1	External vaginal bleeding present. Uterine tenderness and tetany may be present. No sign of maternal shock or fetal distress
2	External vaginal bleeding may or may not be present. No signs of maternal shock, but fetal distress is present
3	External bleeding may or may not be present. Marked uterine tetany, a board-like rigidity on palpation. Persistent abdominal pain, maternal shock and fetal distress are present. Coagulopathy may become evident in 30% of cases

Risk Factors and Aetiopathogenesis

The exact aetiology of placental abruption is unknown, although haemorrhage at the decidual–placental interface and acute vasospasm of the small blood vessels seems to precede the placental separation. Vascular thrombosis can also lead to decidual necrosis and venous haemorrhage. Recently, reduced expression of RCAS1 placental cell membrane protein has been shown in labours complicated by placental abruption [44].

Direct trauma to the abdomen can cause a shearing force, leading to acute placental separation. This mechanism also explains placental separation with sudden intrauterine decompression, following membrane rupture in cases of polyhydramnios or after the delivery of the first twin. Cocaine and drug abuse cause placental vasoconstriction, leading to abruption. Maternal smoking doubles the risk of abruption, whereas if both parents smoke the risk is increased five-fold [41]. A dose–response relationship has been demonstrated between the number of cigarettes smoked and the risk of placental abruption. In addition, women who stop smoking early in pregnancy have the same risk of placental abruption as women who have never smoked. Other risk factors include bleeding in early pregnancy, an elevated second trimester maternal serum alpha-fetoprotein (ten-fold increased risk of abruption) and second trimester notching of the uterine artery Doppler [45]. Pre-eclampsia is associated with a 2.7-fold increased risk of placental abruption [41], chronic hypertension, pregnancy-induced hypertension, premature rupture of membranes and previous CS are other risk factors. The association between thrombophilias and abruption is controversial; therefore in women with placental abruption without a known cause, thrombophilia screening should be considered.

Clinical Implication

Since the degrees of placental abruption vary from non-substantial vaginal bleeding with minimal or nil consequence to substantive or massive abruption leading to marked perinatal morbidity and mortality, the clinical implication will therefore depend on the severity of the bleeding [46].

Maternal Risks

These include:

1. Maternal mortality: about 1%. In the last *Confidential Enquiry into Maternal Deaths and Morbidity* report (2009–12) [3] from the UK, two maternal deaths were due to placental abruption. Although, severe haemorrhage is usually the cause of mortality, disseminated intravascular coagulation itself can cause severe bleeding, renal failure and death.
2. Hypovolaemic shock: this is due to an underestimation of the blood loss, with concealed bleeding within the myometrium.
3. Disseminated intravascular coagulation.
4. Renal tubular necrosis: this occurs secondary to acute hypovolaemia and cortical necrosis and can result from disseminated intravascular coagulation. This can further lead to chronic renal failure.
5. Postpartum haemorrhage: occurs due to disseminated intravascular coagulation or 'couvelaire uterus', where concealed bleeding has tracked within the myometrium, impairing its ability to contract.
6. Feto-maternal haemorrhage can occur; therefore all Rhesus (D) negative cases should undergo the Kleihauer Betke test and anti-D immunoglobulin administered within 72 hours to prevent sensitization. Repeated doses will be dependent on the size of the feto-maternal bleed, as determined by the Kleihauer Betke test.

7. Recurrence is greatest (11.9%) when a previous pregnancy is affected by placental abruption [47]. The risk was shown to be increased 15- to 20-fold after an earlier pregnancy complicated by abruption [48].

Fetal Risks

These include:

1. Increased perinatal mortality (OR = 30.0 [95% CI 19.7–45.6]) [38]. In a US population-based cohort, the perinatal mortality in pregnancies complicated by placental abruption was shown to be 14-fold higher than all other births [49]. This is attributed primarily to preterm births, as abruption is an important indication for iatrogenic preterm delivery. In a fetus delivered after an abruption, there is a ten-fold increased risk of developing periventricular leukomalacia [50].
2. Fetal growth restriction has been reported in about 80% of the fetus born before 36 weeks' gestation [8].
3. Major congenital malformations are increased three-fold and most involve the central nervous system.
4. Fetal anaemia can occur due to severe fetal bleeding, and transient coagulopathies have been noted in neonates born to women with placental abruption.

Diagnosis

Clinical

The diagnosis is usually made based on the clinical symptoms and signs. In milder forms it is made after delivery when a retro-placental clot is identified or reported after placental histology. The classical presentation is with vaginal bleeding, abdominal pain and uterine contractions. Vaginal bleeding is seen in 70–80% of cases, although the amount of revealed bleeding correlates poorly with the degree of abruption. In about 50% of cases vaginal bleeding occurs after the 36th week of gestation, and as labour is a precipitating factor nearly 50% of patients with placental abruption are in established labour. Abdominal pain probably indicates extravasation of blood into the myometrium. In posteriorly located placenta, backache might be the only symptom, whereas in severe cases the pain may be sudden, sharp and severe. Patients may present with symptoms of shock, including nausea, thirst, anxiety and restlessness. At times abdominal pain due to placental abruption can be difficult to differentiate from uterine contractions, which in placental abruption are frequent, with a rate of over five in ten minutes. In addition to the above symptoms, the patient may complain of absent or reduced fetal movements.

Examination, in severe cases, may demonstrate features of hypovolaemic shock with marked tachycardia. Pre-existing hypertension may mask true hypovolaemia, therefore blood pressure reading in itself is not a reliable sign. Abdominal palpation may reveal a woody-hard, tender uterus, with high-frequency, low-amplitude uterine contractions. There may be difficulty in palpating the fetus and locating the fetal heart in such cases. Depending upon the degree of placental separation, the fetal heart rate may be normal, show signs of distress or absent where the fetus is dead. The cardiotocogram can show recurrent variable or late decelerations, reduced variability, a sinusoidal pattern or even bradycardia. Stillbirths have been reported where there is greater than 50% placental separation [39]. Vaginal examination is likely to reveal blood and the presence of blood clots; in cases complicated with coagulopathy (35–38%), there may be dark-coloured blood with absence of clotting. With ruptured membranes, blood-stained liquor can be seen and, more often, labour tends to proceed rapidly [51].

Ultrasonography

The role of ultrasound in the diagnosis of placental abruption is controversial. In cases of acute revealed abruption there may be no specific ultrasound findings. Where the placental site is not known, it has a role in identifying coincident placenta praevia. It can also be a useful tool in monitoring cases managed expectantly, and help with the timing of delivery. The parameters that can be assessed are location of haematoma, variation in size and fetal growth. Nyberg et al. [52] have described the appearances of an acute phase abruption as varying from hyperechoic to isoechoic when compared to the placenta. As the clot resolves, the appearances become hypoechoic within a week, and sonolucent within two weeks. Certain ultrasound features have been described with a sensitivity of 80% and specificity of 92% [53]. These include preplacental collection under the chorionic plate, jello-like movement of the chorionic plate with fetal activity, retro-placental collection, marginal haematoma, sub-chorionic haematoma, increased heterogeneous placental thickness of more than 5 cm in the perpendicular plane and intra-amniotic haematoma.

Management Options

As the clinical presentation is variable, management options need to be individualized and are guided by the severity of abruption, gestational age and the maternal and fetal condition. While aggressive management is needed for more severe cases, a conservative approach should be adopted for milder forms. After the general management described earlier in this chapter, specific measures to be considered are as described below.

Expectant Management

For mild abruption presenting between 24 and 34 weeks' gestation, and where the maternal–fetal condition is stable, conservative management should be the option of choice. Preterm delivery is a major cause of perinatal death, and if possible all attempts should be made to prolong the gestation at delivery. These patients need close monitoring for signs of worsening abruption and deterioration in fetal well-being. Steroids should be administered for fetal lung maturity and serial ultrasound scans performed to assess fetal growth and, in cases with retro-placental clot, the size of the haematoma. For expectant management, initial hospitalization and assessment of the maternal and fetal condition is reasonable; further outpatient management has a role provided the maternal–fetal condition remains stable. Timing of delivery depends upon vaginal bleeding, fetal condition and the gestational age. With recurrent bleeding episodes and a satisfactory fetal assessment, induction at 37–38 weeks' gestation is recommended. Delivery should be organized at centres with appropriate neonatal facilities and the parents should be counselled regarding the potential treatments and outcomes for the neonate.

In cases of prematurity, mild abruption and uterine contractions, the use of tocolytics is controversial. Their use has traditionally been contraindicated as they can worsen the process of abruption [54]. Some studies have used tocolytics with abruption, achieving a mean latency period to delivery of 12.4 and 18.9 days respectively [55]. It seems reasonable to use tocolytics with caution in mild and stable cases of placental abruption that are remote from term. As newer tocolytics with milder side-effect profiles are available, β-sympathomimetics can be avoided. Tocolytics may allow time for steroid administration to promote fetal lung maturity.

Immediate Delivery

This depends upon the severity of the placental abruption and fetal survival. In cases of fetal death, regardless of the gestation, and in the absence of other contraindications, it is prudent to aim for a vaginal delivery. Once the initial resuscitation has been initiated, amniotomy is frequently sufficient to induce labour and delivery is achieved fairly rapidly. In some cases Syntocinon augmentation may be needed, which must be administered cautiously because of the risk of hyper-stimulation and consequent uterine rupture.

When the fetus is alive, at or near term, prompt delivery is indicated. The decision regarding the mode of delivery is guided by fetal and maternal well-being. In addition, in severe cases the fetal outlook is poor not only for immediate survival; about 15.4% of live-born infants do not survive.

Where there is evidence of fetal compromise and delivery is not imminent, CS should be performed immediately once maternal resuscitation has been commenced. Longer decision-delivery intervals have been associated with poor perinatal outcomes [56]. Some studies have suggested better perinatal outcomes with CS rather than vaginal delivery [56,57]. However, emphasis must be placed on stabilizing the maternal condition as the presence of coagulopathy contributes to considerable maternal morbidity and mortality, especially with surgery.

In mild to moderate cases of placental abruption at term, with no fetal compromise, vaginal delivery is a reasonable option. Prostaglandins can be used for cervical ripening with extreme caution in order to avoid tetanic uterine contractions. Where possible, amniotomy is performed to hasten delivery, with Syntocinon augmentation if needed. Continuous electronic fetal monitoring should be performed to identify early abnormal fetal heart rate patterns, as it has been shown that perinatal mortality is higher with vaginal delivery in the absence of continuous fetal monitoring.

Management of complications

Major complications include haemorrhagic shock, disseminated intravascular coagulation, ischaemic necrosis of distal organs and postpartum haemorrhage.

Haemorrhagic Shock

Haemorrhagic shock usually occurs when the blood loss is in excess of 1000–1500 ml. Blood loss is often underestimated as a result of concealed haemorrhage and variation in clinical judgement. For guidance, trebling the volume of visible blood clot provides a rough estimate of the blood loss. Resuscitation is aimed at restoring the circulating blood volume for adequate tissue perfusion. Four to six units of blood should be cross-matched and urgent blood sent for full blood count, coagulation profile, renal and liver function tests. The initial haemoglobin and haematocrit can be deceptively high because of haemoconcentration. While awaiting cross-matched blood, colloids can be used as plasma expanders; dextrose is avoided as it interferes with clotting and blood cross-matching. In emergent situations, uncrossed O negative blood can be transfused. Fluid replacement should be monitored closely to avoid overloading. This can be done by monitoring maternal pulse, blood pressure, jugular venous pulse and hourly urine output. An indwelling urethral catheter should be passed and urinary output should be at least 30 ml/h. With severe haemodynamic compromise, especially in the presence of pre-eclampsia, the central venous pressure line (CVP) should be used. Measurement of the pulmonary capillary wedge pressure via a Swan-Ganz catheter reflects circulatory adequacy better than CVP, but its use depends upon the expertise and facilities. It is necessary to be alert to complications from massive blood transfusion (transfusion in excess of one and a half times the patient's blood volume or ten or more units). These can be hyperkalaemia, hypocalcaemia, thrombocytopenia and other clotting disorders. Hyperkalaemia presents clinically with confusion, lethargy and cardiac monitoring showing bradycardia, characteristic T wave changes with conduction defects and ultimately ventricular arrest. Hypocalcaemia presents with tingling in hands and feet, painful cramps and positive Trousseau's and Chvostek's sign. Platelet transfusion is considered if the platelet count is less than 50 000/mm^3 and fibrinogen replacement if levels fall below 100 mg/ml.

Disseminated Intravascular Coagulation

Disseminated intravascular coagulation (DIC) occurs more commonly with severe abruption and is seen in 10% of cases. The mechanism involves release of tissue thromboplastin from the site of placental injury, which activates widespread coagulation with consumptive coagulopathy. Fibrinolysis of the clots increases the fibrin degradation products which also act as anticoagulants.

Based on the coagulation profile, Letsky [57] has classified DIC into three stages. In stage 1 (compensated phase) there are raised fibrinogen degradation products (FDP) and increased soluble fibrin complexes. In stage 2 (uncomplicated progression) there is a fall in fibrinogen levels, platelet count and factor V and VII. In stage 3 (complicated phase, with haemostatic failure) the fibrinogen levels and platelet count are very low, with high fibrinogen degradation products. The findings are of a normal bleeding time, abnormal clot retraction, thrombocytopenia, elevated FDP levels, normal to prolonged prothrombin time (PT) and partial thromboplastin time (PTT), low fibrinogen levels and short thrombin time.

The ultimate treatment in the presence of DIC is delivery of the fetus and the placenta, as spontaneous resolution can occur only after delivery. After the initial diagnosis, management involves liaising with the haematologists and anaesthetists, and replacing the lost blood volume and the consumed clotting factors. Fresh frozen plasma, cryoprecipitate and platelets are the products of choice. Fresh plasma is preferred as it is rich in factor V and VII, the fibrinogen content of fresh frozen plasma (1 g per unit) is four times that of cryoprecipitate (0.25 g per unit). Cryoprecipitate is rich in factor VII and XII. If the patient needs to undergo surgery, platelets can be given if the count is less than 50 000/mm^3. In addition, use of heparin in DIC is controversial. In early stages and in cases where there is distal organ microvascular plugging, heparin can be used, whereas in severe cases heparin is contraindicated. Similarly, antifibrinolytic agents can precipitate unchecked intravascular coagulation. Where surgery is required, general anaesthesia is preferred as opposed to regional anaesthesia for the risk of haemorrhage in the dural and epidural space, and the worsening of shock secondary to sympathetic outflow blockade leading to hypotension.

Renal Failure

Tubular renal necrosis occurs secondary to hypovolaemia, and cortical necrosis can be caused by microvascular clotting in the renal vasculature. Oliguria in the first 12 hours after placental abruption is common and is not necessarily associated with renal damage. Fluid replacement should be monitored closely and renal function assessed by serum biochemistry. Diuretics should be used with caution in consultation with renal physicians.

Postpartum Haemorrhage

Postpartum haemorrhage complicates 25% of cases and a contributing factor is poor myometrial contractility secondary to couvelaire uterus and the presence of DIC. Initial management involves the use of oxytocics, ergometrine, prostaglandins, blood transfusion and rapid correction of coagulopathy. If these measures fail, intrauterine balloon compression, uterine brace suture, internal iliac artery ligation and hysterectomy are other available treatment options.

Subsequent Pregnancy After Placental Abruption

Optimal counselling and support through subsequent pregnancy should be provided in cases with previous placental abruption. There is a ten-fold increased risk of recurrence [57] in a subsequent pregnancy. In addition, there is an increased risk of recurrence for other pregnancy complications. Pre-conception counselling is essential to encourage smoking and cocaine cessation, and to obtain good blood pressure control where needed. With previous severe abruption, use of low-dose aspirin from as early as five weeks of pregnancy has shown some benefit in reducing the complications. In cases with confirmed inherited thrombophilias, relevant thrombo-prophylaxis is indicated in subsequent pregnancies. It has been estimated that up to 7% of women with placental abruption severe enough to kill the fetus have the same outcome in subsequent pregnancies and, furthermore, that approximately 30% of all future pregnancies in women who have had an abruption do not produce a living child [2].

References

1. Bottomley V. House of Commons Hansard Col 173 (1990).

2. McShane PM, Heye PS, Epstein ME. Maternal and perinatal mortality resulting from placental praevia. *Obstet Gynecol.* 1985; 65: 176–82.

3. Knight M, Kenyon S, Brocklehurst P, *et al.* (eds). *Saving Lives, Improving Mothers' Care: Lessons Learned to Inform Future Maternity Care from the UK and Ireland Confidential Enquiries into Maternal Deaths and Morbidity 2009–2012.* Oxford: National Perinatal Epidemiology Unit, University of Oxford; 2014.

4. AbouZahr C. Global burden of maternal death and disability. *Br Med Bull.* 2003; 67: 1–11.

5. Faiz AS, Ananth CV. Etiology and risk factors for placenta previa: an overview and meta-analysis of observational studies. *J Matern Fetal Neonatal Med.* 2003; 13: 175–90.

6. Naeye RL. Abruptio placenta and placenta previa: frequent, perinatal mortality and cigarette smoking. *Obstet Gynecol.* 1980; 55: 701–4.

7. Hershkowitz R, Fraser D, Mazor M, Leiberman JR. One or multiple cesarean sections are associated with similar increased frequency of placenta previa. *Eur J Obstet Gynecol Reprod Biol.* 1995; 62: 185–8.

8. Hibbard BM. Bleeding in late pregnancy. In Hibbard BM (ed.), *Principles of Obstetrics* (pp. 96–104). London: Butterworths; 1988.

9. Cotton DB, Read JA, Paul RH, *et al.* The conservative aggressive management of placenta previa. *Am J Obstet Gynecol.* 1980; 137: 687–95.

10. Papinniemi M, Keski-Nisula L, Heinonen S. Placental ratio and risk of velamentous umbilical cord insertion are increased in women with placenta previa. *Am J Perinatol.* 2007; 24: 353–57.

11. Naeye ER. Placenta previa: predisposing factors and effects on the fetus and the surviving infants. *Obstet Gynecol.* 1978; 52: 150–5.

12. Rasmussen S, Irgrens KM, Dalaker K. The occurrence of placenta abruption in Norway 1967–1991. *Acta Obstetrica et Scandinavica.* 1996; 75: 222–8.

13. Navti OB, Konje JC. Bleeding in late pregnancy. In James D, Steer PJ, Weiner CP, Gonik B (eds), *High-Risk Pregnancy: Management Options*, 4th edition (pp. 1037–52). St Louis, MO: Saunders/Elsevier; 2011.

14. Taipale P, Hiilesmaa V, Ylostalo P. Transvaginal ultrasonography at 18–23 weeks in predicting placenta previa at delivery. *Ultrasound Obstet Gynecol.* 1998; 12: 422–5.

15. Becker R, Vonk R, Vollert W, Entezami M. Doppler sonography of uterine arteries at 20–23 weeks: risk assessment of adverse pregnancy outcome by quantification of impedance and notch. *J Perinat Med.* 2002; 30: 388–94.

16. Oppenheimer L, Holmes P, Simpson N, *et al.* Diagnosis of low-lying placenta: can migration in the third trimester predict outcome? *Ultrasound Obstet Gynecol.* 2001; 18: 100–2.

17. Ghourab S. Third-trimester transvaginal ultrasonography in placenta previa: does the shape of the lower placental edge predict clinical outcome? *Ultrasound Obstet Gynecol.* 2001; 18: 103–8.

18. Laing FC. Placenta previa: avoiding false-negative diagnoses. *J Clin Ultrasound.* 1981; 9: 109–13.

19. Rosen DMB, Peek MJ. Do women with placenta previa without antepartum hemorrhage require hospitalization? *A N Z J Obstet Gynaecol.* 1994; 34: 130–4.

20. RCOG. *Antepartum Haemorrhage.* London: RCOG Press; 2011.

21. Brenner WE, Edelman DA, Hendricks CH. Characteristics of patients with placenta previa and results of 'expectant management'. *Am J Obstet Gynecol.* 1978; 132: 180–91.

22. Towers CV, Pircon RA, Heppard M. Is tocolysis safe in the management of third trimester bleeding? *Am J Obstet Gynecol.* 1999; 180: 1572–8.

23. Besinger RE, Moniak CW, Paskiewicz LS *et al.* The effect of tocolytic use in the management of symptomatic placenta previa. *Am J Obstet Gynecol.* 1978; 172: 1770–5.

24. Bhide A, Prefumo F, Moore J, *et al.* Placental edge to internal os distance in the late third trimester and mode of delivery in placenta praevia. *BJOG* 2003; 110: 860–4.

25. ACOG. Committee opinion no. 266: antepartum hemorrhage. *Obstet Gynecol.* 2002; 99: 169–70.

26. Royal Australian and New Zealand College of Obstetricians and Gynaecologists. Placenta acreta; 2014. www.ranzcog.edu.au/.../954-placenta-accreta-c-obs-20.html (accessed 20 May 2016).

27. Myerscough PR (ed.). *Munro Kerr's Operative Obstetrics*, 10th edition. London: Bailliere Tindall; 1982.

28. Kayem G, Davy C, Goffinet F, *et al.* Conservative versus extirpative management in cases of placenta accreta. *Obstet Gynecol.* 2004; 104: 531–6.

29. Lee W, Kirk JS, Comstock CH, *et al.* Vasa previa: prenatal detection by three-dimensional ultrasonography. *Ultrasound Obstet Gynecol.* 2000; 16: 384–7.

30. Derbala Y, Grochal F, Jeanty P. Vasa previa. *J Perinat Med.* 2007; 1: 2–13.

31. RCOG *Placenta Praevia, Placenta Praevia Accreta and Vasa Praevia: Diagnosis and Management.* London: RCOG Press; 2011.

32. Oyelese Y, Catanzarite V, Prefumo F, *et al.* Vasa previa: the impact of prenatal diagnosis on outcomes. *Obstet Gynecol.* 2004; 103: 937–42.

33. Knight M. Peripartum hysterectomy in the UK: management and outcomes of the associated haemorrhage. *BJOG.* 2007; 114: 1380–7.

34. Yang JI, Lim YK, Kim HS, *et al.* Sonographic findings of placenta lacunae and the prediction of adherent placenta in women with placenta previa totalis and prior cesarean section. *Ultrasound Obstet Gynecol.* 2006; 28: 178–2.

35. Chou MM, Tseng JJ, Ho ES. The application of three-dimensional color power Doppler ultrasound in the depiction of abnormal uteroplacental angioarchitecture in placenta previa percreta. *Ultrasound Obstet Gynaecol.* 2002; 19: 625–7.

36. Confidential Enquries into Maternal and Child Health. *Saving Mothers Lives: Reviewing Maternal Deaths to Make Motherhood Safer 2003–2005.* London: CEMACH; 2007.

37. Warshak CR, Eskander R, Hull AD, *et al.* Accuracy of ultrasonography and magnetic resonance imaging in the diagnosis of placenta accreta. *Obstet Gynecol.* 2006; 108: 573–81.

38. Sheiner E, Shoham-Vardi I, Hallak M, *et al.* Placental abruption in term pregnancies: clinical significance and obstetric risk factors. *J Matern Fetal Neonatal Med.* 2003; 13: 45–9.

39. Ananth CV, Berkowitz GS, Savitz DA, Lapinski RH. Placental abruption and adverse perinatal outcomes. *JAMA.* 1999; 282: 1646–51.

40. Ananth CV, Oyelese Y, Yeo L, Pradhan A, Vintzileos AM. Placental abruption in the United States, 1979 through 2001: temporal trends and potential determinants. *Am J Obstet Gynecol.* 2005; 192: 191–8.

41. Tikkanen M, Nuutila M, Hiilesmaa V, *et al.* Clinical presentation and risk factors of placental abruption. *Acta Obstet Gynecol Scand.* 2006; 85: 700–5.

42. Fox H (ed.), *Pathology of the Placenta.* London: Saunders; 1978.

43. Oyelese Y, Ananth CV. Placental abruption. *Obstet Gynecol.* 2006; 108: 1005–16.

44. Wicherek L, Klimek M, Dutsch-Wicherek M, *et al.* The molecular changes during placental detachment. *Eur J Obstet Gynecol Reproduct Biol.* 2006; 125: 171–5.

45. Harrington K, Fayyad A, Thakur V, Aquilina J. The value of uterine artery Doppler in the prediction of uteroplacental complications in multiparous women. *Ultrasound Obstet Gynecol.* 2004; 23: 50–5.

46. Toivonen S, Heinonen S, Anttila M, Kosma VM, Saarikoski S. Obstetric prognosis after placental abruption. *Fetal Diagn Ther.* 2004; 19: 336–41.

47. Ananth CV, Savitz DA, Williams MA. Placental abruption and its association with hypertension and prolonged rupture of membranes: a methodologic review and meta-analysis. *Obstet Gynecol.* 1996; 88: 309–18.

48. Ananth CV, Demissie K, Smulian JC, Vintzileos AM. Relationship among placenta previa, fetal growth restriction, and preterm delivery: a population-based study. *Obstet Gynecol.* 2001; 98: 299–306.

49. Gibbs JM, Weindling AM. Neonatal intracranial lesions following placental abruption. *Eur J Pediatr.* 1994; 153: 195–7.

50. Niswander KR, Friedman EA, Hooer DB, *et al.* Fetal morbidity following potentially ataxigenic obstetric conditions: I, abruption placentae. *Am J Obstet Gynecol.* 1996; 95: 838–55.

51. Ananth CV, Oyelese Y, Srinivas N, Yeo L, Vintzileos AM. Preterm premature rupture of membranes, intrauterine infection, and oligohydramnios: risk factors for placental abruption. *Obstet Gynecol.* 2004; 104: 71–7.

52. Nyberg DA, Cyr DR, Mack LA, *et al.* Sonographic spectrum of placental abruption. *Am J Roentgenol.* 1987; 148: 161–4.

53. Besinger RE, Niebyl JR. The safety and efficacy of tocolytic agents for the treatment of preterm labor. *Obstet and Gynecol Surv.* 1990; 45: 415–40.

54. Towers CV, Pircon RA, Heppard M. Is tocolysis safe in the management of third-trimester bleeding? *Am J Obstet Gynecol.* 1999; 180: 1572–8.

55. Kayani SI, Walkinshaw SA, Preston C. Pregnancy outcome in severe placental abruption. *BJOG.* 2003; 110: 679–83.

56. Rasmussen S, Irgens LM, Dalaker K. Outcome of pregnancies subsequent to placental abruption: a risk assessment. *Acta Obstet Gynecol Scand.* 2000; 79: 496–501.

57. Letsky EA. Disseminated intravascular coagulation. *Best Pract Res Clin Obstet Gynaecol.* 2001; 15: 623–44.

Management of the Third Stage of Labour

Hajeb Kamali and Pina Amin

The third stage of labour is defined as the time from the birth of the baby to the delivery of the placenta and membranes. In the majority of cases, the third stage is uneventful. However, complications of the third stage lead to significant mortality and morbidity, especially so in the developing nations. Worldwide, postpartum haemorrhage leads to approximately 130 000 deaths annually, accounting for 10.5% of all births [1]. It is the leading cause of maternal death in Africa and Asia, accounting for up to half of these [2]. The death rate in the UK from postpartum haemorrhage (PPH) had not significantly changed in the last Confidential Enquiry into maternal death [3], at 0.49 per 100 000. However, this still places obstetric haemorrhage as the third highest cause of direct maternal death. In total, it accounted for 17 maternal deaths in the UK during the period of 2009–12 and still accounts for 25% of maternal deaths in the developing world [4].

Physiology of the Third Stage of Labour

Placental Separation

During birth of the baby, there is a rapid and significant reduction in uterine size. The average of this diminution in length from onset of birth to its completion is 6.5 inches in 5 min. This is achieved by myometrial retraction, which is a unique characteristic of the uterine muscle, involving all three muscle fibre layers, allowing maintenance of the shortened length following each successive contraction. This continued retraction results in thickening of the myometrium, reduction of uterine volume and shrinkage of placental bed. The non-contractile placenta is undermined, detached and propelled into the lower uterine segment. This process is usually completed within 4.5 min

of delivery of the baby [5]. The second mechanism involved in uterine separation is haematoma formation, which occurs secondary to venous occlusion and vascular rupture in the placental bed caused by uterine contractions.

Signs of Placental Separation

1. The most reliable sign is the lengthening of the umbilical cord as the placenta separates and is pushed into the lower uterine segment by progressive uterine contractions. Placing a clamp on the cord near the perineum allows for a more reliable appreciation of this lengthening. Traction on the cord should not be applied without counter-traction or guarding of the uterus above the symphysis, otherwise cord lengthening as a result of uterine prolapse or inversion could be mistaken for placental separation.

2. The uterus takes on a more globular shape and becomes firmer. This occurs as the placenta descends into the lower segment and the body of the uterus continues to retract. This change may be difficult to appreciate clinically, especially in an obese mother.

3. A gush of blood occurs. The retro-placental clot is able to escape as the placenta descends to the lower uterine segment. The retro-placental clot usually forms centrally and escapes following complete separation. However, if the blood can find a path to escape, it may do so before complete separation and thus is not a reliable indicator of complete separation. This occurrence is sometimes associated with increased bleeding and a prolonged third stage, with the delivery of the leading edge of the placenta and maternal surface

first (the Matthews Duncan method), rather than the cord insertion and fetal surface, which is more common (the Schultze method).

Haemostasis

The placental bed at term is perfused with a blood flow of 500–700 ml/min. The blood vessels penetrating the uterus to supply the placental bed are surrounded by the interlacing muscle fibre of the myometrium. Contraction of these muscle fibres compresses the blood vessels like 'living ligatures'. Retraction of the muscle fibre keeps the vessels closed. A vivid demonstration of this physiological control of bleeding is seen at caesarean section (CS) when the emptied uterus becomes thick, firm and pale. In addition to uterine muscle contraction, fibrinous thrombi formation occurs in maternal sinuses, contributing to haemostasis by sealing the small sinuses in the uterine wall.

Vaginal Examination and Assessment of the Perineum After the Birth of the Baby

Although an assessment of the vagina and perineum can be carried out prior to delivery of the placenta, a more thorough, detailed look should be undertaken following placental delivery. The labia and perineum should be evaluated for any lacerations or haematomas. This examination is especially important following an operative delivery, in which case a rectal examination should also be routinely performed to assess for third- or fourth-degree tears. Instrumental delivery should also prompt the routine assessment of vagina and cervix. If there are lacerations around the urethra, consideration should be given to insertion of an indwelling urinary catheter. Consideration for an indwelling catheter should also be given in the case of instrumental delivery involving regional analgesia.

Third Stage Management

Expectant Management

This is often described as physiological. It involves omission of routine use of uterotonic agents, delaying cord clamping/cutting until umbilical pulsations have ceased and delivery of the placenta by maternal effort. Mothers wanting to delay cord clamping for greater

Table 14.1 Risks of physiological vs. active third stage [6]

	Physiological third stage	Active third stage
Nausea and vomiting	1/20	1/10
Blood loss >1000 ml	29/1000	13/1000
Need for blood transfusion	40/1000	14/1000

than five minutes should be supported in this decision as long as there is no fetal or maternal reason to expedite this process [6].

Active Management

This involves the administration of oxytocic drugs (10 IU oxytocin IM [6] or 10 IU IV/IM [7]) following delivery of the anterior shoulder or immediately after the birth of the baby, before the cord is clamped and cut. This is followed by delayed cord clamping and controlled cord traction (CCT) once there are signs of placental separation.

Women should be advised to have an active third stage as it reduces rates of PPH or blood transfusion, although low-risk mothers wanting a physiological third stage should be supported in their decision as long as they have been counselled regarding the risks (Table 14.1). Unless there are concerns about cord integrity or newborn well-being, the cord should not be clamped earlier than 1 min [6]. Controlled cord traction should take place after 5 min during active management [6]. Current WHO recommendations [7] are for delayed cord clamping of 1–3 min for all births while undertaking simultaneous newborn care. This can reduce rates of neonatal anaemia and is especially relevant in resource-poor settings [6,7]. Some modern resuscitaires can be kept alongside the mother's bedside during vaginal delivery or at time of CS. This allows significantly delayed cord clamping/cutting and a resultant continuation of cord circulation and transfer of maternal oxygen to the newborn until such time that external resuscitation has taken effect. Delaying cord clamping does not lead to increased rates of PPH, length of the third stage or rates of retained placenta [6].

Uterotonic Drugs Used in the Third Stage of Labour (Table 14.2)

Oxytocin is usually given IV or IM as a bolus. There are no adverse maternal haemodynamic responses to an

Table 14.2 Drugs used for the third stage of labour

Agent	Dose	Route	Side-effects	Contraindications	Comments
Oxytocin	10 IU 5 IU	IM IV	Few	None	Effective, relatively cheap, can be repeated. Needs cold storage conditions and protection from light
Ergometrine	250 mcg	IM or IV	Nausea, vomiting, hypertension	Pre-eclampsia, hypertension, cardiac, migraine	Needs cold storage conditions and protection from light
Syntometrine®	5 IU Syntocinon®/0.5 mg ergometrine	IM	Nausea, vomiting, hypertension	Pre-eclampsia, hypertension, cardiac, migraine	Needs cold storage conditions and protection from light
Carbetocin	100 mcg	IV			Long-acting
Carboprost	250 mcg	IM	Bronchospasm	Asthma	Can be given into the myometrium
Misoprostol	600 mcg	PO for prophylaxis	GI disturbance, shivering, pyrexia		Cheap, stable, no special storage conditions
	800 mcg	Sublingual for treatment of PPH			
Intraumbilical oxytocin	10 IU in 20 ml saline	Umbilical	None	None	May reduce manual removal, uncertain effect on PPH

IV bolus of 5 IU or an IM bolus of 10 IU. Infusion is less effective at preventing PPH, but may be used following an initial bolus for prophylaxis or treatment of PPH. It is a well-tolerated drug that can be safely used for all women. Given IV, it is the recommended uterotonic drug for the treatment of PPH [6,7].

Ergot alkaloids (ergometrine, methylergometrine) are usually given intravenously (IV) or intramuscularly (IM) as the oral forms are unstable and have unpredictable side-effects. The usual dose is 250–500 mcg. They are effective in reducing PPH, but are associated with increased vomiting, pain and elevation of blood pressure. Both agents cause smooth muscle contraction, affecting uterine muscle and vessel wall muscle, leading to vasoconstriction. As such, they are contraindicated in the presence of hypertension, cardiac disease and other vascular conditions such as migraine [8].

Syntometrine® combines 5 IU oxytocin with 0.5 mg ergometrine and is given IM. It is associated with a small reduction in the risk of PPH at 500–1000 ml compared to oxytocin alone at any dose [6]. However, there is also an increase in maternal side-effects (increased blood pressure, nausea and vomiting) [9]. Ergometrine/methylergometrine and fixed drug combinations of oxytocin and ergometrine (e.g.

Syntometrine®) should be given as first line uterotonics in settings where oxytocin alone is not available [7].

Carbetocin is a long-acting synthetic oxytocin analogue. Its effect is related to dose, but the licensed dose is 100 mcg IV. It is commonly used following delivery by CS. In comparison to 5 IU oxytocin it is associated with less need for additional uterotonic agents and uterine massage. However, current evidence does not suggest that it is better than oxytocin alone at preventing PPH [10,11].

Misoprostol is an analogue of prostaglandin E1. There has been much interest in this as an uterotonic agent as it is cheap, heat-stable, does not require refrigeration and can be given orally. It has been shown to be effective at preventing PPH, but rates of severe PPH and additional need for uterotonics are higher than injectable uterotonics [12]. It is also associated with side-effects including shivering and pyrexia [13]. These side-effects are reduced when it is given rectally [14]. It can also be used in women where ergometrine is contraindicated. The recommended dose is 600 mcg orally for prophylaxis and 800 mcg sublingually for treatment of PPH [7]. It is an ideal agent in the management of the third stage and reduction in the rates of PPH in the developing world, but is unlikely to become a first line uterotonic drug in those settings where oxytocin is available. Current recommendations are for the use of misoprostol in settings where oxytocin is not available to women for the third stage [7].

Carboprost is an analogue of prostaglandin F2α that stimulates uterine contraction. It is usually given IM and in theory can also be administered directly into the myometrium, although this is clearly a more invasive route. The dose is 250 mcg repeated every 15 min to a maximum dose of 2 mg. Studies have suggested that carboprost is more effective than oxytocin for the prevention of PPH [15] and its use as a first line agent for active management of the third stage has also shown encouraging results [16]. However, lack of convincing evidence and a significant side-effect profile have prevented its routine use for the third stage as prophylaxis, although it continues to have a role in the treatment of PPH.

Intraumbilical oxytocin is usually given as a bolus of 10 IU oxytocin diluted to 20 ml with normal saline and given into the proximal umbilical cord. There have been a number of trials looking at prevention of PPH that have shown no significant benefit, although there is some evidence that it reduces the need for manual removal of the placenta when delivery of the placenta is delayed [17,18]. The current NICE guidance on intrapartum care [6] recommends that intraumbilical oxytocin should not be routinely used in active management of the third stage and this finding is supported by a recent systematic review [19] that concluded that the use of umbilical vein oxytocin has little or no effect.

In conclusion, management of the third stage should be active, with 10 IU oxytocin IM at delivery of anterior shoulder or immediately after birth, delayed cord clamping of at least 1 min and CCT [6] by the Brandt Andrews method.

Delayed Cord Clamping

There is increasing evidence that delayed cord clamping and enhanced placental transfusion provides improved neonatal outcomes (Table 14.3). In situations where urgent obstetric intervention is required, umbilical cord milking may facilitate more rapid neonatal resuscitation, although there is no strong evidence for this. Studies have also shown that delayed cord clamping has minimal, if any, effect on rates of polycythaemia or need for phototherapy [20].

The benefits of delayed cord clamping are of particular value in preterm infants and have been shown

Table 14.3 Delayed cord clamping

Advantages	Disadvantages
Higher haematocrits [21,22]	Delay to critical resuscitation attempts [31,32,33]
Improved haemodynamic stability [23,24]	
Reduced need for blood transfusion [25,26]	
Reduced rates of necrotizing enterocolitis [27,28]	
Reduced rates of sepsis [29]	
50% reduction in rates of intraventricular haemorrhage [29,30]	

to lead to improved neonatal outcomes, including a reduction in neonatal mortality in this group [34].

Gravity is also thought to play a role in the degree of placental transfusion. For term births where the cord is intact, the baby should not be lifted higher than the mother's abdomen or chest [35].

Controlled Cord Traction

There are two methods of CCT. The Brandt Andrews manoeuvre is most commonly employed in UK practice. This involves one hand on the lower abdomen, which secures the uterine fundus to prevent inversion, and steady traction on the cord with the other hand. The second is the Crede manoeuvre in which the hand holding the cord is fixed and the hand on the lower abdomen applies upward traction. Use of fundal pressure to deliver the placenta is also described, although this may cause pain, haemorrhage and increase the risk of uterine inversion [36]. In situations where a birth attendant trained in CCT is not present, CCT should not be undertaken [7]. There is very little increase in the risk of severe PPH (>1000 ml) associated with omission of CCT (RR 1.09 [37]). CCT as part of active management should not be undertaken until oxytocin has been administered and there are signs of placental separation [6].

Management at Caesarean Section

Delivery of the placenta at CS should be by CCT following administration of oxytocic drugs [7]. Manual removal is associated with increased risk of PPH and endometritis.

Retained Placenta

The third stage of labour is diagnosed as prolonged if not completed within 30 min of the birth of the baby with active management and 60 min with physiological management [6]. Severe PPH is related to a prolonged third stage of labour of more than 30 min. A prospective study [5] of 6588 women delivered vaginally showed that a third stage longer than 18 min is associated with significant risk of PPH. After 30 min the odds of having PPH are six times higher than before 30 min.

Aetiology of Retained Placenta

Retained placenta can have three underlying aetiologies:

1. **Trapped placenta:** there has been complete separation of the placenta but it has not been delivered spontaneously or with gentle cord traction. This is often because the cervix has begun to constrict.
2. **Adherent placenta:** a placenta that is superficially adherent to the myometrium but that will come away easily with manual separation.
3. **Placenta accreta:** a placenta that is histologically invading the myometrium and cannot be simply separated. This cause carries with it the highest morbidity.

Immediately after birth, there is myometrial contraction. It is thought that there is a slight delay in retro-placental myometrial contraction. In cases where there is inadequate retro-placental contraction, for example secondary to uterine fatigue in those with prolonged uterine contraction or failure to progress, there will be an adherent placenta.

The pathogenesis of placenta accreta, however, is very different and occurs during pregnancy. Its aetiology is not fully understood but there are several theories. Previous surgery or an anatomical defect can cause defective decidualization that allows direct placental attachment to the myometrium. Previous CS, myomectomy and endometrial curettage account for up to 80% of cases of accreta [27].

Other possibilities are that there is aggressive over-invasion of extravillous trophoblastic tissue or defective placental vascular remodelling at the site of previous uterine surgery. It is also possible that early partial or complete wound dehiscence 'opens the door' for extravillous trophoblast to invade the myometrium [27].

Placenta accreta has an affinity for multiparous women with advanced age. The two most important risk factors for placenta accreta are a known placenta praevia and a prior caesarean delivery.

Risk Factors for Retained Placenta

- Previous uterine surgery, e.g. caesarean delivery, curettage, myomectomy;
- history of uterine infection;
- uterine fibroids;
- previous manual removal of placenta;
- preterm delivery;
- congenital uterine anomaly;
- pre-eclampsia, intrauterine growth restriction and other consequences of defective placentation.

Management of Retained Placenta

The retained or partially detached placenta interferes with uterine contraction and retraction and leads to bleeding. The decision for method of analgesia, whether it is regional block or a general anaesthetic, is based on the level of clinical urgency, and following discussion and consent by the patient. Uterine relaxants or the cessation of oxytocin infusion to aid uterine exploration is likely to lead to increased bleeding and is therefore not advisable.

Once a diagnosis of retained placenta is made, an initial assessment should be made to elicit the degree of resuscitation required. Intravenous access should always be secured in women with retained placenta, and blood taken for full blood count and group and save serum. If there is any evidence of haemodynamic compromise or hypovolaemic shock, resuscitation of the patient takes priority over manual removal of the placenta. This should occur in conjunction with an experienced anaesthetist. It is reasonable for resuscitation to take place in conjunction with preparations for and transfer to theatre in cases where there is ongoing bleeding refractory to initial measures.

Ensuring the bladder is empty may speed the delivery of the placenta and aid in the assessment and control of the bleeding. If the placenta does not deliver spontaneously, a second dose of 10 IU oxytocin can be administered in combination with CCT [7]. Current NICE guidance [6] does not recommend use of either intraumbilical oxytocin or intravenous administration of oxytocin in cases of retained placenta.

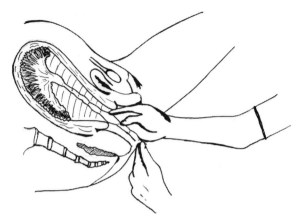

Figure 14.1 Insertion of hand into the uterus following the umbilical cord.

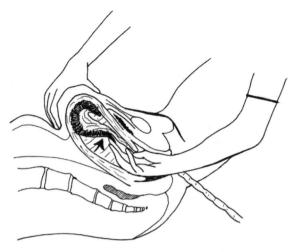

Figure 14.2 Creating plane between placenta and uterus.

However, intravenous oxytocic agents are recommended in those patients where there is a retained placenta and active bleeding. An appropriate anaesthetic agent should be in place prior to uterine exploration or attempt at manual removal [6].

Technique of Manual Removal of the Placenta

The procedure should be carried out in a sterile operating theatre with the patient in lithotomy. Once, scrubbed and gowned, an elbow-length glove or gauntlet glove is worn with a focus on aseptic technique to minimize the risk of subsequent endometritis. The perineum should be prepared with a sterile solution and bladder emptied at this point with an in/out catheter. The vaginal hand should be lubricated with an antiseptic cream to facilitate entry. The hand first passes through the vagina and then cervix. Often, the cervix will have begun to constrict back down and will be at the stage where direct entry is not always immediately possible. The fingers and thumb should be positioned into a conical shape to minimize the profile and volume of the hand. Entry through the cervix may require continuous gentle pressure against the cervix until it has dilated back up enough to allow access. As the procedure is done blindly, the cord can be used to guide the hand towards the placenta (Figure 14.1).

It is crucial that the uterine fundus is controlled with the other hand in order to minimize the risk of uterine rupture or trauma secondary to excessive force. This manipulation of the fundus will also aid in orientation and positioning. If the placenta has already sep-

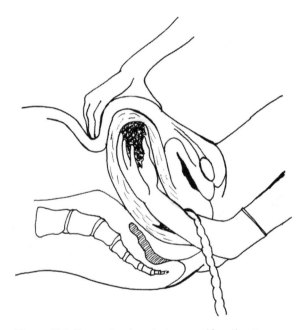

Figure 14.3 Placenta in palm prior to removal from the uterus.

arated and is sat in the lower segment, this can simply be removed. However, if still attached, the placental edge is located and the operator's fingers used to gently and slowly shear the placenta away from the uterus (Figure 14.2).

The placenta is pushed to the palmar aspect of the hand and when it is entirely separated, the hand is withdrawn with the placenta in the palm, as in Figure 14.3. Effort should not be made to remove the placenta until the obstetrician is confident there are still no attached areas, as this will increase the likelihood of an incomplete placenta and undiagnosed retained placenta. If the placenta does not separate from the uterine surface by gentle lateral movement of the fingertips at the line of cleavage, suspect placenta accreta. Call for expert help to confirm the findings. If the placenta is adherent and difficult to remove, consider laparotomy with a view to hysterectomy if there is massive bleeding of concern. If there is no bleeding it may be possible to cut the cord as high as possible and consider conservative management. Such management needs antibiotics and close observation for bleeding and infection.

An oxytocin infusion should be ready and running prior to completion of the process in order to maintain uterine tone following complete removal. Concurrent bimanual massage can be performed. It is crucial that the membranes and placenta are carefully examined and uterine cavity examined to make sure it is empty and the uterus is hard and contracted. There should be a low threshold for further exploration if the placenta and membranes were found to be incomplete or there is ongoing significant bleeding. A vessel leading to the edge of the membrane suggests a likelihood of retained succenturiate lobe of the placenta. As a rule of thumb, the membranes should be large enough to cover the placenta one and a half times. Whenever manual removal of placenta is undertaken, a single prophylactic dose of antibiotics should be administered [7].

Retained Placenta Under Special Circumstances

Morbidly adherent placentae, such as placenta accreta, placenta increta and placenta percreta as mentioned earlier, occur due to abnormal placentation and a defective basalis layer due to previous scarring [38]. The incidence of morbidly attached placenta is rising due to the rising rate of caesarean delivery.

Placenta accreta shares many of the risk factors for a retained placenta. The risk of placenta accreta rises sharply in mothers who have had two or more previous CSs who are aged 35 years or over and have an anterior or central placenta praevia. Women with previous uterine trauma in the form of uterine curettage and uterine perforation are also at risk of morbidly adherent placenta.

Placenta accreta is usually diagnosed when difficulty is encountered during delivery of the placenta and manual removal has to be performed. With a high index of suspicion, placenta accreta and its variants can be diagnosed antenatally in the aforementioned high-risk women. When a diagnosis of placenta accreta is suspected, colour flow Doppler ultrasonography should be performed, as it has higher sensitivity and specificity compared to magnetic resonance imaging [39]. Where antenatal imaging is not possible locally, such women should be managed as if they have placenta accreta until proven otherwise. Bilateral internal iliac artery occlusion balloons can be placed prior to commencement of CS. At CS, after delivery of the baby, uterine arterial embolization could be carried out via pre-inserted catheters and hysterectomy performed if there is continued blood loss. This complex management clearly requires a high level of organization and a multidisciplinary approach with involvement of obstetricians, anaesthetists, midwives, radiologists, haematologists, vascular surgeons and theatre staff.

Placenta increta/accreta/percreta can be managed conservatively in highly selected cases, where there is minimal bleeding and the woman desires to preserve her fertility. This involves delivering the baby via an upper segment vertical incision and leaving the placenta behind. This conservative management requires rigorous follow-up until complete resorption of the placenta occurs. Undetectable βhCg values do not seem to guarantee complete resorption of retained placental tissue. Close monitoring for signs and symptoms of infection and coagulopathy are mandatory. In the case of major haemorrhage, which usually [39] occurs 10–14 days after delivery, hysterectomy should not be delayed. Careful counselling of the woman is crucial in these cases.

Placenta percreta can invade the urinary bladder and usually requires surgery, which may include partial resection of the bladder. More detailed accounts on the management of morbidly adherent placenta are given in Chapter 16.

Women at Risk of Postpartum Haemorrhage

Women with risk factors for postpartum haemorrhage (PPH) should be advised to deliver in an obstetric unit where more advanced options and resources are at hand for the management of a significant PPH. Close observation for signs of bleeding following delivery is vital in such women.

Risk Factors for PPH [6]

Antenatal risk factors

- Previous retained placenta or PPH;
- maternal haemoglobin <85 g/l at start of labour;
- BMI >35 kg m^2;
- grand multiparity (parity four or more);
- antepartum haemorrhage;
- overdistension of the uterus (e.g. multiple gestation, polyhydramnios, macrosomia);
- current uterine abnormality, e.g. fibroids;
- low-lying placenta; or
- maternal age 35 or older.

Intrapartum risk factors

- Induction of labour;
- prolonged first, second or third stage;
- use of oxytocin;
- precipitate labour; or
- operative birth or CS.

In two-thirds of cases, PPH occurs without any risk factors. Therefore, it is important units and staff are equipped and prepared for this eventuality.

Prevention of Postpartum Haemorrhage is Much Easier than its Treatment

Every birth attendant needs to have the knowledge, skills and clinical judgement to carry out active management of the third stage of labour as well as having access to the necessary supplies and equipment. Incorporation of guidelines for the active management of the third stage of labour and prevention of PPH into local guidance is also essential. The skills in the management of a complicated third stage of labour should be updated regularly by conduction of 'obstetric drills' similar to other obstetric emergencies. National professional associations and government bodies play an important role in addressing legislative and other barriers that impede the prevention and treatment of PPH. It is also important to provide adequate education to the public (mothers and their families) for prevention of PPH.

Postpartum Care

Maternal postpartum observation should be tailored to the need for timely identification of signs of excessive blood loss, including hypotension and tachycardia. Maternal vital signs and the amount of vaginal bleeding should be evaluated continuously alongside massage of uterine fundus to identify size and degree of contraction, which should be noted [40].

Women with anaemia are particularly vulnerable, since they may not tolerate even a moderate amount of blood loss. Women with inherited coagulopathies require individualized management plans, as their risks for bleeding extend beyond the first 24 hours after delivery. In women with infective risks or where infection may worsen the maternal condition, a single dose of prophylactic antibiotics is given [41] according to trust policy.

Errors in the Management of the Third Stage and their Sequelae

Attempts to deliver a placenta that is not completely separated may cause partial separation and retained products. Inappropriate management of the third stage of labour with excessive cord traction and fundal pressure is responsible for uterine inversion in the majority of cases.

There is an ever-present danger of uterine rupture during the manual removal of a placenta. This usually occurs if the operator fails to push the fundus down onto the vaginal hand. The inexperienced operator may mistake the lower segment for the uterine cavity and grasp the upper segment, mistaking it for the placenta. Further trauma to the lower segment may be the result of trying to force the hand through the retraction ring of the cervix.

Conclusion

The majority of women will have an uneventful third stage of labour. However, it can be associated with significant morbidity and mortality and requires careful and effective management by an experienced clinician.

References

1. AbouZahr C. Global burden of maternal death and disability. In Rodeck C (ed.), *Reducing Maternal Death and Disability in Pregnancy* (pp. 1–11). Oxford: Oxford University Press; 2003.
2. Khan KS, Wojdyla D, Say L, Gümezoglu AM, Look PFA. WHO analysis of causes of maternal death: a systematic review. *Lancet*. 2006; 367: 1066–74.

3. Knight M, Kenyon S, Brocklehurst P, *et al.* (eds). *Saving Lives, Improving Mothers' Care: Lessons Learned to Inform Future Maternity Care from the UK and Ireland Confidential Enquiries into Maternal Deaths and Morbidity 2009–12.* Oxford: National Perinatal Epidemiology Unit, University of Oxford; 2014.

4. World Health Organization. *Maternal Mortality in 2005.* Geneva: WHO; 2007.

5. Magann EF, Evans S, Chauhan SP, *et al.* The length of the third stage of labor and the risk of postpartum hemorrhage. *Obstet Gynecol.* 2005; 105: 290–3.

6. NICE. *Intrapartum Care: Care of Healthy Women and their Babies during Childbirth*: Clinical Guideline 190. London: NICE; 2014.

7. World Health Organization. *WHO Recommendations for the Prevention and Treatment of Postpartum Haemorrhage*: Geneva: WHO; 2013.

8. Liabsuetrakul T, Choobun T, Peeyananjarassri K, Islam QM. Prophylactic use of ergot alkaloids in the third stage of labour. *Cochrane Database Syst Rev.* 2007; 2: CD005456.

9. McDonald S, Abbott JM, Higgins SP. Prophylactic ergometrine–oxytocin versus oxytocin for the third stage of labour. *Cochrane Database Syst Rev.* 2004; 1: CD000201.

10. Attilakos G, Psaroudakis D, Ash J, *et al.* Carbetocin versus oxytocin for the prevention of postpartum haemorrhage following caesarean section: the results of a double-blind randomised trial. *BJOG.* 2010; 117: 929–36.

11. Su LL, Chong YS, Samuel M. Oxytocin agonists for preventing postpartum haemorrhage. *Cochrane Database Syst Rev.* 2007; 3: CD005457.

12. Abalos E. Choice of uterotonic agents in the active management of the third stage of labour: RHL commentary. Geneva: World Health Organization; 2009.

13. Gulmezoglu AM, Forna F, Villar J, Hofmeyr GJ. Prostaglandins for preventing postpartum haemorrhage. *Cochrane Database Syst Rev.* 2007; 3: CD000494.

14. Khan RU, El-Refaey H. Pharmacokinetics and adverse-effect profile of rectally administered misoprostol in the third stage of labor. *Obstet Gynecol.* 2003; 101: 968–74.

15. Bai Jing, Sun Qian, Zhai Hui. A comparison of oxytocin and carboprost tromethamine in the prevention of postpartum hemorrhage in high-risk patients undergoing cesarean delivery. *Exp Ther Med.* 2014; 7(1): 46–50.

16. Vaid A, Dadhwal V, Mittal S, *et al.* A randomized controlled trial of prophylactic sublingual misoprostol versus intramuscular methyl-ergometrine versus intramuscular 15-methyl PGF2alpha in active management of third stage of labor. *Arch Gynecol Obstet.* 2009; 280: 893–7.

17. Habek D, Franicevic D. Intraumbilical injection of uterotonics for retained placenta. *Int J Gynaecol Obstet.* 2007; 99: 105–9.

18. Ghulmiyyah LM, Wehbe SA, Saltzman SL, Ehleben C, Sibai BM. Intraumbilical vein injection of oxytocin and the third stage of labor: randomized double-blind placebo trial. *Am J Perinatol.* 2007; 24: 347–52.

19. Nardin JM, Weeks A, Carroli G. Umbilical vein injection for management of retained placenta. *Cochrane Database Syst Rev.* 2011; 5: CD001337.

20. Andersson O, Hellström-Westas L, Andersson D, Domellöf M. Effect of delayed versus early umbilical cord clamping on neonatal outcomes and iron status at 4 months: a randomised controlled trial. *BMJ.* 2011; 343: d7156.

21. Strauss RG, Mock DM, Johnson KJ, *et al.* A randomized clinical trial comparing immediate versus delayed clamping of the umbilical cord in preterm infants: short-term clinical and laboratory endpoints. *Transfusion.* 2008;48: 658–65.

22. Kaempf JW, Tomlinson MW, Kaempf AJ, *et al.* Delayed umbilical cord clamping in premature neonates. *Obstet Gynecol.* 2012; 120: 325–30.

23. Sommers R, Stonestreet BS, Oh W, *et al.* Hemodynamic effects of delayed cord clamping in premature infants. *Pediatrics.* 2012; 129: e667–72.

24. Takami T, Suganami Y, Sunohara D, *et al.* Umbilical cord milking stabilizes cerebral oxygenation and perfusion in infants born before 29 weeks of gestation. *J Pediatr.* 2012; 161: 742–7.

25. Ibrahim HM, Krouskop RW, Lewis DF, Dhanireddy R. Placental transfusion: umbilical cord clamping and preterm infants. *J Perinatol.* 2000; 20: 351–4.

26. Kinmond S, Aitchison TC, Holland BM, *et al.* Umbilical cord clamping and preterm infants: a randomised trial. *BMJ.* 1993; 306: 172–5.

27. Rabe H, Diaz-Rossello JL, Duley L, Dowswell T. Effect of timing of umbilical cord clamping and other strategies to influence placental transfusion at preterm birth on maternal and infant outcomes. *Cochrane Database Syst Rev.* 2012, 8: CD003248. doi: 10.1002/14651858.CD003248.pub3.

28. Aziz K, Chinnery H, Lacaze-Masmonteil T. A single-center experience of implementing delayed cord clamping in babies born at less than 33 weeks' gestational age. *Adv Neonatal Care.* 2012; 12: 371–6.

29. Mercer JS, Vohr BR, McGrath MM, *et al.* Delayed cord clamping in very preterm infants reduces the incidence of intraventricular hemorrhage and late-onset sepsis: a randomized, controlled trial. *Pediatrics.* 2006; 117: 1235–42.

30. American College of Obstetricians and Gynecologists. Timing of umbilical cord clamping after birth: committee opinion no. 543. *Obstet Gynecol.* 2012; 120: 1522–6.

31. Saigal S, O'Neill A, Surainder Y, Chua LB, Usher R. Placental transfusion and hyperbilirubinemia in the premature. *Pediatrics.* 1972; 49: 406–19.

32. Saigal S, Usher RH. Symptomatic neonatal plethora. *Biol Neonate.* 1977; 32: 62–72.

33. Yao AC, Lind J, Vuorenkoski V. Expiratory grunting in the late clamped normal neonate. *Pediatrics.* 1971; 48: 865–70.

34. Backes CH, Rivera BK, Haque U, *et al.* Placental transfusion strategies in very preterm neonates. *Obstet Gynecol.* 2014; 124: 47–56.

35. Royal College of Obstetricians and Gynaecologists. Clamping of the Umbilical Cord and Placental Transfusion. Scientific Impact Paper No. 14, 2015.

36. Pena-Marti G, Comunian-Carrasco G. Fundal pressure versus controlled cord traction as part of the active management of the third stage of labour. *Cochrane Database Syst Rev.* 2007; 4: CD005462.

37. Gulmezoglu AM, Lumbiganon P, Landoulsi S, *et al.* Active management of the third stage of labour with and without controlled cord traction. *Lancet.* 2012; 379: 1721–7.

38. Tantbirojn P, Crum CP, Parast MM. Pathophysiology of placenta creta: the role of decidua and extra villous trophoblast. *Placenta.* 2008; 29: 639–45.

39. RCOG. *Placenta Praevia and Placenta Praevia Accreta: Diagnosis and Management.* London: RCOG Press; 2005.

40. ACOG. *Guideline for Perinatal Care*, 6th edition. Washington, DC: ACOG; 2007.

41. WHO. *Managing Complications in Pregnancy and Childbirth. A Guide for Midwives and Doctors.* Geneva: WHO; 2003.

Postpartum Haemorrhage

Anushuya Devi Kasi and Edwin Chandraharan

Postpartum haemorrhage (PPH) is the world's leading preventable cause of maternal mortality. It affects 2% of all women who give birth and still accounts for 27% of maternal deaths globally. More than half of these deaths occur within 24 hours of delivery. It is estimated that worldwide 140 000 women die of PPH each year – one every four minutes – and PPH remains a cause of maternal death in the UK [1].

PPH is defined as the loss of 500 ml or more of blood from the genital tract within 24 hours of the birth of a baby. PPH can be minor (500–1000 ml) or major (more than 1000 ml). Major could be divided into moderate (1000–2000 ml) or severe (more than 2000 ml). Secondary PPH is defined as abnormal or excessive bleeding from the birth canal between 24 hours and 12 weeks postpartum [2]. There is no single satisfactory definition for PPH as a blood loss of 1000 ml following caesarean has been used for diagnosis. A drop of 10% of haematocrit has also been used to define PPH.

Although young and fit pregnant women tolerate mild to moderate blood loss well, loss of more than 40% of total blood volume is often life threatening. Clinical signs and symptoms of blood loss, including weakness, sweating and tachycardia, might not appear until 15–25% of total blood volume is lost; haemodynamic collapse occurs only at losses between 35% and 45%.

Complications of massive blood loss include haemorrhagic shock, disseminated intravascular coagulopathy (DIC), adult respiratory distress syndrome, renal failure, hepatic failure, loss of fertility, pituitary necrosis (Sheehan's syndrome) and maternal death [3].

Pathophysiology

Uterine blood flow increases from approximately 30–50 ml at the onset of pregnancy to approximately 1000 ml at term. Haemodynamic and haematologic changes during pregnancy are designed to be protective against blood loss that may result from bleeding from the large placental site after the delivery of the placenta. Maternal blood volume increases by 45%; this is approximately 1200–1600 ml above non-pregnant values, thereby creating a hypervolaemic state during pregnancy by increase in both the plasma volume (40%) and the red cell mass (25%) [4]. This provides a 'protective cushion' against rapid decompensation following blood loss.

Progressive hyperplasia and hypertrophy of uterine muscle fibres (myometrium) and their special 'criss-cross' arrangement create the 'living ligatures' to rapidly squeeze blood vessels supplying the placenta by effective contraction and retraction of muscle fibres. In addition, changes in the coagulation system during pregnancy result in a hypercoagulable state enabling rapid clotting in the placental bed following placental expulsion. Therefore, a pregnant woman is generally protected against hypovolaemic shock arising from rapid blood loss following delivery.

Haemodynamic compensatory response to ongoing blood loss includes tachypnoea and tachycardia. Women may lose up to 20–25% of their blood volume before displaying symptoms of hypovolaemia (Table 15.1), and clinical symptoms of hypovolaemia follow a predictable sequence (Table 15.2), although the speed of the blood loss, the woman's original haematocrit, the extent of her blood volume expansion and her hydration status will affect the individual response [5].

Best Practice in Labour and Delivery, Second Edition, ed. Sir Sabaratnam Arulkumaran. Published by Cambridge University Press. © Cambridge University Press 2016.

Table 15.1 Risk Factors for PPH

Antepartum	Age Ethnicity (Black African, Asian) BMI Previous PPH Assisted conception (multiple pregnancy or abnormal placentation)
During pregnancy	Multiparity Multiple pregnancy Polyhydramnios uterine fibroids Pre-eclampsia
Intrapartum	Operative vaginal delivery Chorioamnionitis Prolonged labour Augmented labour Precipitate labour Episiotomy

Table 15.2 The 4 'T's: the mechanisms by which bleeding occurs include the 4 'T's

Tone of uterus (80%) – abnormalities of uterine contractions
Tissue – retained tissue inside the uterus
Trauma – lacerations to any part of the genital tract
Thrombin – abnormalities of coagulation

Table 15.3 Aetiology of PPH

Hypotonia/atonia (80%)	Uterine atony (grand multipara) Placenta praevia (poor contractility of the lower segment) Uterine inversion Uterine overdistension – polyhydramnios, multiple pregnancy, fibroids
Trauma	Genital tract injury including broad ligament haematoma Uterine rupture Surgical – caesarean sections, angular extensions, episiotomy
Tissue	Retained placenta or products of conception
Coagulation failure	Placental abruption Pre-eclampsia Septicaemia/intrauterine sepsis Existing coagulation abnormalities

The severe loss of blood leads to inadequate tissue oxygenation, a release of epinephrine and nore-pinephrine, and increased vasoconstriction. This catecholamine response increases the heart rate, vascular tone and myocardial contractility to compensate for the decreased volume [6].

Risk Factors for PPH

Risk factors for PPH are given in Table 15.1. Abnormalities of one or a combination of four basic processes (four Ts): uterine atony (tone); retained placenta, membranes or blood clots (tissue); genital tract trauma (trauma); or coagulation abnormalities (thrombin) usually account for PPH.

Causes of PPH

Causes of primary PPH are due to the 4 Ts (Table 15.2) and the vast majority (80%) are due to poor tone of the uterine myometrium (Table 15.3). Secondary PPH occurs due to infection (endometritis), which is usually associated with retained placenta and membranes or, rarely, secondary to uterine arteriovenous malformations in the placental bed.

Young and fit pregnant women with no pre-existing co-morbidities (such as severe anaemia or cardiac disease) may tolerate 10–15% of loss of blood volume without demonstrating significant alteration in haemodynamic parameters. However, with progressive blood loss (15–30%) hypotension may be evidenced and loss of >40% of blood volume may result in CNS and myocardial decompensation (Table 15.4). An acute and severe blood loss can lead to rapid

decompensation and cardiovascular failure. Severity depends on body weight (i.e. BMI), pre-haemorrhage haemoglobin level and the presence of other co-morbidities. A window of opportunity often exists in which, if treatment is commenced, the outcome may be optimal. This is often termed 'the golden hour' and refers to the time in which resuscitation must begin to ensure the best chance of survival. The probability of survival decreases sharply after the first hour if the patient is not effectively resuscitated.

Role of the 'Rule of 30' and 'Obstetric Shock Index' in Estimation of Blood Loss

Visual estimation of blood loss is notoriously inaccurate and is fraught with inter- and intra-observer variation. In continuing PPH, it may not be possible to accurately document the exact volume of ongoing blood loss. The Rule of 30 (Table 15.5) and Obstetric Shock Index (OSI) have been proposed to aid the estimation of blood loss in obstetric haemorrhage. The OSI refers to the pulse rate divided by systolic blood pressure; this should be less than 0.9 during pregnancy.

Table 15.4 Symptoms and signs of hypovolaemic shock

Signs and symptoms	Aetiology
Compensation	
Tachypnoea	Increasing in the rate and depth of respiration is often the first compensatory response to increase oxygen intake so as to maintain arterial oxygen level. In late stages, laborious breathing may indicate the onset of metabolic acidosis.
Tachycardia	Reflects catecholamine response to increase cardiac output and constrict the peripheral vasculature so as to divert blood from non-essential to essential (central) organs. Progressive tachycardia indicates worsening haemodynamic instability.
Skin: cold, clammy, pale	Peripheral vasoconstriction and sympathetic activity leading to increased sweating.
Capillary filling time	Takes more than 2 sec due to peripheral vasoconstriction. Therefore, pulse oximetry may not accurately reflect tissue oxygen perfusion.
Oliguria	Decreased renal perfusion secondary to catecholamine surge and renal vasoconstriction. In severe cases, acute renal failure may ensue.
Decompensation	
Hypotension	Reflects onset of decompensation secondary to decreased blood volume; in severe cases it may be due to metabolic acidosis resulting in peripheral vasodilatation and myocardial dysfunction.
Hypothermia	Initial intense peripheral vasoconstriction due to catecholamine surge followed by peripheral vasodilatation due to ensuing metabolic acidosis.
Altered mental status: anxiety, restlessness, confusion and decreased level of consciousness	Reflects progressive reduction in cerebral perfusion and hypoxia to central nervous system.
Cardiac arrest	Myocardial hypoxia and acidosis leading to systolic and diastolic dysfunction.

Table 15.5 'Rule of 30' for massive obstetric haemorrhage

Systolic blood pressure	Falls by 30 mmHg
Pulse	Increased by 30 beats/min
Haemoglobin	Falls by 30% (approx 3 g/dl)
Haematocrit	Falls by 30%
Estimated blood loss	30% of the estimated blood volume (70 ml/kg in adults) (100 ml/kg during pregnancy)

If OSI is >1 (i.e. pulse rate is more than the systolic blood pressure), then it has been reported that there is a need for intensive resuscitation and up to 70% may require blood transfusion [7].

Management

Management of PPH involves timely recognition of severity of blood loss, effective multidisciplinary communication, prompt resuscitation to ensure maternal haemodynamic stability (ABC – airway, breathing, circulation) and identification and treatment of the underlying cause of PPH. In reality, all these actions should occur simultaneously to improve outcomes. In massive PPH, a multidisciplinary approach is essential and the presence and advice of a senior obstetrician, midwife, anaesthetist and haematologist are vital.

It is good practice to involve colleagues with gynaecological surgical experience to assist in complex surgical procedures that may be required to arrest bleeding. Similarly, transfer to a tertiary hospital should be considered early once the woman is haemodynamically stable, if further complex treatment is anticipated.

An initial assessment regarding the degree of blood loss and the severity of the haemodynamic instability is vital and it is always better to overestimate the blood loss and to anticipate the possibility of further bleeding. However, caution should be exercised as overtreatment with excessive intravenous fluid and oxytocics may be equally harmful.

The degree of pallor, level of consciousness, vital signs (pulse, blood pressure, respiration and temperature) and, if facilities are available, oxygen saturation should be monitored. Management algorithms are useful for this serious and potentially fatal condition. 'HEMOSTASIS' (Table 15.6) is one such algorithm that spells out the suggested actions that may facilitate the management of atonic PPH in a logical and stepwise manner. It has been reported that this enables a

Table 15.6 Management algorithm for postpartum haemorrhage 'HEMOSTASIS'

H – Ask for HELP and hands on the uterus (uterine massage)

E – Establish aetiology, ensure availability of blood and ecbolics (oxytocin or ergometrine IM), assess vital parameters (ABC) and resuscitate (IV fluids and blood and blood products)

M – Massage uterus

O – Oxytocin infusion/prostaglandins – IV/per rectal/IM/intramyometrial

S – Shift to theatre – aortic pressure or anti-shock garment/bimanual compression as appropriate

T – Tamponade balloon/uterine packing – after exclusion of tissue and trauma, tranexamic acid

A – Apply compression sutures – B-Lynch/modified

S – Systematic pelvic devascularization – uterine/ovarian/quadruple/internal iliac

I – Interventional radiology and, if appropriate, uterine artery embolization

S – Subtotal/total abdominal hysterectomy

logical and stepwise management with a low peripartum hysterectomy rate.

Resuscitation of the patient and identification of the specific causes of PPH to institute immediate appropriate management should be carried out simultaneously, so as to avoid any delay in correcting of hypovolaemia.

Resuscitation

Resuscitation should follow a simple structured 'ABC' approach, with resuscitation taking place simultaneously with evaluation and preparations for definitive treatment. The urgency and measures undertaken to resuscitate and arrest haemorrhage need to be altered according to the degree of shock.

A and B: Assess Airway and Breathing

A high concentration of oxygen (10–15 l/min) via a facemask should be administered, regardless of maternal oxygen concentration. If the airway is compromised owing to impaired consciousness, anaesthetic assistance should be sought urgently. Securing the airway and ensuring adequate oxygenation are paramount. This should be followed by replacement of blood volume to restore the oxygen-carrying capacity of blood. Investigations to determine the degree of blood loss and the integrity of the coagulation system, as well as monitoring of the vital signs, should

be carried out. Usually, level of consciousness and airway control improve rapidly once the circulating volume is restored.

C: Circulation

Two large-bore (14 G) intravenous cannulae should be inserted and blood should be taken for investigations. These include full blood count (FBC), clotting profile, urea and electrolytes, and grouping and cross-matching. Rapid fluid infusion with crystalloids and colloids should be carried out until cross-matched blood is available. Crystalloids (0.9% normal saline or Hartmann's solution) are preferred over colloids, as the latter are associated with a 4% increase in the absolute risk of maternal mortality compared with crystalloids [8]. Colloids may also interfere with cross-matching and platelet function. If they are used, the maximum recommended dosage of colloids is 1500 ml in 24 hours.

By consensus, total volume of 3.5 l of clear fluids (up to 2 l of warmed Hartmann's solution as rapidly as possible, followed by up to a further 1.5 l of warmed colloid if blood is still not available) comprises the maximum that should be infused while awaiting compatible blood. There is controversy as to the most appropriate fluids for volume resuscitation. The nature of fluid infused is of less importance than rapid administration and warming of the infusion. The woman needs to be kept warm using appropriate measures.

It is vital to try to identify a cause of ongoing PPH while resuscitation is being carried out to save valuable time. The single most common cause of haemorrhage is uterine atony, which accounts for about 80% of PPH. Hence, the bladder should be emptied to aid uterine contractions and a bimanual pelvic examination should be performed. The finding of the characteristic soft, poorly contracted (boggy) uterus suggests atony as a causative factor. The uterine contractions can be enhanced by uterine massage or bimanual compression. Both of these may help reduce blood loss, expel blood and clots, and allow time for other measures to be implemented. Once atonic uterus has been identified as the cause of PPH, measures should be taken to ensure optimum uterine contraction and retraction. These include the use of pharmacologic agents, use of uterine balloon tamponade, interventional radiology (uterine artery embolization) and surgical measures (exploratory laparotomy, uterine compression sutures,

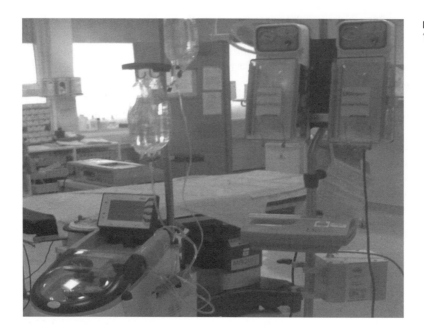

Figure 15.1 Cell-saver for 'auto-transfusion'.

ligation of blood vessels and total or subtotal hysterectomy), if needed.

If bleeding persists despite measures to correct uterine atony, other causes must be considered. Even if atony persists, there may be other contributing or co-existing factors such as a retained placenta, a tear of the vaginal wall or cervix, a vulval or paravaginal haematoma, a uterine scar rupture, DIC and, rarely, amniotic fluid embolism.

One should be aware of possible concealed bleeding, which may be intrauterine or 'BAD' (within the broad ligament, abdominal cavity or deeper tissue planes such as the paravaginal tissues). Lacerations should be ruled out by careful visual assessment of the lower genital tract.

Restoration of the oxygen-carrying capacity of the blood and correction of any derangements in coagulation by blood transfusion and the use of blood products should be considered. This is especially so in cases of massive PPH, where more than 30% of blood volume is lost, as further bleeding may result in hypoxia and metabolic acidosis that may affect the vital organs. Furthermore, the clotting factors may be lost along with excessive blood loss ('washout phenomenon'). Until cross-matched blood is available, O negative or uncross-matched group-specific blood may be transfused, if there were no abnormal antibodies in the recipient's blood. In special circumstances, auto-transfusion (or cell salvaging) may be considered,

although during a caesarean section (CS) this carries a theoretical risk of amniotic fluid embolism and infection. Auto-transfusion involves collection of maternal blood and the use of a cell-saver device (Figure 15.1) to wash and filter the blood to remove the leukocytes and re-infuse the red cells.

Apart from intravenous (IV) crystalloids, colloids, blood and oxytocin, the infusion of blood products needs to be considered. In massive obstetric blood loss, rapid infusion of fresh frozen plasma (FFP) may be required to replace clotting factors other than platelets. It is recommended that with every six units of blood transfusion, 1 l of FFP should be administered (15 ml/kg). Hence, 4–5 bags of FFP are required, as each bag contains about 200–250 ml of FFP. Platelet count should be maintained above 50 000 by infusing platelet concentrates, if indicated. Cryoprecipitate may also be needed if the patient develops DIC and her fibrinogen drops to less than 1 g/dl (10 g/l) [9].

Pharmacological Treatment of Postpartum Haemorrhage

Current evidence suggests that uterotonics including oxytocin, ergometrine and 15-methyl prostaglandin F2 alpha (intramyometrial or intramuscular) are effective measures to achieve haemostasis and to avoid surgical intervention in the majority of cases of atonic PPH [10]. Syntocinon (ten units) can be administered as a slow IV bolus. Syntometrine is considered to be more effective than oxytocin in causing tonic uterine contraction to arrest bleeding, but is associated with more side-effects. Carbetocin, a more heat-stable oxytocin agonist, appears to be a promising agent for the prevention of PPH. The potential advantage of intramuscular carbetocin over intramuscular oxytocin is its longer duration of action. Its relative lack of gastrointestinal and cardiovascular side-effects may also prove advantageous, as compared with Syntometrine [11].

Syntocinon 40 units can be added to 500 ml of normal saline and infused at a rate of 125 ml/h (i.e. 10 units of Syntocinon per hour). Fluid overload and dilutional hyponatraemia has been reported with injudicious use of oxytocin. Hence, careful monitoring of fluid input and output is essential to avoid fatal pulmonary and cerebral oedema if oxytocin is infused in large amounts.

Prostaglandins cause smooth muscle contraction and are invaluable in the management of atonic PPH. They are not recommended as prophylaxis of PPH due to their adverse gastrointestinal side-effects. Hemabate (15-methyl prostaglandin F2 alpha) 250 mg can be administered intramuscularly. The dose can be repeated every 15 min for a maximum of eight doses (2 mg). However, it is advisable to move the patient to the theatre if profuse bleeding persists after three doses of hemabate. Intramyometrial injection of hemabate has been tried [11], but recent studies have questioned its effectiveness. Serious complications, including severe hypotension and cardiac arrest, have been reported with intramyometrial prostaglandin administration; likely to be due to inadvertent injection into uterine veins. Hence, the plunger of the syringe should be withdrawn to ensure that the needle is not inside a vein prior to injection. If the PPH is unresponsive to ergometrine or oxytocin, or in the absence of these drugs, sublingual misoprostol 800 mcg has been recommended by the WHO [12]. This is a valuable option in developing countries due to its low cost and relatively easier storage. Four tablets (200 mcg each) of misoprostol are administered sublingually. Rigors, fever, diarrhoea and other gastrointestinal side-effects are common complications.

Surgical Management of Intractable Postpartum Haemorrhage

When medical treatment fails, surgical treatment should be considered and transfer of the woman to the operating theatre should be ensured. These include balloon tamponade, uterine compression suture, uterine artery embolization and internal iliac artery ligation. A recent systematic review of management of PPH has found no statistical difference in the outcome of various conservative surgical methods, with equal efficacy rates between 84% and 91% in avoiding a peripartum hysterectomy [13]. Simple surgical techniques should be undertaken before coagulopathy sets in or with simultaneous correction of coagulopathy.

Uterine Tamponade

Tamponade of the uterus can be effective in decreasing haemorrhage secondary to uterine atony, especially when uterotonics fail to cause sustained uterine contractions and satisfactory control of haemorrhage after vaginal delivery or CS. Balloon tamponade has been very popular, with a success rate of over 80%, and is now the first line approach in the management of PPH when medical management fails. Senior obstetric input should be sought at this stage as further surgical measures may be necessary if uterine tamponade fails to arrest haemorrhage.

Uterine packing has a long history and has been described in early editions of many textbooks, usually using gauze as a packing material. Uterine packing was stopped in the 1950s due to concealed haemorrhage and infection. However, a review conducted in 1993 concluded that uterine packing was an effective method of controlling haemorrhage when performed correctly. It requires careful layering of the gauze, back and forth from one cornua to the other using a sponge stick, and ending with the extension of the gauze through the cervical os. A modification of this method was the use of Sengstaken–Blakemore tube by Katesmark and colleagues in 1994 to control PPH [14].

Balloon tamponade was initially described using a 30 cc Foley balloon that led to the development of commercially available products such as the Bakri balloon in 2001. Uterine tamponade works by exerting counter pressure on the uterine cavity, reducing capillary and venous bleeding from the endometrium. This also gives the opportunity to correct coagulopathy by replacement of blood products. The balloon could be inflated with 200–600 ml of sterile water or saline, depending on the size of the uterine cavity. Insertion of the balloon is easy and does not require anaesthesia. Once inserted, the patient must be monitored continually and a broad-spectrum antibiotic and an oxytocin infusion should be administered. The balloon can be deflated gradually and withdrawn without the need for anaesthesia. If the tamponade test is positive (i.e. the uterine bleeding stops with uterine tamponade), it has been reported there is an 85% chance the woman does not require a laparotomy [15].

In developing countries, if these catheters are not freely available, uterine packing could be tried with sterile gauze. Success with a condom used as a balloon tied to a plastic or Foley catheter has been reported from Bangladesh [16].

Compression Sutures

Uterine compression sutures exert external tamponade by opposing the anterior and posterior walls of the uterus. Overall the success rates vary between 75% and 90%, irrespective of the technique used. Lynch was the first to highlight this technique. Other techniques include horizontal and vertical brace sutures by Hayman *et al.*, multiple square technique by Cho *et al.* and various medications – the reader is referred to 'Surgical aspects of postpartum haemorrhage' [17]. The simplest technique is the placing of vertical compression sutures on either side of the uterus, medial to the cornua (Figure 15.2). The advantages of compression sutures include ease of placement and fertility preservation.

Systematic Pelvic Devascularization

If the compression sutures fail to achieve haemostasis, ligation of blood vessels supplying the uterus could be tried in a systematic manner. These include ligation of both uterine arteries, followed by tubal branches of both ovarian arteries proximal to the ovarian ligament (called the 'quadruple ligation'). Uterine artery ligation is straightforward once the uterovesical fold of peritoneum is incised and the bladder is reflected down. If bleeding continues, tubal branches of both ovarian arteries can be ligated medial to the ovarian ligament. The needle should be passed through a 'clear' area of the mesosalpinx on either side of the blood vessels.

Internal iliac artery ligation is an option if bleeding persists. This requires an experienced surgeon who is familiar with the anatomy of the lateral pelvic wall. In many centres, it is standard practice to involve the gynaecological oncologists as they are more familiar

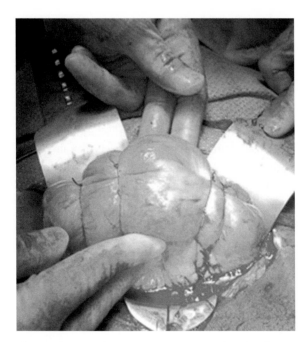

Figure 15.2 Vertical compression sutures. Note the atonic 'floppy and flabby' uterus.

with this procedure. Identification of the internal iliac vessels and the ureters during elective hysterectomies may help obstetricians to build up confidence when faced with an emergency. Bilateral internal iliac artery ligation has been shown to reduce the pelvic blood flow by 49% and pulse pressure by 85% in arteries distal to the ligation. This translates to an acute reduction in the blood flow by about 50% in the distal vessels and the reported success rate of this procedure has been between 40% and 100%. Due to extensive collateral circulation within the pelvis, acute ischaemic necrosis of the uterus or other pelvic organs does not occur.

Potential complications of bilateral internal iliac artery ligation include haematoma formation in the lateral pelvic wall, injury to the ureters and laceration of the iliac vein, and accidental ligation of the external iliac artery. Ligation of the main trunk of the internal iliac artery may result in intermittent claudication of the gluteal muscles due to ischaemia. Fortunately, these complications are rare and may be prevented by accurate identification of anatomical structures and ligating the anterior division of the internal iliac artery, and by examining the femoral pulse prior to tightening the ligature to identify inadvertent ligation of the external iliac artery.

Selective Arterial Embolization

Interventional radiology can be considered in women who are not haemodynamically compromised and the clinical condition permits the placement of uterine artery catheters. Arterial embolization requires a radiologist with special skills in interventional radiology. The procedure involves placement of arterial catheter under a fluoroscopic guidance and injection of an 'embolus'. Embolic materials available for vascular occlusion include: gelfoam (gelatin), polyvinyl alcohol particles, steel coils and *n*-butyl-2-cyanoacrylate glue. Most radiologists prefer gelfoam pledgets as these result in temporary distal occlusion of the uterine arterial bed for approximately four weeks' duration. The reported success rate is approximately 90–95%. Menstruation typically returns within three months and subsequent pregnancies have been reported. Complications include vessel perforation, haematoma, infection and bladder and rectal wall necrosis. Embolization can be used for bleeding that continues after hysterectomy.

Subtotal or Total Abdominal Hysterectomy

Hysterectomy is a radical surgical option to save life when all other conservative measures have failed, or if the patient is haemodynamically very unstable. A senior obstetrician should take a decision to perform this procedure and the patient and her next of kin should be informed, if possible. If the bleeding is predominantly from the lower uterine segment (as in PPH following a major degree placenta praevia, accreta or, rarely, extension of uterine angles during CS), a total abdominal hysterectomy is warranted. A subtotal hysterectomy may be performed if the bleeding is mainly from the upper segment and the aetiology is 'unresponsive' uterine atony. Subtotal hysterectomy has lower morbidity and mortality rates and requires less time to perform. The likelihood of ureteric or bladder injury is lower than for a total abdominal hysterectomy. It is important to realize that hysterectomy is the 'last resort' in the management of atonic PPH.

Hysterectomy is reserved for when all other available surgical modalities have been exhausted, when bleeding continues with a severely shocked patient and in cases of coagulopathy in which no replacement blood products are available. Obstetric hysterectomy to control PPH should be performed by the most senior obstetrician, as a 15-year experience of obstetric hysterectomy from a tertiary centre in Nigeria revealed a maternal mortality rate of 26.3% and urinary tract injury rate of 7.5% after this procedure [18].

The immediate postoperative care should be in a high-dependency area with adequate monitoring (pulse, blood pressure, oxygen saturation, vaginal loss, urine output, haemoglobin, renal function, coagulation and central venous pressure). Intravenous antibiotics and thrombo-prophylaxis should be considered.

Current Concepts and New Developments

Systemic Haemostatic agents

Tranexamic Acid

Tranexamic acid is a potent inhibitor of fibrinolysis. It can be used in prevention and treatment of PPH in a dose of 1 g intravenously either as a single or as multiple doses. It has a high affinity for the lysine binding sites of plasminogen, blocks these sites and prevents binding of activated plasminogen to the fibrin surface, thus exerting its antifibrinolytic effect. It is an inexpensive drug and easy to administer. It has a short half-life of two hours. A systematic review and a meta-analysis including 453 participants identified only two clinical trials of tranexamic acid for the prevention of PPH [19]. The use of tranexamic acid was associated with a reduction of mean blood loss, but the difference was not statistically significant [20]. A recent CRASH-2 trial has shown that the early administration of tranexamic acid significantly reduces mortality in bleeding trauma patients [21]. Based on this trial tranexamic acid has been included in the WHO list of essential medicines.

In addition, blood loss of more than 400 ml after vaginal or caesarean delivery was less common in women receiving tranexamic acid. The WOMAN (World Maternal Antifibrinolytic) trial is currently underway to determine the effect of early administration of tranexamic acid on death, hysterectomy and other morbidities in women with PPH.

Recombinant Activated Factor VII

Intractable PPH may require human recombinant factor VIIa (rFVIIa), which has been shown to be effective in controlling severe, life-threatening haemorrhage by acting on the extrinsic pathway. rFVIIa is available as a room-temperature stable product in 1 mg and 2 mg strengths, and it is administered at the dose of 90 mcg/kg as intravenous bolus over three to five minutes. A second dose of 90 mcg/kg should be considered after 20 minutes if there is no response. Cessation of bleeding ranges from 10 to 40 min after administration. It is estimated that it may avoid an emergency hysterectomy in about 76% of patients with massive PPH [22]. rFVIIa may be considered as a treatment for life-threatening PPH in conjunction with a haematologist. However, it should not be considered as a substitute for a life-saving procedure such as embolization or surgery, and it should not delay such treatment or a transfer to a referral centre. It may not be widely available due to its cost, as a single treatment may cost up to £3500. Administration also requires a minimum fibrinogen level of 100 mg/dl, INR ratio of <1.5, platelet counts >50 000/m^3 and haemoglobin level of >7 g/dl. In case of any derangements, all these parameters are optimized before injection. Also hypothermia and metabolic acidosis should be corrected for maximum effectiveness. Concerns have been raised because of the apparent risk of subsequent thromboembolic events following rFVIIa use.

Cell Salvage

Recovering, purifying and re-circulating the patient's blood is especially useful in patients who refuse blood and blood products, such as Jehovah's Witnesses. It is important to discuss this procedure during the antenatal consultation, prior to signing the 'Advance Directive'. Auto-transfusion, using the patient's own blood, using a cell salvage mechanism (Figure 15.1), may be acceptable for some patients.

Non-pneumatic Anti-shock Garment (NASG)

The NASG is a low-technology first-aid device for stabilizing women suffering hypovolaemic shock secondary to PPH. It is a lightweight, re-usable lower-body compression garment made of neoprene and Velcro™. This is predominantly a first-aid device (Figure 15.3). The NASG plays a unique role in haemorrhage and shock management by reversing shock and decreasing blood loss; thereby stabilizing the woman until definitive care is accessed. The NASG increases blood pressure by decreasing the vascular volume and increasing vascular resistance within the compressed region of the body, but does not exert pressure sufficient for tissue ischaemia. The advantage of

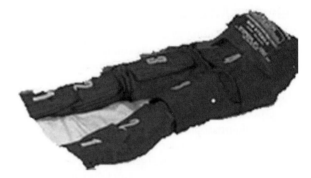

Figure 15.3 Non-pneumatic anti-shock garment (NASG).

this device is that it can be applied by individuals with minimal training.

Blood and Blood Products

Based on experience in battlefields, it is now recommended that the ratio of blood transfusion to blood products should be 1:1 rather than the previously accepted 4:1. This is because the risk of mortality was reported to be reduced by 30% with a 1:1 regime.

The Triple P Procedure for Morbidly Adherent Placentae

The Triple P procedure has been developed as a conservative alternative for peripartum hysterectomy for women with morbidly adherent placenta [23]. It is aimed at avoiding the complications of a peripartum hysterectomy, minimizing perioperative blood loss and reducing intentional and unintentional injury to the urinary bladder. It is a three-step procedure aimed at avoiding incising the placenta prior to delivery of the fetus and avoiding forcible separation of the morbidly adherent placenta from its underlying myometrial bed after reducing uterine blood supply. An analysis of outcomes of the first 16 cases of the Triple P procedure reported a reduction in blood loss and maternal morbidity with no cases of peripartum hysterectomy [24]. A recent comparative study is suggestive of a reduced incidence of PPH and inpatient hospital stay [25].

Conclusion

Although the recent CMACE report indicates that the numbers of deaths due to PPH are decreasing in the UK, substandard care still contributes to approximately 70% of all maternal deaths due to PPH. Postpartum haemorrhage remains a leading cause of severe maternal morbidity and mortality in developing countries. The Confidential Enquiries have re-emphasized that deaths caused by PPH are due to 'too little done too late'. Primary PPH may be due to atonic uterus, genital tract trauma, coagulopathy or retained products of conception. Secondary PPH occurs after the first 24 hours of delivery and is due to infection, often secondary to retained products of conception. Morbidly adherent placenta (accreta, increta or percreta) may sometimes cause profuse haemorrhage after delivery that may necessitate a hysterectomy. Rare complications of PPH include Sheehan's syndrome (pituitary necrosis secondary to massive PPH and resultant hypovolaemia and hypoperfusion) that may present with failure of lactation, secondary amenorrhoea and features of hypothyroidism.

References

1. Centre for Maternal and Child Enquiries (CMACE). Saving Mothers' Lives: Reviewing Maternal Deaths to Make Motherhood Safer: 2006–08. The Eighth Report on Confidential Enquiries into Maternal Deaths in the United Kingdom. *BJOG*. 2011; 118(suppl. 1): 1–203.

2. RCOG. *Postpartum Haemorrhage, Prevention and Management*. London: RCOG Press; 2011.

3. ACOG. Practice bulletin: clinical management guidelines for obstetrician-gynecologists number 76, October 2006: postpartum hemorrhage. *Gynecol*. 2006; 108(4): 1039–47.

4. Chesley LC. Plasma and red cell volumes during pregnancy. *Am J Obstet Gynecol*. 1972; 112: 440–50.

5. Robbins KS, Martin SR, Wilson WC. Intensive care considerations for the critically ill parturient. In Creasy RK, Resnik R, Iams JD, *et al.* (eds), *Creasy and Resnik's Maternal-Fetal Medicine: Principles and Practice*, 7th edition. Philadelphia, PA: Elsevier; 2014.

6. Ruth D, Kennedy BB. Acute volume resuscitation following obstetric hemorrhage. *J Perinat Neonatal Nurs*. 2011; 25(3): 253–60.

7. Le Bas A, Chandraharan E, Addei A, Arulkumaran S. Use of the 'obstetric shock index' as an adjunct in identifying significant blood loss in patients with massive postpartum hemorrhage. *Int J Gynaecol Obstet*. 2014; 124(3): 253–5.

8. Hofmeyr GJ, Mohlala BK. Hypovolaemic shock. *Best Pract Res Clin Obstet Gynaecol*. 2001; 15: 645–62.

9. Santosa JT, Lin DW, Miller DS. Transfusion medicine in obstetrics and gynecology. *Obstet Gynecol Surv*. 1995; 50: 470–81.

10. Mousa HA, Wilkinshaw S. Major postpartum haemorrhage. *Curr Opin Obstet Gynecol*. 2001; 13: 593–603.

11. Chong YC, Su LL, Arulkumaran S. Current strategies for the prevention of postpartum haemorrhage in the third stage of labour. *Curr Opin Obstet Gynecol*. 2004; 16: 143–50.

12. WHO. *WHO Recommendations for the Prevention and Treatment of Postpartum Haemorrhage*. Geneva: WHO; 2012.

13. Doumouchtsis SK, Papageorghiou AT, Arulkumaran S. Systematic review of conservative management of postpartum hemorrhage: what to do when medical treatment fails. *Obstet Gynecol Surv*. 2007; 62: 540–7.

14. Katesmark M, Brown R, Raju KS. Successful use of a Sengstaken–Blakemore tube to control massive postpartum haemorrhage. *Br J Obstet Gynaecol*. 1994; 101(3): 259–60.

15. Condous GS, Arulkumaran S, Symonds I, *et al.* The 'tamponade test' in the management of massive postpartum hemorrhage. *Obstet Gynecol*. 2003; 101(4): 767–72.

16. Akhter S, Begum M, Kabir Z, *et al.* Use of a condom to control massive postpartum hemorrhage. *MedGenMed*. 2003; 5(3).

17. Chandraharan E, Arulkumaran S. Surgical aspects of postpartum haemorrhage: review article. *Best Pract Res Clin Obstet Gynaecol*. 2008; 22(6): 1089–102.

18. Jimoh AAG, Saidu R, Olatinwo AWO, *et al.* Emergency peripartum hysterectomy and its outcome in Ilorin, Nigeria. *The Internet Journal of Gynecology and Obstetrics*. 2010; 15.

19. Novikova N, Hofmeyr GJ. Tranexamic acid for preventing postpartum haemorrhage. *Cochrane Database Syst Rev*. 2010; 7(7): CD007872. doi: 10.1002/14651858.CD007872.pub2.

20. Franchin M, Mauzato F, Salvaguno GL, Lipp G. Potential role for recombinant activated factor VII for the treatment of severe bleeding associated with DIC: a systematic review. *Blood Coagul Fibrinolysis*. 2007; 18(7): 589–93.

21. Roberts I, Shakur H, Coats T, *et al.* The CRASH-2 trial: a randomised controlled trial and economic evaluation of the effects of tranexamic acid on death, vascular occlusive events and transfusion requirement in bleeding trauma patients. *Health Technol Assess*. 2013; 17(10): 1–79.

22. Searle E, Pavord S, Alfirevic Z. Recombinant factor VIIa and other prohaemostatic therapies in primary postpartum haemorrhage. *Best Pract Res Clin Obstet Gynaecol*. 2008; 22: 1075–88.

23. Chandraharan E, Rao S, Belli AM, Arulkumaran S. The Triple-P procedure as a conservative surgical alternative to peripartum hysterectomy for placenta percreta. *Int J Gynaecol Obstet*. 2012; 117(2): 191–4.

24. Chandraharan E, Moore J, Hartopp R, Belli A, Arulkumaran S. Effectiveness of the 'Triple P Procedure for percreta' as a conservative surgical alternative to peripartum hysterectomy: outcome of first 16 cases. *BJOG*. 2013; 120(s1): 30.

25. Teixidor Viñas M, Belli A, Arulkumaran S, Chandraharan E. Prevention of postpartum haemorrhage and hysterectomy in patients with morbidly adherent placenta: a cohort study comparing outcomes before and after introduction of the Triple-P procedure. *Ultrasound Obstet Gynecol*. 2014; 46(3): 350–5.

Management of Morbidly Adherent Placenta

Rosemary Townsend and Edwin Chandraharan

What is Morbidly Adherent Placenta?

Disorders of placentation can be classified into two groups – placenta praevia, which refers to an abnormally sited placenta, and morbid adherence (placenta accreta, increta and percreta), which refers to abnormal placental invasion into the uterine wall.

Placenta praevia refers to a placenta partially or completely lying in the lower segment of the uterus, with an overall incidence at term of around 0.4–0.8%. Incidence increases with maternal age, smoking, multiple pregnancy, parity, previous caesarean sections (CSs) and previous uterine instrumentation [1]. Morbidly adherent placenta (MAP) encompasses a group of disorders: placenta accreta (placenta abnormally adherent to the inner half of the myometrium), placenta increta (placenta invading into the outer half of the myometrium) and placenta percreta (placenta penetrating through the myometrium and the uterine serosa). MAP may be associated with placenta praevia, but can also occur in a normally sited placenta. In fact, any factor that damages the uterine decidua can lead to a morbidly adherent placenta.

The site of placental implantation is determined by the position of the trophoblast at 8–10 weeks' gestation. If this is initially 'low lying', the leading edge of the placenta often appears to migrate upwards as the lower segment of the uterus develops. It is thought that scar tissue in the lower segment of the uterus may prevent the normal growth that usually leads to the placenta 'migrating' upwards, resulting in a higher incidence of placenta praevia in women with a previous CS. In particular, previous CS increases the likelihood of a low-lying placenta detected at the 20–22 week anomaly scan to become a placenta praevia at term from 11% to 50% [2]. The risk of abnormal placentation increases with every uterine operation, such that after four or more CSs, the risk of placenta praevia in any subsequent pregnancies is 10% while the risk of placenta accreta at the fourth CS is 2.13% [3].

What Causes MAP?

Morbidly adherent placentae are a result of excessive penetration of the trophoblast through the endometrium (i.e. decidua of pregnancy). The decidua basalis may be deficient in the lower segment or in the presence of scarring from previous operations. This increases the risk of trophoblast invading to the myometrium and beyond [4], especially in cases of damage secondary to previous CS, uterine curettage, endometritis, resection of submucous leiomyoma, endometrial ablation [5] and uterine artery embolization [6].

Why is MAP Important?

Morbidly adherent placenta is associated with severe maternal and fetal morbidity and mortality. The maternal morbidity is largely secondary to massive obstetric haemorrhage and the surgical complications of removing a placenta that may be invading other pelvic organs. The average blood loss is 3000–5000 ml [7] and around 90% of cases require blood transfusion. Morbidity includes hysterectomy, ureteric, bladder, bowel and neurovascular injury at laparotomy, intensive care admission and the risks associated with massive transfusion. Major obstetric haemorrhage is also known to be associated with psychological sequelae, including post-traumatic stress disorder (PTSD) as well as intensive care admission. As the frequency of these conditions increases, the long-term mental health implications are likely to become more significant. Maternal mortality is reported to be in the range of 7–10% of

Best Practice in Labour and Delivery, Second Edition, ed. Sir Sabaratnam Arulkumaran. Published by Cambridge University Press. © Cambridge University Press 2016.

all cases globally [8]. Fetal morbidity is mainly associated with preterm delivery, which may be elective or as an emergency in the context of major haemorrhage and exposure of the fetus to complications of maternal hypotension and a technically complicated delivery.

Can MAP be Prevented or Predicted?

The overall incidence of MAP in the UK is quoted as 1.7 per 10 000 maternities [1] and it is rising in line with increasing CS rates. Other risk factors include increasing maternal age and shorter intervals between previous CS and current pregnancy, multiparity, placenta praevia, female fetus in the current pregnancy, submucosal leiomyomas, IVF pregnancies, smoking, hypertensive disease and any previous uterine surgery [1]. Since many of these risk factors may be determined pre-pregnancy, attempts have been made to give women individualized risk estimates in the future to help when planning further pregnancies. For example, as many as 65% of women with a history of CS have a deficient scar identifiable on transvaginal ultrasound [9]. However, such a predictive model has not been developed so far due to the complexity of this condition. Rather than pre-pregnancy screening, ultrasound and biochemical markers that may help predict or diagnose invasive placenta at earlier gestations are currently being attempted, albeit without success.

The most common risk factor for MAP is unquestionably CS, and prevention of MAP must include prevention of unnecessary CS, particularly the first one. There is considerable interest in determining whether surgical technique at closure of the uterus can impact on the future risk of MAP, i.e. single or double layers, continuous or interrupted, or the suture material used [10]. It seems plausible that the technique chosen could have an impact, but all the studies so far have been underpowered to detect a difference and it would be challenging to recruit sufficient women to provide robust evidence on what is a relatively uncommon outcome.

Antenatal Care of Women with MAP

Presence of advanced maternal age, placenta praevia in index pregnancy and previous uterine scars should raise suspicion of MAP, and it is reported that approximately 50% of cases of MAP are suspected antenatally in the UK, but this is based on a cohort from 2010–11 in which a substantial number of women who had a previous CS and placenta praevia did not receive investigation for possible invasive placenta [11]. This group of women represents a missed opportunity for early diagnosis and the subsequent benefit to mother and child in outcomes.

How is MAP Diagnosed?

It has been reported that placental mRNA may be isolated from maternal serum and is significantly elevated from an early gestation in pregnancies affected by MAP [12]. At the time of first trimester screening, AFP has been found to be elevated in women who go on to develop MAP [13], and is particularly interesting because it is already routinely checked as part of the screening for chromosomal abnormalities. Creatine kinase [14] has also been proposed as a marker. None of these tests meet sensitivity or specificity thresholds for clinical utility and there is no established early diagnostic test.

The focus of care is on management of women after ultrasound diagnosis in the second and third trimesters, and the only way to make that diagnosis is to have an appropriate degree of clinical suspicion in women with a number of risk factors, particularly women with a low placenta overlying a uterine scar.

Ultrasound imaging can be used to detect invasive placentae with a high sensitivity and specificity. In addition to routine ultrasound scan to demonstrate classical features of placental lacunae (Figure 16.1), thinning of the myometrial border and disruption of bladder posterior wall, use of colour Doppler may help in the diagnosis [15]. Ultrasound can be used to detect bladder invasion but performs less well at estimating the invasion of the placenta into the pelvic sidewall and other organs.

MRI has been shown to be equivalent to ultrasound in the diagnosis of invasive placenta [16] but may provide additional information in terms of the degree of invasion. There will be a small subset of women, especially with a posterior placenta praevia in whom invasive placenta is not apparent on ultrasound scan. MRI may provide additional information; however, neither test is fully sensitive and surgeons should proceed with caution even with negative findings on imaging.

A high index of clinical suspicion should remain in the situation of placenta praevia with previous CS. In these patients the risk of MAP is as high as 1 in 20 and in the UK the RCOG recommends preparing for

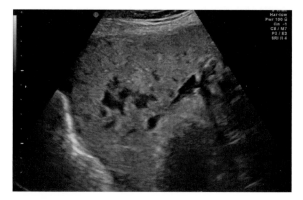

Figure 16.1 Placenta percreta with presence of placental lacunae on ultrasound scan. Note the 'moth-eaten' appearance.

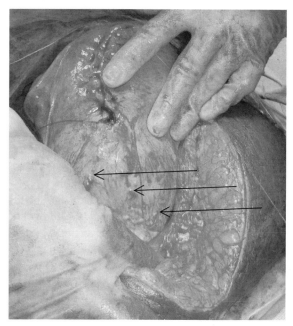

Figure 16.2 Classical caesarean section for IRP. Note the invading placental tissue (arrows).

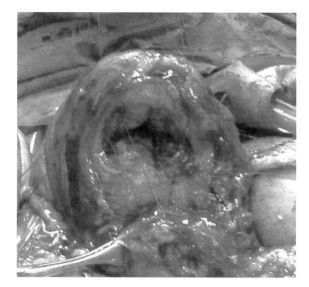

Figure 16.3 Anterior uterine myometrial defect after placental non-separation and myometrial excision, prior to closure.

the delivery of a woman with placenta praevia and one previous CS as if they had known invasive placental disease.

Antenatal Monitoring and Place of Care

Once a diagnosis has been made, a multidisciplinary discussion with the woman at the centre of care should begin. It is important for patients to be alert to bleeding and present early to hospital with even minor bleeding if outpatient management has been chosen. If managed as outpatients, patients need to be able to attend hospital rapidly and should have close vigilance at

home. Prolonged inpatient admissions carry significant psychosocial morbidity for women and their families in addition to the added risk of venous thromboembolism and hospital-acquired infections. It is paramount that women and their families are fully informed of the reasons for recommending inpatient admission and participate in making the final decision in order to minimize the psychosocial harm.

Empathetic and supportive midwifery care for these women is critical as there will be many complex discussions and possibly protracted antenatal admissions that will be challenging for families preparing for birth. Women may feel cut off from the experience of 'normal pregnancy' and can benefit from regular one-to-one midwifery care in addition to their obstetric visits. A named midwife for each patient is the gold standard of care, so that the woman has a single contact point for questions and concerns. Ideally this midwifery team would also perform the postnatal care of these women as they would have an appreciation of the special needs of these patients.

Women who experience major haemorrhage, particularly if that leads to hysterectomy and/or critical care admission, are at risk of postnatal depression, PTSD and anxiety [17]. Therefore, they need support from an experienced team with a low threshold for referral for counselling and mental health support.

Planning the timing and place of birth should begin antenatally with the earliest suspicion of MAP, and the focus of care shifted from emergency management of massive unexpected haemorrhage to antenatal diagnosis and careful multidisciplinary planning. The multidisciplinary team should comprise experienced obstetricians, midwives, anaesthetists, neonatologists, haematologists and interventional radiologists. All units should develop a robust multidisciplinary care pathway for these patients, reflecting the interventions and expertise available in their local units.

Preoperative counselling by the surgeon should cover the choice between elective hysterectomy and uterine sparing techniques such as leaving the placenta *in situ* or the Triple P procedure. Some women may be interested in preserving the uterus in order to pursue future fertility. Although pregnancies have been reported after conservative management of MAP, there is a marked risk of recurrent MAP and women should be counselled regarding this, and bilateral tubal ligation (BTL) at the time of surgery should be offered. In our regional referral centre for placenta percreta, where the Triple P procedure is routinely performed, over 60% of patients have chosen to undergo simultaneous BTL. The options of cell salvage and interventional radiology either as prophylaxis or as treatment should be discussed, depending on local availability. If a patient with known invasive placenta is booked for antenatal care at a facility without these services, a transfer of care to a tertiary centre should be instituted.

If bladder invasion is known or suspected the urological surgical team should be incorporated in predelivery planning and may choose to participate in the delivery or site ureteric stents preoperatively. General surgery involvement is not often indicated but in the situation of known complex intra-abdominal adhesions and/or bowel involvement surgical help may be warranted.

Discussion with the anaesthetic team should include the likelihood of blood transfusion as it is estimated that over 90% of all women being delivered for MAP will need a blood transfusion and consent should be obtained for this prospectively. Women who would refuse blood should be identified and sensitively counselled by the full multidisciplinary team and a specific 'Advance Directive' should be prepared covering blood, cell salvage and all the available blood fractions

Table 16.1 NPSA/RCOG care bundle for morbidly adherent placenta

Consultant obstetrician planned and directly supervising delivery
Consultant obstetric anaesthetist planned and directly supervising anaesthesia at delivery
Blood and blood products available on-site
Multidisciplinary involvement in preoperative planning
Discussion and consent includes possible interventions (such as hysterectomy, leaving placenta *in situ*, cell salvage and interventional radiology)
Local availability of level 2 critical care bed

and products. In addition, invasive monitoring via arterial and central lines should be discussed.

If delivery is planned prior to 36 weeks, the neonatology team should be involved in the pre-delivery discussions. Because of the high risk of haemorrhage if these patients labour, elective delivery at 36–37 weeks' gestation after administration of corticosteroids may be planned. In practice, any woman with persistent vaginal bleeding or abdominal pain would be delivered at 34 weeks. Earlier elective delivery may be appropriate but should be carefully considered by the multidisciplinary team, taking into account the individual factors of each case.

The haematologist should be notified well in advance of any planned elective delivery and as soon as the decision to deliver is made in an emergency. It would be prudent to have cross-matched blood in the theatre prior to commencing surgery. Other blood products including platelets, fresh frozen plasma and cryoprecipitate should be readily available.

Management of Delivery in Patients With MAP

The delivery of patients with MAP is the subject of an NPSA/RCOG patient safety care bundle [18] comprising the minimum expected standards of care (Table 16.1). Immediately prior to delivery, regardless of the planned surgical approach, it is helpful to perform ultrasound assessment of the placental site to plan a uterine incision away from the placental site. Incision of the placenta will provoke heavy bleeding, may limit the surgical options and compromise the fetus by exsanguination.

Peripartum Hysterectomy

The traditional approach to MAP has been to perform a caesarean hysterectomy either as an emergency procedure in response to a massive obstetric haemorrhage or as a planned procedure. This peripartum total abdominal hysterectomy is a radical approach that may also involve resection of affected organs to remove invading placenta, for example a portion of the urinary bladder.

Elective peripartum hysterectomy has the advantage of avoiding attempts to separate the placenta, which are likely to provoke massive haemorrhage. Significantly reduced short-term morbidity (admission to intensive care unit, massive blood transfusion, coagulopathy, urological injury, return to theatre) has been demonstrated by avoiding all attempts at removing the placenta and proceeding straight to 'elective' hysterectomy [19]. This strategy also has the advantage of ensuring in most cases complete removal of all placental tissue at the time of delivery.

The disadvantages of peripartum hysterectomy are that bleeding may continue even after hysterectomy as the placenta may derive its blood supply from adjacent organs into which it has invaded. This may also result in damage (intentional or otherwise) to adjacent organs like the bladder, ureters or bowel into which the placenta has invaded. It also inadvertently leads to loss of fertility that may be associated with long-term psychological consequences for women.

With the advent of more conservative techniques it has become clear that hysterectomy in itself increases the psychological trauma associated with delivery, increasing blood loss, risk of ureteric and bowel injury and postoperative complications.

Uterine Conserving Measures

The main objective of conservative surgical management is to avoid the risks of intra-operative massive obstetric haemorrhage and resultant morbidity and mortality as well as avoidance of inadvertent injury to the urinary tract (or the bowel). Some women may opt for conservative surgery to preserve future fertility.

Intentional Retention of the Placenta (IRP)

Expectant management involves delivery of the fetus through an incision on the uterus above the placental border so as to avoid cutting through the placenta. In most cases, such an incision should be placed at the fundus of the uterus, in the midline and above the upper border of the placenta through a supra-umbilical midline skin incision.

Once the baby is delivered, the umbilical cord is clamped and cut very close to the placenta and ligated with an absorbable suture material. The placenta is then left inside the uterus, undisturbed. The uterine incision is closed in two layers as usual. Syntocinon is not used after the delivery of the fetus to prevent partial separation of an adherent placenta due to contraction and retraction of the uterine myometrium. Intentionally retained placenta is likely to be reabsorbed or expelled within the next 16–20 weeks. Conservative management was tried as early as 1933 because there has always been a significant demand from women for uterine sparing management options, and the evidence is building that it may in fact be physiologically less traumatic than even a planned hysterectomy.

Meyer et al. described a cohort of 12 cases of morbidly adherent placenta, which were managed by intentional retention of placenta with adjunctive interventional radiology. They used transabdominal ultrasound to identify the upper border of the placenta and the uterus was incised away from the placental site. If bleeding persisted despite inflating uterine artery balloons, the interventional radiology team performed uterine artery embolization after CS. In their series of 12 women, where interventional radiology was used with intentional retention of the placenta, only one patient needed a hysterectomy [20].

The main disadvantage of intentional retention of the placenta is the long follow-up required and the fact that as long as placental tissue is left *in situ* women remain at risk of secondary postpartum haemorrhage or sepsis, and may eventually undergo secondary hysterectomy for that reason. Timmermans *et al.* reviewed 60 case reports with successful preservation of uterus in all but 12 women, suggesting that the risk of hysterectomy in women with intentional retention of placenta is approximately 20% [21]. Antibiotics are essential and methotrexate is not recommended, as placenta at term does not have significant rapidly dividing cells.

Most clinicians recommend prolonged use of antibiotics for up to two weeks after surgery where the placenta remains *in situ*. Although there is little scientific evidence to support the effectiveness of this

Table 16.2 Steps of the Triple P procedure for morbidly adherent placentae

1. *Perioperative placental localization* and delivery of the fetus via transverse uterine incision above the upper border of the placenta, which is determined preoperatively by a transabdominal ultrasound.
2. *Pelvic devascularization*: once the fetus is delivered, uterine blood supply is reduced by inflation of pre-positioned occlusion balloons in the anterior division of the internal iliac artery.
3. *Placental non-separation with myometrial excision* and reconstruction of the uterine wall (see Figure 16.3). The entire myometrial wall overlying the placental bed is excised together with the adherent placenta and the ensuing myometrial defect is repaired.

practice over the single-dose prophylaxis that is commonly used in other elective or emergency caesarean deliveries; leaving the placenta *in situ* theoretically increases the risk of infection. Hence, at the Regional Referral Service for Morbidly Adherent Placenta at St George's Healthcare NHS Trust, London, antibiotics are administered for ten days for all cases of intentional retention of the placenta.

Serial ultrasound scans and βhCG may be used to document resolution of placental tissue but do not predict infection or haemorrhage. Falling levels of βhCG do not guarantee complete placental resolution and therefore measurements should be supplemented by ultrasound imaging. Although there is no scientific evidence to support the beneficial role of ultrasound for the assessment of placental involution, our experience shows that the use of colour Doppler helps to determine vascularity and may assist in assessing the overall clinical picture.

Although as previously stated, it is usual to advise women who have suffered from MAP to approach another pregnancy with caution, there are cases of future pregnancies progressing to term. In these cases, a closer antenatal surveillance as well as a planned CS should be advised.

Triple P Procedure

The Triple P procedure is a form of uterine conserving surgery bringing together a number of steps to minimize blood loss and risk of intrapartum injury to the mother [22]. It is a three-step conservative surgical alternative to peripartum hysterectomy for women with morbidly adherent placentae (Table 16.2) and early results show benefits in morbidity and maternal outcomes.

This procedure combines the benefits of avoiding attempts at separating the placenta with the removal of as much placental tissue as possible and makes routine use of prophylactic interventional radiology balloon insertion.

It is usually possible to remove the placenta in its entirety using the myometrial excision technique, but where the placenta has invaded significantly into the urinary bladder this may not be possible. In this case, the small portion of invading placenta (approximately 2 cm) is left undisturbed. In performing the myometrial excision, it is important to ensure that an approximately 2 cm margin of myometrium is retained in the lower portion of the uterine incision to facilitate closure of the uterus.

Blood loss from the separated and adherent part of the placenta is controlled by suturing the placental bed. In cases of placenta percreta in which trophoblastic invasion into the posterior wall of the urinary bladder is seen, haemostatic sutures are placed along the line of invasion of the placental tissue into the posterior wall of the bladder to achieve haemostasis.

A local haemostatic agent (PerClot) is useful in achieving haemostasis. This is followed by closure of the myometrial defect in two layers, as is usual in CS. Cell salvage and autologous transfusion are useful in maintaining blood volume during surgery.

We reported good outcomes of the first 16 cases of the Triple P procedure at our regional referral centre, with no peripartum hysterectomy [23]. Maternal morbidity is minimized because there is no extensive surgery involving resection of the urinary bladder and risk to bowel and ureters. Avoiding hysterectomy and separation of the placenta reduces intra-operative blood loss (average 1.5 l).

Standard postnatal follow-up for women who have undergone a Triple P procedure includes seven days of antibiotics and an ultrasound scan at eight weeks to confirm complete resorption of placental tissue invading the urinary bladder. All women undergoing the Triple P procedure are counselled to avoid subsequent pregnancy and a majority (>60%) choose to undergo simultaneous BTL. No pregnancies after Triple P have yet been reported.

Other Uterine Conserving Approaches

Other surgical approaches designed to avoid hysterectomy while achieving haemostasis have been described. It is possible to simply excise the placental site – this is done by inverting the uterus in order to provide access to the placental bed. If the area of placental attachment is focal and the majority of the placenta has separated, then a wedge resection of the area can be performed.

The other conservative option involves resecting the invaded area together with the placenta and performing the reconstruction as a one-stop procedure, described initially by Palacios-Jaraquemada et al. in a large case series of women with anterior percreta. They performed a large retrovesical and parametrial dissection in all cases. The anterior wall defect was repaired using a myometrial suture, fibrin glue and polyglycolic mesh before a non-adherent cellulose layer was applied over this reconstruction. Out of 50 patients with anterior placenta percreta, 18 women needed a hysterectomy, 16 of which were required because of massive defects unsuitable for reconstruction and two were secondary to coagulopathies. This procedure was associated with intra-abdominal postoperative haemorrhage, coagulopathy, uterine infection, low ureteral ligations and postoperative sepsis due to collections [24].

Role of Interventional Radiology

The aim of balloon catheter occlusion or arterial embolization is to reduce blood flow to the uterus and to prevent or arrest postpartum haemorrhage. Arterial catheters may be inserted prophylactically or in an emergency in response to haemorrhage. Emergency insertion is technically more complex and requires that IR facilities are available in the operating theatre or that the patient can be made stable for transfer to an interventional radiology suite. In our centre, we reported that embolization had a success rate of 90% in avoiding a hysterectomy [25].

Elective pelvic arterial catheterization and prophylactic balloon occlusion is superior to emergency embolization for anticipated massive postpartum haemorrhage. The prophylactic insertion of interventional radiology arterial catheters is recommended by the RCOG in diagnosed cases of MAP, and could be considered in cases with a high clinical suspicion of MAP. The main risks are rare recognized vascular complications of thrombosis, critical limb ischaemia and vascular rupture [26]. In a recent series, we reported very good outcomes among women who underwent prophylactic pelvic arterial balloon placement at our regional referral centre [27].

Management of Significant Bladder or Ureteric Invasion

Management of patients with bladder or ureteric involvement requires careful preoperative planning and involvement of the urologists. Preoperative ureteric stenting may help to reduce ureteric injuries in such cases and facilitate repair. The placenta may invade the broad ligament and pelvic sidewall, jeopardizing the ureters without necessarily invading the bladder itself, and care must be taken when dissecting in this area. Ureteric injury may in some cases be unavoidable, but early identification is crucial and stenting may be of benefit in this situation.

Care must be taken during surgery not to attempt to dissect the bladder off the lower uterine segment that may result in heavy bleeding, and also to avoid lacerations of the bladder, urinary fistula, frank haematuria, ureteric transaction and reduced bladder capacity. Partial cystectomy may be indicated. Intentional anterior bladder wall incision may be helpful in defining dissection planes and the location of the ureters [28]. In view of the serious morbidities described above, the role of conservative management, including the Triple P procedure, should be discussed with a woman in such cases.

Key Learning Points

- Morbidly adherent placenta is increasing in incidence and all obstetricians should be familiar with the management of these patients.
- Prevention at present is focused on prevention of primary CSs.
- Early diagnosis is facilitated by improvements in antenatal imaging. It facilitates in-depth multidisciplinary planning for delivery.
- The cornerstone of safe and effective management is early, senior, multidisciplinary involvement and delivery in a centre with facilities for interventional radiology and critical care.
- Safe uterine conserving alternatives such as the Triple P procedure seem to offer benefits compared with the traditional peripartum hysterectomy in terms of less surgical complications and maternal morbidity.

- Holistic care of these women includes an appreciation of the psychological and emotional impact of a diagnosis of MAP on women and their families, along with prolonged antenatal admission and highly medicalized delivery.

References

1. Fitzpatrick KE, Sellers S, Spark P, *et al*. Incidence and risk factors for placenta accreta/increta/percreta in the UK: a national case-control study. *PloS One*. 2012;7(12): e52893.

2. Dashe JS, McIntire DD, Ramus RM, Santos-Ramos R, Twickler DM. Persistence of placenta previa according to gestational age at ultrasound detection. *Obstet Gynecol*. 2002;99(5 Pt 1): 692–7.

3. Silver RM, Landon MB, Rouse DJ, *et al*. Maternal morbidity associated with multiple repeat cesarean deliveries. *Obstet Gynecol*. 2006;107(6): 1226–32.

4. Garmi G, Goldman S, Shalev E, Salim R. The effects of decidual injury on the invasion potential of trophoblastic cells. *Obstet Gynecol*. 2011;117(1): 55–9.

5. Hamar BD, Wolff EF, Kodaman PH, Marcovici I. Premature rupture of membranes, placenta increta, and hysterectomy in a pregnancy following endometrial ablation. *J Perinatol*. 2006;26(2): 135–7.

6. Pron G, Mocarski E, Bennett J, *et al*. Pregnancy after uterine artery embolization for leiomyomata: the Ontario multicenter trial. *Obstet Gynecol*. 2005;105(1): 67–76.

7. Hudon L, Belfort MA, Broome DR. Diagnosis and management of placenta percreta: a review. *Obstet Gynecol Surv*. 1998;53(8): 509–17.

8. O'Brien JM, Barton JR, Donaldson ES. The management of placenta percreta: conservative and operative strategies. *Am J Obstet Gynecol*. 1996;175(6): 1632–8.

9. van der Voet LF, Bij de Vaate AM, Veersema S, Brolmann HA, Huirne JA. Long-term complications of caesarean section: the niche in the scar. A prospective cohort study on niche prevalence and its relation to abnormal uterine bleeding. *BJOG*. 2014;121(2): 236–44.

10. Sumigama S, Sugiyama C, Kotani T, *et al*. Uterine sutures at prior caesarean section and placenta accreta in subsequent pregnancy: a case-control study. *BJOG*. 2014;121(7): 866–74.

11. Fitzpatrick KE, Sellers S, Spark P, *et al*. The management and outcomes of placenta accreta, increta, and percreta in the UK: a population-based descriptive study. *BJOG*. 2014;121(1): 62–70.

12. El Behery MM, Rasha LE, El Alfy Y. Cell-free placental mRNA in maternal plasma to predict placental invasion in patients with placenta accreta. *Int J Gynaecol Obstet*. 2010;109(1): 30–3.

13. Hung TH, Shau WY, Hsieh CC, *et al*. Risk factors for placenta accreta. *Obstet Gynecol*. 1999;93(4): 545–50.

14. Ophir E, Tendler R, Odeh M, Khouri S, Oettinger M. Creatine kinase as a biochemical marker in diagnosis of placenta increta and percreta. *Am J Obstet Gynecol*. 1999;180(4): 1039–40.

15. Riteau AS, Tassin M, Chambon G, *et al*. Accuracy of ultrasonography and magnetic resonance imaging in the diagnosis of placenta accreta. *PloS One*. 2014;9(4): e94866.

16. Dwyer BK, Belogolovkin V, Tran L, *et al*. Prenatal diagnosis of placenta accreta: sonography or magnetic resonance imaging? *J Ultrasound Med*. 2008;27(9): 1275–81.

17. Thompson JF, Roberts CL, Ellwood DA. Emotional and physical health outcomes after significant primary post-partum haemorrhage (PPH): a multicentre cohort study. *A N Z J Obstet Gynaecol*. 2011;51(4): 365–71.

18. RCOG/NPSA. Placenta praevia after caesarean section care bundle: background information for healthcare professionals, 2010.

19. Eller AG, Porter TF, Soisson P, Silver RM. Optimal management strategies for placenta accreta. *BJOG*. 2009;116(5): 648–54.

20. Meyer NP, Ward GH, Chandraharan E. Conservative approach to the management of morbidly adherent placentae. *Ceylon Med J*. 2012;57(1): 36–9.

21. Timmermans S, van Hof AC, Duvekot JJ. Conservative management of abnormally invasive placentation. *Obstet Gynecol Surv*. 2007;62(8): 529–39.

22. Chandraharan E, Rao S, Belli AM, Arulkumaran S. The Triple-P procedure as a conservative surgical alternative to peripartum hysterectomy for placenta percreta. *Int J Gynaecol Obstet*. 2012;117(2): 191–4.

23. Chandraharan E, Moore J, Hartopp R, Belli A, Arulkumaran S. Effectiveness of the 'Triple P Procedure for percreta' as a conservative surgical alternative to peripartum hysterectomy: outcome of first 16 cases. *BJOG*. 2013;120(1): 30.

24. Palacios Jaraquemada JM, Pesaresi M, Nassif JC, Hermosid S. Anterior placenta percreta: surgical approach, hemostasis and uterine repair. *Acta Obstet Gynecol Scand*. 2004;83(8): 738–44.

25. Ratnam LA, Gibson M, Sandhu C, *et al*. Transcatheter pelvic arterial embolisation for control of obstetric and gynaecological haemorrhage. *J Obstet Gynaecol*. 2008;28(6): 573–9.

26. Dilauro MD, Dason S, Athreya S. Prophylactic balloon occlusion of internal iliac arteries in women with placenta accreta: literature review and analysis. *Clin Radiol.* 2012;67(6): 515–20.

27. Teixidor Viñas M, Chandraharan E, Moneta MV, Belli AM. The role of interventional radiology in reducing haemorrhage and hysterectomy following caesarean section for morbidly adherent placenta. *Clin Radiol.* 2014;69(8): e345–51.

28. Konijeti R, Rajfer J, Askari A. Placenta percreta and the urologist. *Rev Urol.* 2009;11(3): 173–6.

Acute Illness and Maternal Collapse in the Postpartum Period

Jessica Hoyle, Guy Jackson and Steve Yentis

Introduction

For most new mothers the postpartum period is a time of celebration and relief, but it can also represent a time of great danger, even in apparently straightforward cases.

For the purposes of this chapter we have defined 'acute illness' as the onset of a new condition, or worsening of an existing one, within a few hours of delivery, that might present with maternal collapse or lead to it; 'postpartum period' is defined as the first 24 hours after delivery.

Several aspects of this chapter may also be covered in other chapters in this book.

Incidence

The true incidence of postpartum collapse is impossible to estimate since the definitions and clinical presentations vary enormously and data collection is difficult. In 2013 the World Health Organization estimated that there were 289 000 maternal deaths worldwide during pregnancy, childbirth or in the postpartum period [1]. In the UK, the reports into *Confidential Enquiries into Maternal Deaths* (Maternal Death Enquiry; MDE) have estimated an incidence of 10.12 deaths per 100 000 maternities [2], but it is not possible to ascertain the proportion of women who die within the first 24 hours following delivery or those who become acutely unwell during this time. Studies of obstetric morbidity are even more varied in their methodology and variability of definitions, but many of the conditions described may present or become more severe shortly after delivery [3–5].

Certain conditions with the potential to cause acute illness and/or death are common enough that every unit might expect to experience them regularly,

while others might only occur once every few years. It is important, therefore, that every unit is equipped to deal with both common and rare causes of postpartum collapse.

Causes

Acute postpartum illness can result from a wide range of underlying pathologies (Table 17.1). Although the incidences of different causes are difficult to determine, the leading causes of maternal death as reported by the MDE report for 2009–11 are listed in Table 17.2.

Presentation

The timing, speed of onset and presentation depend on the underlying pathology and may even suggest the cause. However, conditions that typically develop relatively slowly in the non-obstetric setting may do so much faster in pregnancy or after delivery. For example, it is unusual for non-pregnant patients to suffer rapidly progressing, overwhelming sepsis, whereas the MDE reports describe many cases in which an apparently healthy woman becomes moribund and dies of sepsis within hours of the first symptoms [2,6]. This may be related to an impaired ability to withstand infection associated with pregnancy itself, or it may reflect the ability of young, fit patients to compensate for physiological challenges very effectively until just before their compensatory mechanisms become overwhelmed. A classic example of this in obstetrics is the response to haemorrhage, in which the mother maintains blood pressure and perfusion relatively well until sudden, catastrophic collapse.

Since mothers may be discharged from the delivery suite to other wards or into the community soon after delivery, those who develop an acute illness may

---

Best Practice in Labour and Delivery, Second Edition, ed. Sir Sabaratnam Arulkumaran. Published by Cambridge University Press. © Cambridge University Press 2016.

Table 17.1 Causes of acute illness and/or collapse in the postpartum period

Obstetric	Hypertensive disorders	Eclampsia, pre-eclampsia/HELLP syndrome with haemorrhage, liver rupture, stroke
	Postpartum haemorrhage	
	Genital tract/abdominal sepsis	
	Amniotic fluid embolism	
	Peripartum cardiomyopathy	
Non-obstetric	Thromboembolic disease	Pulmonary embolism, cerebral vein thrombosis
	General anaesthesia	Aspiration pneumonitis, atelectasis, respiratory depression, airway obstruction
	Regional anaesthesia	Hypotension, high block, local anaesthetic toxicity, meningitis, spinal haematoma/abscess
	Cardiac disease	Cardiac failure, myocardial infarction, aortic dissection, arrhythmias
	Respiratory disease	Asthma, pneumonia
	Adverse drug reactions	Anaphylaxis*, toxicity/side-effects, drug withdrawal
	Metabolic	Hypo/hyperglycaemia; hyponatraemia
	Primary neurological	Epilepsy, stroke
	Other	Air embolus, vasovagal syncope, splenic artery rupture, mesenteric infarction

Note:
* Remember latex allergy.
The list is not exhaustive and there is some overlap, i.e. more than one may co-exist.

Table 17.2 Leading causes of maternal death as reported by the MDE report for 2009–11 and 2010–12 [2]

Condition	Rate per 100 000 maternities	
	2009–2011	2010–2012
Direct causes		
Genital tract sepsis	0.63	0.5
Pre-eclampsia and eclampsia	0.42	0.38
Thromboembolism	1.26	1.08
Amniotic fluid embolism	0.29	0.33
Early pregnancy deaths	0.17	0.33
Haemorrhage	0.59	0.46
Anaesthetic	0.12	0.17
Other direct	–	–
Indirect causes		
Cardiac	2.14	2.25
Neurological	1.26	1.29
Psychiatric	0.55	0.67
Malignancies	0.17	0.13
Other indirect	3.03	2.54

do so in a variety of locations. It is important, therefore, that staff who might encounter such cases (e.g. general practitioners, emergency department doctors and nurses) are aware of the immediate problems they may pose, and that the women themselves have ready access to clinical services if they are not in hospital.

Presentation ranges from non-specific mild symptoms to sudden collapse with loss of consciousness. It is important that all symptoms are taken seriously and, if appropriate, investigated and treated as early as possible, the aim being to prevent clinical deterioration leading to severe systemic collapse. Successive MDE reports abound with tales of women whose condition's severity was not recognized until it was too late, and the 2005 report first emphasized the potential value of early warning systems based on deviations from pre-determined physiological limits (e.g. heart rate, blood pressure, respiratory rate, temperature, urine output and neurological response), to alert staff to clinical deterioration [7]. Such early warning systems have now been widely implemented and a number of studies have suggested a high sensitivity and specificity in the identification of obstetric patients at risk of deterioration, but a low positive predictive value [8,9,10].

Management

The basic principles of management are the same as for any patient presenting acutely, and can be divided into immediate and subsequent.

Immediate Management

The two initial priorities are, first, resuscitation and stabilization of the patient and, second, assessment and immediate investigations to determine the differential

Table 17.3 Main points of current resuscitation guidelines [11] with comments related to specific aspects relevant to pregnancy and the immediate postpartum period

	General	**Obstetric**
A – Airway	• Open airway • Give high-flow oxygen • Call for help	• May be oedema, e.g. in pre-eclampsia • Risk of regurgitation/aspiration of gastric contents ever-present; cricoid pressure should be applied if unconscious • Incidence of difficult intubation in obstetrics in the UK is ∼1:200–1:300 [12]
B – Breathing	• Assess saturations, respiratory rate and auscultate	
C – Circulation	• Assess pulse – presence, rate and rhythm • Large-bore intravenous access and fluid resuscitation	• Aorto-caval compression must be avoided with lateral tilt/uterine displacement. Even after delivery the uterus remains bulky • O negative blood should always be available in case of emergency
D – Disability	• Assess Glasgow Coma Score (see Table 17.4) • Blood glucose	
E – Exposure	• Ensure no obvious pathology missed	• Postpartum haemorrhage may be concealed
Reversible causes in cardiac arrest	• Hypovolaemia • Hypo/hyperkalaemia • Hypothermia • Hypoxia • Tension pneumothorax • Tamponade, cardiac • Toxins • Thrombosis – coronary or pulmonary	
Monitoring	• Electrocardiogram • Pulse oximeter • Non-invasive blood pressure	• Normal changes of pregnancy may include: left axis deviation; depressed ST segments and flattened/inverted T waves ± Q waves in lead III • Use appropriately sized cuff for obese patients
Investigations	• Basic blood tests including full blood count, blood sugar, urea/electrolytes, liver function tests, clotting studies and blood cultures • Arterial blood gas sample • Chest X-ray	

diagnosis. In practice, a focused history and examination, in the context of any known specific issues relating to the recent pregnancy, can be undertaken during immediate resuscitation.

Resuscitation and Stabilization

Guidelines for basic and advanced adult life support are now well established and all clinical staff should be familiar with them [11]. However, in the obstetric setting there are three factors that may make it more difficult to keep up both individual and team skills: (1) the physiological changes accompanying pregnancy and the particular aspects of resuscitation, especially in late pregnancy, many of which continue into

the early postpartum period (Table 17.3) [3,12]; (2) the rarity of cardiac arrest in this patient population; and (3) a relatively high turnover of large numbers of staff (especially junior) that is typical of most delivery units.

Assessment

Assessment should be directed towards the most likely causes (see Table 17.1 and below). Level of consciousness is most usefully assessed using the Glasgow Coma Score (GCS), which although originally introduced for the assessment of patients with head injury, has been adopted as a convenient and useful tool in most clinical settings (Table 17.4).

	Urgency	Definition	Category
	Maternal or fetal compromise	Immediate threat to life of woman or fetus	1
		No immediate threat to life of woman or fetus	2
	No maternal or fetal compromise	Requires early delivery	3
		At a time to suit the woman and maternity services	4

Table 3.2 Classification relating the degree of urgency to the presence or absence of maternal or fetal compromise

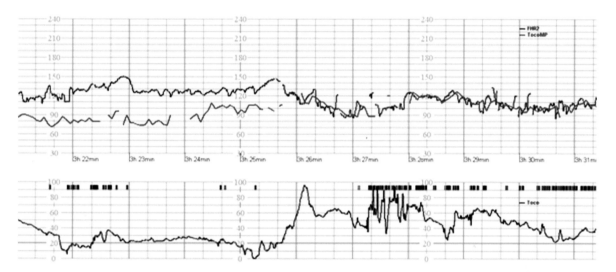

Figure 5.2 CTG recording that shows contractions, FHR and MHR.

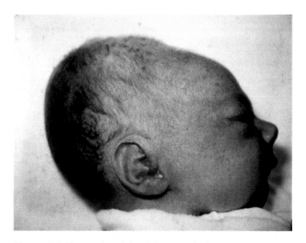

Figure 9.2 The newborn's head showing the larger suboccipito-bregmatic diameter well above the position of the ear.

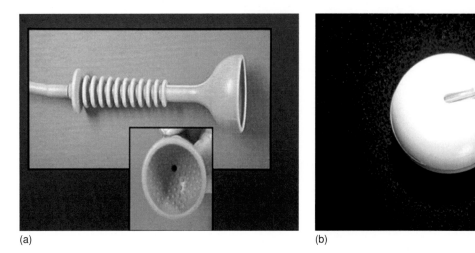

(a)   (b)

Figure 9.3 (a) Silk cup; (b) Kiwi^{TM} posterior cup (Omnicup) showing the tubing used for creating suction and also used for traction, going through a groove to the centre of the cup.

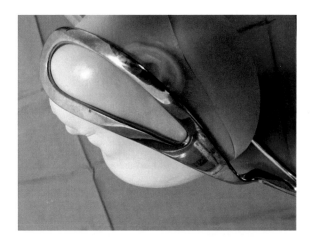

Figure 9.6 Bimalar–biparietal application of the forceps which when checked before traction will allow one finger between the head and heel of the blade on either side, the sagittal suture would be perpendicular to the shank and the occiput would be 3 cm above the shank, allowing the traction on a flexed head with the line of pull along the flexion point.

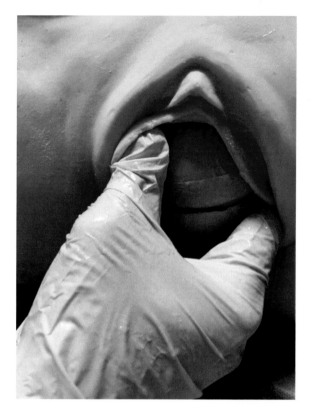

Figure 9.7 Manual rotation of the fetal head from left occipito-transverse to occipito-anterior position.

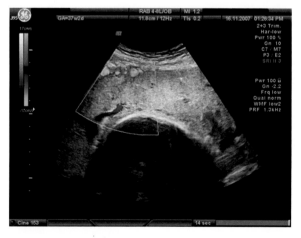

Figure 13.2 Placenta praevia approximately 18 mm from the cervical os.

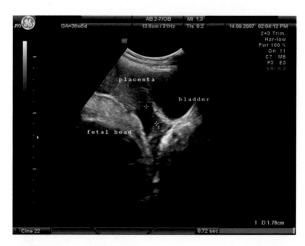

Figure 13.3 Placenta accreta: note the increased vascularity at the poorly defined placenta–uterine interface.

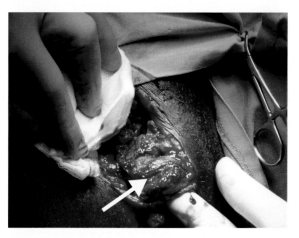

Figure 18.3 A partial tear (arrow) along the length of the external anal sphincter [6, with permission].

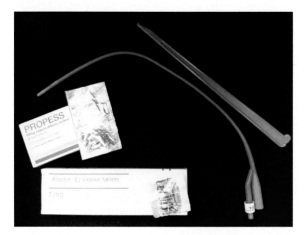

Figure 19.1 Commonly used methods of cervical ripening/induction of labour (includes slow-release PGE2 pessary, PGE2 pessary, PGE1 tablets, Foley balloon catheter and amniohook).

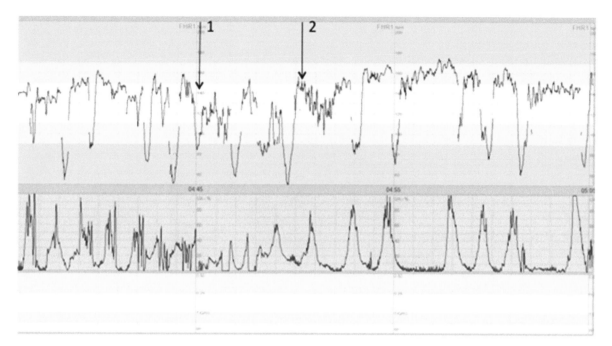

Figure 21.1 Non-reassuring preterm cardiotocographic trace. A nulliparous woman presented with contractions and spontaneous rupture of the membranes with maladorous amniotic fluid at 34 + 2/7 weeks' gestation. The cervical dilatation was 4–5 cm and the fetus was presenting cephalically with the presenting part above the ischial spines. Electronical fetal monitoring was established and at 04:45 h (arrow 1 on CTG trace) an intravenous injection of 0.25 mg of terbutaline was given for acute tocolysis to correct tachysystole and a non-reassuring CTG trace (complicated variable decelerations). Ten minutes later a fetal scalp blood sample (FBS – arrow 2) was performed with a pH of 7.17. An emergency caesarean section was carried out. The baby was born with a birth weight of 1960 g, with Apgar scores of 5[1] and 8[5] and umbilical cord artery pH of 7.07 and standard base excess of 12.6.

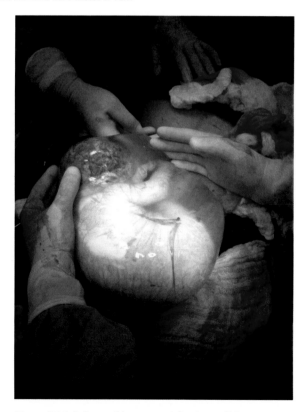

Figure 21.2 Delivery of the preterm infant 'en caul'. Caesarean section with 'en caul' delivery of the preterm infant within an intact amniotic sac with gentle and blunt removal from the uterine cavity to prevent pressure trauma to the head, abdominal viscera or injuries to the limbs and skin of the infant (with kind permission

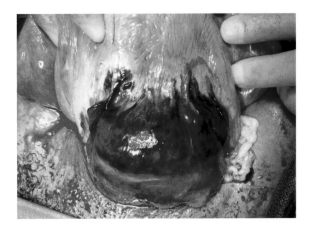

Figure 24.2 Uterine scar dehiscence during second stage of labour with a haematoma under the visceral peritoneum during laparotomy.

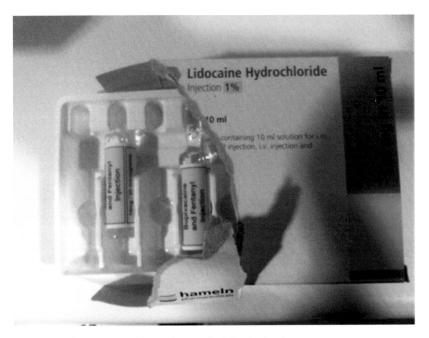

Figure 29.1 Bupivacaine and fentanyl returned to lidocaine box in error.

Performance and Governance Scorecard:
Always Aiming for Excellence

St George's Maternity Unit
The 'Maternity Dashboard' 2013

			Goal	Red Flag	Comment	Data Source	2008 Nov	2009 Nov	2010 Nov	2011 Nov	2012 Nov	JAN	FEB	MAR	APR	MAY	JUN	JUL	AUG	SEP	OCT	NOV	DEC	COMMENTS / ACTION THIS MONTH
Clinical Activity	Births	Benchmarked to 5000 per annum	5000 (425)	>433 (5200)	Review 3 monthly	Maternity System	498	447	459	431	452	458	380	359	421	402	405	434	413	445	415	402		
	Scheduled Bookings	Bookings (1st visit) scheduled	5880 (500)	>5225(6300)		Maternity System	442	512	541	516	407	481	338	457	504	458	477	516	481	469	476	520		
	Bookings <12W+6		>90%	>90%		Maternity Diary	NA	NA	86	92.8	85	79	83	81	81	81	80	76	75	73	76	75		
	Carmen Suite	Benchmarked 500 year	>60/Month	>50/month	Review 6 monthly	Maternity System	NA	NA	58	49	59	68	47	43	46	46	52	56	54	56	54	57		
	Transfers to D/Suite for reasons other than	Calculated based on National Data	<40	<41%		Lead Midwife Carmen Suite	NA	39	20.5	44	32	24	24	27	23.8	31%	35	38	41	41	38	25		Epid (32%), Mec (29%), Failure to progress (24%), Fetal cpompromise 9%
	Normal Vaginal Births	50 % (based on National Average of 48%)	>60%	<45% (<60%)	Review 6 monthly	Maternity System	NA	34.4	69.3	57.6	60.1	60	54.1	59.1	59.7	60.7	60	61.3	57.4	60.7	59.8	64.1		
	Home Births		>3%	<1%			Not monitored during this Period				2.2	0.9	3	1.1	1.9	1.5	1.7	0.2	1.4	2	1.2	1.2		
	Instr. Vag Del	Ventouse & Forceps	10-18%	>5%or >20%		Maternity System	NA	13.1	15	15.1	12	18.8	18.9	14	15.8	17.5	15.3	15	18.2	14.6	15.1	16.1		
	Induction of Labour	Percentage of total birth /	<28%	>30.5 %	According to NICE. IOL	Maternity System	10.7	17.5	16.9	23	22	22.9	21.9	30	25.9	26.6	26.2	29	23.6	24.3	27.5	32.6		
	Postponed IOL due to overcapacity	Planned induction rebooked due to staffing/activity issues	<4/month	>5/month		D/Suite Escalation	NA	N/A			1	4	4	3	4	4	3	4	3	4	4	2		
	C- Section	Total rate (planned & unscheduled)	<28%	>30%	Rate based on other	Maternity System	25.2	24.4	24.0	23.4	22.1	22.2	26.9	25.6	24.2	20.6	22.7	20.7	21.9	21.5	25	18.9		Maternal Request C Section - 18% of all elective C sections and 44 %, inciding declining VBAC
	Emergency C-Sections	Excluding 'No Labour Emergency LSCS')	14 (aspirational goal 12)	>16%		Maternity System	NA	NA	10.3	11.6	10	6.1	9.6	7.5	8.2	8.7	8.6	8.5	7.2	8.3	8.2	6.2		
	Maternal Request C. Section	No medical or obstetric indication	5%	10%	% of total number of	Electronic Diary	Not monitored during this Period				9.1	8	18	8.6	9.2	8.4	9	8.6	8.8	9.1	10.8	9		
	Vaginal Birth After Caesarean Section	UK Sentinel Audit 33%	<33%	< 30 %		Labour Ward Book	Not monitored during this Period				66.7	66.7	60.5	60.7	63.6	65.7	53.6	68	71.4	43.3	61.3	76.5		
	Refusal of NNU Transfers	Awaiting guidance from NNU Team	<4	>6		Maternity System	Not monitored during this Period				6	5	0	4	17	13	5	3	2	3	2	0		
	GA C.Sections		<7%	>10%		Maternity System	NA	NA	NA	6	1.3	0.4	1.3	0.6	1.4	1.5	2.7	0.7	1.3	1.3	2.4	1.2		
Workforce		Locally Agreed Weekly hours of Labour Ward consultant cover	>98 hours/wk	<92 hours/wk	Per week	Delivery Suite Consultant Rota	NA	58	73	86	86	90	98	98	98	98	98	98	98	98	98	98		
		Safer Childbirth Requirement Weekly hours of labour ward	>168	<168		Consultant & SR Rota	NA	66	129	104	102	104	116	118	122	124	128	124	116	116	118	116		
		Midwife/birth ratio	<1.30	>1.40	Per week	Head of Midwifery	1.36	1.33	1.33	1.3	1.31		1.26			1.26			1.27					Being monitored quarterly - Q4 11/12
		Supernumerary Midwife in Labour Ward	>90%	>75%		Maternity System							95			97.7			98.7	Quarterly		Quarterly		
	Staffing levels	Mandatory Training for CNST Midwives	>75%	<70%	CNST Training	Practice Educator	NA	NA	89	89	88	88	88	88	88	88	88	88	88	88	88	87		
		Mandatory Training for CNST Doctors	>75%	<70%	CNST Training	Practice Educator	NA	NA	92	92	94	92	92	90	92	92	92	92	92	90	92	90		

Figure 29.3 Maternity Dashboard: a clinical governance monitoring tool.

	Indicator	Target	Review	System																		Comments
Clinical Indicators — Maternal morbidity	All Readmissions	<1%	Review 6 monthly	Maternity System	N/A					2.7	0.5	0.8	0.4	0.5	0.5	0.8	0.7	0.6	0.5	0.5	
	Retained Products/ Sepsis	>2%			New for 2013					10	1	0	0	0	0	0	1	0	0	0	
	Life Threatening PPH >2.0L	<2%	Review 6 monthly		3	3	0.3	0.7	1.1	0.9	0.6	0.8	1.9	0.7	1.7	2.4	2	0.6	1.7	1.2	Home birth - admitted with cerebellar infarction to Neuro-ITU
	Unexpected Admission to ITU		ITU, Medical, Surgery,	Maternity System	Not monitored during this Period	0				2	1	0	0	1	1	0	0	1	1	1	
	BMI > 30 Kg/m2		% from Database	Maternity System	New for 2013					16.8	13.1	18.4	12.5	14.7	16	12.5	15.6	11.4	16.5	14.6	
	Severe Pre-Eclampsia / eclampsia (MgSO4)			Maternity System	N/A	0	1	2	0	1	1	0	0	1	0	0	0	1	0		
	Number of cases of meconium aspiration			Neonatal Team	NA	1	0	1	0	0	0	0	0	0	0	1	0	0	2		
	Number of cases of hypoxic encephalopathy (Grade 2/3)	cases every 6 months	Review 6 monthly	Neonatal Team	NA	3	0	0	1	1	0	1	1	0	1	1	0	1	1		
Peri-natal morbidity & Mortality	Term Stillbirths	<2	Review 6 monthly	Maternity System	1	1	0	1	1	0	0	0	1	0	0	0	0	0	0		
	Preterm Stillbirths 28-36	<2		Maternity System	0	NA	NA	2	1	0	1	2	0	1	5	1	1	1	2	Fetal abnormalities & severe growth restriction
	Preterm Stillbirths <28	3	Review 3 monthly	Maternity System	NA	NA	NA	NA	1	0	1	0	0	0	2	0	0	0	1		
	Early Neonatal Deaths	<2	Review 6 monthly	Maternity System	NA	NA	NA	NA	1	0	0	0	3	1	0	0	0	0	0		
	Risk Incidents involving Fetal Monitoring / Syntocinon	>4 (2)	Review 6 monthly	Risk Management	NA	NA	NA	0	2	0	0	0	0	1	0	0	0	0	1		
	Failed Instrumental Delivery	<1%	Erb's palsy 14%, #	Maternity System	0.7	0.1	0.6	0.5	0.4	0.4	0	0	1.2	1	0.5	0.7	0.5	0	0.2	0.2	
	Morbidity Shoulder dystocia	> 3 / month	Total Number as per revised	Physio Department	NA	NA	0	0.4	0.4	0	0	0	1	1	1	1	0	0	0		
Risk Management	Total number of SUIs	<2 / month		Risk Management	NA	NA	0	0	0	2	3	1	1	0	2	2	2	2	4		
	SUIs where Clinical Care / Organisational Issues identified	<4/month		Risk Management	Not monitored during this Period	1	0	0	1	0	0	1	0	0	0	0	1		
	3rd degree tear	<5%	1.5% of deliveries	Maternity System	4.1	2.7	6	4.2	2.8	2.6	3.6	3.4	3.1	3.5	4.2	3.6	2.7	2.2	2.8	2.7	
Responsive Care — Formal Complaints					4	4	3	5	5	5	3	4	2	3	4	3	3	6	4	3	
	Attitude	0			1	1	1	1	0	0	2	0	0	1	1	0	0	1	0		
	Clinical Care	>0			2	2	1	2	1	3	3	1	2	2	2	1	1	3	1	1	Requesting the patient to book after miscarriage, poor environment in pre-op area
	Organisational				1	1	1	2	3	2	0	1	0	1	1	1	3	2	2		
	Commendations				1	3	2	3	2	5	11	2	3	6	6	7	6	2	3	7	

Figure 29.3 (cont.)

Table 17.4 Glasgow Coma Score

	Response	Score
Eye opening	Spontaneous	4
	Eye opening to speech	3
	Eye opening to pain	2
	No eye opening	1
Verbal	Orientated, spontaneous speech	5
	Confused conversation	4
	Inappropriate words	3
	Incomprehensible sounds/grunts	2
	No verbal response	1
Motor	Obeys commands	6
	Localizes to pain	5
	Withdraws limb from painful stimuli	4
	Abnormal flexion or decorticate posture to pain	3
	Extensor response, decerebrate posture to pain	2
	No motor response	1

After the immediate 'ABC' assessment, a systematic assessment is then required.

- *Obstetric:* see other chapters.
- *Respiratory:* breathlessness is a common feature of acute illness, but the degree may indicate the severity. Chest pain may suggest pulmonary embolism or pneumonia if pleuritic, or cardiac causes if central. Wheeze may indicate aspiration of gastric contents, anaphylaxis or pulmonary oedema; crepitations may indicate aspiration, pneumonia or pulmonary oedema. Tachypnoea is a relatively non-specific symptom and can occur in most illnesses; it is an important feature of early warning systems and frequently mentioned in MDE reports as a clinical sign that merits more attention [2,6]. Hypoxaemia (on saturation monitoring or blood gas analysis) is also non-specific but important to detect, so early use of a pulse oximeter is vital. One potential problem with the pulse oximeter is that in hypoventilation, once oxygenation has been treated by administering oxygen, the saturation may be restored to near-normal even though the patient may only be taking a few breaths each minute. In such situations there may be severe hypercapnia despite reassuring oxygen saturation. Therefore, it is important to monitor respiratory rate and, if low, to monitor carbon dioxide tension by taking blood gas samples. A chest X-ray may be useful, although many conditions (e.g. amniotic or thromboembolism, bronchospasm) are typically not associated with early signs.
- *Cardiovascular:* breathlessness is a non-specific symptom, as discussed above. Cardiac pain is typically central and may indicate myocardial ischaemia or aortic dissection (classically severe and radiating through to the back). Hypertension may indicate pre-eclampsia or be related to pain/anxiety. Rarely it may indicate raised intracranial pressure. Hypotension may reflect loss of circulating volume, a pump problem (heart failure, pulmonary embolism) or a dilated vasculature, e.g. in sepsis. Tachycardia is relatively non-specific but, like tachypnoea, important. Bradycardia may suggest vasovagal syncope (which does not exclude other conditions), but it may also indicate severe hypovolaemia or hypoxaemia, in which sudden severe slowing of the heart rate may indicate imminent cardiac arrest. Heart murmurs can either reflect simple flow murmurs that often develop in pregnancy due to an increased cardiac output, or structural disease. If a cardiac condition is suspected, electrocardiography (ECG) is vital, and a cardiological referral and echocardiogram should be considered.
- *Neurological:* the GCS is a useful overall assessment tool, as discussed above. A reduced conscious level may result from a primary neurological disorder, such as stroke, or be secondary to other pathology, such as severe hypotension. Hypoglycaemia should always be sought as a cause of unconsciousness. Limb weakness may indicate stroke, although residual neuraxial blockade may confuse the clinical picture. Visual disturbances may be seen in primary hypertension, secondary to pre-eclampsia or due to raised intracranial pressure. A headache might be innocent in nature, but might also suggest post-dural puncture headache, intracranial haemorrhage or thrombosis, or severe hypertension/pre-eclampsia. Convulsions may be due to previously diagnosed epilepsy, or result from eclampsia or local anaesthetic toxicity.
- *Other:* bleeding may be obvious from operative site or vagina but may be concealed. Bleeding from puncture sites suggests a coagulopathy. Pyrexia may indicate an infective process. Skin rash may indicate allergic reaction or sepsis.

203

Subsequent Management

Clearly, this will depend on the underlying cause and may involve further investigation and/or treatment that may involve other specialists and units. Labour wards are busy clinical areas, and this presents difficulties in coordinating care of the acutely unwell mother. It may be difficult to devote adequate attention to her while other priorities continue to present, and organizing invasive procedures and investigations may take longer in an area unfamiliar to them. It is important that specialists from other acute areas, especially the critical care/high-dependency unit, be involved early, and that all staff appreciate that the patient does not physically have to be in the intensive care unit in order to receive high-level care.

Specific Conditions

Hypertensive Disorders

Pre-eclampsia can deteriorate after delivery, leading to acute collapse with pulmonary oedema, cerebral haemorrhage, coagulopathy or convulsions. Oedema may also affect the airway leading to respiratory collapse. In the UK almost 40% of eclamptic fits occur after delivery [13].

This topic is covered in more detail in Chapter 25.

Postpartum Haemorrhage

Acute blood loss is a major cause of collapse in the immediate and early postpartum period. It is defined as blood loss >500 ml after delivery of the placenta. The degree of blood loss is frequently underestimated and sometimes unnoticed when attention is focused on the baby. In addition, young patients are often able to compensate until hypovolaemia is severe.

Because of the tendency to underestimate hypovolaemia, it is important that administration of intravenous fluids is prompt and that appropriately sized cannulae are used. Below is an estimate of flow rates through different sizes of cannula:

- 20 G = 40–80 ml/min
- 18 G = 75–120 ml/min
- 16 G = 130–220 ml/min
- 14 G = 250–360 ml/min

Postpartum haemorrhage is covered in more detail in Chapter 15.

Genital Tract/Abdominal Sepsis

'Sepsis' is a non-specific term that refers to the systemic inflammatory response to infection. Systemic inflammatory response syndrome (SIRS) is defined as a clinical state including two or more of the following:

- temperature >38 °C or <36 °C;
- heart rate >90 bpm;
- respiratory rate >20/min or $PaCO_2$ <4.3 kPa;
- white cell count >12 × 10^9/L

The clinical condition defined as 'SIRS' is very non-specific and occurs commonly, especially in pregnancy. Furthermore, it may be caused by many other conditions than infection alone.

In severe sepsis, organ dysfunction develops as a result of hypotension and hypoperfusion. 'Septic shock' is defined as severe sepsis with hypotension, despite adequate fluid resuscitation, along with perfusion abnormalities such as lactic acidosis, oliguria and mental disturbance.

The clinical presentation of sepsis is very variable and often insidious, with rapid clinical deterioration. Typically the patient presents with pyrexia >38 °C, tachycardia and tachypnoea, progressing to hypotension and hypoxaemia. There may be other symptoms such as abdominal pain, nausea and vomiting, and abdominal features are common in deaths associated with pregnancy [2,6].

A high index of suspicion should be maintained with early implementation of broad-spectrum antibiotics after screening for sources of sepsis, and early referral to critical care services if severe. Management of sepsis involves the use of the Surviving Sepsis care bundles [14]. These bundles are a selected set of evidence-based clinical interventions. The care bundles for the first three and six hours are:

- To be completed within three hours:
  - measure lactate level;
  - obtain blood cultures before administering broad-spectrum antibiotics;
  - if patient is hypotensive or blood lactate >4 mmol/l, give IV crystalloid (30 ml/kg).

- To be completed within six hours:
  - aim for a MAP >65 mmHg. If patient does not respond to IV fluids, give vasopressors;
  - if patient is persistently hypotensive/lactate >4 mmol/l, measure CVP and central venous oxygen saturation (aim for CVP >8 mmHg and ScvO2 >70%).

Amniotic Fluid Embolus

The mortality rate from amniotic fluid embolism in the UK is estimated at 0.57 per 100 000 maternities, with women from ethnic minorities at increased risk [2,15].

The traditional explanation is that amniotic fluid enters the maternal circulation following forceful contractions, causing pulmonary vascular obstruction and thence right ventricular failure and cardiovascular collapse, although this has been questioned [16].

It is traditionally diagnosed by the presence of fetal squames and lanugo hair in the pulmonary vasculature at autopsy. In the case of survival, the diagnosis remains clinical.

Amniotic fluid embolus can present at any point from early labour until the early postpartum period. Classically, symptoms include sweating, cyanosis, cardiovascular collapse, confusion, convulsions and disseminated intravascular coagulation (DIC). These symptoms typically progress quickly, with rapid deterioration in clinical condition [15,16].

Management remains supportive with early recognition, prompt resuscitation and early involvement of critical care. There are no specific therapies that have been shown to improve survival.

Peripartum Cardiomyopathy

Peripartum cardiomyopathy (PPCM) develops between the last month of pregnancy and up to five months after delivery [17]. Typical symptoms include breathlessness, oedema and orthopnoea with tachycardia and tachypnoea. A wheeze is often mistaken for asthma but may result from heart failure.

Classically, PPCM results in a dilated cardiomyopathy with reduced cardiac contractility and raised right-sided pressures. In the majority of cases, symptoms develop after delivery, with only 9% presenting in the month before delivery [17].

Treatment of PPCM includes inotropes (dobutamine or dopamine acutely) and reduction in afterload with diuretics and vasodilators. Anticoagulation is advised because of the risk of thromboembolic disease.

PPCM often recurs in subsequent pregnancies and carries significant maternal mortality.

Thromboembolic Disease

There are many risk factors in pregnancy for thromboembolic disease and successive MDE reports have highlighted its importance [2,6].

Pulmonary Embolism

Pulmonary emboli (PE) present in many ways, often depending on their size. Micro- or small emboli might initially be asymptomatic but present subtle, increasing symptoms such as worsening exertional dyspnoea, tiredness or syncope. Small and medium emboli occlude segmental arteries causing pleuritic chest pain, haemoptysis and tachypnoea. Massive emboli become lodged in the proximal pulmonary arteries and chambers of the right heart, resulting in acute and massive reduction in cardiac output with hypotension, right heart failure and major disruption in pulmonary perfusion.

Arterial blood gas measurement classically, but not always, reveals hypoxaemia and hypocapnia. Metabolic acidosis may be present if there is shock. An ECG most often shows sinus tachycardia; however, other signs can be present. A chest radiograph should be performed, although only ~50% of confirmed PE exhibit signs. Most commonly, non-specific features are present such as cardiac enlargement, pleural effusions and localized infiltrates.

An echocardiogram is often useful, indicating right ventricular size and function, although it is poor at excluding PE. The choice for further imaging is usually between a ventilation–perfusion lung scan or computed tomography pulmonary angiogram, depending on local availability and clinical condition.

Management should involve a multidisciplinary resuscitation team including senior physicians, obstetricians, radiologists and anaesthetists [18].

The management of PE depends on the patient's clinical state. Massive PE with clinical compromise justifies more immediate and invasive treatment, including thrombolysis, which may be instituted on clinical grounds alone if cardiac arrest is imminent. Current recommendations suggest a 50 mg bolus of alteplase. Invasive approaches, such as thrombus fragmentation and placement of an inferior vena caval filter, can be considered where facilities and expertise are readily available. In non-massive PE, heparin at therapeutic dosage is recommended instead of thrombolysis, before any imaging is undertaken [19].

Cerebral Vein Thrombosis

Pregnancy predisposes to cerebral vein thrombosis. It is likely to present as either headache, focal neurological signs or reduced consciousness (see below).

General Anaesthesia

Aspiration Pneumonitis

Pregnant patients present particular problems when undergoing general anaesthesia, in particular increased risk of difficult intubation and acid regurgitation. Often the anaesthetic is urgent. Aspiration of gastric contents might occur and present at induction, intra-operatively or postoperatively. Features include bronchospasm, hypoxaemia, raised airway pressure, tachypnoea, tachycardia and pyrexia. Management is largely supportive, as prophylactic antibiotics and steroids are no longer advocated. Chest radiographs may be useful to assess evidence of aspiration and monitor progression.

Atelectasis, Respiratory Depression and Airway Obstruction

During general anaesthesia, patients usually receive opioids for postoperative analgesia. Their potent respiratory depressant effects can be exacerbated by the anaesthetic agents during early recovery, leading to airway obstruction and respiratory depression. The situation is made worse if there is weakness caused by residual neuromuscular blockade. The development of special recovery areas with staff who are familiar with postoperative recovery care is important in preventing such complications. Simple airway manoeuvres can be tried and oxygen administered while anaesthetic help is summoned. Naloxone can be titrated to effect if respiratory depression is due to opioids.

Basal atelectasis commonly follows general anaesthesia and describes small airway collapse due to poor regional ventilation and/or mucous plugging. Patients typically are hypoxaemic with reduced tidal volumes and raised respiratory rates. Effective analgesia must be ensured to allow deep breathing and coughing. Physiotherapy may be useful in encouraging adequate lung expansion and effective removal of secretions.

Regional Anaesthesia

The physiological effects of regional anaesthesia extend into the postpartum period and can present problems for both the anaesthetist and for those caring for the patient after the procedure.

A residual regional block can result in hypotension due to the sympathetic block that accompanies the sensory blockade. This is exacerbated by any hypovolaemia already present or that develops after delivery, and by bradycardia that may occur if the block extends up to the cardiac sympathetic fibres at thoracic spinal segments T2–T4. If the block extends to the cervical segments (C3–C5), there is risk of diaphragmatic weakness, leading to hypoventilation. There may also be inability to talk/swallow, weakness of the arms/hands, and sedation (which may be put down to simple tiredness). Any patient who has received a spinal or epidural anaesthetic must be monitored carefully to exclude a dangerously high block, which may only develop 30–60 min after the procedure.

Following epidural anaesthesia, in which larger volumes of local anaesthetic are used than for spinal anaesthesia, local anaesthetic toxicity may be encountered. Typically the signs and symptoms progress from mild features such as circumoral tingling, tinnitus and visual disturbances, to cardiac arrhythmias, convulsions and reduced consciousness. The use of lipid suspension is now recommended as treatment for local anaesthetic toxicity [20,21].

Both trauma and infection may be caused during regional anaesthesia. Epidural/spinal haematomas can present acutely with acute cord compression. Investigation of any suspected lesion should be prompt with referral to an appropriate neurosurgical centre. Meningitis is a rare complication; classic signs include headache, neck stiffness, photophobia, vomiting, fever and leukocytosis. Lumbar puncture should be considered, and broad-spectrum antibiotics started pending the result. Spinal abscesses and other rare neurological complications such as arachnoiditis are unlikely to present in the early postpartum period.

Cardiac Disease

Cardiac disease is becoming more common due to increasing maternal age, improved survival of women with complex congenital heart disease and the influx of immigrant women with pre-existing uncorrected conditions. Risk factors associated with ischaemic heart disease include obesity, smoking, older age, higher parity, diabetes, pre-existing hypertension and a family history.

The early postpartum period is associated with large fluid shifts that potentially contribute to haemodynamic instability. Most cardiac disease is sensitive to these changes, hence this period can be associated with cardiac complications such as heart failure, arrhythmias and ischaemia [22]. Systolic 'flow' heart murmurs are common in normal pregnancy, as are ECG changes (see Table 17.3).

Myocardial Infarction

Myocardial infarction (MI) in the postpartum period is rare. Typically, chest pain occurs at rest and is described as central, crushing or heavy, radiating to the arm or neck, although presentation is often 'atypical'. Early management includes aspirin 300 mg orally and cardiological referral. The choice between thrombolysis and primary coronary angioplasty will depend on local availability as well as other factors, such as risk of haemorrhage following delivery and surgical procedures.

Aortic Dissection

Typically, severe sudden anterior chest pain radiates to the interscapular area, often associated with hypertension. Sudden death or profound shock is usually due to aortic rupture or cardiac tamponade. Patients can also present with other features, including cardiac failure, stroke, acute limb ischaemia, paraplegia, MI, renal failure or abdominal pain.

The ECG may be normal or show left ventricular hypertension or even acute MI. A chest radiograph may show a widened upper mediastinum with enlargement of the aortic knuckle. An echocardiogram may show aortic root dilatation or aortic regurgitation. CT or angiography may also be indicated.

Management will depend on the type of dissection. If the aortic arch is affected, surgical repair is usually required. If medical management is indicated, then control of blood pressure is the main goal of therapy to stop the spread of intramural haematoma and prevent rupture.

Arrhythmias

The incidence of cardiac arrhythmias is increased in the pregnant population, and presentation ranges from mild symptoms to severe hypotension and even cardiac arrest. The most common rhythms include supraventricular tachycardia and atrial fibrillation. Evidence of deranged electrolytes or hypovolaemia should be sought and treated accordingly. Supraventricular tachycardias may respond to vagal manoeuvres, adenosine or amiodarone, but may require direct current cardioversion in severe compromise.

Respiratory Disease

Asthma

Acute exacerbations of asthma are uncommon in the peripartum period, but the physiological changes of pregnancy may potentially lead to misinterpretation of the signs and symptoms of disease severity – for example, hyperventilation. Asthma can be exacerbated by general anaesthesia and some drugs, such as non-steroidal anti-inflammatories. The classical symptoms include wheeze, breathlessness and cough, and patients can present with either gradually worsening symptoms or acute severe bronchospasm.

The severity of the attack should be assessed along with the cause of the exacerbation (drugs, infection). Immediate management includes oxygen, nebulized salbutamol (bronchodilator), and ipratropium bromide, hydration, antibiotics and steroids. Intravenous aminophylline, salbutamol and adrenaline can be considered in life-threatening attacks.

Pneumonia

Patients typically present with cough, fever, breathlessness, chest pain and abnormal chest radiograph. Appropriate broad-spectrum antibiotics should be started along with oxygen, adequate hydration and chest physiotherapy.

Adverse Drug Reactions

Anaphylaxis

Anaphylactic reactions are IgE-mediated type-B hypersensitivity reactions to an antigen resulting in histamine and serotonin release from mast cells and basophils. *Anaphylactoid* reactions produce indistinguishable clinical features, but are IgG-mediated, with complement activation, and require no previous exposure to the stimulus. Recent guidelines have emphasized that the distinction, while of interest in terms of aetiology, is irrelevant during an acute severe reaction, and therefore advocate the term 'anaphylaxis' to describe the clinical condition, whatever the mechanism [23].

The most common cause is drugs, especially antibiotics and some anaesthetic drugs, although there are many other possible causes including intravenous colloids, latex and some foods. Reactions against blood or blood components must also be remembered.

Anaphylaxis typically presents with cardiovascular collapse, erythema, bronchospasm, angio-oedema and rash. However, skin lesions may not be present and features (which may include abdominal pain) may be confusing, especially against a background of recent delivery, and a high index of suspicion is required.

Management involves removal of the suspected antigen and immediate supportive care with adrenaline 0.5–1 mg boluses IM (or 50 mcg increments IV if the doctor is familiar with this route of injection and there is ECG monitoring) repeated until symptoms improve. Antihistamines (chlorphenamine 10 mg IV) and corticosteroids (hydrocortisone 200 mg IV) should be given to lessen the subsequent inflammatory response. Bronchodilators may also be considered if bronchospasm is persistent.

All patients with a suspected anaphylactic reaction should have blood taken for mast cell tryptase levels. These samples should be taken immediately (do not delay resuscitation) 1–2 hours following the start of the reaction and approximately 24 hours after the reaction. A raised tryptase level will confirm mast cell degranulation, although other measurements (e.g. complement) may also be useful. All patients should be followed up after the event and allergy testing arranged [23].

Toxicity/Side-Effects

Most drugs have side-effects, even at normal doses, while in overdose many have significant untoward effects. Opioids can cause respiratory depression, hypotension, bradycardia and reduced consciousness. Naloxone can be used to reverse the effects, but care should be taken to titrate to effect, and the antagonist's effect may be shorter than the duration of action of the original opioid so that repeated dosage or an infusion may be required.

Syntocinon® may cause profound hypotension and tachycardia, although this should not preclude its careful administration in a patient who is hypovolaemic from haemorrhage. Ergometrine may cause hypertension and severe vomiting. Antiemetics such as metoclopramide and cyclizine may cause severe tachycardia and, rarely, dystonic reactions. Beta-adrenergic agonists used for tocolysis may cause tachycardia and pulmonary oedema. Early signs of magnesium toxicity include nausea, vomiting and flushing. Later signs include ECG changes, loss of tendon reflexes, respiratory depression, apnoea and cardiac arrest. Toxicity is reversed by intravenous calcium gluconate (10 ml of 10% solution IV).

Drug Withdrawal

The proportion of pregnant women who abuse drugs is difficult to determine and varies depending on the socioeconomic area. While patients are unlikely to present with acute intoxication in the immediate postpartum period, symptoms of withdrawal may occur. Withdrawal from alcohol typically is worst about 24–36 hours after cessation of intake, resulting in aggression, confusion and tremor. Opioid withdrawal occurs within 6–12 hours of the last dose and may cause problems with postoperative analgesia as well as hypertension, tachycardia, sweating, abdominal pain and vomiting. Myocardial ischaemia, arrhythmias and convulsions can occur with both cocaine withdrawal and acute intoxication.

Metabolic

Diabetes can be particularly difficult to manage during pregnancy, with significant increases in insulin requirements. Following delivery, requirements fall dramatically, and hypoglycaemia can occur if the infusion rates of insulin are not reduced. Hypoglycaemia can present with symptoms ranging from mild (nausea, anxiety, tremor, pallor) to more severe (personality change, confusion, ataxia, coma). Any acute illness in a diabetic mother should prompt a glucose level check and treatment of hypoglycaemia. Initial treatment includes a glucose bolus (50 ml of 50% glucose IV). Hyperglycaemia in a poorly controlled diabetic can also present with a range of symptoms including ketoacidosis and coma. Treatment involves recognition and treatment with insulin.

The potential danger of hyponatraemia from excessive administration of hypotonic intravenous fluids is well described, and this may occur in the delivery suite [24]. Parturients may be at increased risk because of the dilution of oxytocics in hypotonic solutions and the antidiuretic action of oxytocin.

Rarely, there may be other, unexpected, metabolic causes of collapse or acute illness (e.g. severe abnormalities of potassium or calcium status) and the usefulness of routine electrolyte analysis should not be forgotten.

Primary Neurological

Epilepsy

Convulsions due to epilepsy may present for the first time in the postpartum period or may occur in a patient with known epilepsy. Control of epilepsy in pregnancy may become poorer due to altered pharmacokinetics and pharmacodynamics, as well as reduced compliance with and alteration of normal medication. In some epileptics, convulsions are triggered by pain, anxiety and hyperventilation, all of which may occur during or after delivery. There are, of course, other causes of seizures on the labour ward (particularly eclampsia), and other pathology should always be excluded. Typical treatment includes diazepam 5–10 mg followed by phenytoin 10–15 mg/kg (with ECG monitoring) if seizures continue.

Stroke/Cerebrovascular Accident (CVA)

The most common type of haemorrhagic CVA is subarachnoid haemorrhage. Typically, patients present with sudden onset severe headache with photophobia, neck stiffness, vomiting and sometimes reduced conscious level. Management involves early consultation with neurosurgeons regarding surgical intervention along with supportive treatment. There is usually underlying pathology, such as an arteriovenous malformation or berry aneurysm. Rarely, subdural haemorrhage has followed dural puncture (spinal anaesthesia, diagnostic lumbar puncture or accidental dural tap during epidural analgesia/anaesthesia).

Patients may also present with focal neurological signs due to ischaemic or haemorrhagic stroke affecting the cortex. Again, this may be accompanied by reduced conscious level. Stroke is a common feature in deaths due to hypertensive diseases of pregnancy, and focal neurological features may be a presentation of cerebral venous thrombosis, so that these diagnoses must be considered.

Posterior Reversible Encephalopathy Syndrome (PRES)

This syndrome was first described in 1996 and is characterized by headaches, altered mental status, seizures and visual disturbances. Diagnostic MRI shows a classical pattern of white matter changes suggestive of posterior cerebral oedema. PRES has been associated with many conditions, including eclampsia; and in one recent series 100% of patients with eclampsia were found to have neuroradiological evidence of PRES [25].

Management mainly focuses on correcting the underlying cause, so treatment of eclampsia with magnesium sulphate and blood pressure control with antihypertensives is advised. The treatment of cerebral oedema with IV dexamethasone has also been suggested.

Other Non-Obstetric

Air Embolus

Air emboli may occur for a variety of reasons. Subclinical entry of air into the circulation has been shown to occur in caesarean sections, and this is more likely if the uterus is exteriorized and held above the level of the heart; positioning the patient head-up may reduce this [26]. In the postpartum period, the most likely mechanism of air embolism is entrainment into the circulation on insertion or manipulation of central venous catheters or peripheral cannulae where the pressure within the vein is negative relative to atmospheric pressure. Accidental injection of air into venous lines can also occur in the form of small bubbles, or as large boluses when pressure devices are used with air-containing bags of fluid.

The clinical features are usually non-specific (hypotension, tachycardia, reduced arterial saturation) and the diagnosis is not always clear. Chest pain with ST segment depression may suggest air in the coronary circulation. Larger volumes of air may cause reduced cardiac output due to obstruction of right ventricular output. If a patent foramen ovale is present (seen in about 30% of the population) air can pass into the arterial circulation and cause systemic lesions such as stroke or MI. In the case of massive air embolism, auscultation of the heart may reveal 'mill wheel' or churning noises.

Management includes prevention of further entrainment of air followed by supportive care. It has been suggested that aspiration of air from the right ventricle is possible, but in practice this is rarely successful or practical. Positioning the patient in the left lateral position may reduce right ventricle outflow obstruction.

Vasovagal Syncope

Vasovagal syncope may be associated with chronic autonomic instability or occur de novo. Triggers include stress, prolonged standing, dehydration, painful or unpleasant procedures and hyperthermia. Collapse is usually preceded by prodromal symptoms such as feeling faint, nausea, sweating and visual disturbance.

The underlying mechanism involves increased activity of the parasympathetic nervous system ±

reduced sympathetic activity. The common feature is usually hypotension due to either a bradycardia (vagal effect) or vasodilatation (sympathetic effect).

Specific treatment is usually not required other than lying the patient down with legs elevated to increase venous return. In the postpartum period, dehydration as well as the other common triggers may be more prevalent.

Other Vascular

MDE reports have contained cases of splenic artery rupture and mesenteric infarction; although rare, such conditions may be more common in pregnancy. Rare causes of postpartum collapse should always be considered during resuscitation, especially if the patient is unresponsive to initial management.

Other Considerations

The effect of acute illness/collapse on the mother's partner/relatives and on other women around her should not be forgotten. The typical maternity suite is not an area where acute critical illness is commonly seen, and the psychological impact of a sudden deterioration, compounded by the lack of familiarity of the attending staff, may be considerable. If time permits it might be appropriate to transfer the patient to an area more familiar with acute medical management, such as the recovery area or even the labour ward operating theatre; alternatively, screens/curtains should be used and other patients even moved away from the area. Counselling for other patients, relatives and even staff may be appropriate after the event.

Summary

The causes of postpartum collapse are varied, but the initial approach to the management remains the same. A systematic approach (*Airway, Breathing, Circulation*) helps to address the immediate issues while helping to establish the underlying cause and therefore allowing appropriate treatment.

A large number of patients present with acute illness in the postpartum period, although exact numbers are difficult to establish. Most of these patients have a good outcome, but a few remain severely unwell and require management by a combination of obstetric, anaesthetic and intensive care staff. Systems should be in place for the recognition, monitoring and referral of these patients, as well as for the training of staff who might be involved in their management.

References

1. World Health Organization. *Trends in Maternal Mortality: 1990–2013*. Geneva: WHO; 2014. www.who.int/reproductivehealth/publications/monitoring/maternal-mortality-2013/en (accessed 1 October 2014).

2. Knight M, Kenyon S, Brocklehurst P, *et al.* (eds). *Saving Lives, Improving Mothers' Care: Lessons Learned to Inform Future Maternity Care from the UK and Ireland Confidential Enquiries into Maternal Deaths and Morbidity 2009–12*. Oxford: National Perinatal Epidemiology Unit, University of Oxford; 2014. www.npeu.ox.ac.uk/mbrrace-uk/reports (accessed 9 December 2014).

3. RCOG. *Maternal Collapse in Pregnancy and the Puerperium*. London: RCOG Press; 2011. www.rcog.org.uk/globalassets/documents/guidelines/gtg56.pdf (accessed 1 October 2014).

4. Bateman BT, Mhyre JM, Hernandez-Diaz S, *et al.* Development of a comorbidity index for use in obstetric patients. *Obstet Gynecol*. 2013; 122: 957–65.

5. Campbell KH, Savitz D, Werner EF, *et al.* Maternal morbidity and risk of death at delivery hospitalization. *Obstet Gynecol*. 2013; 122: 627–33.

6. Lewis G (ed.). Special Issue: Saving Mothers' Lives – Reviewing Maternal Deaths to Make Motherhood Safer: 2006–2008. The Eighth Report of the Confidential Enquiries into Maternal Deaths in the United Kingdom. *B J Obstet Gynaecol*. 2011; 118: 1–203.

7. Lewis G (ed.). *The Confidential Enquiries into Maternal and Child Health (CEMACH): Saving Mothers' Lives – Reviewing Maternal Deaths to Make Motherhood Safer – 2003–2005. The Seventh Report on Confidential Enquiries into Maternal Deaths in the United Kingdom*. London: CEMACH; 2005. www.hqip.org.uk/assets/NCAPOP-Library/CMACE-Reports/21.-December-2007-Saving-Mothers-Lives-reviewing-maternal-deaths-to-make-motherhood-safer-2003-2005.pdf (accessed 1 October 2014).

8. Singh S, McGlennan A, England A, Simons R. A validation study of the CEMACH recommended modified early obstetric warning system (MEOWS). *Anaesthesia*. 2012; 67: 12–18.

9. Isaacs RA, Wee MYK, Bick DE, *et al.* A national survey of obstetric early warning systems in the United Kingdom: five years on. *Anaesthesia*. 2014; 69: 687–92.

10. McGlennan A, Sherratt K. Charting change on the labour ward. *Anaesthesia*. 2013; 68: 338–42.

11. Resuscitation Council (UK). *The Resuscitation Guidelines 2010*, 6th edition. London: Resuscitation Council (UK); 2010. www.resus.org.uk/pages/guide.htm (accessed 1 October 2014).

12. Quinn AC, Milne D, Columb DM, Gorton H, Knight M. Failed tracheal intubation in obstetric anaesthesia: 2 yr national case-control study in the UK. *Br J Anaesth*. 2013; 110: 74–80.

13. Knight M. Eclampsia in the United Kingdom 2005. *Br J Obstet Gynaecol*. 2007; 114: 1072–8.

14. Dellinger RP, Levy MM, Rhodes A, *et al.* Surviving Sepsis Campaign: international guidelines for management of severe sepsis and septic shock, 2012. *Intensive Care Med*. 2013; 39: 165–228.

15. Knight M, Tuffnell D, Brocklehurst P, Spark P, Kurinczuk JJ. Incidence and risk factors for amniotic fluid embolism. *Obstet Gynecol*. 2010; 115: 910–17.

16. Tuffnell DJ. Amniotic fluid embolism. *Curr Opin Obstet Gynecol*. 2003; 15: 119–22.

17. Sliwa K, Hilfiker-Kleiner D, Petrie MC, *et al.* Current state of knowledge on aetiology, diagnosis, management, and therapy of peripartum cardiomyopathy: a position statement from the Heart Failure Association of the European Society of Cardiology Working Group on peripartum cardiomyopathy. *Eur J Heart Failure*. 2010; 12: 767–8.

18. Greer IE, Thompson AJ. *The Acute Management of Thrombosis and Embolism During Pregnancy and the Puerperium*. London: RCOG Press; 2007. www.rcog.org.uk/globalassets/documents/guidelines/gtg37b_230611.pdf (accessed 1 October 2014).

19. NICE. *Venous Thromboembolic Diseases: The Management of Venous Thromboembolic Diseases and the Role of Thrombophilia Testing*. London: National Clinical Guidelines Centre; 2012. www.nice.org.uk/guidance/cg144 (accessed 1 October 2014).

20. Weinberg GM. Lipid emulsion infusion: resuscitation for local anaesthetic and other drug overdose. *Anesthesiology*. 2012; 117: 180–7.

21. Association of Anaesthetists of Great Britain and Ireland. *Management of Severe Local Anaesthetic Toxicity 2*. London: AAGBI; 2010. www.aagbi.org/sites/default/files/la_toxicity_2010_0.pdf (accessed 1 October 2014).

22. RCOG. *Cardiac Disease and Pregnancy: Good Practice No. 13*. London: RCOG Press; 2011. www.rcog.org.uk/en/guidelines-research-services/guidelines/good-practice-13/ (accessed 1 October 2014).

23. Association of Anaesthetists of Great Britain and Ireland. *Suspected Anaphylactic Reactions Associated with Anaesthesia*. London: AAGBI; 2009. www.aagbi.org/sites/default/files/anaphylaxis_2009.pdf (accessed 1 October 2014).

24. Ophir E, Solt I, Odeh M, Bornstein J. Water intoxication: a dangerous condition in labor and delivery rooms. *Obstet Gynecol Surv*. 2007; 62: 731–8.

25. Brewer J, Owens MY, Wallace K, *et al.* Posterior reversible encephalopathy syndrome in 46 of 47 patients with eclampsia. *Am J Obstet Gynecol*. 2013; 208 (468): e1–e6.

26. Fong J, Gadalla F, Druzin M. Venous emboli occurring caesarean section: the effect of patient position. *Can J Anesth*. 1991; 38: 191–5.

Chapter 18

Episiotomy and Obstetric Perineal Trauma

Ranee Thakar and Abdul H. Sultan

Perineal repair after childbirth affects millions of women worldwide. In the UK, approximately 85% of women sustain some form of perineal trauma during vaginal delivery; of these, 69% will require stitches [1]. The prevalence of perineal trauma is dependent on variations in obstetric practice, including rates and types of episiotomies, which not only vary between countries but also within the same country and the same provider groups [2].

The overall risk of obstetric anal sphincter injuries (OASIS) is approximately 2% of all vaginal deliveries. A recent study conducted in the UK showed that the OASIS rate in England tripled from 1.8% to 5.9% between 2000 and 2012 [3]. However, 'occult' anal sphincter injury (i.e. defects in the anal sphincter detected by anal endosonography that was not recognized clinically) has been identified in 33% of primiparous women following vaginal delivery [4]. The most plausible explanation for an 'occult' injury is either an injury that has been missed, recognized but not reported or wrongly classified as a second-degree tear [5,6]. With increased awareness and training, there appears to be an increase in detection of anal sphincter injuries [7]. In centres where mediolateral episiotomies are practised, the rate of OASIS occurs in 1.7% (2.9% in primiparae) compared to 12% (19% in primiparae) in centres practising midline episiotomy [8].

The majority of women experience some form of short-term discomfort or pain following perineal repair, and up to 20% will continue to have long-term problems, such as superficial dyspareunia. Short- and long-term morbidity associated with perineal repair can lead to major physical, psychological and social problems affecting the woman's ability to care for her newborn baby and other members of the family [9]. The morbidity associated with perineal trauma depends on the extent of perineal damage, the technique and materials used for suturing, and the skill of the person performing the procedure. It is important that practitioners ensure that routine procedures, such as perineal repair, are evidence-based in order to provide care which is effective, appropriate and cost-efficient.

Applied Anatomy

An understanding of the anatomy of the pelvic floor, anal sphincters and perineum is essential for healthcare providers managing and suturing perineal trauma.

Anatomy of the Perineum

The perineum corresponds to the outlet of the pelvis and is somewhat lozenge-shaped. The perineum can be divided into two triangular parts by drawing a line transversely between the ischial tuberosities. The anterior triangle, which contains the urogenital organs, is known as the *urogenital triangle*, and the posterior triangle, which contains the termination of the anal canal, is known as the *anal triangle* [10].

Urogenital Triangle

The urogenital triangle has been divided into two compartments, the superficial and deep perineal spaces, separated by the perineal membrane, which spans the space between the ischiopubic rami. Just beneath the skin and subcutaneous fat lie the superficial perineal muscles: superficial transverse perineal, bulbospongiosus and ischiocavernosus. The superficial transverse perineal muscle is a narrow slip of muscle which arises from the inner and forepart of the

Best Practice in Labour and Delivery, Second Edition, ed. Sir Sabaratnam Arulkumaran. Published by Cambridge University Press. © Cambridge University Press 2016.

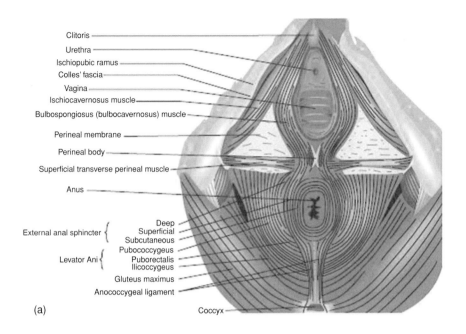

(a)

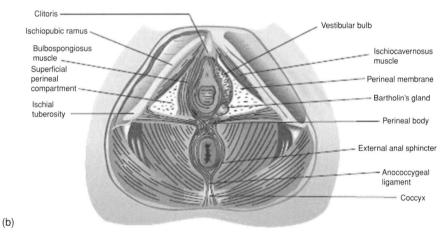

(b)

Figure 18.1 (a) The superficial muscles of the perineum; namely, the superficial transverse perineal muscle, the bulbospongiosus and the ischiocavernosus form a triangle on either side of the perineum. (b) The left bulbospongiosus muscle has been removed to demonstrate the vestibular bulb [10, with permission].

ischial tuberosity and is inserted into the central tendinous part of the perineal body. The bulbospongiosus muscle runs on either side of the vaginal orifice, covering the lateral aspects of the vestibular bulb anteriorly and the Bartholin's gland posteriorly. The ischiocavernosus muscle is situated on the side of the lateral boundary of the perineum. The deep transverse perineal muscle lies in the deep perineal space. It is thin and difficult to delineate, and hence some authors deny the existence of this muscle (Figure 18.1).

Anal Triangle

The anal triangle includes the anal canal, the anal sphincters and ischioanal fossae. The anal canal is approximately 3.5 cm long and is attached posteriorly to the coccyx by the anococcygeal ligament, a midline fibromuscular structure which runs between the posterior aspect of the EAS and the coccyx. The anus is surrounded laterally and posteriorly by loose adipose tissue within the ischioanal fossae. The pudendal nerves pass over the ischial spines and can be accessed

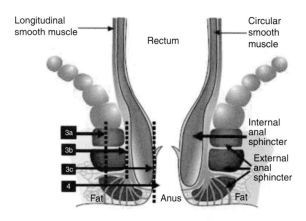

Figure 18.2 Classification of perineal trauma depicted in a schematic representation of the anal sphincters [6, with permission].

EAS, the IAS has a pale appearance to the naked eye. As shown in Figure 18.2, the subcutaneous EAS lies at a lower level than the IAS, but during regional or general anaesthesia the paralysed EAS lies at almost the same level as the IAS. The conjoint longitudinal coat lies between the EAS and IAS and consists of a fibromuscular layer, longitudinal muscle and intersphincteric space with its connective tissue elements. Traced downwards, it separates opposite the lower border of the IAS, and the fibrous septae fan out to pass through the EAS and ultimately attach to the skin of the lower anal canal and perianal region. As a result of tonic circumferential contraction of the sphincter, the skin is arranged in radiating folds around the anus, and this is called the anal margin. These folds appear to be flat or ironed out when there is underlying sphincter damage [10].

digitally at this site for measurement of pudendal nerve terminal motor latency using a modified electrode. The perineum can also be anaesthetized by injection of local anaesthetic into the pudendal nerve at this site. Anteriorly, the perineal body separates the anal canal from the vagina. The anal canal is surrounded by an inner epithelial lining, a vascular subepithelium and the anal sphincter complex. The lining of the anal canal varies along its length due to its embryologic derivation. The proximal anal canal is lined with rectal mucosa (columnar epithelium) and is separated by the dentate line from the distal anoderm, which consists of modified squamous epithelium. Since the epithelium in the lower canal is well supplied with sensory nerve endings, acute distension or invasive treatment of haemorrhoids in this area causes profuse discomfort, whereas treatment can be carried out with relatively few symptoms in the upper canal lined by insensate columnar epithelium. The anal sphincter complex consists of the external anal sphincter (EAS) and internal anal sphincter (IAS) separated by the conjoint longitudinal coat (Figure 18.2). The striated EAS is subdivided into subcutaneous, superficial and deep, and is responsible for voluntary squeeze and reflex contraction pressure. It is innervated by the pudendal nerve, which is a mixed sensory and motor nerve. However, these subdivisions are not easily demonstrable during anatomical dissection or surgery, but may be of relevance during imaging. To the naked eye, the EAS appears like red meat. The IAS, which is a thickened continuation of the circular smooth muscle of the bowel, contributes about 70% of the resting pressure and is under autonomic control. In contrast to the

Perineal Body

The perineal body is the central point of the perineum and is situated between the urogenital and the anal triangles of the perineum. Its three-dimensional form has been likened to that of the cone of the red pine, with each 'petal' representing an interlocking structure, such as an insertion site of fascia or a muscle of the perineum. Within the perineal body there is interlacing of muscle fibres from the bulbospongiosus, superficial transverse perineal and EAS muscles. Above this level, there is a contribution from the longitudinal rectal muscle and the medial fibres of the puborectalis muscle.

Levator Ani

The pelvic floor (pelvic diaphragm) is a musculotendineous sheet that spans the pelvic outlet and consists mainly of the symmetrically paired levator ani. The levator ani is a broad muscular sheet of variable thickness attached to the internal surface of the true pelvis and is subdivided into parts according to their attachments and pelvic viscera to which they are related, namely iliococcygeus, puborectalis and pubovisceralis. The pubovisceralis is subdivided into separate parts according to the pelvic viscera to which they relate (i.e. puboanalis, pubovaginalis, pubourethralis and puboperinealis). The levator ani is innervated largely by direct nerves from the pelvic plexus, while the muscles of the perineum are innervated by the pudendal nerve.

Classification

Perineal trauma may occur spontaneously during vaginal birth, or intentionally when a surgical incision (episiotomy) is made to facilitate delivery. It is also possible to have both an episiotomy and a spontaneous tear either as an extension of the episiotomy or as a separate tear. Anterior perineal trauma is defined as injury to the labia, anterior vagina, urethra or clitoris. Posterior perineal trauma is defined as any injury to the posterior vaginal wall, perineal muscles or anal sphincters, and may include disruption of the anal sphincter.

In order to standardize the classification of perineal trauma (Figure 18.2), Sultan proposed the following classification that has been adopted by the Royal College of Obstetricians and Gynaecologists and also recommended by the International Consultation on Incontinence [7,11]:

- First degree: laceration of the vaginal epithelium or perineal skin only.
- Second degree: involvement of the perineal muscles (bulbocavernosus, transverse perineal), but not the anal sphincter. If the trauma is very deep, the pubococcygeus muscle may be disrupted.
- Third degree: disruption of the anal sphincter muscles, which should be further subdivided into:
  - 3a: <50% thickness of external sphincter torn;
  - 3b: >50% thickness of external sphincter torn;
  - 3c: internal sphincter also torn.
- Fourth degree: a third-degree tear with disruption of the anal epithelium as well.

If there is any doubt about the grade of a third-degree tear involving the external sphincter, it is advisable to classify it to the higher degree to avoid underestimation [6]. Isolated tears of the anal epithelium (buttonhole) without involvement of the anal sphincters are rare. In order to avoid confusion, they are not included in the above classification but are referred to as such.

Episiotomy

An episiotomy is a surgical incision made with scissors or a scalpel into the perineum in order to increase the diameter of the vulval outlet and facilitate delivery. There are two main types of episiotomy incisions: midline and mediolateral. A midline episiotomy is an incision from the mid-point of the posterior fourchette directed vertically towards the anus, while with a mediolateral episiotomy the incision is directed 40–60 degrees away from the midline. It is claimed that the midline incision is easier to repair and that it is associated with less blood loss, better healing, less pain and earlier resumption of sexual intercourse. However, there is no reliable evidence to support these claims. Limited evidence from one quasi-randomized trial suggested that the midline incision may increase the risk of third- and fourth-degree tears compared with the mediolateral incision. However, these data should be interpreted with caution, as there may be an increased risk of selection bias due to quasi-random treatment allocation, and also analysis was not by intention to treat [12].

There is evidence accumulating that episiotomies angled too close to the midline are at a higher risk of causing OASIS [13,14,15]. This risk reduces by 50% for every six degrees the episiotomy is angled away from the midline [14]. However, if the episiotomy angle becomes nearly horizontal (90°), the pressure on the perineum is not relieved and OASIS incidence increases nine-fold [15]. The current recommendation is to cut an episiotomy at 45–60° from the midline originating from the vaginal fourchette [16]. It is important to note that the angle of a mediolateral episiotomy will reduce significantly after the baby is born, i.e. a 40° episiotomy incision results in a suture angle of 22° from the midline [17]. If an episiotomy is performed at a 60° angle when the perineum is distended, this will result in a suture angle of 45°, which is associated with a lower incidence of anal sphincter tears, anal incontinence and perineal pain [18].

Indications for Episiotomy

Episiotomy is still performed routinely in many parts of the world in the belief that it protects the pelvic floor. However, evidence from randomized controlled trials (RCTs) suggests that routine episiotomy does not prevent severe posterior perineal tears. Carroli and Belizan have conducted the most recent systematic review of randomized clinical trials using the Cochrane Collaboration methodology to determine the possible benefits and risks of restrictive episiotomy versus routine episiotomy. This revealed that compared with routine use, restrictive use of episiotomy resulted in less severe perineal trauma, less suturing and fewer healing complications. There were no significant differences in severe vaginal/perineal trauma, dyspareunia, urinary incontinence or severe pain measures. The only disadvantage shown in restrictive use of episiotomy was an increased risk of anterior perineal trauma. The systematic review concluded that there is evidence to support the restrictive use of episiotomy compared to routine episiotomy (irrespective of the type of episiotomy performed) [12].

There is currently an absence of clear, evidence-based clinical indications for the use of episiotomy. However, it is reasonable to suggest that an episiotomy should be performed to accelerate vaginal delivery in cases of fetal distress, to facilitate manoeuvres during shoulder dystocia, to minimize severe perineal trauma during a forceps delivery, to reduce the occurrence of multiple lacerations in the presence of a thick or rigid perineum, and in situations where prolonged 'bearing down' may be harmful for the mother (e.g. severe hypertensive or cardiac disease).

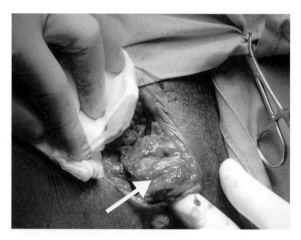

Figure 18.3 A partial tear (arrow) along the length of the external anal sphincter [6, with permission]. See the colour plate section for a colour version of this figure.

Diagnosis of Perineal Trauma

1. Before assessment for genital trauma, the healthcare professional should [16]:

   - explain to the woman what they plan to do and why;
   - offer inhalational analgesia or ensure that epidural analgesia is effective;
   - ensure good lighting; and
   - position the woman so that she is comfortable and the genital structures can be seen clearly, and if this is not possible then the woman should be placed in lithotomy.

2. Informed consent should be obtained for a vaginal and rectal examination.

3. If the examination is restricted because of pain, adequate analgesia must be given prior to examination.

4. Following a visual examination of the genitalia, the labia should be parted and a vaginal examination should be performed to establish the full extent of the vaginal tear. When multiple or deep tears are present it is best to examine and repair in lithotomy. The apex of the vaginal laceration should always be identified.

5. A rectal examination should then be performed to exclude OASIS. Figure 18.3 shows a partial tear along the EAS which would have been missed if a rectal examination was not performed. The vagina should be exposed by parting the labia with the index and middle fingers of the other hand. Every woman should have a rectal examination prior to suturing in order to avoid missing isolated tears such as 'buttonhole' of the rectal mucosa [6]. Furthermore, a third- or fourth-degree tear may be present beneath apparently 'intact' perineal skin, highlighting the need to perform a rectal examination in order to exclude OASIS following every vaginal delivery [6]. Following diagnosis of the tear, it should be graded according to the recommended classification [6].

6. In order to diagnose OASIS, clear visualization is necessary, and the injury should be confirmed by palpation. By inserting the index finger in the anal canal and the thumb in the vagina, the anal sphincter can be palpated by performing a pill-rolling motion. If there is still uncertainty, the woman should be asked to contract her anal sphincter and if the anal sphincter is disrupted, there will be a distinct gap felt anteriorly. If the perineal skin is intact there will be an absence of puckering on the perianal skin anteriorly. This may not be evident under regional or general anaesthesia. As the EAS is in a state of tonic contraction, disruption results in retraction of the sphincter ends [6].

7. The IAS is a circular smooth muscle that appears paler (similar to raw fish) than the striated EAS (similar to raw red meat). If the IAS or anal epithelium is torn, the EAS will invariably be torn.

Management and Repair of Perineal Trauma

Basic principles prior to repairing perineal trauma include [6–8] the following:

- The skills and knowledge of the operator are important factors in achieving a successful repair. The woman should be referred to a more experienced healthcare professional if uncertainty exists as to the nature or extent of trauma sustained [16].
- Repair of the perineum should be undertaken as soon as possible to minimize the risk of bleeding and oedematous swelling of the perineum, as this makes it more difficult to recognize tissue structures and planes when the repair eventually takes place.
- Perineal trauma should be repaired using aseptic techniques.
- Equipment should be checked and swabs and needles counted before and after the procedure.
- Good lighting is essential to visualize and identify the structures involved.
- A repair undertaken on an uncooperative patient, due to pain, is likely to result in a poor repair. Ensure that the wound is adequately anaesthetized prior to commencing the repair. It is recommended that 20 ml of lidocaine 1% is injected evenly into the perineal wound. If the woman has an epidural it may be 'topped-up' and used to block perineal pain during suturing instead of injecting local anaesthetic [16]. Repair of obstetric anal sphincter trauma should be undertaken in theatre, under general or regional anaesthesia. In addition to providing pain relief, this provides the added advantage of relaxing the muscles, enabling the operator to retrieve the ends of the torn sphincter while performing an overlap repair [8].

First-Degree Tears and Labial Lacerations

Women should be advised that in the case of first-degree trauma, the wound should be sutured in order to improve healing, unless the skin edges are well opposed [16]. If the tear is left unsutured, the midwife or doctor must discuss the implications with the woman and obtain her informed consent. Details regarding the discussion and consent must be fully documented in the woman's case notes.

Labial lacerations are usually very superficial but may be very painful. Some practitioners do not recommend suturing, but if the trauma is bilateral the lacerations can sometimes adhere together over the urethra and the woman may present with voiding difficulties. It is important to advise the woman to part the labia daily during bathing to prevent adhesions from occurring.

Episiotomy and Second-Degree Tears

Women should be advised that in the case of second-degree trauma, the muscle should be sutured in order to improve healing [16]. A recent Cochrane systematic review [9] of 16 studies involving 8184 women showed that continuous suture techniques compared with interrupted sutures for perineal closure (all layers or perineal skin only) was associated with less pain up to ten days postpartum. Furthermore, there was a greater reduction in pain when the continuous suturing technique was used for all layers. There was an overall reduction in analgesia use associated with the continuous subcutaneous technique versus interrupted stitches for repair of perineal skin. Subgroup analysis showed some evidence of reduction in dyspareunia experienced by participants in the groups that had continuous suturing of all layers. There was also a reduction in suture removal in the continuous suturing groups versus those with interrupted sutures, but no significant differences were seen in the need for re-suturing of wounds or long-term pain. The authors concluded that compared to interrupted methods, the continuous suturing technique for perineal closure, is associated with less short-term pain.

Apart from the technique, suture material used to repair perineal trauma needs to be taken into consideration. A Cochrane systematic review of 18 randomized controlled trials [19] involving 10 171 women was carried out to assess the effects of different suture materials on short- and long-term morbidity following perineal repair. The pooled results from nine of the included studies showed that absorbable synthetic material (polyglycolic acid and polyglactin 910) when compared with catgut suture material was associated with less pain up to three days after delivery and required less analgesia up to ten days postpartum. Compared with synthetic sutures, more women with catgut sutures required re-suturing.

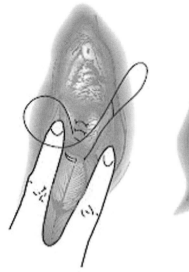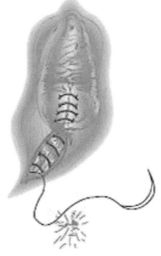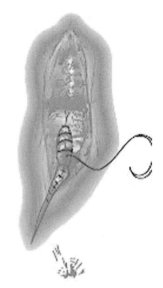

a. Loose, continuous, non-locking stitch to vaginal wall

b. Loose, continuous, non-locking stitch to perineal muscles

c. Closure of skin using a loose subcutaneous stitch

Figure 18.4 Continuous suturing technique for mediolateral episiotomy [20, with permission].

Furthermore, more women with standard synthetic sutures required the removal of unabsorbed suture material compared to the rapidly absorbing synthetic sutures. Currently, the use of catgut has been largely superseded in developed countries by absorbable suture material.

The following steps should be adopted [20] (Figure 18.4).

1. *Suturing the vagina.* The first stitch is inserted above the apex of the vaginal trauma to secure any bleeding points that might not be visible. Close the vaginal trauma with a loose, continuous, non-locking technique, making sure that each stitch is inserted not too wide otherwise the vagina may be narrowed. Continue to suture down to the hymenal remnants and insert the needle through the skin at the fourchette to emerge in the centre of the perineal wound.

2. *Suturing the muscle layer.* Check the depth of the trauma and close the perineal muscle (deep and superficial) with continuous non-locking stitches. If the trauma is deep, the perineal muscles can be closed using two layers of continuous stitches. A crown stitch is inserted to re-approximate the bulbocavernosus muscles. Realign the muscle so that the skin edges can be re-approximated

without tension, ensuring that the stitches are not inserted through the rectum or anal canal.

3. *Suturing the perineal skin.* At the inferior end of the wound, bring the needle out just under the skin surface reversing the stitching direction. The skin sutures are placed below the skin surface in the subcutaneous tissue, thus avoiding the profusion of nerve endings. Continue to take bites of tissue from each side of the wound edges until the hymenal remnants are reached. Secure the finished repair with a loop or Aberdeen knot placed in the vagina behind the hymenal remnants.

Third- and Fourth-Degree Tears

1. Repair should be conducted in the operating theatre where there is access to good lighting, appropriate equipment and aseptic conditions. In our unit we have a specially prepared instrument tray containing a Weitlander self-retaining retractor, four Allis tissue forceps, McIndoe scissors, tooth forceps, four artery forceps, stitch scissors and a needle holder (www.perineum.net). In addition, deep retractors (e.g. Deavers) are useful when there are associated paravaginal tears.

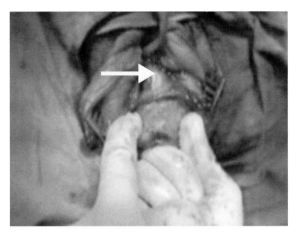

Figure 18.5 A buttonhole tear of the rectal mucosa (arrow) with an intact external anal sphincter demonstrated during a digital rectal examination [6, with permission].

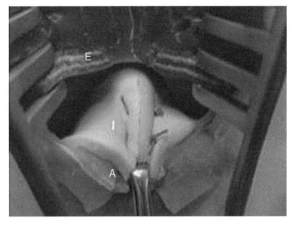

Figure 18.6 Internal anal sphincter (I) end-to-end repair using mattress sutures demonstrated on a model. This same technique is used to perform an end-to-end repair of the external sphincter. (E, external sphincter; A, anal epithelium) [8, with permission].

2. On rare occasions an isolated 'buttonhole' type tear can occur in the rectum without disrupting the anal sphincter or perineum (Figure 18.5). This is best repaired transvaginally using interrupted Vicryl (polyglactin) sutures. To minimize the risk of a persistent rectovaginal fistula, a second layer of tissue should be interposed between the rectum and vagina by approximating the rectovaginal fascia. A colostomy is rarely indicated unless there is a large tear extending above the pelvic floor or there is gross faecal contamination of the wound.

3. In the presence of a fourth-degree tear, the torn anal epithelium is repaired with interrupted Vicryl 3/0 sutures with the knots tied in the anal lumen. This technique has been widely described and proponents of this technique argue that by tying the knots outside, the quantity of foreign body within the tissue would be reduced, and hence the risk of infection reduced. However, this concern probably applies to the use of catgut that dissolves by proteolysis as opposed to the newer synthetic material, such as Vicryl or Dexon (polygylcolic acid) that dissolve by hydrolysis. We currently prefer a continuous suture technique with the knots secured on the vaginal aspect.

4. The sphincter muscles are repaired with either monofilament fine sutures such as 3/0 PDS (polydioxanone) or modern braided sutures such as 2/0 Vicryl (polyglactin) as these may cause less irritation and discomfort with equivalent outcome. To minimize suture migration, care

should be taken to cut suture ends short and ensure that they are covered by the overlying superficial perineal muscles. Women should be warned of the possibility of knot migration to the skin surface with the long-acting and non-absorbable suture materials.

5. The IAS should be identified and, if torn, repaired separately from the EAS. The ends of the torn muscle are grasped with Allis forceps and an end-to-end repair is performed with interrupted sutures (3/0 PDS or 2/0 Vicryl) [8] (Figure 18.6).

6. As the EAS is normally under tonic contraction, it tends to retract when torn. The torn ends of the EAS therefore need to be identified and grasped with Allis tissue forceps. When the EAS is only partially torn (Grade 3a and some 3b), then an end-to-end repair should be performed using two or three mattress sutures instead of haemostatic 'figure-of-eight' sutures. If there is a full-thickness EAS tear (some 3b, 3c or fourth-degree), either an overlapping (Figure 18.7) or end-to-end method can be used with equivalent outcome [8]. A recent Cochrane review showed that at one-year follow-up, immediate primary overlap repair of the external anal sphincter compared with immediate primary end-to-end repair appears to be associated with lower risks of developing faecal urgency and anal incontinence symptoms. At the end of 36 months there appears to be no difference in flatus or faecal incontinence between the two techniques. However, since this evidence

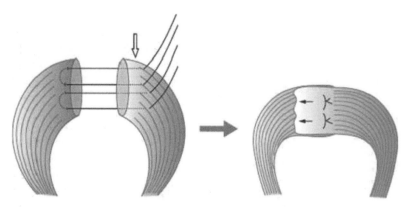

Figure 18.7 Repair of a fourth-degree tear using the overlap repair technique for the external anal sphincter. The arrow in the figure on the left indicates the first suture at 1.5 cm from the edge. The small arrows on the figure on the right indicate the site of the second set of sutures at 0.5 cm from the edge.

is based on only two small trials, more research evidence is needed in order to confirm or refute these findings [21].

7. After repair of the sphincter, the perineal muscles should be sutured to reconstruct the perineal body in order to provide support to the repaired anal sphincter. Furthermore, a short, deficient perineum would make the anal sphincter more vulnerable to trauma during a subsequent vaginal delivery. Finally, the vaginal skin should be sutured and the perineal skin approximated with a Vicryl 2/0 subcuticular suture [8].

8. Basic principles after repair of perineal tears [7,8]:

   - Check that complete haemostasis is achieved and confirm that the finished repair is anatomically correct.
   - A rectal and vaginal examination should be performed to confirm adequate repair so as to ensure that no other tears have been missed, and that a suture is not inadvertently placed through the rectal mucosa.
   - Confirm that all tampons or swabs have been removed.
   - A Foley catheter should be inserted for 12–24 hours to prevent urinary retention, particularly following regional anaesthesia.
   - Detailed notes should be made of the findings and repair. Completion of a pre-designed proforma and a pictorial representation of the tears prove very useful when notes are being reviewed following complications, audit or litigation.
   - An accurate detailed account of the repair should be documented in the woman's case notes following completion of the procedure, including details of the suture method and

materials used. It is also useful to include a simple diagram illustrating the structures involved.

- The woman should be informed about the use of appropriate analgesia, hygiene and the importance of a good diet.
- It is important that the woman is given a full explanation of the injury sustained and contact details if she has any problems during the postnatal period. Special designated clinics should be available for women with perineal problems to ensure that they receive appropriate, sensitive and effective treatment.
- Women should be advised that the prognosis following EAS repair is good, with 60–80% asymptomatic at 12 months. Most women who remain symptomatic describe incontinence of flatus or faecal urgency [8].

Postoperative Care

Ensure adequate analgesia by prescribing analgesics such as Diclofenac 75 mg slow release 12 hourly on a regular basis.

- Broad-spectrum antibiotics are given intra-operatively (intravenously) and continued orally for three days.
- All women should be prescribed stool softeners (lactulose 15 ml BD or enough to keep stools soft) for ten days as straining to pass a bolus of hard stool may disrupt the repair. This must be explained to the woman and the community midwife needs to ensure that normal bowel action has occurred within three days if the patient is discharged. It is recommended that women with OASIS are called by a healthcare provider 24 or

48 hours after hospital discharge to ensure bowel evacuation has occurred.

- The woman must be given a detailed explanation of the extent of trauma and advised that if there is any concern about infection or poor bowel control they must present to either their midwife or GP.
- Pelvic floor exercises can be commenced when the woman finds it comfortable to do so.

Follow-up

All women who sustain OASIS should be assessed by a senior obstetrician 6–12 weeks after delivery [7]. If facilities are available, follow-up of women with obstetric anal sphincter injuries should be in a dedicated clinic with access to endoanal ultrasonography and anal manometry, as this can aid decision on future mode of delivery [7,22].

In the clinic, a genital examination should be performed, looking specifically for scarring, residual granulation tissue and tenderness. All women should undergo anal manometry and endosonography. The women are advised to continue pelvic floor exercises, while others with minimal sphincter contractility may need electrical stimulation.

If a perineal clinic is not available, women with OASIS should be given clear instructions, preferably in writing, before leaving the hospital. In the first six weeks following delivery, they should look for signs of infection or wound dehiscence. They should contact the clinic if there is an increase in pain or swelling, rectal bleeding or purulent discharge. Any incontinence of stool or flatus should also be reported. Under such circumstances, referral to a specialist gynaecologist or colorectal surgeon for endoanal ultrasound and manometry should be considered [7].

Management of Subsequent Pregnancy

There are no randomized studies to determine the most appropriate mode of delivery following OASIS. In order to counsel women with previous OASIS appropriately, it is useful to have a symptom questionnaire along with anal ultrasound and manometry results. Tests should be performed during the current pregnancy unless performed previously and found to be abnormal. Figure 18.8 provides a flow diagram demonstrating the management of subsequent pregnancy following OASIS.

If there are no facilities for anal manometry and endosonography, then the management will depend on symptoms and clinical evaluation. Asymptomatic women without any clinical evidence of sphincter compromise as determined by assessment of anal tone could be allowed a vaginal delivery. All women who are symptomatic should be referred to a centre with facilities for anorectal assessment, and should be counselled for caesarean section (CS). Current evidence suggests that if a sonographic defect (>one hour or 30°) is present, and if the squeeze pressure increment is less than 20 mmHg, then the risk of impaired continence is increased after a subsequent delivery. These women should be counselled and, particularly those who have mild symptoms, offered a CS. There is evidence that when this protocol is followed, there is no deterioration in symptoms in both the vaginal delivery and CS group [23]. Figure 18.9 demonstrates the four-layered ultrasound appearance of an intact anal sphincter, in contrast to Figure 18.10 which demonstrates endosonography of an extensive tear following vaginal delivery involving both the internal and external sphincters between 9 and 2 o'clock. Mild incontinence (faecal urgency or flatus incontinence) may be controlled with dietary advice, constipating agents (loperamide or codeine phosphate), physiotherapy or biofeedback. Asymptomatic women who do not have compromised anal sphincter function can be allowed a normal delivery by an experienced accoucher [8]. If an episiotomy is considered necessary, e.g. because of a thick, inelastic or scarred perineum, a mediolateral episiotomy should be performed. There is no evidence that routine episiotomies prevent recurrence of OASIS [7]. The threshold at which these women may be considered for a CS may be lowered if a traumatic delivery is anticipated, e.g. in the presence of one or more additional relative risk factors, e.g. big baby, shoulder dystocia, prolonged labour, difficult instrumental delivery. However, in deciding the mode of delivery, counselling (and its clear documentation) is extremely important. Some of these women who have sustained OASIS may be scarred both physically and emotionally and may find it difficult to cope with the thought of another vaginal delivery. These women will require sympathy, psychological support and consideration to their request for CS [7].

Women who sustained a previous OASIS with subsequent severe incontinence should be offered secondary sphincter repair by a colorectal surgeon, and all subsequent deliveries should be by CS. Some women

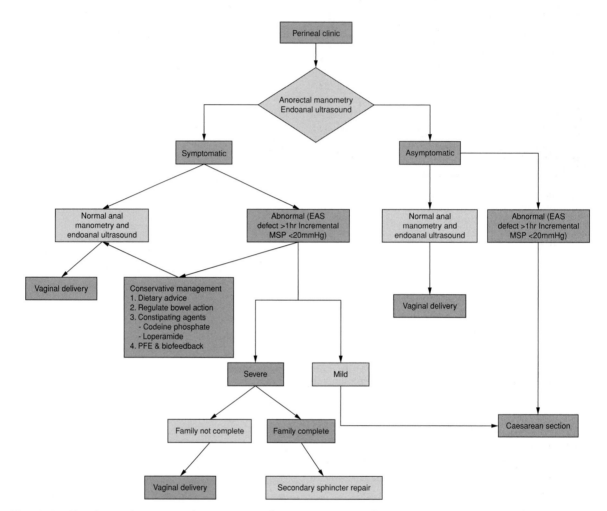

Management of pregnancy after OASIS

Figure 18.8 Flow diagram demonstrating the management of subsequent pregnancy following OASIS (EAS = external anal sphincter; MSP = maximum squeeze pressure; PFE = pelvic floor exercises). From: Croydon Integrated Continence Care Group (version 4, reviewed by Ranee Thakar and Abdul Sultan, 2014).

with faecal incontinence may choose to complete their family before embarking on anal sphincter surgery. It remains to be established whether these women should be allowed a vaginal delivery, as it could be argued that damage has already occurred and risk of further damage is minimal and possibly insignificant in terms of outcome of surgery. The benefit, if any, should be weighed against the risks associated with CS for all subsequent pregnancies. Women who have had a

previous successful secondary sphincter repair for faecal incontinence should be delivered by CS [8].

Medico-legal Considerations

Although creating a third- or fourth-degree tear is seldom found to be culpable, missing a tear is considered to be negligent. It is essential that a rectal examination is performed before and after any perineal repair

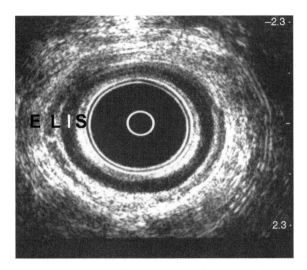

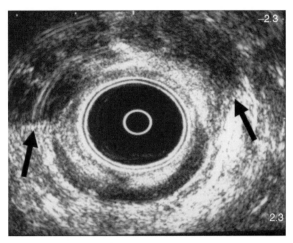

Figure 18.9 The normal four-layer pattern of the anal canal on axial endosonography in the normal orientation. The subepithelium (S) is moderately reflective; the internal sphincter (I) is a well-defined, low reflective ring; the longitudinal layer is a mixture of muscle (L) and fibroelastic tissue, so of varying reflectivity; and the external sphincter (E) is of mixed but predominantly high reflectivity.

Figure 18.10 Endosonography of an extensive tear following vaginal delivery involving both the internal and external sphincters between 9 and 2 o'clock (arrows).

and findings are carefully documented in the notes. A recent report of maternity claims from 1 April 2000 to 31 March 2010 compiled by the NHS Litigation Authority (NHSLA) found that claims due to perineal trauma ranked as the fourth highest cause, with the total value of claims amounting to £3.2 million. On review of the claims, criticisms were made of the following standards of care: failure to consider CS, failure to perform or extend the episiotomy, failure to diagnose the true extent and grade of injury, including failure to perform a rectal examination, the adequacy of the repair and failure to perform a repair. It appears that the claims focus on events which take place immediately following delivery by the way of examination and repair, rather than on the delivery itself [24].

Training

As more than two-thirds of doctors practising obstetrics feel inadequately trained, it is important that focused and intensive training is available. In this regard, Sultan and Thakar have introduced an ongoing course using video presentations, specially designed models and fresh animal specimens to demonstrate anatomy and techniques of repair (www.perineum. net). The feedback from attendees is that this type of

training has resulted in a change in practice and should become an essential part of the modular training for specialist registrars [25].

Prevention

The case for prevention of perineal trauma and its consequences is compelling. How to achieve this is less than clear. The incidence of perineal trauma can be reduced by modifying some of the risk factors, such as episiotomy and instrumental delivery. Episiotomy should only be performed when indicated, and a mediolateral episiotomy is preferable to a midline episiotomy [12]. Fewer women with vacuum delivery have anal sphincter trauma compared to forceps delivery [26]. The use of warm compresses on the perineum is associated with a decreased occurrence of OASIS [27]. A recent Cochrane review has concluded that antenatal perineal massage reduces the likelihood of perineal trauma (mainly episiotomies) and the reporting of ongoing perineal pain, and is generally well-accepted by women. As such, women should be made aware of the likely benefit of perineal massage and provided with information on how to do it [28]. Other interventions such as water birth, position during labour and birth, delayed pushing with an epidural, second stage pushing advice, perineal stretching massage during the second stage and perineal support at delivery have not been shown to reduce the risk of perineal trauma in randomized studies [29].

Conclusions

The majority of women undergoing vaginal delivery sustain perineal trauma. While CS is the only alternative available to bypass vaginal delivery, it is associated with increased morbidity and mortality [30]. It is therefore mandatory that every effort is made to minimize injury and make vaginal delivery safer. In this chapter we have endeavoured to highlight safe obstetric practice and preventative measures in the light of the best available evidence to minimize perineal and anal sphincter trauma.

References

1. McCandlish R, Bowler U, van Asten H, *et al*. A randomised controlled trial of care of the perineum during second stage of normal labour. *Br J Obstet Gynaecol*. 1998; 105: 1262–72.

2. Graham DD, Carroli G, Davis C, Medves JM. Episiotomy rates around the world: an update. *Birth*. 2005; 32: 219–23.

3. Gurol-Urganci I, Cromwell D, Edozien L, *et al*. Third- and fourth-degree perineal tears among primiparous women in England between 2000 and 2012: time trends and risk factors. *BJOG*. 2013; 120: 1516–25.

4. Sultan AH, Kamm MA, Hudson CN, Thomas JM, Bartram CI. Anal sphincter disruption during vaginal delivery. *New Engl J Med*. 1993; 329: 1905–11.

5. Andrews V, Thakar R, Sultan AH. Occult anal sphincter injuries: myth or reality. *Br J Obstet Gynaecol*. 2006; 113: 195–200.

6. Sultan AH, Kettle C. Diagnosis of perineal trauma. In Sultan AH, Thakar R, Fenner D (eds), *Perineal and Anal Sphincter Trauma* (pp. 13–19). London: Springer-Verlag; 2007.

7. RCOG. *Management of Third and Fourth Degree Perineal Tears Following Vaginal Delivery*. London: RCOG Press; 2007.

8. Sultan AH, Thakar R. Third and fourth degree tears. In Sultan AH, Thakar R, Fenner D (eds), *Perineal and Anal Sphincter Trauma* (pp. 33–51). London: Springer-Verlag; 2007.

9. Kettle C, Dowswell T, Ismail KMK. Continuous and interrupted suturing techniques for repair of episiotomy or second-degree tears. *Cochrane Database Syst Rev*. 2012; 11: CD000947. doi: 10.1002/14651858.CD000947.pub3.

10. Thakar R, Fenner DE. Anatomy of the perineum and the anal sphincter. In Sultan AH, Thakar R, Fenner D (eds), *Perineal and Anal Sphincter Trauma* (pp. 1–12). London: Springer-Verlag; 2007.

11. Norton C, Christensen J, Butler U, *et al. Anal Incontinence*, 2nd edition, pp. 985–1044. Plymouth: Health Publication Ltd; 2005.

12. Carroli G, Mignini L. Episiotomy for vaginal birth. *Cochrane Database Syst Rev*. 2009; 1: CD000081. doi: 10.1002/14651858.CD000081.pub2.

13. Andrews V, Thakar R, Sultan AH, Jones PW. Are mediolateral episiotomies actually mediolateral? *BJOG*. 2005; 112: 1156–8.

14. Eogan M, Daly L, O'Connell, PRO'Herlihy C. Does the angle of episiotomy affect the incidence of anal sphincter injury? *BJOG*. 2006; 113: 190–4.

15. Stedenfeldt M, Pirhonen J, Blix E, *et al*. Episiotomy characteristics and risks for obstetric anal sphincter injury: a case-control study. *BJOG*. 2012; 119: 724–30.

16. NICE. *Intrapartum Care: Care of Healthy Women and their Babies During Childbirth*: Cinical Guidline 190. London: NICE; 2014.

17. Kalis V, Karbanova J, Horak M, *et al*. The incision angle of mediolateral episiotomy before delivery and after repair. *Int J Gynaecol Obstet*. 2008; 103: 5–8.

18. Kalis V, Karbanova J, Bukacova Z, *et al*. Evaluation of the incision angle of mediolateral episiotomy at 60 degrees. *Int J Gynecol Obstet*. 2011; 112: 220–4. doi: 10.1016/j.ijgo.2010.09.015.

19. Kettle C, Dowswell T, Ismail KMK. Absorbable suture materials for primary repair of episiotomy and second degree tears. *Cochrane Database Syst Rev*. 2010; 6: CD000006. doi: 10.1002/14651858.CD000006.pub2.

20. Kettle C, Fenner D. Repair of episiotomy, first and second degree tears. In Sultan AH, Thakar R, Fenner D (eds), *Perineal and Anal Sphincter Trauma* (pp. 20–32). London: Springer; 2007.

21. Fernando RJ, Sultan AH, Kettle C, Thakar R. Methods of repair for obstetric anal sphincter injury. *Cochrane Database Syst Rev*. 2013; 12: CD002866. doi: 10.1002/14651858.CD002866.pub3.

22. Thakar R, Sultan A. Postpartum problems and the role of a perineal clinic. In: Sultan AH, Thakar R, Fenner D (eds), *Perineal and Anal Sphincter Trauma* (pp. 65–79). London: Springer-Verlag; 2007.

23. Scheer I, Thakar R, Sultan AH. Mode of delivery after previous obstetric anal sphincter injuries (OASIS): a reappraisal? *Int Urogynecol J*. 2009; 20: 1095–101.

24. NHS Litigation Authority *Ten Years of Maternity Claims: An Analysis of NHS Litigation Authority Data*, pp. 49–60. London: NHSLA; 2012.

25. Andrews V, Thakar R, Sultan AH. Structured hands-on training in repair of obstetric anal sphincter

injuries (OASIS): an audit of clinical practice. *Int Urogynecol J*. 2009; 20(2): 193–9.

26. O'Mahony F, Hofmeyr GJ, Menon V. Choice of instruments for assisted vaginal delivery. *Cochrane Database Syst Rev*. 2010; 11: CD005455. doi: 10.1002/14651858.CD005455.pub2.

27. Aasheim V, Nilsen ABV, Lukasse M, Reinar LM. Perineal techniques during the second stage of labour for reducing perineal trauma. *Cochrane Database Syst Rev*. 2011; 12: CD006672. doi: 10.1002/14651858. CD006672.pub2.

28. Beckmann MM, Stock OM. Antenatal perineal massage for reducing perineal trauma. *Cochrane Database Syst Rev*. 2013; 4: CD005123. doi: 10.1002/14651858.CD005123.pub3.

29. Thakar R, Eason E. Prevention of perineal trauma. In Sultan AH, Thakar R, Fenner D (eds), *Perineal and Anal Sphincter Trauma* (pp. 52–64). London: Springer-Verlag; 2007.

30. Sultan AH, Stanton SL. Preserving the pelvic floor and perineum during childbirth: elective caesarean section? *BJOG*. 1996; 103: 731–4.

Chapter 19

Induction of Labour

Vikram Sinai Talaulikar and Sabaratnam Arulkumaran

The rates of induction of labour (IOL) are rising all over the world. The availability of prostaglandins, which act as both cervical ripening as well as inducing agents, has improved the success rates of IOL in the presence of an unfavourable cervix. Mechanical methods such as intracervical balloon catheters appear to be equally effective as compared to pharmacological agents and have fewer adverse effects. The process of IOL is associated with significant risks such as hyperstimulation, rupture of the uterus and increased risk of operative deliveries. There should be a clear indication for IOL based on best available evidence, with benefits to either mother or fetus, which outweigh the perceived risks. The World Health Organization (WHO), National Institute for Health and Clinical Excellence (NICE) and Royal College of Obstetricians and Gynaecologists (RCOG) have produced guidelines to assist clinicians in decision making regarding IOL in various obstetric situations. The process of IOL should be tailored to meet the expectations or preferences of women in their unique circumstances.

Introduction

Acquisition of the ability to artificially induce labour to control the timing of birth has been one of the most striking accomplishments in the field of obstetrics and it has contributed to reduction in maternal and perinatal morbidity and mortality. The past few decades have witnessed a rise in rates of IOL throughout the world, with one out of every four babies in developed countries being born following IOL at term [1].

Despite recent improvements in the safety and efficacy of methods of IOL, there is a need for further research and development in many related areas. The search for the ideal agent for IOL (one which is highly effective yet has no major risks for the mother and fetus) continues. There is a long-felt need to develop tests that can accurately identify those fetuses most at risk of morbidity or stillbirth who are likely to benefit from early intervention such as IOL. Further research is also required to assess the cost-effectiveness of policies of routine IOL for prolonged pregnancies and for identification of those women most likely to have a successful induction.

Definition

Induction of labour is defined as a process of artificial initiation of uterine contractions after the age of fetal viability and before spontaneous onset of labour, with the aim of achieving cervical effacement and dilatation leading to vaginal delivery. IOL is indicated when it is felt that the risks to mother or fetus of continuing pregnancy outweigh the risks of induction and delivery. Induction rates vary greatly between obstetric units depending on incidence of high-risk pregnancies, local hospital protocols and the resources available. It has been estimated that more than 22% of all gravid women undergo IOL in the USA and the overall rate of IOL in the USA doubled between 1990 and 2006 [2]. Every year in the UK about one in five labours is induced [3]. It is clear that the decision to induce labour should not be taken lightly because the process of induction is associated with risks to mother and baby. There should be a clear indication based on best available evidence, with benefits to either mother or fetus that outweigh the perceived risks. The process of IOL should be tailored to meet the expectations or preferences of women in their unique circumstances.

Best Practice in Labour and Delivery, Second Edition, ed. Sir Sabaratnam Arulkumaran. Published by Cambridge University Press. © Cambridge University Press 2016.

Table 19.1 Modified Bishop cervical score

Score	0	1	2	3
Cervical dilatation (cm)	0	1–2	3–4	>4
Cervical length (cm)	>4	3–4	1–2	<1
Station of presenting part	–3	–2	–1, 0	+1 or more
Consistency	Firm	Medium	Soft	
Position	Posterior	Mid	Anterior	

Table 19.2 Median total uterine activity by parity and cervical score (scored from 0–10) with an automatic infusion system and manually controlled infusion system during induction of labour

Parity	Cervical score	Total uterine activity (kPa)	
		Manually controlled infusion system	Automatic infusion system
Nulliparous women	≤5	56 878	61 685
	≥6	27 065	35 619
Multiparous women	≤5	27 633	35 155
	≥6	15 632	14 488

Factors Determining Success of Induction of Labour

Success of IOL mainly depends on: (1) parity; (2) cervical score; (3) position of vertex (occipito-anterior versus occipito-posterior); (4) body mass index (BMI); and (5) method of induction.

Parity and Cervical Status

Changes in the Cervix

In the first trimester of pregnancy, half of the dry weight of the cervix is tightly aligned collagen (predominantly type 1 and 3) and the rest is composed of smooth muscle and ground substance that includes fibronectin, elastin and glycosaminoglycans (heparin sulphate, dermatan sulphate and hyaluronic acid) [4,5]. As pregnancy advances, hyaluronic acid increases whereas dermatan, chodroitin and collagen decrease. Collagenase and elastase enzymes progressively increase along with the vascularity and water content of the cervix [4]. These changes in the cervix, which prepare it for dilatation in labour, are collectively known as cervical ripening and they result from a series of biochemical reactions involving various hormones, cytokines, enzymes and other bioactive factors. A ripe cervix that is soft and pliable increases the success of IOL. Various pharmacological and mechanical agents are in use to achieve cervical ripening before IOL. However, these agents may themselves induce labour during the process of ripening and the boundary between ripening and induction often becomes clinically indistinguishable. In clinical practice, the ripeness of the cervix is commonly assessed using a modified Bishop score (Table 19.1). A score of 5 or less represents an unfavourable cervix, while 6 or above

indicates a ripe cervix. Bishop cervical scoring still remains the simplest yet a cost-effective method of evaluating the cervix before IOL.

Uterine Contractions

During the process of IOL, the uterus performs work in the form of myometrial contractions to bring about cervical effacement and dilatation along with descent of the head, overcoming cervical and pelvic tissue resistance. The higher the resistance offered, the more work is needed by the myometrium and hence the greater chance of failure to reach full cervical dilatation in labour. Resistance offered by the cervix and pelvic floor is less in multiparous women who have had previous vaginal delivery because these structures have undergone thinning and stretching in previous labour.

Clinical experience as well as studies which have evaluated the total uterine work needed to achieve full cervical dilatation suggest that labour is difficult when induction is attempted with a poor cervical score. Nulliparous women with a cervical score of 3 out of 10 or less had a 65.4% caesarean section (CS) rate, of which more than two-thirds were for failed IOL (with artificial rupture of membranes and oxytocin infusion) [6]. A study on total uterine activity (TUA) to achieve full cervical dilatation in induced labour (with oxytocin infusion and artificial rupture of membranes) in patients with vertex presentation provided information according to parity, cervical score and mode of oxytocin infusion [7] (Table 19.2). TUA progressively declined from the highest level required in nulliparous women with a poor cervical score to the lowest level in multiparous women with a good score. The study confirmed that the uterus has to achieve a target total uterine activity in induced labour to effect full cervical dilatation and vaginal delivery of the baby. It was estimated that nulliparous women with a poor cervical score had to perform nearly four times the uterine activity compared with multiparous women with a good score.

Position of Vertex

Persistent occipito-posterior position has been associated with increased chance of failure of IOL [8].

Body Mass Index

For reasons still not fully understood, high BMI is a risk factor for failed induction and increases the risk of caesarean delivery [9].

Role of Cervical Length Measurement by Ultrasound and Fetal Fibronectin

Several studies have assessed the predictive accuracy of ultrasound for successful IOL. A study compared transvaginal sonography to Bishop scoring for predicting successful IOL and suggested that cervical length is a better predictor than the cervical score [10]. Cervical length (greater than 20 mm) has been found useful in prediction of the need for CS delivery following IOL. Fetal fibronectin is a basement membrane glycoprotein present in high concentrations in amniotic fluid. It is found in the vaginal fluid before labour and studies have suggested that its presence can predict successful IOL. A study ($n = 90$) compared cervical clinical data, ultrasound parameters and fetal fibronectin assessment in the prediction of the duration of induced labour when the cervix was unfavourable [11]. Cervical dilatation as assessed by digital examination appeared to be the best predictor of the duration of the latent phase and of that of the whole of labour. Ultrasound measurement of cervical length was not more accurate at predicting the duration of labour than clinical data.

Methods of Induction of Labour

In modern obstetrics, prostaglandins (PGE2 or PGE1), balloon catheters and oxytocin with amniotomy are the most commonly used methods of IOL (Figure 19.1).

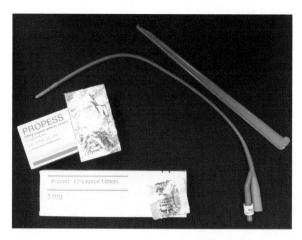

Figure 19.1 Commonly used methods of cervical ripening/induction of labour (includes slow-release PGE2 pessary, PGE2 pessary, PGE1 tablets, Foley balloon catheter and amniohook). See the colour plate section for a colour version of this figure.

Pharmacological Methods

Dinoprostone (PGE2)

This is a vaginal prostaglandin that is the most commonly recommended method of IOL with an unfavourable cervix in the absence of any contraindications or risk of hyper-stimulation. PGE2 may be administered as a gel, tablet or slow-release pessary. Each 3 g of gel contains 1 or 2 mg dinoprostone, while tablets contain 3 mg dinoprostone. The first dose is inserted high into the posterior fornix. The patient is then instructed to remain recumbent for at least 30 min. A second and, if required, third dose may be administered at intervals of six hours following cervical assessment. Adverse reactions are uncommon and include vomiting, nausea and diarrhoea. Rarer adverse reactions include uterine hyper-stimulation, fetal distress, maternal hypertension, bronchospasm, backache, rash and, extremely rarely, amniotic fluid embolism. NICE guidelines recommend one cycle of vaginal PGE2 tablets or gel: one dose, followed by a second dose after six hours if labour is not established (up to a maximum of two doses) or one dose of vaginal PGE2 controlled-release pessary over 24 hours [3]. If oxytocin is used after PGE2, six hours should elapse after the last dose of PGE2 to reduce the risk of hyper-stimulation.

Evidence

A Cochrane systematic review in 2014 determined the effects of vaginal prostaglandins E2 and F2α for third trimester cervical ripening or induction of labour in comparison with placebo/no treatment or other vaginal prostaglandins (except misoprostol) [12]. Seventy randomized controlled trials (RCTs) (11 487 women) were included. Overall, vaginal PGE2 compared with placebo or no treatment probably reduced the likelihood of vaginal delivery not being achieved within 24 hours. The risk of uterine hyper-stimulation with fetal heart rate (FHR) changes was increased (4.8% versus 1.0%; risk ratio (RR) 3.16; 95% confidence interval (CI) 1.67 to 5.98; 15 trials, 1359 women). The CS rate was probably reduced by about 10% (13.5% versus 14.8%; RR 0.91; 95% CI 0.81 to 1.02; 36 trials, 6599 women). The overall effect on improving maternal and fetal outcomes (across a variety of measures) was uncertain. PGE2 tablets, gels and pessaries (including sustained-release preparations) appeared to be as effective as each other. The authors concluded that prostaglandin PGE2 probably increased the chance of vaginal delivery in 24 hours. There was an increase in uterine hyper-stimulation with fetal heart changes but this did not affect the CS rates. There was increased likelihood of cervical change, with no increase in operative delivery rates. Another Cochrane review in 2008 that included 56 trials (7738 women) reported that intracervical prostaglandins were effective compared to placebo, but appeared inferior when compared to intravaginal prostaglandins [13].

Recent WHO guidelines also provided further evidence in support of PGE2 and confirmed that PGE2 preparations are more effective than placebo for IOL at term [1]. Low-dose PGE2 has been compared with high-dose protocols and the use of lower doses seems to have comparative advantages like: (a) lower risk of uterine hyper-stimulation with FHR changes; and (b) a trend towards reduced risk of neonatal admission to an intensive care unit. The WHO thus recommends low doses of vaginal prostaglandins for IOL.

Gel versus Tablets

A UK-based RCT involving 165 women compared vaginal PGE2 gel versus tablets for IOL. The mean induction to delivery interval was significantly shorter in women who received the gel (1400 min, 690–2280 min, versus 1780 min, 960–2640 min; $p = 0.03$). The rate of failed IOL was significantly higher in women who received tablets (10.84 versus 1.22%; $p = 0.01$). There were no differences in adverse maternal and neonatal outcomes. The authors concluded that PGE2 vaginal gel is superior to vaginal tablets for IOL [14].

Misoprostol (PGE1)

Misoprostol is a PGE1 prostaglandin available for use as tablets, which may be administered through oral, vaginal or rectal routes for IOL. It is available in the form of 200 mcg tablets. While WHO recommends oral misoprostol in a dose of 25 mcg, two-hourly, other authors have advocated use of low-dose vaginal misoprostol, i.e. 25 mcg 3–6 hourly [15]. It is suggested that rather than breaking the 200 mcg tablet into eight pieces using a pill cutter, the tablet should be dissolved into 200 ml of water and 25 ml of that solution be administered as a single dose [1]. In the third trimester, in women with a dead or an anomalous fetus, oral or vaginal misoprostol are recommended for IOL [1]. Misoprostol is, however, not recommended for IOL in women with previous CS. The United States Food and Drug Administration has not yet approved use of misoprostol for induction of labour.

Common side-effects of misoprostol include diarrhoea, vomiting, shivering and pyrexia.

Evidence

Compared with either placebo or expectant management, vaginal misoprostol has been associated with a reduced risk of not achieving vaginal birth within 24 hours of labour induction (RR 0.51; 95% CI 0.37–0.71; five trials, 769 participants) [1]. When compared with intravenous oxytocin alone, vaginal misoprostol has a reduced risk of vaginal births not being achieved within 24 hours (RR 0.62; 95% CI 0.43–0.9; nine trials, 1200 participants), fewer CSs (RR 0.76; 95% CI 0.60–0.96; 25 trials, 3074 participants) and fewer infants with Apgar score below 7 at five minutes of life (RR 0.56; 95% CI 0.34–0.92; 13 trials, 1906 participants) [1]. Compared with other prostaglandins, vaginal misoprostol is associated with a higher chance of vaginal birth achieved within 24 hours (vaginal and intracervical PGE2), fewer CSs (vaginal PGE2) and increased risk of uterine hyper-stimulation with FHR changes, but without increased risk of other adverse perinatal outcomes (vaginal and intracervical PGE2). Compared with higher doses of vaginal misoprostol, lower doses (25 mcg six-hourly) are associated with a reduced risk of uterine hyper-stimulation with FHR changes. When oral and vaginal routes of administration were compared, oral misoprostol was associated with lower risk of poor Apgar score at five minutes of life [1]. A 2010 Cochrane review which included 121 trials also concluded that compared to placebo, misoprostol was associated with reduced failure to achieve vaginal delivery within 24 hours. Uterine hyper-stimulation, without FHR changes, was increased. Compared with vaginal PGE2, intracervical PGE2 and oxytocin, vaginal misoprostol was associated with less epidural analgesia use, fewer failures to achieve vaginal delivery within 24 hours and more uterine hyper-stimulation. Compared with vaginal or intracervical PGE2, oxytocin augmentation was less common with misoprostol and meconium-stained liquor more common [16].

Oral versus Vaginal Misoprostol

A Cochrane review in 2014 assessed the use of oral misoprostol for IOL [17]. Seventy-six trials were included. Oral misoprostol as an induction agent was effective at achieving vaginal birth. It appeared to be more effective than placebo, as effective as vaginal misoprostol and resulted in fewer CSs than vaginal dinoprostone or oxytocin. If using oral misoprostol, the evidence suggests that the dose should be 20–25 mcg in solution. Given that safety is the primary concern, the evidence supports the use of oral regimens over vaginal regimens.

Oxytocin

Commercially used oxytocin is a synthetic form of the posterior pituitary hormone. The WHO recommends that when prostaglandins are not available, intravenous oxytocin alone should be used for induction of labour [1]. However, NICE guidelines do not support the use of intravenous oxytocin alone for IOL. Both guidelines acknowledge that there is a higher chance of vaginal birth within 24 hours with use of prostaglandins as compared to oxytocin alone. In clinical practice, in the case of ruptured membranes, intravenous oxytocin is often recommended as an alternative initiating agent to prostaglandins. Oxytocin is used as an intravenous infusion of a dilute solution (10 mU/ml) and has a time to uterine response of 3–4 min. Steady levels are achieved by 40 min. Generally, the dose is titrated with increasing doses administered every 30 min until regular contractions occur of approximately 45 sec to 1 min duration and are three or four in number every 10 min (Table 19.3).

Evidence

A Cochrane review in 2009 included 61 trials (12 819 women) and found that when oxytocin inductions were compared with expectant management, fewer

Table 19.3 Commonly used regimen of oxytocin infusion

Time (min)	Dose of oxytocin (milliunits/ min)	Dilution 30 IU oxytocin in 500 ml normal saline (ml/hr)	Dilution 10 IU oxytocin in 500 ml normal saline (ml/hr)
0	1	1	3
30	2	2	6
60	4	4	12
90	8	8	24
120	12	12	36
150	16	16	48
180	20	20	60
210	24	24	72
240	28	28	84
270	32	32	96

women failed to deliver vaginally within 24 hours (8.4% versus 53.8%; RR 0.16; 95% CI 0.10–0.25) [18]. There was a significant increase in the number of women requiring epidural analgesia (RR 1.10; 95% CI 1.04–1.17). Fewer women were dissatisfied with oxytocin induction in the one trial reporting this outcome (5.9% versus 13.7%; RR 0.43; 95% CI 0.33–0.56). Compared with vaginal prostaglandins, oxytocin increased unsuccessful vaginal delivery within 24 hours in the two trials reporting this outcome (70% versus 21%; RR 3.33; 95% CI 1.61–6.89). There was a small increase in epidurals when oxytocin alone was used (RR 1.09; 95% CI 1.01–1.17). When oxytocin was compared with intracervical prostaglandins, there was an increase in unsuccessful vaginal delivery within 24 hours (50.4% versus 34.6%; RR 1.47; 95% CI 1.10–1.96) and an increase in CS (19.1% versus 13.7%; RR 1.37; 95% CI 1.08–1.74) in the oxytocin group. The reviewers concluded that prostaglandin agents probably increase the chances of achieving vaginal birth within 24 hours as compared to oxytocin.

Non-Pharmacological Methods

Mechanical Methods

Mechanical methods for IOL include insertion of a balloon catheter, extra amniotic saline infusion and hygroscopic dilators. The advantages of mechanical methods include a low risk of FHR abnormalities, low risk of hyper-stimulation and other systemic side-effects, and convenient storage; the disadvantages include discomfort during insertion and the potential to cause antepartum haemorrhage due to a low-lying placenta. It appears that in the absence of prelabour rupture of membranes, mechanical methods for IOL do not result in an increased risk of ascending infection and chorioamnionitis.

Insertion of intracervical 30–50 ml Foley catheter filled with saline is the commonest mechanical mode of IOL. The catheter may be inserted using a ring forceps; the balloon is then inflated and the catheter is retracted firmly against the cervix. The balloon results in pressure to the lower segment of the uterus and the cervix, resulting in local release of prostaglandins. Generally, the catheter is inserted, inflated and left *in situ* for 12–24 hours.

Several other models of balloon catheters have been introduced based on the same principle.

Evidence

A Cochrane review in 2012 determined the effects of mechanical methods for third trimester cervical ripening or induction of labour in comparison with placebo/no treatment, prostaglandins (vaginal and intracervical PGE2, misoprostol) and oxytocin [19]. The review included 71 RCTs (total of 9722 women). Induction of labour using mechanical methods resulted in similar CS rates as prostaglandins, for a lower risk of hyper-stimulation. Mechanical methods did not increase the overall number of women not delivered within 24 hours; however, the proportion of multiparous women who did not achieve vaginal delivery within 24 hours was higher when compared with vaginal PGE2. Compared with oxytocin, mechanical methods reduced the risk of CS.

The WHO recommends the use of balloon catheter for IOL and cites evidence in its support, including a systematic review which evaluated comparison of the balloon catheter with prostaglandins, oxytocin and placebo [1]. Compared with prostaglandins, the balloon catheter was associated with a lower risk of uterine hyper-stimulation with FHR changes (RR 0.51; 95% CI 0.30–0.86; seven trials, 823 participants), and the risk of CS with the two methods was similar (RR 1.01; 95% CI 0.88–1.17; 19 trials, 2050 participants). Compared with oxytocin, the balloon catheter was associated with a lower risk of CS (RR 0.43; 95% CI 0.22–0.83; two trials, 125 participants). In the comparison of balloon catheter plus oxytocin with misoprostol, the combination approach was associated with

a higher chance of vaginal birth achieved within 24 hours [1].

PROBAAT – an open-label RCT published in 2011 – aimed to compare the effectiveness and safety of Foley catheter versus vaginal prostaglandin E2 gel for IOL at term [20]. There were 824 women allocated to IOL with a Foley catheter ($n = 412$) or vaginal prostaglandin E2 gel ($n = 412$). Caesarean section rates were much the same between the two groups. It was concluded that in women with an unfavourable cervix at term, induction of labour with a Foley catheter is similar to induction of labour with prostaglandin E2 gel, with fewer maternal and neonatal side-effects.

The opinion of professional organizations differs with regard to the use of mechanical methods of IOL. The balloon catheter is recommended by WHO for induction of labour. The combination of balloon catheter plus oxytocin is recommended as an alternative method of IOL when prostaglandins are not available or are contraindicated [1]. NICE guidelines, however, recommend that mechanical procedures (balloon catheters and laminaria tents) should not be used routinely for the IOL, citing limited evidence for their efficacy and possibly increased risk of neonatal infection [3].

Other Methods of Mechanical Induction

These include hygroscopic dilators like laminaria tents which are placed in the cervix and dilate secondary to water absorption. Several dilators may be inserted into the cervix and they expand over 12–24 hours. The evidence regarding the use of hygroscopic dilators is limited and they do not appear to improve the outcome of IOL. Other methods include castor oil, hot baths, enemas, sexual intercourse, breast stimulation, acupuncture, acupressure and transcutaneous nerve stimulation. All of these lack evidence for safety and efficacy.

Amniotomy (ARM – Artificial Rupture of Membranes)

This involves deliberate rupturing of the membranes using an amniohook. This simple procedure may avoid the need for pharmacological intervention. Amniotomy works best when the cervix is dilated at least 3 cm or more and is favourable. In the past amniotomy was often used to prime the cervix and to induce labour. About 60–80% of women may enter labour within 24 hours of rupture of membranes. Amniotomy alone or in combination with oxytocin should not be used as a method for induction of labour

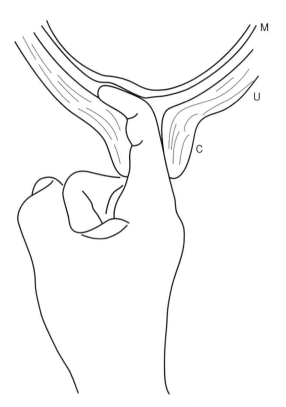

Figure 19.2 Sweeping of membranes (M) from the cervix (C) and lower uterine segment (U) being performed by the index finger of the examiner.

unless the use of PGE2 is contraindicated as per NICE guidelines [3].

Sweeping Membranes

This is recommended for reducing formal IOL. The membranes can be stripped from the internal os and the lower uterine segment by passing a finger and sweeping the membranes around the presenting part leading to release of local prostaglandins (Figure 19.2). Membrane sweeping is associated with a shorter time between treatment and spontaneous labour, a reduction in the incidence of prolonged pregnancy and the need for formal induction. It is estimated that to avoid one formal IOL, membrane sweep must be performed in eight women. The membrane sweep is usually offered at 41 weeks in the antenatal clinic before a planned IOL. Some women may find this procedure uncomfortable and they should be aware of the possibility of having blood-stained vaginal discharge for the next 2–3 days. There is no evidence of increased

risk to the mother or fetus from this procedure. A systematic review consisting of 22 studies suggested that routine use of sweeping of membranes from 38 weeks of pregnancy onwards does not seem to produce clinically important benefits. When used as a means for IOL, the reduction in the use of more formal methods of induction needs to be balanced against women's discomfort and other adverse effects [21].

Mifepristone

Mifepristone is a very effective antiprogesterone and antiglucocorticoid. Randomized trials have shown it to be effective in inducing labour. The use of mifepristone is only recommended following intrauterine fetal death.

The following methods for IOL are not presently recommended for routine clinical practice: oral or intravenous or intracervical PGE2, hyaluronidase, relaxin, corticosteroids, oestrogen and vaginal nitric oxide donors. There is also insufficient evidence to recommend any of the following non-pharmacological methods of IOL: herbal supplements, acupuncture, castor oil, homeopathy, sexual intercourse, curries, enemas and hot baths. It is suggested that nipple stimulation may reduce the number of women not in labour within 72 hours compared to no treatment, but is less effective than oxytocin for this outcome. More research is needed to evaluate the safety of nipple stimulation [22].

Indications for Induction of Labour

Some of the common indications for IOL are listed in Table 19.4. There are also some 'soft' indications for IOL, including: previous rapid delivery, poor obstetric history, psychosocial factors or relative geographic isolation. Most recent clinical studies argue against IOL for these indications, citing lack of good-quality evidence of benefit for the fetus or the mother. Caution is advised when considering IOL in cases of multiple pregnancies, unstable lie, polyhydramnios, grand multiparous women and previous low transverse CS. The last two are associated with increased risk of uterine rupture (especially with use of prostaglandins). These pregnancies require close fetal and maternal monitoring throughout the induction process. In some women with a transverse or oblique lie, there may be an indication for IOL. In such cases, external cephalic version should be performed and the head guided over the pelvic brim. An intravenous infusion of oxytocin

Table 19.4 Common indications and contraindications for IOL

Indications for induction of labour	• Prolonged pregnancy • Preterm/prelabour rupture of membranes • Intrauterine growth restriction • Maternal conditions like pre-eclampsia, diabetes, cholestasis or SLE • Abnormal antenatal fetal surveillance test
Contraindications for induction of labour	
Maternal contraindications	• Previous classical or multiple CS • Infections like HIV, active genital herpes • Previous traumatic delivery • Major placenta praevia
Fetal contraindications	• Malpresentations such as transverse lie, face or brow • Severe fetal compromise (preterminal CTG or severe Doppler abnormalities) • Cord prolapse • Vasa praevia

Table 19.5 Risks associated with induction of labour

Maternal discomfort and increased need for analgesia
Failure of induction and need for caesarean delivery (about 20%)
Water retention and hyponatraemia with prolonged use of oxytocin
Uterine rupture
Placental abruption
Postpartum haemorrhage
Iatrogenic prematurity
Amniotic fluid embolism
Fetal compromise due to uterine hyper-stimulation
Cord prolapse
Chorioamnionitis
Neonatal jaundice with prolonged use of oxytocin

should be started and, when contractions are established, amniotomy should be performed. Such 'stabilizing induction' may reduce chances of cord prolapse. Intrauterine fetal death or major fetal anomalies can necessitate IOL. Mifepristone and misoprostol are the agents of choice for IOL in these situations.

Risks Associated with Induction of Labour

It is critical to ensure that women are counselled adequately regarding the risks and benefits of the process prior to IOL and that this is documented appropriately in the notes. Risks associated with IOL are listed in Table 19.5.

A fundamental requirement before embarking on IOL is confirmation of the gestational age (to avoid unsuspected fetal prematurity). Uterine hyperstimulation can potentially lead to fetal hypoxia, maternal amniotic fluid embolism and even death. Signs and symptoms of hyper-stimulation include: five uterine contractions or more in 10 min without CTG changes, contractions lasting more than 120 sec without CTG changes, and uterine hyper-stimulation syndrome (excessive uterine activity with CTG abnormalities). In case of prostaglandin induction, FHR should be closely monitored during uterine activity. If there is hyper-stimulation, the prostaglandin gel or pessary should be removed or washed out of the vagina (or oxytocin infusion stopped) and if necessary tocolysis in the form of subcutaneous terbutaline 0.25 mg

administered together with turning the woman on to her side. Cord prolapse is a potential risk, especially when the amniotomy is attempted with the presenting part still poorly applied to the lower uterine segment and cervix. Amniotomy in cases of polyhydramnios can lead to sudden uterine decompression and placental abruption. Slow release of amniotic fluid by controlling the fetal head with one hand and stabilizing it over the pelvic brim may help prevent such complication.

Induction of labour is a known risk factor for amniotic fluid embolism (AFE). As per the recent *UK and Ireland Confidential Enquiries into Maternal Deaths and Morbidity (2009–12)*, labour was induced or augmented in six of the women who died from AFE and the reviewers considered that different choices around induction might have led to a different outcome for several women [23]. In some instances, inappropriate uterotonics were used to induce labour, including dinoprostone (Propess) in women of high parity; the manufacturers state that it should not be used in women who have had three or more full-term deliveries. AFE contributed to the death of another woman who was induced with mifepristone and misoprostol following late fetal death.

Place of Induction of Labour

WHO guidelines stress that wherever IOL is carried out, facilities should be available for assessing maternal and fetal well-being and women receiving oxytocin, misoprostol or other prostaglandins should not be left unattended [1]. It is good practice to carry out electronic fetal monitoring (EFM) for a short period to get a reassuring CTG trace prior to induction and at least for another one hour after introduction of vaginal prostaglandins or throughout labour if oxytocin is used. Wherever possible, IOL should be carried out in facilities where CS can be performed [1]. The data available to evaluate the efficacy or potential hazards of outpatient IOL are limited. It is, therefore, not yet possible to determine whether induction of labour is effective and safe in outpatient settings.

Evidence for IOL in Various Obstetric Situations

Given the risks associated with the process of IOL and likelihood of one in five inductions ending up with a caesarean delivery, it is mandatory that benefits from IOL outweigh the associated risks. Analysis of indications for IOL has revealed that while there is high-quality evidence for IOL in cases of prolonged pregnancies or prelabour rupture of membranes (PROM) at term, a fair number of inductions have debatable obstetric indications [24].

Prolonged Pregnancy

Prolonged gestation complicates 5–10% of all pregnancies and has been associated with increased risk to both the mother and fetus. Postterm pregnancy (beyond 42 completed weeks) has been associated with higher rates of stillbirth, macrosomia (birth weight >4000 g), birth injury and meconium aspiration syndrome. The risk of stillbirth has been estimated as 1 per 3000 at 37 weeks to 3 per 3000 at 42 weeks and 6 per 3000 at 43 weeks. Maternal risks include dysfunctional labour, shoulder dystocia, obstetric trauma, increased operative delivery rates and postpartum haemorrhage. Prolonged pregnancy is one of the commonest indications for IOL throughout the world and the rates vary between different countries and birthing units based on their individual induction policies and patient populations.

A Cochrane review evaluated the benefits and harms of a policy of labour induction at term or postterm compared with awaiting spontaneous labour or later induction of labour [25]. It included 22 trials (9383 women) and found that a policy of labour induction compared with expectant management is associated with fewer perinatal deaths and fewer CSs. Some

infant morbidities such as meconium aspiration syndrome were also reduced with a policy of postterm labour induction, although no significant differences in the rate of neonatal intensive care unit (NICU) admission were seen. However, the absolute risk of perinatal death is small and the number needed to treat to benefit (NNTB) with induction of labour in order to prevent one perinatal death was 410 (95% CI 322–1492). Although there have been arguments that there is no conclusive evidence that prolongation of pregnancy per se is the major risk factor for perinatal deaths and that other specific risk factors like intrauterine growth restriction (IUGR) and fetal malformations may play a significant role [26], the current best evidence suggests that induction of labour in the clinical settings of postterm pregnancy reduces meconium aspiration syndrome and perinatal deaths. NICE guidelines recommend that women with uncomplicated pregnancy should be offered induction of labour between 41 and 42 weeks' gestation. Should a woman decline induction of labour following 42 weeks' gestation, it is recommended that the woman be offered at least twice weekly FHR monitoring and ultrasound assessment of the maximum amniotic fluid pool depth [3]. WHO recommends IOL for women who are known with certainty to have reached 41 weeks [1].

Prelabour Rupture of Membranes (PROM) at Term

Prelabour rupture of membranes occurs in 6–19% of term pregnancies. A Cochrane review which assessed the effects of planned early birth versus expectant management for women with term PROM included 12 trials (total 6814 women) and detected no differences for mode of birth between planned and expectant groups: RR of CS 0.94, 95% CI 0.82–1.08 (12 trials, 6814 women); RR of operative vaginal birth 0.98, 95% CI 0.84–1.16 (seven trials, 5511 women) [27]. Significantly fewer women in the planned compared with expectant management groups had chorioamnionitis (RR 0.74, 95% CI 0.56–0.97; nine trials, 6611 women) or endometritis (RR 0.30, 95% CI 0.12–0.74; four trials, 445 women). No difference was seen for neonatal infection (RR 0.83, 95% CI 0.61–1.12; nine trials, 6406 infants). However, fewer infants under planned management went to NICU compared with expectant management (RR 0.72, 95% CI 0.57–0.92, NNTB

20; five trials, 5679 infants). In a single trial, significantly more women with planned management viewed their care more positively than those expectantly managed (RR of 'nothing liked' 0.45, 95% CI 0.37–0.54; 5031 women). Induction of labour for prelabour rupture of membranes at term reduced chorioamnionitis, endometritis and NICU admissions without increasing caesarean deliveries. NICE guidelines recommend that women presenting with prelabour rupture of the membranes at term should be advised that the risk of serious neonatal infection is 1%, rather than 0.5% for women with intact membranes. Sixty per cent of women with prelabour rupture of the membranes will go into labour within 24 hours and induction of labour is appropriate approximately 24 hours after rupture of the membranes [28]. Both prostaglandins and oxytocin can be used for IOL in PROM. Prostaglandins may be preferred as they allow women to be more mobile and are associated with increased chance of successful vaginal delivery within 24 hours. Oxytocin is preferred if a woman with PROM is at high risk or has clinical signs suggestive of clinical infection. Oxytocin induction is preferable for women positive for group B *Streptococci* with PROM at term.

Fetal Macrosomia

Based on current evidence, induction of labour does not improve outcomes in the setting of suspected fetal macrosomia but may increase caesarean deliveries. Unreliability of ultrasound estimation of the fetal weight adds to the complexity of decision making in this situation.

Overt Diabetes and Gestational Diabetes Mellitus (GDM)

Women with diabetes should generally be offered IOL prior to the estimated date of delivery. A Cochrane systematic review, which included one RCT that assigned 200 women with insulin-requiring GDM or pre-existing type 2 diabetes to either induction at 38 weeks of gestation or expectant care found no difference in the rate of caesarean delivery between these approaches, but found that fetal macrosomia, defined as birth weight >4000 g, was significantly reduced by induction of labour (relative risk 0.56; 95% CI 0.32–0.98, NNTB 8) [29,30]. The birth weight of 23% of the babies born to expectantly managed women was at or above the 90th percentile compared with 10% of the babies born to induced women. There were more cases of shoulder dystocia in the expectantly managed group, but this difference was not statistically significant. There were no differences in other fetal or maternal morbidities. There was very little evidence to support either elective delivery or expectant management at term in pregnant women with insulin-requiring diabetes. In cases of GDM with good glycaemic control, no significant differences in perinatal outcomes or caesarean rates have been observed when expectant management up to expected date of delivery and IOL are compared. However, IOL is generally recommended if there is evidence of associated placental insufficiency or poor glycaemic control.

Pre-eclampsia

Severe pre-eclampsia can cause significant mortality and morbidity for both mother and child, particularly when it occurs remote from term, between 24 and 34 weeks' gestation. A systematic review compared the effects of a policy of interventionist care and early delivery with a policy of expectant care and delayed delivery for women with early onset severe pre-eclampsia [31]. Four trials, with a total of 425 women, were included in this review. It was found that an expectant approach to the management of women with severe early onset pre-eclampsia may be associated with decreased morbidity for the baby. However, this evidence was based on data from only four trials. It has been suggested that expectant management for severe pre-eclampsia remote from term increases birth weight and reduces neonatal morbidity and that IOL in this situation is associated with high rates of intrapartum CS but no increased harm when compared with elective caesarean [24]. Labour induction is a reasonable option for patients with severe pre-eclampsia beyond 34 weeks' gestation. The management of mild hypertensive disease in pregnancies at term remains unclear. Many obstetricians will induce labour in women after 37 weeks with pregnancy-induced hypertension to prevent maternal and neonatal complications at the expense of increased operative delivery rates.

Intrauterine Growth Restriction (IUGR)

It has been suggested that in preterm pregnancies with suspected IUGR, induction of labour does not reduce perinatal deaths or overall long-term disability;

however, more evidence is needed to make strong recommendations [24]. When considering IOL in fetuses beyond 34 weeks' gestation with IUGR, it must be remembered that the fetus may have lower reserve than normal and is at increased risk of intrapartum hypoxia. IOL is unlikely to be successful in the presence of fetal compromise or abnormal fetal Dopplers. The DIGITAT multi-centre randomized trial allocated 321 pregnant women to induction and 329 to expectant monitoring [32]. Induction group infants were delivered ten days earlier (mean difference −9.9 days, 95% CI −11.3 to −8.6) and weighed 130 g less (mean difference −130 g, 95% CI −188 g to −71 g) than babies in the expectant monitoring group. A total of 17 (5.3%) infants in the induction group experienced the composite adverse neonatal outcome, compared with 20 (6.1%) in the expectant monitoring group (difference −0.8%, 95% CI −4.3% to 3.2%). Caesarean sections were performed on 45 (14.0%) mothers in the induction group and 45 (13.7%) in the expectant monitoring group (difference 0.3%, 95% CI −5.0% to 5.6%). The authors concluded that in women with suspected IUGR at term, there were no important differences in adverse outcomes between induction of labour and expectant monitoring. Patients who are keen on non-intervention can safely choose expectant management with intensive maternal and fetal monitoring; however, it is rational to choose induction to prevent possible neonatal morbidity and stillbirth.

Vaginal Birth After Caesarean (VBAC)

The NICE guidelines recommend that if delivery is indicated, women who have had a previous CS may be offered induction of labour with vaginal PGE2, CS or expectant management on an individual basis, taking into account the woman's circumstances and wishes [3]. The risk of stillbirth at or after 39 weeks is between 1.5- and 2-fold higher in women with previous caesarean delivery compared to women without prior caesarean delivery (absolute risks – 11 per 10 000 vs. 5 per 10 000). The reduction in risk of perinatal death that occurs by delivering from 41 weeks is likely to be greater among women with previous caesarean delivery. However, both induction and augmentation of VBAC labour are associated with a 2–3-fold increased risk of uterine rupture and around 1.5-fold increased risk of CS compared to spontaneous VBAC labour. A consultant-led review should therefore be planned for women at 41 weeks who wish to have VBAC and in

whom spontaneous onset of labour has not ensued. Based on large studies, the risk of uterine rupture appears to be 3–5 per 1000 in spontaneous labour, 8 per 1000 in oxytocin augmented or induced labour and still higher (about 25 per 1000) when prostaglandins are used. Induction of labour for VBAC should only be considered when the indication is compelling. If the cervix is favourable, amniotomy is the method of choice and adds no extra risk to spontaneous labour. If amniotomy fails to induce labour, oxytocin may be cautiously used with slight increase in the risk of uterine rupture. Mechanical methods of induction such as trans-cervical Foley catheter are preferable to other methods of induction of labour as they are less likely to cause uterine hyper-stimulation. Given the risks associated with induction of labour in a woman attempting VBAC, it is important not to exceed the safe recommended limit for prostaglandin priming in women with prior caesarean birth. Due consideration should be given to restricting the dose and adopting a lower threshold of total prostaglandin dose exposure. The risk of uterine rupture associated with misoprostol has been shown to be very high and this agent should ideally be avoided.

Intrauterine Fetal Death (IUFD)

Vaginal birth can be achieved within 24 hours of induction of labour for IUFD in about 90% of women. The Royal College of Obstetricians and Gynaecologists (RCOG) has provided obstetricians with detailed guidance to assist with IOL in this situation [33]. A combination of mifepristone (200 mg single dose) and a prostaglandin preparation should usually be recommended as the first line intervention for induction of labour. Mifepristone is ideally given 48–72 hours prior to prostaglandin. Misoprostol can be used in preference to PGE2 because of equivalent safety and efficacy with lower cost, but at doses lower than those currently marketed. Women should be advised that vaginal misoprostol is as effective as oral therapy but associated with fewer adverse effects. The addition of mifepristone appears to reduce the time interval to induction and delivery. It is recommended that misoprostol dose should be adjusted according to gestational age (100 mcg six-hourly before 26 + 6 weeks, 25–50 mcg four-hourly at 27 weeks or more up to 24 hours). If delivery does not occur after the first course of misoprostol, the following may be considered as the next options: (1) repeat a course of misoprostol

24 hours or more after starting treatment; (2) oxytocin infusion on intact membranes; (3) amniotomy and oxytocin; (4) surgical uterine evacuation below 24 weeks and hysterotomy or CS. In cases with one previous CS, mifepristone can be used alone to increase the chance of labour significantly within 72 hours (avoiding the use of prostaglandin). Misoprostol may be used for induction of labour in women with a single previous CS; however, it should be used at lower doses than those marketed currently. Women with two previous CSs should be advised that in general the absolute risk of induction of labour with prostaglandin is only a little higher than for women with a single previous CS. Women with more than two caesarean deliveries or atypical scars should be advised that the safety of induction of labour is unknown.

Other Indications

Induction of labour for macrosomia, social circumstances, maternal request or precipitate labour does not have a strong evidence base support. These inductions for 'social indications' are often undertaken electively at 38–39 weeks of gestation when IOL can be harmful to both mother (increased chances of failure and operative interventions) and the baby (higher risk of respiratory morbidity). A study analysed 7430 women with a single baby in vertex presentation, and delivering between 38 and 40 weeks of pregnancy [34]. Among these women, 3546 were excluded for prelabour pregnancy complications. Relative risks adjusted for parity were computed to compare 3353 women who went into labour spontaneously with 531 women whose labour was induced. Induction of labour was found to be associated with a higher risk of CS (RR = 2.4, 95% CI 1.8–3.4). Use of non-epidural and of epidural analgesia was more frequent after labour induction. Resuscitation (RR = 1.2, 95% CI 1.0–1.5), admission to the intensive care unit (RR = 1.6, 95% CI 1.0–2.4) and phototherapy (RR = 1.3, 95% CI 1.0–1.6) were more frequent after induction of labour. Results were similar when controlling simultaneously for parity, maternal age, gestational age, birth weight and the physician in charge of delivery in a logistic regression analysis. The results suggested that induction of labour is associated with a higher risk of CS and of some perinatal adverse outcomes. Induction of labour should therefore be reserved for cases where maternal and perinatal benefits outweigh the risk of these complications. Although there are few studies

suggesting benefits, there is lack of robust evidence to guide practice in cases of oligohydramnios, twin pregnancy, preterm prelabour rupture of membranes (pPROM) and intrahepatic cholestasis of pregnancy (IHCP) and further research is necessary to identify appropriate timing as well as potential risks and benefits of IOL in these settings.

Failed Induction of Labour

With rising rates of induction of labour, the concept of 'failed induction of labour' has grown in importance. There is a need for uniformity in its definition and management. It is very important that prior to IOL, women should be counselled regarding this possibility.

Definition

Over the years, there have been several definitions of failed IOL proposed by various authors. MacVicar defined failed induction as those cases where the uterus failed to contract after amniotomy and adequate stimulation, or the uterus contracted abnormally and the cervix did not dilate completely [35]. Duff *et al.* defined failed induction as the failure to enter the active phase of labour after 12 hours of regular uterine contractions [36]. A few other definitions include: failure to achieve dilatation ≥4 cm after trial of oxytocin to a maximum of 20 mU/min; failure to enter the active phase of labour within 12 hours after IOL was begun; failure to enter the active phase of labour (Bishop score <8) after 24 hours of IOL; failure to achieve the active phase (3 cm and completely effaced) after a maximum of 12 hours of oxytocin administration; and failure of sufficient ripening of the cervix to allow amniotomy following the use of repeated doses of prostaglandin, leading to delivery by CS. The sheer variety of definitions demonstrates the clinical uncertainty in diagnosis of failed induction. Lin and Rouse, in their review, indicated that a definition for induction of labour failure should maximize the number of women progressing to the active phase of labour (and ultimately delivering vaginally) while maintaining a low incidence of adverse maternal and neonatal outcomes. Their proposed definition was the inability to achieve a cervical dilatation of 4 cm and 90% effacement, or at least 5 cm (regardless of effacement) after a minimum of 12–18 hours of membrane rupture and oxytocin administration (with a goal of 250 Montevideo units or five contractions in 10 min) [37].

In current practice, failed induction is diagnosed when the woman does not enter active labour, or the cervical score does not improve or the cervix does not dilate >3 cm after a 12-hour period of artificial rupture of membranes and good uterine activity with oxytocin infusion. Failed induction of labour needs to be differentiated from failure of progress in active phase of labour due to cephalo-pelvic disproportion or malposition.

Reasons for Failed Induction of Labour

1. Cervical and pelvic factors: induction of labour with an unfavourable cervix is likely to fail more often than ripe cervix. As discussed previously, the uterine work needed to overcome resistance offered by a firm cervix is much higher, consequently increasing chances of failure of induction.
2. Fetal factors: fetal macrosomia.
3. Persistent occipito-posterior position has been associated with increased chance of failure of IOL.
4. High body mass index (BMI): a secondary analysis of combined data from three prospective randomized trials (905 women) comparing cervical ripening methods in singleton pregnancies with an unfavourable cervix identified risk factors for caesarean delivery [9]. Risk factors for caesarean delivery in women undergoing an indicated induction include a low Bishop score, high BMI, nulliparity and diabetes.
5. Improper assessment of gestation may contribute to failure of induction: this is a major problem in developing countries where early pregnancy scan may not be available to confirm gestation accurately. Induction below 41 weeks may thus lead to failure of IOL. The use of ultrasound for assessment of gestational age has been shown to decrease the incidence of postterm pregnancy from 12% to 3% [38].

Failed Induction of Labour: Suggestions to Improve the Vaginal Delivery Rates

As discussed previously, a number of common indications for IOL do not have a strong evidence base from which to guide practice, while many others have shown no major benefits for women. A strict policy of IOL for indications where benefits clearly outweigh the risks can contribute to reduction in the induction rates. Sweeping membranes is recommended for reducing formal IOL. A membrane sweep should be offered to all women unless there are specific clinical concerns like a low-lying placenta or if the woman does not wish to have it. Tailoring IOL to the parity, cervical score and indication might reduce the CS rate for failed IOL. Cervical ripening is crucial before the process of induction, and the use of PGE2 or PGE1 to ripen cervix and further induce labour has already been shown to be a more successful approach over the traditional methods like amniotomy or oxytocin infusion. Once the woman enters active labour, appropriate management to ensure adequate uterine activity and, if required, augmentation with oxytocin is equally important. Adequate pain relief should be discussed with women undergoing induction of labour. Transvaginal ultrasound assessments of cervical length, biochemical markers (such as fetal fibronectin) and Bishop score have all been shown to be useful in predicting the success of induction of labour. However, further research is needed, including cost–benefit analyses, before such tests can be routinely recommended.

Antenatal Counselling

Failed IOL does not necessarily indicate CS. The mother and fetus should be completely reassessed. A repeat attempt at IOL after a variable length of time may be considered. The repeat induction can be attempted either with the same or different prostaglandin or mechanical method of induction. The woman should be appropriately counselled about the options of repeat IOL versus CS and her choice should be respected at all times. Advanced antenatal education of the possibility of repeat induction may help more women to accept repeat induction and improve chances of vaginal birth.

Management Options after Failed Primary Induction

These options mainly apply to failed induction after IOL for prolonged pregnancy in absence of any obvious fetal or maternal complications. If IOL was performed for medical indications, the severity of fetal or maternal compromise will determine which option takes priority.

1. **Expectant management:** perform CTG and USG scan for liquor volume. If both are reassuring, the woman may be given an option of expectant management for up to three days based on her

preference. She then follows up for CTG and liquor volume assessment in 72 hours if spontaneous labour has not set in by this time. Reconsideration of all the options may be done based on cervical score at the next visit and a decision for repeat induction or caesarean be made, taking the woman's wishes on board.

2. **Repeat induction with same PG regime:** perform CTG and USG scan for liquor volume. If both are reassuring, repeat induction with same prostaglandin (usually PGE2) after an interval of 48 hours.

3. **Repeat induction with alternative PG regime:** perform CTG and USG scan for liquor volume. If both are reassuring, repeat induction with alternative prostaglandin (e.g. PGE1) after a gap of 48 hours.

4. **Repeat induction with mechanical method:** perform CTG and USG scan for liquor volume. If both are reassuring, repeat induction with mechanical method after a gap of 48 hours (Foley balloon catheter is inserted into the cervix and the balloon distended). The patient is then allowed home and instructed to come back if the catheter falls off, she starts contracting or notes leakage of fluid/blood per vaginum or any other concerns. If there are no concerns, she follows up after a further 48 hours for reassessment of cervical status.

5. **Caesarean section if induction is not acceptable:** perform CTG and USG scan for liquor volume. If both are reassuring, repeat CTG and USG scan after 48–72 hours to assess chance of success of repeat induction based on assessment of cervical length and position of occiput. For women not willing for conservative management or repeat prostaglandins with a poor cervical score and unfavourable ultrasound findings, CS may be offered. A study that used an alternative method (intracervical Foley catheter) for repeat IOL after failure of primary induction with PGE2 tablets found that 75% of these patients delivered vaginally [39].

Summary

IOL is becoming increasingly common. The availability of prostaglandins, which act as both cervical ripening as well as inducing agents, has improved the success rates of inductions as compared to the traditional approaches of amniotomy and oxytocin infusion. Prolonged pregnancy is one of the commonest indications for induction of labour. Up to 20% of inductions fail and need delivery by CS. The process of induction itself is associated with significant risks of complications like hyper-stimulation, ruptured uterus and increased risk of operative deliveries. The decision to induce labour therefore should not be taken lightly and the woman should be involved in the decision-making process after appropriate counselling. Adequate pain relief should be offered to women undergoing induction of labour. Induction for borderline indications not justified by current evidence should be avoided. The increasing rates of CSs are a cause for concern and the issue of failed induction needs to be addressed as a priority. Uniformity in its definition and management strategies is necessary. Failed primary induction does not necessarily indicate a CS. In the absence of fetal or maternal complications, either a repeat attempt at induction with prostaglandins/mechanical methods after 48 hours or expectant management with fetal surveillance for an additional 48–72 hours may be worth considering to improve the vaginal delivery rates in women with failed induction.

References

1. WHO. WHO recommendations for induction of labour. 2011. www.who.int/reproductivehealth/ publications/maternal_perinatal_health/9789241501156/ en/index.html (accessed 11 January 2015).

2. Martin JA, Hamilton BE, Sutton PD et al. Births: final data for 2006. *Natl Vital Stat Rep*; 2009; 57: 1–102.

3. NICE. *Induction of Labour:* Clinical Guideline 70. London: NICE; 2008.

4. McCarthy FP, Kenny LC. Induction of labour. *Obstet Gynaecol Reproduct Med*; 2011; 21(1): 1–6.

5. Hofmeyr GJ. Induction of labour with an unfavourable cervix. *Best Pract Res Clin Obstet Gynaecol*; 2003; 17(5): 777–94.

6. Arulkumaran S, Gibb DMF, TambyRaja RL et al. Failed induction of labour. *Aus NZ J Obstet Gynaecol*; 1985; 25(3): 190–3.

7. Arulkumaran S, Gibb DMF, Ratnam SS et al. Total uterine activity in induced labour: an index of cervical and pelvic tissue resistance. *BJOG*; 1985; 92: 693–97.

8. Rane SM, Guirgis RR, Higgins B et al. The value of ultrasound in the prediction of successful induction of labor. *Ultrasound Obstet Gynecol*; 2004; 24(5): 538–49.

9. Ennen CS, Bofill JA, Magann EF *et al.* Risk factors for cesarean delivery in preterm, term and post-term patients undergoing induction of labor with an unfavorable cervix. *Gynecol Obstet Invest*; 2009; 67(2): 113–17.

10. Gabriel R, Darnaud T, Chalot F *et al.* Transvaginal sonography of the uterine cervix prior to labour induction. *Ultrasound Obstet Gynaecol*; 2002; 19(3): 254–7.

11. Roman H, Verspyck E, Vercoustre L *et al.* The role of ultrasound and fetal fibronectin in predicting the length of induced labor when the cervix is unfavorable. *Ultrasound Obstet Gynecol*; 2004; 23(6): 567–73. See comment in PubMed Commons below this article.

12. Thomas J, Fairclough A, Kavanagh J *et al.* Vaginal prostaglandin (PGE2 and PGF2a) for induction of labour at term. *Cochrane Database Syst Rev*; 2014; 6: CD003101. doi: 10.1002/14651858.CD003101.pub3.

13. Boulvain M, Kelly A, Irion O. Intracervical prostaglandins for induction of labour. *Cochrane Database Syst Rev*; 2008; 1: CD006971.

14. Taher S, Inder J, Soltan S *et al.* Prostaglandin E2 vaginal gel or tablets for the induction of labour at term: a randomised controlled trial. *BJOG*; 2011; 118: 719–25.

15. ACOG. Induction of labour. Practice bulletin. Clinical Management Guidelines for Obstetrician-Gynecologists 107; 2009.

16. Hofmeyr GJ, Gulmezoglu AM, Pileggi C. Vaginal misoprostol for cervical ripening and induction of labour. *Cochrane Database Syst Rev*; 2010; 10: CD000941.

17. Alfirevic Z, Aflaifel N, Weeks A. Oral misoprostol for induction of labour. *Cochrane Database Syst Rev*; 2014; 6: CD001338. doi: 10.1002/14651858.CD001338.pub3.

18. Alfirevic Z, Kelly AJ, Dowswell T. Intravenous oxytocin alone for cervical ripening and induction of labour. *Cochrane Database Syst Rev*; 2009: CD003246. doi: 10.1002/14651858.CD003246.pub2.

19. Jozwiak M, Bloemenkamp KW, Kelly AJ. Mechanical methods for induction of labour. *Cochrane Database Syst Rev;*. 2012; 3: CD001233. doi: 10.1002/14651858.CD001233.pub2.

20. Jozwiak M, Oude Rengerink K, Benthem M, *et al.* Foley catheter versus vaginal prostaglandin E2 gel for induction of labour at term (PROBAAT trial): an open-label, randomised controlled trial. *Lancet*; 2011; 378(9809): 2095–103.

21. Boulvain M, Stan CM, Irion O. Membrane sweeping for induction of labour. *Cochrane Database Syst Rev*; 2005; 1: CD000451. doi: 10.1002/14651858.CD000451.pub2.

22. Mozurkewich EL, Chilimigras JL, Berman DR *et al.* Methods of induction of labour: a systematic review. *BMC Pregnancy and Childbirth*; 2011; 11: 84.

23. Knight M, Kenyon S, Brocklehurst P *et al. Saving Lives: Improving Mothers' Care – Lessons Learned to Inform Future Maternity Care from the UK and Ireland Confidential Enquiries into Maternal Deaths and Morbidity 2009–2012.* Oxford: National Perinatal Epidemiology Unit; 2014.

24. Mozurkewich E, Chilimigras J, Koepke E *et al.* Indications for induction of labour: a best-evidence review. *BJOG*; 2009; 116: 626–36.

25. Gülmezoglu AM, Crowther CA, Middleton P *et al.* Induction of labour for improving birth outcomes for women at or beyond term. *Cochrane Database Syst Rev*; 2012; 6: CD004945. doi: 10.1002/14651858. CD004945.pub3.

26. Mandruzzato G, Alfirevic Z, Chervenak F *et al.* Guidelines for the management of post term pregnancy. *J Perinat Med*; 2010; 38: 111–19.

27. Dare MR, Middleton P, Crowther CA *et al.* Planned early birth versus expectant management (waiting) for prelabour rupture of membranes at term (37 weeks or more). *Cochrane Database Syst Rev*; 2006; 1: CD005302.

28. NICE. *Intrapartum Care: Care of Healthy Women and their Babies during Childbirth:* Clinical Guideline 190. London: NICE; 2014.

29. Boulvain M, Stan C, Irion O. Elective delivery in diabetic pregnant women. *Cochrane Database Syst Rev*; 2001; 2: CD001997.

30. Kjos S, Henry OA, Montoro M *et al.* Insulin requiring diabetes in pregnancy: a randomized trial of active induction of labour and expectant management. *Am J Obstet Gynecol*; 1993; 169: 611–15.

31. Churchill D, Duley L, Thornton JG *et al.* Interventionist versus expectant care for severe pre-eclampsia between 24 and 34 weeks' gestation. *Cochrane Database Syst Rev*; 2013; 7: CD003106. doi: 10.1002/14651858.CD003106.pub2. See comment in PubMed Commons below this article.

32. Boers KE, Vijgen SM, Bijlenga D *et al.* Induction versus expectant monitoring for intrauterine growth restriction at term: randomised equivalence trial (DIGITAT). *BMJ*; 2010; 341: c7087. doi: 10.1136/bmj.c7087.

33. RCOG. *Late Intrauterine Fetal Death and Stillbirth.* London: RCOG Press; 2010.

34. Boulvain M, Marcoux S, Bureau M *et al.* Risks of induction of labour in uncomplicated term pregnancies. *Paediatr Perinat Epidemiol*; 2001; 15: 131–8.

35. MacVicar J. Failed induction of labour. *J Obstet Gynaecol Br Commonw*; 1971; 78: 1007–9.

36. Duff P, Huff RW, Gibbs RS. Management of premature rupture of membranes and unfavourable cervix in term pregnancy. *Obstet Gynaecol*; 1984; 63: 697–702.

37. Lin MG, Rouse DJ. What is a failed labor induction? *Clin Obstet Gynaecol*; 2006; 49: 585–93.

38. Savitz DA, Terry JW Jr, Dole N *et al.* Comparison of pregnancy dating by last menstrual period, ultrasound scanning, and their combination. *Am J Obstet Gynecol*; 2002; 187: 1660–6.

39. Mazhar SB, Jabeen K. Outcome of mechanical mode of induction in failed primary labour induction. *J Coll Physicians Surg Pak*; 2005; 15: 616–19.

Chapter 20

Preterm Prelabour Rupture of Membranes (pPROM)

Austin Ugwumadu

Introduction

Preterm prelabour rupture of membranes (pPROM) may be defined as the spontaneous rupture of fetal membranes at least an hour prior to the onset of labour, in a viable fetus (≥ 23 weeks), and before 37 completed weeks of gestation. It complicates 2–3% of all pregnancies, thus affecting some 14 000 pregnancies in the UK and 140 000 in the USA each year. Preterm prelabour rupture of membranes accounts for 30–40% of preterm deliveries, and is an independent risk factor for neonatal morbidity and mortality from prematurity, sepsis and pulmonary hypoplasia. Infants born after prolonged periods of pPROM have an excess risk of long-term neurological deficits and pulmonary disease. Subclinical intrauterine infection is a major aetiological factor in the pathogenesis of pPROM. Studies of transabdominal amniocentesis following pPROM show that the frequency of positive culture for infection of the amniotic fluid is 25–40%. The risk of a positive culture is inversely related to the gestational age at which pPROM occurred. Women with intrauterine infection have shorter latency than non-infected women, and infants born with sepsis have a fourfold increase in mortality compared to infants born without sepsis [1]. These findings fuelled interest in the use of antibiotics to prevent pPROM in at-risk women, increase latency after pPROM and as prophylaxis against neonatal morbidity such as oxygen dependency, intraventricular haemorrhage, necrotizing enterocolitis, neonatal sepsis and mortality. In one study, women with a prior history of pPROM had a 13.5% risk of subsequent preterm birth due to pPROM compared to 4.1% risk among their peers without such a history (RR 3.3, $p < 0.01$) [2]. These women also had a 14-fold higher risk of pPROM at less than 28 weeks

in the subsequent pregnancy (1.8% versus 0.13%, $p < 0.01$), raising the question of whether antibiotics may reduce this risk of pPROM. McGregor and colleagues showed that in women who are at increased risk of pPROM, prophylactic antibiotics significantly reduced the incidence of pPROM in the subsequent pregnancy [3].

Aetiology and Pathophysiology

The tensile strength of the membranes is resident mostly in the amnion, an avascular structure consisting of five distinct histological layers. The epithelial cells of the amnion layer secrete types 3 and 4 collagen, and non-collagenenous glycoproteins including fibronectins [4]. The chorion, on the other hand, provides the feto-maternal interface through the interaction between the cytotrophoblasts and the maternal decidua. Our understanding of the cellular and molecular factors that govern the structural integrity of fetal membranes and their regulation has increased in recent years and it is now evident that only a proportion of cases of pPROM are attributable to infection. Evidence has also accumulated that other pathologic processes unrelated to infection may play a role including choriodecidual fusion defects [5], fetal growth dysregulation [6], activation of membrane apoptosis [7], up-regulation of matrix metalloproteinases, and inhibition of tissue inhibitors of matrix metalloproteinases [8], nutritional factors [9] and smoking [10]. A detailed review of these factors and processes is outside the scope of this chapter, but these observations suggest that routine antibiotics for pPROM may be a simplistic response to a very complex problem.

Diagnosis and Initial Assessment

The diagnosis of pPROM is made by clinical suspicion, maternal history, speculum examination and simple bedside tests. Although it is stated that maternal history has an accuracy of 90% for the diagnosis of pPROM [11], the management and prognosis of a pregnancy complicated by pPROM is so drastically different from the one without that it is critically important to confirm the diagnosis before initiating interventions for pPROM. The presence of a pool of amniotic fluid in the posterior fornix on speculum examination is confirmatory of pPROM. Whether this fluid needs to be tested for confirmation is debatable. There may be a role for nitrazine pH paper testing when there is a very small amount of fluid in the posterior fornix and the observer is uncertain. However, the nitrazine test is not specific, and has a false-positive rate of 17% [11]. The pH of vaginal fluid changes towards the alkaline range in the presence of bacterial vaginosis, other vaginitis, contamination with cervical secretion, blood, semen or urine. In doubtful cases, the clinician should visualize the external cervical os with a Cusco's speculum and ask the patient to cough gently. Amniotic fluid may be observed trickling down through the os. An extended pad test is also useful. A panel of newer tests has been evaluated for pPROM, including fetal fibronectins and insulin-like growth factor binding protein-1 (IGFBP-1) in cervico-vaginal secretions. These have sensitivities of 94% and 75% respectively, and specificities of 97% [12,13]. Spontaneous rupture of membranes during the second and early third trimesters is usually associated with a near total loss of the entire amniotic fluid pool. Therefore, ultrasound scan evidence of marked oligohydramnios or anhydramnios is highly suggestive in women suspected of a diagnosis of pPROM [14]. Such an ultrasound examination should also evaluate the fetal presentation, growth and estimated fetal weight.

A digital vaginal examination should be avoided following a diagnosis of pPROM unless there is a strong suspicion of labour or imminent delivery. If one or two digital vaginal examinations were done after pPROM, this should not constitute an indication to abandon conservative management or pursue an immediate induction of labour for fear of increased risk of feto-maternal infectious morbidity. Studies have shown that two or fewer digital examinations were associated with a shorter latency period but no increase in fetal or maternal infectious morbidity [15,16].

Current State of the Management of pPROM

In many units, women with a diagnosis of pPROM are admitted into hospital and managed conservatively until 37 completed weeks of gestation in an attempt to increase fetal maturity. Conservative management may include Trendelenburg (head-down tilt) position, four-hourly measurements of maternal temperature, heart rate, respiratory rate and blood pressure, daily cardiotocographs (CTG), weekly, twice or thrice weekly maternal white cell counts, C-reactive protein measurements and culture of vaginal swabs, all in an effort to detect intrauterine infection or chorioamnionitis. However, chorioamnionitis is a fetal disease, not maternal, and maternal inflammatory markers are raised in only 10–15% of cases of proven histological chorioamnionitis [17], suggesting that maternal markers are not sufficiently sensitive to guide clinical decisions. The intrauterine compartment is sequestrated and not necessarily contiguous with the maternal systemic circulation. Furthermore, the bacterial species that commonly participate in chorioamnionitis are frequently subpathogenic, non-pyrogenic and are often not detected on routine microbiological culture methods. Prognostically, it is fetal rather than maternal host response to infection that is predictive of adverse neonatal outcome. However, the search for evidence of fetal inflammation by amniocentesis and/or cordocentesis is not routinely done, and its role in reducing the risk of neonatal complications has not been evaluated.

Appropriate Setting for Management

The value of inpatient management beyond five days is dubious. The majority of women with infection-driven pPROM will deliver within this time frame. Outpatient care with instruction for the patient to take her own temperature and be reviewed once or twice weekly in hospital is reasonable. She should, however, be discouraged from vaginal intercourse, protected or not, and any form of intravaginal cleansing. Immersion in bath water is not associated with an increase in infectious morbidity. A one-off vaginal swab for pathogens and specifically for group B *Streptococcus* (GBS) will suffice. There is little or no correlation between the organisms that cause amniotic fluid infection/chorioamnionitis and those isolated from the lower genital tract. Nursing women with pPROM in a head-down tilt position is unnecessary, and may encourage a stagnant pool of amniotic fluid and cervico-vaginal secretions, potentially encouraging bacterial growth and multiplication. Although fetal CTG is recommended as part of the surveillance, there are no specific or reliable CTG patterns that are predictive of fetal inflammation or sepsis until very late, and neurological injuries may occur without significant CTG changes. Clinical chorioamnionitis defined as maternal fever (temperature $\geq 38\,^{\circ}$C) and the presence of any two or more of maternal or fetal tachycardia, uterine tenderness, foul-smelling or purulent vaginal discharge, maternal leukocytosis or raised C-reactive protein is poorly predictive of histologic chorioamnionitis, which has been shown to be more predictive of abnormal neonatal outcomes including periventricular echodensity/echolucency, ventriculomegaly, intraventricular haemorrhage and seizures [18].

Biophysical profile scores have been proposed and in some centres used for the prediction of intrauterine infection. There is conflicting evidence that abnormal biophysical profile scores or Doppler studies of the placenta or fetal circulation provided accurate distinction between infected and non-infected fetuses [14,19,20].

Timing of Delivery

The practice of expectant management until 37 completed weeks of gestation to improve fetal maturity is historical and based on the assumption that the prolongation of pregnancy automatically translated to better perinatal outcome. The risks of acute cord compression, cord prolapse and ascending infection are not insignificant. It is well established that the risks of prematurity-related morbidity, including respiratory distress syndrome, necrotizing enterocolitis and high-grade intraventricular haemorrhage and mortality, diminish significantly beyond 32–34 weeks, and that neonatal survival at ≥ 34 weeks in tertiary units is similar to 37–40 weeks. The increase in survival per additional week of conservative management is less than 1%. Furthermore, studies evaluating the risk–benefit analysis of induction of labour at 34 weeks found similar vaginal delivery rates, and no increase in the risk of obstetric intervention such as instrumen-

tal vaginal or caesarean delivery [21]. On the other hand, these studies documented an excess incidence of ascending infection, neonatal sepsis, cord prolapse or compression, fetal demise and longer hospital stay in cases managed conservatively [21,22]. They concluded that the benefits of delivery at 34 weeks' gestation outweigh the risks of conservative management without increasing obstetric intervention. This balance, however, is in favour of expectant management prior to 32 completed weeks. Delivery before 32 weeks' gestation is associated with a significant risk of gestational age-related morbidity and mortality. Therefore, unless there are concerns regarding fetal well-being, clinical and/or biochemical evidence of infection, women with pPROM remote from term (≤ 32–34 weeks) should be managed conservatively to prolong gestation and reduce the risk of gestational age-dependent morbidity and mortality in the newborn. Even with conservative management, 70–80% of women with preterm prelabour rupture of membranes deliver within one week of membrane rupture, leaving a smaller subset of fetuses to remain and mature in utero. The potential benefit has to be balanced against the risk of amnionitis, abruption, umbilical cord compression or prolapse and fetal demise.

Antibiotic Therapy to Prolong Latency and Prevent Neonatal Morbidity After pPROM

Evidence from meta-analysis of 22 randomized trials including 6872 mother–infant pairs suggests that antibiotic therapy following pPROM significantly reduced chorioamnionitis (RR 0.66, 95%CI 0.46–0.96), delayed preterm birth within 48 hours (RR 0.71, 95%CI 0.58–0.87), oxygen therapy (RR 0.88, 95% CI 0.81–0.96) and abnormal cerebral imaging prior to discharge from the hospital (RR 0.81, 95% CI 0.68–0.98) [23]. Co-amoxiclav was associated with an increased risk of neonatal necrotizing enterocolitis (RR 4.72, 95% CI 1.57–14.23) and should be avoided. The antibiotic of choice is still unclear. There was no significant reduction in perinatal mortality or evidence of longer-term benefit in childhood. However, the advantages on short-term morbidities were thought to justify recommendation of routine antibiotics in women with pPROM. A follow-up study evaluated the children's health at seven years of age and found that antibiotics had little effect [24], but increased the risk of functional impairment among those who were exposed to erythromycin with intact membranes [25].

Questions have persisted regarding the methodology and interpretation of the primary studies, and the choice of antibiotic. Published meta-analyses are dominated by the larger, multi-arm, multi-centre, placebo-controlled ORACLE (Overview of the Role of Antibiotics in Curtailing Labour and Early delivery) trial [26]. Although the role of bacterial vaginosis in spontaneous preterm delivery and pPROM was known at the time of the ORACLE trial, none of the antibiotics used (co-amoxiclav and erythromycin) was effective against bacterial vaginosis organisms. Other methodological flaws in the design, analyses and interpretation were outlined in an accompanying lead commentary [27].

Widespread use of broad-spectrum antibacterial drugs may lead to the emergence of antibiotic-resistant organisms. There had been an increase in erythromycin-resistant organisms even in the years leading up to the publication of the ORACLE trial [28–30]. This trend was attributed to increased use of erythromycin for prophylaxis against GBS for women who were allergic to penicillin, and is likely to escalate with its increased use for pPROM. Broad-spectrum antibiotics may eliminate protective commensal flora, especially in the gut, encourage antimicrobial resistance and the emergence of unusual and more pathogenic species. Furthermore, early-life exposures are recognized as an important factor in the immunological health of children. It has been suggested that the significant rise in childhood allergy in developed countries may be related to abnormal initial gut colonization of infants as a result of obstetric and neonatal practices, including antibiotic exposure [31]. Routine antibiotic therapy presumes an infectious aetiology and is based on the belief that antibiotics somehow prevent or reverse fetal damage. This is not necessarily the case and indeed the reverse may well be true [32]. A significant number of mother–fetus pairs whose pPROM were unrelated to infection are exposed to broad-spectrum antibiotics and no studies have yet examined the risk versus benefit equation of mass antibiotic therapy for pPROM.

Tocolysis

Tocolysis may be applied prophylactically to prevent the onset of uterine contractions/labour in women with pPROM, or used therapeutically to abolish uterine contractions/labour after pPROM. Randomized trials of prophylactic [33,34] and therapeutic tocolysis [35,36], including case control studies [37], failed to show prolongation of pregnancy or reduction in perinatal morbidity or mortality. Therefore, the use of tocolysis should be individualized and restricted to those situations where there is no clinical or biochemical evidence of infection and a course of corticosteroids needed to be completed, or to allow the transfer of the woman to a tertiary centre. The choice of a tocolytic agent in this setting is a matter for local guidelines. The efficacies of the available agents on the market are broadly similar. The β-adrenoceptor agonists have become less popular because of their marked cardiovascular side-effects.

Antenatal Corticosteroids Administration

Initial concerns that corticosteroids may increase the risks of chorioamnionitis, postpartum endometritis and neonatal sepsis are not supported by current evidence. A meta-analysis of 15 randomized controlled trials (RCTs) including over 1400 women with pPROM showed that antenatal steroids did not increase the risk of maternal (RR 0.86; 95% CI 0.61–1.20) or neonatal infectious morbidity (RR 1.05; 95% CI 0.66–1.68) [38]. On the other hand, it showed that antenatal steroids reduced the risks of respiratory distress syndrome (RR 0.56; 95% CI 0.46–0.70) intraventricular haemorrhage (RR 0.47; 95% CI 0.31–0.70), and necrotizing enterocolitis (RR 0.21; 95% CI 0.05–0.82) [38]. Taken together, these substantial reductions in the risk of major gestational age-related morbidity translate to a significant reduction in neonatal mortality. Data on whether the same dose of corticosteroid translated to similar magnitudes of benefit for twins and other higher-order pregnancies with pPROM, because of greater maternal volume of distribution, are scanty. In diabetic women, the administration of corticosteroids may result in the loss of glycaemic control. This risk has to be carefully balanced with the potential benefit. Therefore, the value of steroid administration is questionable for women with pPROM near term – for example ≥32–34 weeks – or in whom fetal lung maturation can be demonstrated. Below 32 completed weeks of gestation, consideration should be given for sliding scale insulin/glucose infusion for 48–96 hours during the course of antenatal prophylactic steroid. Intramuscular betamethasone 12 mg 24 hours apart is preferable to dexamethasone 12 mg 12 hours apart. Betamethasone has a stronger evidence base and, unlike dexamethasone, it is not associated with necrotizing enterocolitis.

Group B Streptococcal Colonization and pPROM

Approximately 20–30% of pregnant women are GBS carriers, with higher rates of colonization in Black compared to White or Asian women [39]. It is common for women with pPROM to be colonized by GBS. Their babies are at risk of ascending or established intrauterine GBS infection, sepsis, death or intrapartum fetal distress. Very rarely, GBS may be vertically transmitted to the fetus from the mother via the haematogenous route. In this setting, the mother is usually very unwell with GBS sepsis, which may be isolated from her blood cultures. Histopathological examination of the placenta will show villitis rather than the predominant polymorphonuclear cell infiltration of the extraplacental membranes observed in the case of ascending GBS infection. Regardless of whether the fetal infection is of the ascending or haematogenous type, the risk of perinatal death or long-term sequelae is inversely related to gestational age. For optimal detection of GBS, a rectovaginal or vagino-perineal swab inoculated into a selective medium should be obtained [40]. If conservative management is planned following pPROM and the woman is colonized by GBS, consideration should be given to eradication of the GBS with benzyl penicillin for 24–48 hours if appropriate sampling and selective subculture techniques can be applied; otherwise treat for five days. Within 5–6 weeks there is a 5–10% chance of recolonization, and the treatment may be reconsidered. For women who are allergic to penicillin, clindamycin or erythromycin should be used, but sensitivity studies should be undertaken, as GBS strains exhibiting resistance to these antibiotics are on the increase. During labour intrapartum, antibiotic prophylaxis should be offered.

The Role of Amniocentesis

Studies of amniocentesis in pPROM women show that up to 40% will have positive amniotic fluid cultures at presentation, with the proportion increasing with latency. More recent studies using DNA amplification techniques have shown higher rates of amniotic fluid colonization by a variety of organisms. Women with established intrauterine infection deliver soon after pPROM and before amniocentesis can be performed. This situation weakens the accuracy of prevalence studies of intra-amniotic fluid infection and pPROM. Other studies have defined intra-amniotic infection using low glucose levels, elevated amniotic fluid polymorphs, pro-inflammatory cytokines including IL-6, IL-8 or TNF-α, and viral proteins. Amniocentesis and/or cordocentesis are powerful tools in distinguishing pPROM cases with intra-amniotic infection from non-infected cases. However, the isolation of microorganisms from the amniotic fluid does not equate to infection. It is fetal host inflammatory response rather than amniotic fluid colonization or maternal response that is correlated with adverse neonatal outcome. The characterization of cases complicated by infection is critically important because amniotic fluid infection is associated with a shorter latency and a higher risk of adverse perinatal and childhood outcomes, including respiratory distress syndrome, neonatal sepsis, chronic lung disease, periventricular leukomalacia, intraventricular haemorrhage and mortality.

Amniocentesis, culture of amniotic fluid and determination of the presence or absence of fetal host response may allow clinicians to select and triage cases for conservative or aggressive management and indeed test out the subset of cases that may benefit from antibiotic therapy. There is no evidence, however, that adopting this approach to guide management improved perinatal outcome. The timing of fetal injury is unknown, and it is plausible that by the time women present with pPROM, it is already too late to reverse an established inflammatory cascade. Although ampicillin and/or erythromycin therapy delayed preterm delivery, and reduced maternal and neonatal morbidity, the exact mechanism(s) through which antibiotics exert these 'beneficial effects' are unknown. Candidate mechanistic hypotheses including eradication of intrauterine infection, reduction/prevention of host inflammatory response and prevention of ascending infection from the lower genital tract have been proposed. However, Gomez and colleagues studied the microbiologic and inflammatory profiles of the amniotic fluid of 541 women with pPROM admitted to their institution over a period of just under five years [32]. Of the 541 women, 481 (88.9%) delivered within five days. Antibiotics (ceftriaxone, clindamycin and erythromycin for 10–14 days (IV for 48 hours and oral thereafter)) and corticosteroid therapy were initiated from 24 weeks' gestation if there was evidence of microbial invasion of the amniotic cavity (MIAC) or inflammation. Antibiotic therapy was initiated before 24 weeks' gestation if there was evidence of MIAC, but without steroid administration. If there was no evidence of MIAC or inflammation, ampicillin and erythromycin were administered for seven days (IV for 48 hours and oral thereafter). Tocolysis was not used in patient management. Of the 60 women who remained undelivered, 46 had a second amniocentesis after five days. Patients with intra-amniotic inflammation had a lower median gestational age at admission and at delivery than those without intra-amniotic inflammation. The prevalence of intra-amniotic inflammation was 39% (18/46) before antibiotic treatment and increased to 53% (24/45) after antibiotic therapy. The prevalence of a positive amniotic fluid culture was 15% (7/46) at the first amniocentesis, increasing to 28% (13/46) at the second amniocentesis, after completion of antibiotic therapy. Of seven patients with positive amniotic fluid culture for microorganisms at first amniocentesis, six (86%) had persistent positive amniotic fluid culture after antibiotic treatment, while a positive amniotic fluid culture was found in 18% (7/39) of cases with negative amniotic fluid culture at admission. Of 18 patients with intra-amniotic inflammation, 3 (17%) did not have evidence of inflammation after antibiotic therapy. Among 28 patients without intra-amniotic inflammation at admission, 9 (32%) developed inflammation, despite antibiotic treatment. Five of these women also had positive amniotic fluid culture [32].

This study showed that antibiotic treatment did not eradicate MIAC in patients with pPROM. An overwhelming 86% of pPROM patients with positive amniotic fluid culture and 83% with intra-amniotic inflammation maintained the same microbiologic/inflammatory profile, respectively, despite aggressive antibiotic therapy for 10–14 days. This is consistent with data that showed poor transplacental transfer of macrolide antibiotics [41,42]. Therefore, if indeed antibiotic therapy reduced neonatal complications in pregnancies complicated by pPROM, it is unlikely to be as a result of the eradication of MIAC or attenuation of the host inflammatory response. Also disturbing is the study's findings that women with negative amniotic fluid culture or inflammation at admission developed MIAC despite antibiotic therapy. The authors speculated that routine antibiotic therapy currently recommended for pPROM patients may be exerting its beneficial effects by preventing ascending infection or the development of fetal systemic inflammatory response syndrome (FSIRS). Both of these suggestions are unlikely. First, their data suggested that almost 90% of women admitted with pPROM delivered within the first five days, suggesting that in the majority of cases infection/inflammation may be so well established that delivery was imminent. In the undelivered group, the infection may be localized within the choriodecidual interface, where it may provoke pPROM but give a false-negative amniocentesis, which might explain, at least in part, the higher prevalence of positive amniotic fluid culture and inflammation at the second amniocentesis. Second, although both clindamycin and erythromycin exhibit anti-inflammatory properties, there is no evidence that these antibiotics reach the fetal compartment in sufficient amounts to alter its host inflammatory response. The timing of initiation of antibiotic therapy may be important in determining the outcome. In a rabbit model of ascending intrauterine infection, antibiotic administration within 12 hours of inoculation, but not after 18 hours, reduced the rate of preterm delivery and increased neonatal survival [43]. Such a near precise timing of the onset of intrauterine infection is impossible in human pregnancy. Neither our group [44] nor others [45] demonstrated a reduction in the frequency of histologic chorioamnionitis in randomized trials of antibiotic administration early in the second trimester in women at risk of chorioamnionitis, suggesting that even a pre-emptive antibiotic therapy earlier in pregnancy does not prevent histologic chorioamnionitis.

Conclusions

- Preterm prelabour rupture of membranes accounts for over one-third of preterm deliveries and is an independent risk factor for adverse fetal and neonatal outcome.
- Erythromycin and/or ampicillin is currently recommended for pPROM even though a significant proportion of pPROM cases are unrelated to infection, and antibiotic therapy may be raising their risks. More importantly, this intervention has not been shown to improve long-term outcomes.
- Further research is needed to define the natural history of intrauterine infection and what subsets of fetuses may benefit from the use of antibiotic therapy.

- Conservative management should be adopted if pPROM occurred prior to 34 weeks and delivery undertaken at or greater than 34 weeks' gestation.

References

1. Cotton DB, Hill LM, Strassner HT, Platt LD, Ledger WJ. Use of amniocentesis in preterm gestation with ruptured membranes. *Obstet Gynecol.* 1984; 63: 38–43.

2. Mercer BM, Goldenberg RL, Moawad AH, *et al.* The preterm prediction study: effect of gestational age and cause of preterm birth on subsequent obstetric outcome. *Am J Obstet Gynecol.* 1999; 181: 1216–21.

3. McGregor JA, Schoonmaker JN, Lunt BD, Lawellin DW. Antibiotic inhibition of bacterially induced fetal membrane weakening. *Obstet Gynecol.* 1990; 76: 124–8.

4. Parry S, Strauss JF III. Premature rupture of the fetal membranes. *N Engl J Med.* 1998; 338: 663–70.

5. Bryant-Greenwood GD, Millar LK. Human fetal membranes: their preterm premature rupture. *Biol Reprod.* 2000; 63: 1575–9.

6. Cooperstock MS, Tummaru R, Bakewell J, Schramm W. Twin birth weight discordance and risk of preterm birth. *Am J Obstet Gynecol.* 2000; 183: 63–7.

7. Fortunato SJ, Menon R, Bryant C, Lombardi SJ. Programmed cell death (apoptosis) as a possible pathway to metalloproteinase activation and fetal membrane degradation in premature rupture of membranes. *Am J Obstet Gynecol.* 2000; 182: 1468–76.

8. Fortunato SJ, Menon R, Lombardi SJ. MMP/TIMP imbalance in amniotic fluid during PROM: an indirect support for endogenous pathway to membrane rupture. *J Perinat Med.* 1999; 27: 362–8.

9. Barrett BM, Sowell A, Gunter E, Wang M. Potential role of ascorbic acid and beta-carotene in the prevention of preterm rupture of fetal membranes. *Int J Vitam Nutr Res.* 1994; 64: 192–7.

10. Barrett B, Gunter E, Jenkins J, Wang M. Ascorbic acid concentration in amniotic fluid in late pregnancy. *Biol Neonate.* 1991; 60: 333–5.

11. Friedman ML, McElin TW. Diagnosis of ruptured fetal membranes: clinical study and review of the literature. *Am J Obstet Gynecol.* 1969; 104: 544–50.

12. Gaucherand P, Guibaud S, Awada A, Rudigoz RC. Comparative study of three amniotic fluid markers in premature rupture of membranes: fetal fibronectin, alpha-fetoprotein, diamino-oxydase. *Acta Obstet Gynecol Scand.* 1995; 74: 118–21.

13. Rutanen EM, Pekonen F, Karkkainen T. Measurement of insulin-like growth factor binding protein-1 in cervical/vaginal secretions: comparison with the ROM-check Membrane Immunoassay in the diagnosis of ruptured fetal membranes. *Clin Chim Acta.* 1993; 214: 73–81.

14. Carroll SG, Papaioannou S, Nicolaides KH. Assessment of fetal activity and amniotic fluid volume in the prediction of intrauterine infection in preterm prelabor amniorrhexis. *Am J Obstet Gynecol.* 1995; 175: 1427–35.

15. Alexander JM, Mercer BM, Miodovnik M, *et al.* The impact of digital cervical examination on expectantly managed preterm rupture of membranes. *Am J Obstet Gynecol.* 2000; 183: 1003–7.

16. Lewis DF, Major CA, Towers CV, *et al.* Effects of digital vaginal examinations on latency period in preterm premature rupture of membranes. *Obstet Gynecol.* 1992; 80: 630–4.

17. Romero R, Sirtori M, Oyarzun E, *et al.* Infection and labor. V. Prevalence, microbiology, and clinical significance of intraamniotic infection in women with preterm labor and intact membranes. *Am J Obstet Gynecol.* 1989; 161: 817–24.

18. De Felice C, Toti P, Laurini RN, *et al.* Early neonatal brain injury in histologic chorioamnionitis. *J Pediatr.* 2001; 138: 101–4.

19. Carroll SG, Papaioannou S, Nicolaides KH. Doppler studies of the placental and fetal circulation in pregnancies with preterm prelabor amniorrhexis. *Ultrasound Obstet Gynecol.* 1995; 5: 184–8.

20. Lewis DF, Adair CD, Weeks JW, *et al.* A randomized clinical trial of daily nonstress testing versus biophysical profile in the management of preterm premature rupture of membranes. *Am J Obstet Gynecol.* 1999; 181: 1495–9.

21. Naef RW III, Allbert JR, Ross EL, *et al.* Premature rupture of membranes at 34 to 37 weeks' gestation: aggressive versus conservative management. *Am J Obstet Gynecol.* 1998; 178: 126–30.

22. Grable IA. Cost-effectiveness of induction after preterm premature rupture of the membranes. *Am J Obstet Gynecol.* 2002; 187: 1153–8.

23. Kenyon S, Boulvain M, Neilson JP. Antibiotics for preterm rupture of membranes. *Cochrane Database Syst Rev.* 2013; 12: CD001058. doi: 10.1002/14651858.CD001058.pub3.

24. Kenyon S, Pike K, Jones DR, *et al.* Childhood outcomes after prescription of antibiotics to pregnant women with preterm rupture of the membranes: 7-year follow-up of the ORACLE I trial. *Lancet.* 2008; 372: 1310–18. doi: 10.1016/S0140-6736(08)61202-7.

25. Kenyon S, Pike K, Jones DR, *et al.* Childhood outcomes after prescription of antibiotics to pregnant women with spontaneous preterm labour: 7-year follow-up of the ORACLE II trial. *Lancet.* 2008; 372: 1319–27. doi: 10.1016/S0140-6736(08)61203-9.

26. Kenyon SL, Taylor DJ, Tarnow-Mordi W. Broad-spectrum antibiotics for preterm, prelabour rupture of fetal membranes: the ORACLE I randomised trial. ORACLE Collaborative Group. *Lancet.* 2001; 357: 979–88.

27. Hannah M. Antibiotics for preterm prelabour rupture of membranes and preterm labour? *Lancet.* 2001; 357: 973–4.

28. Manning SD, Foxman B, Pierson CL, *et al.* Correlates of antibiotic-resistant group B streptococcus isolated from pregnant women. *Obstet Gynecol.* 2003; 101: 74–9.

29. Manning SD, Pearlman MD, Tallman P, Pierson CL, Foxman B. Frequency of antibiotic resistance among group B Streptococcus isolated from healthy college students. *Clin Infect Dis.* 2001; 33: E137–9.

30. Pearlman MD, Pierson CL, Faix RG. Frequent resistance of clinical group B streptococci isolates to clindamycin and erythromycin. *Obstet Gynecol.* 1998; 92: 258–61.

31. Murch SH. Toll of allergy reduced by probiotics. *Lancet.* 2001; 375: 1057–9.

32. Gomez R, Romero R, Nien JK, *et al.* Antibiotic administration to patients with preterm premature rupture of membranes does not eradicate intraamniotic infection. *J Matern Fetal Neonatal Med.* 2007; 20: 167–73.

33. How HY, Cook VD, Miles DE, Spinnato JA. Preterm prelabour rupture of membranes: aggressive tocolysis versus expectant management. *J Mat Fetal Med.* 1998; 7: 8–12.

34. Levy DL, Warsof SL. Oral ritodrine and preterm premature rupture of membranes. *Obstet Gynecol.* 1985; 66: 621–3.

35. Weiner CP, Renk K, Klugman M. The therapeutic efficacy and cost-effectiveness of aggressive tocolysis for premature labor associated with premature rupture of the membranes. *Am J Obstet Gynecol.* 1988; 159: 216–22.

36. Garite TJ, Keegan KA, Freeman RK, Nageotte MP. A randomized trial of ritodrine tocolysis versus expectant management in patients with premature rupture of membranes at 25 to 30 weeks of gestation. *Am J Obstet Gynecol.* 1987; 157: 388–93.

37. Combs CA, McCune M, Clark R, Fishman A. Aggressive tocolysis does not prolong pregnancy or reduce neonatal morbidity after preterm premature rupture of membranes. *Am J Obstet Gynecol.* 2004; 190: 1723–8.

38. Harding JE, Pang J, Knight DB, Liggins GC. Do antenatal corticosteroids help in the setting of preterm rupture of membranes? *Am J Obstet Gynecol.* 2001; 184: 131–9.

39. Regan JA, Klebanoff MA, Nugent RP. The epidemiology of group B streptococcal colonization in pregnancy: Vaginal Infections and Prematurity Study Group. *Obstet Gynecol.* 1991; 77: 604–10.

40. Jamie WE, Edwards RK, Duff P. Vaginal–perianal compared with vaginal–rectal cultures for identification of group B streptococci. *Obstet Gynecol.* 2004; 104: 1058–61.

41. Witt A, Sommer E, Cichna M, *et al.* Placental passage of clarithromycin surpasses other macrolide antibiotics. *Am J Obstet Gynecol.* 2003; 188: 816–19.

42. Heikkinen T, Laine K, Neuvonen PJ, Ekblad U. The transplacental transfer of the macrolide antibiotics erythromycin, roxithromycin and azithromycin. *BJOG.* 2000; 107: 770–5.

43. Fidel P, Ghezzi F, Romero R, *et al.* The effect of antibiotic therapy on intrauterine infection-induced preterm parturition in rabbits. *J Matern Fetal Neonatal Med.* 2003; 14: 57–64.

44. Ugwumadu A, Reid F, Hay P, Manyonda I, Jeffrey I. Oral clindamycin and histologic chorioamnionitis in women with abnormal vaginal flora. *Obstet Gynecol.* 2006; 107: 863–8.

45. Goldenberg RL, Mwatha A, Read JS, *et al.* The HPTN 024 Study: the efficacy of antibiotics to prevent chorioamnionitis and preterm birth. *Am J Obstet Gynecol.* 2006; 194: 650–61.

Chapter 21

The Management of Preterm Labour

Jan Stener Jørgensen and Ronald F. Lamont

Background

Preterm birth (PTB), particularly at early gestations, is the major cause of death and handicap in newborn babies world-wide. The March of Dimes white paper on PTB demonstrated that, worldwide, 12.9 million PTBs occur annually (9.6% of all births). Approximately 85% of PTBs occur in Africa and Asia, though the rate of PTB in North America is high (10.6%) compared to Europe (6.2%). It is estimated that 28% of the 4 000 000 neonatal deaths that occur worldwide annually are due to PTB. The rate of PTB is increasing and has risen by 36% in the USA in the last 25 years, mostly through late PTB (34–36 completed weeks of gestation). The March of Dimes has called for strategies that reduce death and disability to be given priority. The United Nations Millennium Development Goals number 4 (child survival) and number 5 (improvement of women's health) are directly related to this aim [1].

Mortality and Morbidity Associated with PTB

Mortality and morbidity are inversely related to gestational age at birth, and while 50% of all PTB's occur after 35 completed weeks of gestation, 99% of the mortality and morbidity associated with PTB occurs before this time. In Sweden, babies born at 22, 24 and 26 completed weeks of gestation have an infant mortality rate of 54%, 21% and 2% respectively, and at 365 days of life have a rate of survival without major morbidity of 0.02%, 14.1% and 45.9% respectively. In the UK and Ireland, approximately 65% of babies born between 22 and 26 completed weeks of gestation will die on the delivery suite or neonatal intensive care unit (NICU) and at 30-month follow-up around 50% will

be handicapped, and in 50% of these the handicap will be severe. This means that at 2.5 years of age, only 12–13% remain alive and neurologically intact.

Financial Cost of PTB

In the UK, the cost of hospital readmission during the first five and ten years of life is 20 times greater for those babies born before 28 completed weeks of gestation compared to those born after 37 completed weeks. The cost of neonatal intensive care is approximately £800–1000/day. In 2007, the Institute of Medicine in the USA calculated that the annual cost associated with PTB was $26.2 billion. This comprised medical costs for the baby ($16.9 billion), labour and delivery costs for the mother ($1.9 billion), early intervention programmes for children with disabilities and developmental delays from birth to age three years ($611 million), special education services ($1.1 billion) and lost work and pay for those born preterm ($5.7 billion). The psychosocial cost of PTB remains incalculable.

Diagnosis of Genuine Preterm Labour

The diagnosis of genuine preterm labour is difficult. Spontaneous preterm labour (SPTL) is defined as the onset of regular, prolonged, painful, frequent and synchronous contractions together with progressive effacement and dilatation of the *cervix uteri* occurring before 37 completed weeks of gestation. Accordingly, the diagnosis of genuine SPTL should not be made on contractions alone and must include cervical changes. Using a history of contractions alone, without consideration of cervical change, 50% of patients and 30% of attendant midwives and obstetricians will be wrong in their diagnosis of genuine SPTL. The assessment of uterine contractions and cervical status may be relative

Best Practice in Labour and Delivery, Second Edition, ed. Sir Sabaratnam Arulkumaran. Published by Cambridge University Press. © Cambridge University Press 2016.

or absolute and may be objective or subjective. External electronic cardiotocography (CTG) of contractions is more objective than clinical palpation, and change of Bishop score is more objective than a narrative record. A high Bishop score together with CTG evidence of significantly prolonged, frequent, synchronous and objectively recordable contractions may merit an absolute diagnosis of genuine SPTL. A changing Bishop score together with a progressive increase in the regularity, duration, frequency and synchronicity of uterine contractions can be considered relative evidence of genuine SPTL. Most importantly, early diagnosis is crucial. At a Bishop score of 3.5, the use of tocolytics can prolong gestation by >55 days. Conversely, at a Bishop score of 8, tocolytics can only prolong gestation by <2 days [2]. Accordingly, any intervention study for the management of genuine SPTL should consider using some objective measure like the Bishop score to ensure comparability between intervention and control groups.

The Use of Transvaginal Ultrasound Scanning of Cervical Length or Measurement of Fetal Fibronectin for the Diagnosis of SPTL

The measurement of transvaginal ultrasound scanning (TVUSS) of cervical length (CL) or measurement of fetal fibronectin (fFN) for the diagnosis of genuine SPTL has been advocated, but these may not be clinically practical outside clinical trials or tertiary referral centres. In most studies, these measurements have been applied to asymptomatic women as part of a predictive process rather than diagnostic in symptomatic women. The results of fFn testing are also affected by whether or not sampling was carried out singly or serially, in low- or high-risk women, in singleton or multiple pregnancies, with or without optimal timing (24–27 weeks' gestation). Serial sampling in high-risk women, with multiple pregnancies, between 24 and 27 weeks' gestation, increases sensitivity and decreases specificity. Overall, in asymptomatic women, TVUSS of CL and fFN have a high specificity but lower sensitivity. In symptomatic women, using the combination of fFN and TVUSS between 24 and 34 completed weeks of gestation, a positive fFN together with a CL on TVUSS of ≤26 mm was associated with a risk of birth before 37 weeks of 52.4%. In contrast, a negative fFN together with a CL on TVUSS of

>26 mm was associated with a risk of birth before 37 weeks of 5.6% [3].

Contraindications to Intervention in SPTL

Contraindications to intervention in SPTL will be either relative or absolute. The two major factors which influence the decision as to whether or not to interfere in suspected PTL are: (1) is the patient in labour? And (2) is she preterm? This emphasizes the importance of the diagnosis of genuine preterm labour as discussed above and also the importance of calculating and recalculating the best estimate of the expected date of delivery and hence the current accurate assessment of gestational age. Between 22 and 26 completed weeks of gestation, every day by which delivery is delayed the neonatal survival rate increases by 3% [4]. Conversely, after 30 completed weeks of gestation, it may take many weeks of delay of delivery to demonstrate a 3% increase in survival. This being the case, one week's difference in the calculated gestational age may weigh heavily on the decision of whether or not to intervene. Other contraindications to intervention would include any reason whereby prolongation of the pregnancy would seriously compromise the safety of mother or baby. These might be absolute or relative (as a matter of degree) but would include: significant antepartum haemorrhage, severe intrauterine growth restriction, non-reassuring tracing of the fetal heart rate (FHR), lethal congenital malformations, prolonged prelabour rupture of the membranes (pPROM), fulminating pre-eclampsia and evidence of intrauterine feto-maternal infection. As an aid to such decision making, an ultrasound scan as soon as possible after diagnosis of SPTL would be ideal, but this may only be practical in tertiary referral obstetric units. Such a scan might confirm appropriate or restricted growth in relation to gestational age and estimate of fetal weight, amniotic fluid index, number of fetuses, anatomical normality, fetal presentation and placental site, all of which might affect the decision of whether or not to intervene and the mode of delivery if intervention is contemplated (see below).

Tocolytics for the Inhibition of SPTL and PTB

There is robust evidence which demonstrates that tocolytics are significantly superior to placebo or control for the delay of PTB by 24 hours or seven days. The perfect tocolytic that is uniformly efficacious and completely safe does not exist. No tocolytic has been specifically developed for the treatment of SPTL and only β_2-agonists and atosiban are licensed for use as a tocolytic. Even atosiban, which is the most uterospecific tocolytic, was initially developed as a treatment for dysmenorrhoea. Accordingly, since most tocolytics were developed for other indications but found to inhibit uterine contractions, they are not uterospecific and so have multi-organ side-effects.

Historical Perspective

In the 1960s, bed rest, hydration, opiate analgesia (in some cases to deliberately sedate a very active baby) and alcohol (which is a primitive oxytocin antagonist) were used to prevent or delay PTB. Hydration has scientific merit since intravenous fluid administration will inhibit antidiuretic hormone (vasopressin) secretion by the posterior pituitary and reduce stimulation of vasopressin receptors in the uterus with myometrial relaxation. In the 1970s, β_1-agonists (isoxuprine) and later β_2-agonists were introduced; the 1980s became the decade of β_2-agonists. In 1982 the Food and Drug Administration approved ritodrine for use in the USA, soon after replacing β_1-agonists and alcohol worldwide. Other β_2-agonists such as terbutaline (Scandinavia), salbutamol (France), fenoterol (Germany), hexaprenaline (Austria) and orciprenaline were introduced preferentially in many countries. There followed a marked increase in pulmonary oedema and in 1986 in the USA and Japan, post-marketing surveillance advice recommended the cessation of preloading with intravenous fluids prior to initiation of β_2-agonist treatment. In 1992, the Canadian Preterm Labour Investigators Group reported similar findings to the Keirse meta-analysis, namely that β_2-agonists were able to stop contractions and delay delivery for a short time, albeit that they had not been shown to be associated with a reduction in neonatal mortality or morbidity. In the same issue of the journal, Leveno and Cunningham published an editorial in which they called for a reappraisal of the use of β_2-agonists. There followed a decline in use of β_2-agonists in the USA and Europe, and in 1999 atosiban was launched in Europe (Austria first). Because of the cost of atosiban, there followed a drift towards the use of cheaper tocolytic alternatives such as magnesium sulphate and calcium channel blockers (CCBs), mainly nifedipine.

Alternatively, there followed a drift towards therapeutic nihilism in which, fearful of the adverse effects of tocolytic drugs, clinicians preferred to do nothing when faced with a woman in SPTL. Finally, if tocolytics were to be used, treatment was limited to: (1) 24–34 completed weeks of gestation; (2) no more than 48 hours' duration; (3) not until SPTL had been confirmed (which decreases efficacy); and (4) not for prophylaxis or maintenance.

Tocolytic Myths and Legends

Tocolytics are frequently criticized for: (1) failing to reduce the rate of PTB since their introduction; (2) failing to reduce the rate of neonatal mortality and morbidity; and (3) only being beneficial for 48 hours. While these criticisms have some validity, they should not remain without qualification. The risk factors for PTB, such as multiple pregnancy due to assisted reproduction techniques, pregnancy at the extremes of reproductive age and drug abuse have markedly increased since tocolytic therapy was introduced. In addition, with improvements in neonatal care and neonatal outcomes, the use of iatrogenic PTB as a therapeutic intervention has increased. Finally, with the marked increase in the registration of very early PTBs around the limits of viability, infants that previously would not have been considered in registry statistics are now included.

Between 22 and 26 weeks of gestation, every day gained in utero is associated with a 3% increase in survival [4], and the use of tocolytics (compared to no tocolytics) up to 34 completed weeks of gestation with intact membranes and up to 32 weeks with ruptured membranes does not have a deleterious effect on neonatal mortality and morbidity [5]. The main indications given for the use of tocolytics are: (1) to delay delivery until a full course of antepartum glucocorticoids (APG) can be administered for the prevention of hyaline membrane disease; and (2) to arrange transfer to a centre with NICU facilities. Since both interventions have been demonstrated to result in a reduction in neonatal mortality and morbidity and no tocolytic study has ever been powered by a sample size big enough to demonstrate a significant reduction in neonatal mortality and morbidity, the evidence must be surrogate, so it requires a leap of faith to accept the beneficial effect of tocolytics on neonatal mortality and morbidity. Lack of proof of effect is not the same as proof of lack of effect.

Many consider that tocolytics should only be used for 48 hours. This may be related to the duration of a course of antepartum glucocorticoids or because of Keirse *et al.*'s meta-analysis of β_2-agonists [6] in which he found only 16 studies that were methodologically acceptable. With different outcome parameters, the only outcome that was common to all studies for comparison was the ability to delay delivery for 48 hours. This has erroneously become carved in stone as the optimal period for the use of tocolytics, but many studies have demonstrated that tocolytics are able to delay delivery for much longer.

Maintenance Therapy

While the evidence for the use of maintenance tocolytic therapy is sparse, one well-conducted study has demonstrated that following successful tocolysis with atosiban, the median time from the start of maintenance treatment to the first recurrence of labour was 32.6 days with atosiban and 27.6 days with placebo ($p = 0.02$) [7].

Efficacy of Tocolytics for the Inhibition of Preterm Labour

The evidence supporting the use of magnesium sulphate as a tocolytic is poor, albeit that many of the studies were under-dosed. Nevertheless, in parts of the world where atosiban is not available and where β_2-agonists are out of favour, magnesium sulphate is still used. Similarly, nitric oxide donors are rarely used and though prostaglandin synthetase inhibitors (PGSIs) are used in some units, they are rarely used as first line therapy, which is usually limited to atosiban, nifedipine or a β_2-agonist. The Royal College of Obstetricians and Gynaecologists recommend changing from β_2-agonists to either nifedipine or atosiban, but also provide the option for no tocolytic use, which is practised in some centres. Accordingly, in the UK, most units use either nifedipine or atosiban as first line therapy, with a β_2-agonist or PGSI as second line treatment.

Prostaglandin Synthetase Inhibitors

Haas *et al.*, in a complex simulation using meta-analysis and decision-analysis of 58 tocolytic studies, attempted to determine the optimal first line tocolytic with the highest tolerability and highest proportion

of delay. The outcomes were efficacy (delay of delivery for 48 hours, 7 days or until 37 weeks), tolerability (side-effects) and neonatal outcome (respiratory distress syndrome (RDS) or death). When the simulation demonstrated which treatment was best for delay of delivery by 48 hours or 7 days, PGSIs were considered to be first and oxytocin receptor antagonists were second. The authors concluded that PGSIs should be the first line tocolytic before 32 completed weeks of gestation. However, concerns were expressed about small numbers in the PGSI studies and the risks of premature closure of the fetal ductus arteriosus after 32 weeks' gestation, the risks of necrotizing enterocolitis, intraventricular haemorrhage and persistent patent fetal ductus arteriosus before 30 weeks' gestation [8].

β_2-agonists

β_2-agonists were the first drugs to be licensed for use as a tocolytic. Their evidence base as a tocolytic is robust, but many of the early trials involved women recruited after 34 completed weeks of gestation. This is understandable because it is beyond this gestational age at which most SPTLs and PTBs occur. However, women recruited beyond 36 completed weeks of gestation may be in slightly early physiological term labour where there is a 40% placebo response rate rather than pathological SPTL. In addition, most of the β_2-agonist trials used contractions alone as an inclusion criterion without involving cervical assessment or change. As pointed out above, a history of contractions alone, without consideration of cervical change, will result in 50% of patients and 30% of attendant midwives and obstetricians being wrong in their diagnosis of genuine SPTL. While there is no doubt that β_2-agonists can stop contractions and prolong SPTL, it is their side-effect profile that mitigates against their use, particularly those serious adverse effects such as pulmonary oedema.

Pathophysiology of Pulmonary Oedema with the Use of β_2-agonists

Due to the physiological adaptations of pregnancy, it has been said that 'a pregnant woman is pulmonary oedema waiting to happen' [9]. It is estimated that the incidence of pulmonary oedema in women receiving β_2-agonists under well-controlled conditions is approximately 0.5%. The factors associated with pulmonary oedema with the use of

β_2-agonists are: (1) maternal (plasma expansion); (2) fetal (twins); (3) feto-maternal infections (tissue permeability); and (4) properties of tocolytics themselves – β_2-agonists cause a positive fluid balance through drug-induced fluid retention caused by effects on the renin/aldosterone/angiotensin system and also by iatrogenic fluid overload. Cardiovascular effects include tachycardia that results in a shorter cardiac cycle and therefore less time in diastole to achieve cardiac filling. This results in a damming back of fluid into the lungs and the potential for pulmonary oedema. Finally, β_2-agonists have metabolic effects such as hypokalaemia that can cause arrhythmias and hence pulmonary oedema [9]. Due to the risks of pulmonary oedema and metabolic side-effects with the use of β_2-agonists, the RCOG guidelines prescribe the following monitoring: (1) maternal pulse and blood pressure every 15 min; (2) blood sugar measurement every four hours; (3) strict record of fluid balance (input/output); (4) daily urea and electrolyte measurement; and (5) auscultation of the lung fields every four hours. Few units, even those of high repute, employ such rigorous monitoring.

Calcium Channel Blockers

While nicardipine has been used as a tocolytic, most of the evidence pertaining to the use of CCBs as a tocolytic concerns the use of nifedipine. The evidence supporting the use of nifedipine as a tocolytic is less than robust and nifedipine is not licensed for use in SPTL. The concerns about the evidence base for nifedipine centres around the facts that: (1) no 'good-quality' placebo controlled trials have been conducted; (2) no follow-up studies have been performed; and (3) most of the evidence is therefore from meta-analyses of trials that were unblinded, of small sample size, investigator-led rather than by pharmaceutical companies which are experienced in conforming to regulatory requirements, had no intention to treat analysis, lacked sufficient power, were carried out at late gestations, had no account of randomization and CCBs were used as second line treatment. The first two meta-analyses on nifedipine [10,11] were critical of each other, one citing the other for having included poor-quality studies and receiving the response that if only good-quality studies had been considered there would have been insufficient data to analyse. There followed two systematic reviews [12,13] which, though the Cochrane Library discourages duplication, were

remarkably similar. The Cochrane review addressed the use of nifedipine as a tocolytic for the prevention of PTB for seven days. Four studies were included, three of which showed no benefit of nifedipine. The fourth study by one of the co-authors of the review (a practice discouraged by Cochrane and other bodies) was the only study to support the benefit of nifedipine, but because of a weighting of >60% rendered the conclusions in favour of nifedipine as efficacious in the prevention of PTB [13].

Meta-analyses are retrospective analyses of pooled data that are only as good as the quality of studies included. While they may be suitable for large numbers of good-quality contradictory studies, they may not be suitable for small numbers of poor-quality studies. Accordingly, a systematic review of the quality of nifedipine studies used to assess tocolytic efficacy was undertaken. Using method- and topic-specific items of quality to assess whether or not these were adequate, inadequate or unstated, a high percentage demonstrated selection bias (77%), inadequate concealment of allocation (97%), no stratification of randomization (94%), performance bias (blinding to treatment) (97%), measurement bias (blinding to outcome) (100%) and attrition bias (intention-to-treat analysis) (71%) [14]. If the studies used to assess the efficacy of a therapeutic agent (tocolytic) for the treatment of a specific condition (SPTL) are considered to be of poor quality, they should not be used to provide guidelines, make recommendations for use or initiate immediate change of practice.

Oxytocin Receptor Antagonists

Atosiban, though marketed as an oxytocin receptor antagonist, has far greater affinity for the vasopressin receptor in the uterus, so should correctly be labelled as a vasopressin/oxytocin receptor antagonist. Atosiban, like oxytocin, is a nonapeptide but with four changes to the molecule. Oxytocin binds to cell surface receptors following which there is release of secondary messengers that open voltage channels in the cell membrane through which there is an influx of extracellular Ca^{2+} into the cell. In addition, these secondary messengers cause release of intracellular Ca^{2+} stored within the sarcoplasmic reticulum. It is this increase in intracellular Ca^{2+} that promotes contractions. Atosiban's antagonism to vasopressin and oxytocin stems from competitive inhibition blocking vasopressin and oxytocin binding to the receptor. Accordingly, there is no release of secondary messengers, no increase in intracellular Ca^{2+} and therefore inhibition of contractions. The evidence base for atosiban as a tocolytic is much more robust than any other tocolytic. Lamont offers a detailed overview of the development and introduction of anti-oxytocic tocolytics [15].

The Worldwide Comparative Trial of Atosiban Versus β₂-agonists

This was a multinational, randomized, double-blind, double-dummy, controlled trial, the biggest tocolytic study ever undertaken and completed. However, though the numbers exceeded the combined nifedipine trials, like all other tocolytic studies they were still not powered to demonstrate benefit with respect to neonatal mortality or morbidity. In 15 centres in Canada and Israel, atosiban was compared with ritodrine. In 27 centres in the UK, Sweden, Denmark and Czech Republic, atosiban was compared with terbutaline, and in 37 centres in France and Australia, atosiban was compared with salbutamol. The component studies were published separately, but because the protocol was the same, the data were pooled and published together [16]. The methodology of the study was very strict, addressing and correcting most of the deficiencies of previously conducted β-agonist trials. The worldwide comparative trial required contractions, plus changes in cervical length and dilatation. Women who had received any other tocolytic in the six hours prior to admission were excluded and all the patients were enrolled before 34 completed weeks of gestation. Randomization was stratified above and below 28 weeks' gestation, alternative tocolytic therapy was permitted for failed treatment and retreatment was permitted following relapse after successful treatment, provided all the entry criteria remained intact. With respect to efficacy and tolerability (defined as no alternative tocolytic use and still undelivered after seven days), atosiban fared significantly better than ritodrine ($p = 0.029$) and salbutamol ($p = 0.021$). There was a trend towards benefit with respect to the use of terbutaline but this did not reach statistical significance ($p = 0.079$). The pooled data demonstrated highly statistically significant benefit of atosiban over β₂-agonists ($p = 0.0003$). Using pooled data to assess efficacy alone, 47.7% of those who received β₂-agonists compared to 59.6% of those who received atosiban remained undelivered after seven days ($p = 0.0004$), a 25% increase in efficacy.

The 2005 Cochrane Systematic Review of Oxytocin Receptor Antagonists

In 2005 a Cochrane systematic review was published that was critical of oxytocin receptor antagonists (effectively atosiban) for the treatment of SPTL [17]. The report has been criticized by a number of opinion leaders in the field. Some expressed concerns that there might have been unintentional bias in favour of CCBs and poor choice of language showing a favourable opinion of CCBs. This was particularly poignant bearing in mind the author of the review had been a co-author on the Cochrane CCBs systematic review whose paper most influenced the results alluded to above. The review was also criticized for having no rationale behind which trials were selected to evaluate both safety and efficacy, for making conclusions about CCBs being superior to β₂-agonists when this was not the subject of the review and for exemplifying the drawbacks of meta-analyses with respect to risk of selection bias and absence of quality weighting. Goodwin, much of whose published research occupied the review, expressed his concerns that acknowledgement of his assistance implied that he concurred with the review's conclusions. He felt the analysis was 'flawed' and 'not up to the high standards of Cochrane reviews'. Other groups recorded that the review contained a worrying degree of subjectivism with respect to study inclusion and interpretation that focused on data taken out of their original context and without reference to subject profiles. While space does not permit detailed discussion, this critical evaluation of nifedipine versus atosiban is extremely important and is described in detail elsewhere [18].

Safety of Tocolytics

Some of the safety concerns for β₂-agonists have already been discussed. Due to its uterospecificity, atosiban has placebo-level side-effects. Maternal cardiovascular side-effects occur in 8% of women who receive atosiban (similar to placebo) compared to 80% for those women who receive β₂-agonists. Similarly, 15 times more women are required to discontinue β₂-agonists compared to atosiban because of unacceptable side-effects ($p = 0.0001$) [16]. In a prospective cohort study evaluating the incidence of serious adverse drug reactions following the use of various tocolytic agents used for the treatment of SPTL in routine clinical practice, 1920 women from 28 hospitals in the Netherlands and Belgium were studied. The relative risk of any adverse drug reaction was 3.8 (95% CI = 1.6–9.2) for β_2-agonists compared with 0.07 (95% CI = 0.01–0.4) for atosiban. Serious adverse events occurred in 0/575 (0%) of women who received atosiban compared to 5/542 (0.9%) of women who received nifedipine and 3/175 (1.7%) of women who received β_2-agonists. Of 16 women who experienced severe adverse effects of tocolytic treatment, five had a twin pregnancy. Of six women who experienced serious dyspnoea, two (one of whom needed admission to the intensive care unit) were receiving more than one tocolytic. Similarly, of two other women who required admission to the intensive care unit, one with heart failure and the other with pulmonary oedema, both were receiving more than one tocolytic and one was pregnant with twins [19]. The message is clear: multiple pregnancy and combined tocolytic use is associated with the most serious adverse effects during tocolytic therapy.

Cardiovascular Actions of Nifedipine

The vascular:cardiac ratio of activity of nifedipine is in a proportion of 10:1. In vessels there is vasodilatation and in the heart there is cardio-depression from a negative inotropic and negative chronotropic effect. In healthy individuals, nifedipine-induced vasodilatation is followed by baroreceptor stimulation in the carotid sinus and aortic arch, followed by an increase in sympathetic tone that compensates for the cardio-depression. If nifedipine is used in twin pregnancies or in the presence of infection where there is already maximal vasodilatation, there is no baroreceptor stimulation, no increase in sympathetic tone and no cardiac compensation. If diminished cardiac output from cardiac disease such as pulmonary hypertension or cardiomyopathy is added to this and nifedipine is administered, the superimposed hypotension and negative inotropic and negative chronotropic effects result in serious cardio-depression [20].

Safety Concerns for Nifedipine

With increased use of nifedipine, between 1999 and 2005 there have been at least six reports from France, Holland, Belgium and Australia of serious feto-maternal adverse effects (maternal hypoxia, pulmonary oedema, myocardial infarction and maternal hypotension, and fetal death) following the use of nifedipine [21]. Accordingly, to evaluate the feto-maternal safety of CCBs in pregnancy, a quantitative systematic review was conducted. Of 269 relevant reports, including 5607 women, adverse feto-maternal events varied according to the total dose of nifedipine and study design. Adverse events were highest among women given more than 60 mg total dose of nifedipine (odds ratio (OR) 3.78; 95% confidence interval (CI) 1.27–11.2; $p = 0.017$) and in reports from case series compared to controlled studies (OR 2.45; 95% CI 1.17–5.15; $p = 0.018$). The adverse event rates generated from the study should be used to provide an evidence base for clinical guidelines and informed patient consent for CCB use in pregnancy [21]. For a more detailed account of the safety of tocolytics, the reader is referred to a recent review [36].

Cost of Tocolytic Therapy

Cost is a major factor in the choice of first line tocolytic therapy. Whether this emphasis is right or wrong, the decision should be evidence based and should include consideration of the balance between the costs of safety and efficacy. It is important to consider not simply drug costs, but the total cost of PTB. A course of the most expensive tocolytic (atosiban) is equivalent to the cost of six hours of care on the NICU. The comparison with other hospital drug budgets such as oncology, psychiatry, fertility and cardiology is important and empowering. The need for diagnostic testing, monitoring, need for change of drug and the cost of direct patient care (savings on midwifery time due to drug safety) are also important considerations in the comparison and choice of first line agent. There are also medico-legal implications if serious feto-maternal adverse events occur following the use or abuse of unlicensed drugs with safety concerns, when licensed, safer drugs with comparable efficacy are available.

International Differences in the Choice of First Line Tocolytic

Worldwide, there are significant differences in the choice of first line tocolytic. In 2009, in preparation for a lecture 'What's new in prematurity and tocolytics' at a Symposium on Uterine Contractility at the IX World Conference in Perinatal Medicine in Berlin, a survey of Western European practice was presented, which is

Table 21.1 National guidelines in European countries for first line tocolytic therapy

Countries	Current guidelines and organization	Treatment
United Kingdom	Royal College of Obstetricians and Gynaecologists (RCOG)	If tocolytics are to be used, atosiban or nifedipine are preferable. Atosiban is licensed and nifedipine is not. β-agonists should not be used (2002; revisions in progress).
Germany	DGGG (German Society of Gynecologists & Obstetricians)	No first line recommendation. Atosiban, fenoterol, nifedipine are equivalent. Atosiban has fewer side-effects (2008; revision July 2010).
Austria	OEGGG (Austrian Society GYN/OB)	β-agonists or atosiban. Atosiban first line for certain patient groups (2005; revision May 2010).
Switzerland	No national guidelines	N/A
Belgium	GGOLFB and VVOG	GGOLF atosiban first line treatment (48 hours) with options of 3× repetitive treatments (2005). VVOG atosiban preferred treatment of choice (2007).
Netherlands	Dutch Gynecology Society (NVOG)	Both atosiban and nifedipine a 'first place' position (2004; possible revision 2010).
France	PTL Guidelines CNGOF (College National des Gynecologues et Obstetriciens Francais)	Atosiban, β-agonists and nifedipine first line of treatment. In multiple pregnancies recommended first line: atosiban or nifedipine.
Italy	SLOG	No first line recommendation. Ritodrine and nifedipine are equivalent. Atosiban first line for 'at-risk patient' (2004).
Norway	Norwegian Society of Obstetrics and Gynaecology (NGF)	(1) atosiban; (2) nifedipine; (3) indomethicin; (4) terbutaline.
Denmark	Danish Society of Obstetrics and Gynecology (DSOG)	Recommendation of atosiban as first line of treatment.
Sweden	No national guidelines. Work in progress	80% of the guidelines at level III hospitals are recommending atosiban as first line.
Spain	PTL guideline No. 10 – SEGO (Spanish Society of Gynecology and Obstetrics)	Atosiban to be used as first choice (2004).
Portugal	No national guidelines	Hospitals implemented internal PTL guidelines. Atosiban or nifedipine are the most prescribed tocolytic drug. Atosiban for diabetic patients, multiple pregnancies and women with cardiac pathology.

summarized in Table 21.1. Colleagues from 13 Western European countries responded with details or lack of detail with respect to guidelines from their respective national professional bodies. Not all organizations recommended tocolytic use or nominated a first line choice but those who did suggested mainly atosiban or nifedipine and rarely β_2-agonists. The European guidelines for the management of SPTL including identification of SPTL, diagnosis of pPROM and tocolytic agents have recently been updated [22].

In Utero Transfer

Most clinicians accept that in utero transfer of a fetus at risk of PTB to a level III centre with NICU facilities is associated with a reduction in morbidity and an increase in survival. Of babies born between 26 and 34 completed weeks of gestation, those who were transferred in utero and born in a level III unit had a survival rate of 83% and a rate of intraventricular haemorrhage of 30% compared to those born in a level I or II centre and transferred neonatally (70% and 45% respectively; $p = 0.01$) [23]. The risk of death before 365 days among live-born infants born at a level III hospital was 26% compared with 44% for those that were not born at a level III hospital (OR = 0.49; 95% CI = 0.32–0.75) [24]. Because of its high specificity, the quantitative measurement of fFN may be of help in identifying those women who do not need in utero transfer.

Antepartum Glucocorticoids

There is no doubt that in both singleton and multiple pregnancies a full course of APGs significantly reduces the incidence of idiopathic respiratory distress syndrome, hyaline membrane disease and neonatal death. The recommended regimen is betamethasone 12 mg given intramuscularly in two doses 24 hours apart or dexamethasone 6 mg given intramuscularly in four doses 12 hours apart. In a review of 21 studies comprising 3885 women and 4269 infants, the treatment of women at risk of PTB with a single course of APGs reduced the risk of neonatal death by 31% (95% CI 19–42%), RDS by 44% (95% CI 31–57%) and intraventricular haemorrhage by 46% (95% CI 31–67%). APG use is also associated with a reduction in necrotizing enterocolitis, respiratory support, admission to the NICU and systemic infections in the first 48 hours of life compared with no treatment or treatment with placebo [25]. While the evidence for the use of APGs is most robust for gestational ages between 26 and 34 completed weeks of gestation, there is sufficient evidence to support the use of APGs prior to this gestational age range when senior staff consider that the case for administration has merit. APGs are most effective in reducing RDS in pregnancies that deliver after 24 hours and before seven days following administration of the second dose. While a full course of APGs is optimal, there is sufficient evidence that a partial course in the 24 hours prior to delivery still reduces the risk of neonatal death and should be given if delivery is expected within this time. While a single course of APGs appears to be safe on the basis of a risk–benefit assessment, there are concerns over the use of repeat courses of APGs. Accordingly, the optimal use of a single course is to be encouraged, but if the initial course was administered prior to 26 completed weeks of gestation, with senior staff approval, consideration could be given to repeating the course during the optimum gestational age range. Glucocorticoids have immunosuppressive qualities so their use in clinically suspected feto-maternal infections should only be undertaken following discussion with senior staff. In diabetic women, APGs may disturb diabetic control, particularly when their use is combined with β_2-agonist tocolytic therapy, under which circumstances greater attention should be paid to monitoring of blood sugar.

Intrapartum Monitoring of Preterm Infants

After the prevention of PTB, the next important goal is to deliver the preterm infant in optimal condition using the best possible surveillance during SPTL. The FHR is set by intrinsic mechanisms but is also under the influence of the autonomic nervous system. The sympathetic control of the FHR begins early in pregnancy, whereas the parasympathetic influence is minimal before late third trimester. Accordingly, the typical reactive CTG pattern with the combination of normal variability and accelerations develops from 31–34 weeks of gestation. This being the case, CTG interpretation before 31–32 weeks is more complicated than at term, and episodes of bradycardia and tachycardia are more likely to be due to disturbances of the intrinsic control rather than influence from the autonomic nervous system. What would be interpreted as a non-reassuring or abnormal intrapartum CTG pattern at term could be considered normal or showing no evidence of imminent asphyxia during SPTL. Surprisingly, a standardized and internationally approved intrapartum CTG classification for the preterm fetus has never been established, and to date, very little research has been conducted in this area [26]. Some well-known and recurrent features of the preterm FHR pattern have been described: (1) higher fetal baseline heart rate gradually decreasing with advancing gestational age; (2) frequency, duration and amplitude of accelerations are reduced; (3) FHR decelerations in the absence of uterine contractions are more frequent; (4) variable decelerations are present in up to 75% of all monitored SPTLs; and (5) baseline variability is decreased (including baseline fluctuations). Some iatrogenic factors contribute to changes in the FHR pattern in SPTL. Administration of some tocolytics (β_2-agonists) causes tachycardia, and opioids such as pethidine, steroids and magnesium sulphate reduce baseline variability. Fetal scalp blood sampling (FBS) can and should be used in conjunction with CTG monitoring during SPTL (Figure 21.1). However, the preterm fetus is more susceptible to acidosis and higher scalp pH cut-off levels should be employed. Immediate delivery is recommended if the scalp pH is below 7.25 (compared to 7.20 in term labour), and repeated FBS sampling is not recommended. The use of FBS in PTB has not been adequately validated. The fetal ECG has only been validated above 36 weeks' gestation and is therefore not recommended for use in SPTL before 36 weeks.

Mode of Delivery of the Preterm Infant

In both term and preterm deliveries, vaginal delivery (VD) should be the preferred route as it is associated with lower maternal morbidity and mortality. The reason for complications after preterm caesarean section (CS) is uncertain, as it is often difficult to determine whether it is the CS per se or the underlying

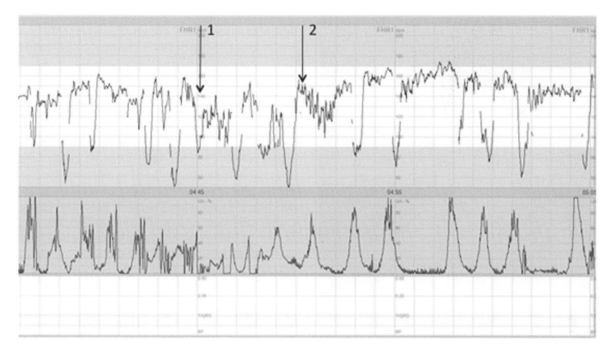

Figure 21.1 Non-reassuring preterm cardiotocographic trace. A nulliparous woman presented with contractions and spontaneous rupture of the membranes with maladorous amniotic fluid at 34 + 2/7 weeks' gestation. The cervical dilatation was 4–5 cm and the fetus was presenting cephalically with the presenting part above the ischial spines. Electronical fetal monitoring was established and at 04:45 h (arrow 1 on CTG trace) an intravenous injection of 0.25 mg of terbutaline was given for acute tocolysis to correct tachysystole and a non-reassuring CTG trace (complicated variable decelerations). Ten minutes later a fetal scalp blood sample (FBS – arrow 2) was performed with a pH of 7.17. An emergency caesarean section was carried out. The baby was born with a birth weight of 1960 g, with Apgar scores of 5[1] and 8[5] and umbilical cord artery pH of 7.07 and standard base excess of 12.6. See the colour plate section for a colour version of this figure.

indication for the CS that causes the complication. At early gestations, the lower segment of the uterus is poorly formed or undeveloped. Accordingly, at the time of preterm CS it may be necessary to perform a low classical uterine incision or a T- or J-incision on the uterus. The higher maternal risks of planned CS compared to VD are shown in Table 21.2. There are a number of factors that influence the decision with respect to mode of delivery of the preterm infant and some of these are listed in Table 21.3. Since the situation may change rapidly and there are two patients to consider, time may be limited to make optimal decisions. Finally, around the limits of viability (22–26 completed weeks of gestation) the decision may be particularly problematic and full discussion with the parents should involve the neonatal paediatricians. There are fetal risks of CS compared to VD. A poorly formed lower uterine segment may cause technical difficulties when delivering the infant. The baby's head is particularly vulnerable, with a risk of intracerebral haemorrhage as well as abdominal visceral injuries

Table 21.2 Greater maternal risks of planned caesarean section compared to vaginal delivery

- Maternal death (3–5-fold)
- Hysterectomy (2-fold)
- Intensive care/hospital stay more than seven days (2-fold)
- Postnatal infections
- Thrombosis and pulmonary embolism
- Excessive blood loss

Table 21.3 Factors affecting the decision with respect to mode of delivery in preterm labour

- Estimated birth weight
- Best estimate of gestational age
- Previous caesarean section
- Parity
- Evidence of IUGR
- Presence or history of antepartum haemorrhage
- Non-reassuring FHR pattern
- Duration of labour
- Descent of the presenting part
- State of the membranes (intact/ruptured/pPROM)
- Signs of intra-amniotic infection
- Presenting part (vertex or breech)

259

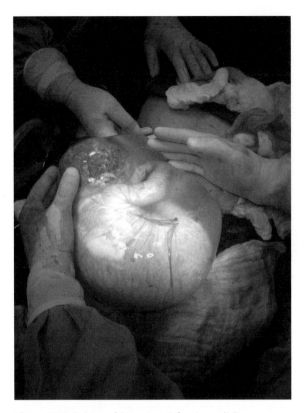

Figure 21.2 Delivery of the preterm infant 'en caul'. Caesarean section with 'en caul' delivery of the preterm infant within an intact amniotic sac with gentle and blunt removal from the uterine cavity to prevent pressure trauma to the head, abdominal viscera or injuries to the limbs and skin of the infant (with kind permission from Dr Aris Tsigris (www.aristsigris.gr/#). See the colour plate section for a colour version of this figure. For a video file of an 'en caul' delivery pleae visit www.cambridge.org/9781107472341.

and injuries to the limbs and skin. Accordingly, one method of delivering the preterm infant by CS to protect against such injuries is birth 'en caul', where the fetus is delivered within an intact amniotic sac (Figure 21.2). With elective CS without labour there is the additional risk of transient tachypnoea of the newborn, as well as idiopathic respiratory distress syndrome. Furthermore, there is a risk of iatrogenic prematurity where a planned CS may be a consequence of misdiagnosed labour (see above). Accordingly, a policy of planned CS for women in SPTL carries a higher risk of increasing numbers of PTBs. To date, only six RCTs to determine the optimum mode of delivery for the very preterm infant have been performed and all six trials were stopped early due to small numbers. These trials did not yield enough evidence to evaluate the use of planned CS vs. VD in SPTL. However, seven cases of major maternal postpartum complications in the CS arm were found compared to none in the VD arm in four of the trials (RR 7.21; 95% CI 1.37–38.08) [27].

Mode of Delivery of the Preterm Infant Presenting Cephalically

In general, VD for the preterm infant presenting cephalically is preferred, but CS can be justified for feto-maternal indications. Based on empirical data, for women presenting in SPTL with a cephalic presentation before 24 completed weeks of gestation, CS for a fetal indication is normally not justified. Between 24 and 26 completed weeks of gestation, CS for a fetal indication can be justified and after 26 completed weeks of gestation, CS for a fetal indication is always justified.

Mode of Delivery of the Preterm Infant Presenting by the Breech

For the preterm infant presenting by the breech, the risk of fetal complications after VD appear to be higher and hence a CS is often preferred. Before 32 completed weeks of gestation and/or with breech presentations with an estimate of fetal weight of <1500 g there is a substantial body of retrospective, descriptive literature that supports CS due to reduced neonatal mortality and morbidity. The risks pertaining to VD include a high incidence of footling breech presentation with greater likelihood of cord accidents and increased risk of asphyxia. Furthermore, there is a higher risk of entrapment of the after-coming head through an incompletely dilated cervix. Infant mortality and morbidity following delivery of the preterm infant presenting by the breech is inversely proportional to gestational age; several (older) reviews confirm this [28]. Large registry studies from the Nordic countries support these findings and report that VD of preterm infants is associated with a small but increased risk of infant death in breech and multiple births. However, in VD of vertex presentations there was no increased risk (excluding cases with pre-eclampsia) [29].

Vaginal Operative Deliveries of the Preterm Infant

It is generally accepted that vacuum extraction (VE) should not be performed before 34 weeks' gestation due to the higher risk of cephalhaematoma and intracranial haemorrhage. The use of forceps or episiotomy does not improve outcome. There are very few studies, most of which are inconclusive, on neonatal outcome after VE for PTB. The conclusions are that, in general, the rate of VE in PTB is very low but is associated with a higher risk of intracranial and extracranial haemorrhage and brachial plexus injury. This is in contrast to CS during SPTL compared with VD, in which there was no increased risk of these outcomes. The authors called for continued caution with use of VE for PTB, especially before 34 weeks' gestation [30].

Preterm Prelabour Rupture of the Membranes

Approximately one-third of all PTBs are preceded by pPROM, which is defined as rupture of the fetal membranes prior to 37 weeks' gestation before the onset of contractions. pPROM complicates only 2% of pregnancies but can result in significant neonatal morbidity and mortality mainly due to sepsis, immaturity and pulmonary hypoplasia. Accordingly, the management of pPROM is a balance between expectant management and the risk of infection versus early intervention and the risk of iatrogenic prematurity. The management of pPROM requires accurate diagnosis and will depend on gestational age. At term, prelabour rupture of the membranes usually results in spontaneous labour within 24 hours. In contrast, in 75% of pPROM before 28 completed weeks of gestation, labour has not started by one week. Traditionally, the diagnosis of pPROM has been clinical (detection of the characteristic pool of liquor on sterile speculum examination), ultrasonographic (oligohydramnios in association with a good history of pPROM), biophysical (the nitrazine test to detect pH change) and microscopic (characteristic crystalline ferning pattern of dried amniotic fluid). Recently, a biochemical method has become commercially available which comprises a rapid immunoassay for placental α-microglobulin-1 with a sensitivity and specificity of 98.9% and 100% respectively for the diagnosis of ruptured membranes. pPROM before 34 completed weeks of gestation is normally managed expectantly with the use of antibiotic prophylaxis and administration of a full course of APGs. The feto-maternal benefits of prophylactic antibiotics for the management of pPROM are well recognized, but the choice of antibiotic is still being debated. Following the findings of the ORACLE I study, most units administer prophylactic erythromycin, but this does not provide cover against many significant pathogens such as mycoplasmas and anaerobes, for which the addition of clindamycin should be considered. Between 34 and 37 completed weeks of gestation, obstetricians differ in their approach to pPROM. Some feel that the benefits of greater maturity outweigh the risks of infection and so follow expectant management. While birth between 34 and 37 completed weeks of gestation is associated with less neonatal mortality and morbidity, there is still a burden of death and handicap for PTBs during this period. Others feel that the risks of infection outweigh the risks of prematurity and so, if labour has not ensued within 48 hours, or when the course of APGs has been completed, they will induce labour and delivery.

Management of SPTL at the Limits of Viability

Around the limits of viability (22–26 completed weeks of gestation) the risk–benefit balance of some interventions may change. The use of interventions in which the risks of adverse events outweigh the theoretical benefits at 34 weeks' gestation may be considered at 24 weeks' gestation in a heroic attempt to improve outcome. Clearly a balance has to be reached between therapeutic nihilism and reckless imprudence, but there is some support for the beneficial use of combined interventions around the limits of viability that would not be considered at later gestations [31]. Parents should know what to expect with respect to obstetric interventions such as CS or neonatal resuscitation. It is therefore vitally important to ensure that midwives, obstetricians and neonatal paediatricians communicate with each other and that the resultant information to the parents on obstetric/neonatal intervention or no intervention is made perfectly clear.

Magnesium Sulphate as a Neuroprotective in the Management of PTB

While the rate of PTB is increasing [32] and the survival rate has improved, especially at very early gestations, the prevalence of cerebral palsy (CP) has increased. Since the incidence of CP is inversely related to gestational age, it would seem obvious to implement treatment strategies to reduce the risk of CP at early gestational ages. Some 15 years ago it was demonstrated that the outcome of infants born to mothers treated with magnesium sulphate, either as a tocolytic or for prophylaxis against eclampsia, caused a reduction in the rate of CP. This putative neuroprotective effect of magnesium sulphate was then demonstrated in RCTs and meta-analyses [33] where intravenous magnesium sulphate was compared to placebo in women at risk of PTB. A Cochrane review from 2009 found enough evidence to conclude the same, with a 32% reduction of CP (RR 0.68; CI 0.54–0.87) [34]. However, despite national guidelines from Australia, Canada and the UK which conclude that antenatal magnesium sulphate reduces the risk of CP in preterm infants, most obstetric departments have not implemented this as standard treatment. The American College of Obstetricians and Gynecologists stated 'the available evidence suggests that magnesium sulphate given before anticipated early PTB reduces the risk of CP in surviving infants. Physicians electing to use magnesium sulphate for fetal neuroprotection should develop specific guidelines regarding inclusion criteria, treatment regimens, concurrent tocolysis, and monitoring in accordance with one of the larger trials' [35]. Such guidelines would typically recommend inclusion at 24–31 completed weeks of gestation for both singletons and multiple pregnancies with pPROM, SPTL or elective PTB with expected delivery within 2–24 hours. A bolus of 5 g magnesium sulphate intravenously is followed by an infusion of 1 g/h in 24 hours or until delivery. Maternal adverse effects of magnesium sulphate like flushing, nausea, vomiting, hypotension and tachycardia are similar to those associated with the use of magnesium sulphate for the prevention of eclampsia.

Conclusions

PTB is the major cause of death and handicap in newborn babies world-wide, and a major drain on healthcare resources. The aetiology of PTB is multifactorial and prediction and prevention is difficult, so SPTL must be managed as it arises. Diagnosis is difficult and opinions differ on the merits or demerits of tocolytic intervention. There are many contraindications to intervention, but even if tocolytics are considered beneficial, there is still debate about the first line choice, based upon efficacy, safety and cost. If there are contraindications to intervention or if interventions are unsuccessful, there is still debate on monitoring and the best way to deliver the preterm infant. While most now accept the benefits of APGs and in utero transfer as means of reducing mortality and morbidity, there remains doubt about the 'who' and 'when' and in the case of APGs, 'how often'. Much more research into this important complication of labour is needed.

References

1. March of Dimes. March of Dimes white paper on preterm birth: the global and regional toll; 2009 (updated 16 December 2009). www.marchofdimes.org/materials/born-too-soon-global-action-report-on-preterm-birth.pdf (accessed 15 May 2016).

2. Downey LJ, Martin AJ. Ritodrine in the treatment of preterm labour: a study of 213 patients. *Br J Obstet Gynaecol.* 1983;90(11): 1046–53.

3. Leitich H. Controversies in diagnosis of preterm labour. *BJOG.* 2005;112(suppl. 1): 61–3.

4. Finnstrom O, Olausson PO, Sedin G, *et al.* The Swedish national prospective study on extremely low birthweight (ELBW) infants: incidence, mortality, morbidity and survival in relation to level of care. *Acta Paediatr.* 1997;86(5): 503–11.

5. Lamont RF, Dunlop PD, Crowley P, Elder MG. Spontaneous preterm labour and delivery at under 34 weeks' gestation. *BMJ.* 1983;286(6363): 454–7.

6. King JF, Grant A, Keirse MJ, Chalmers I. Beta-mimetics in preterm labour: an overview of the randomized controlled trials. *Br J Obstet Gynaecol.* 1988;95(3): 211–22.

7. Valenzuela GJ, Sanchez-Ramos L, Romero R, *et al.* Maintenance treatment of preterm labor with the oxytocin antagonist atosiban: the Atosiban PTL-098 Study Group. *Am J Obstet Gynecol.* 2000;182(5): 1184–90.

8. Haas DM, Imperiale TF, Kirkpatrick PR, *et al.* Tocolytic therapy: a meta-analysis and decision analysis. *Obstet Gynecol.* 2009;113(3): 585–94.

9. Lamont RF. The pathophysiology of pulmonary oedema with the use of beta-agonists. *BJOG.* 2000;107(4): 439–44.

10. Oei SG, Mol BW, de Kleine MJ, Brolmann HA. Nifedipine versus ritodrine for suppression of preterm labor: a meta-analysis. *Acta Obstet Gynecol Scand.* 1999;78(9): 783–8.

11. Tsatsaris V, Papatsonis D, Goffinet F, Dekker G, Carbonne B. Tocolysis with nifedipine or beta-adrenergic agonists: a meta-analysis. *Obstet Gynecol.* 2001;97(5 Pt 2): 840–7.

12. King JF, Flenady V, Papatsonis D, Dekker G, Carbonne B. Calcium channel blockers for inhibiting preterm labour: a systematic review of the evidence and a protocol for administration of nifedipine. *A N Z J Obstet Gynaecol.* 2003;43(3): 192–8.

13. King JF, Flenady VJ, Papatsonis DN, Dekker GA, Carbonne. B. Calcium channel blockers for inhibiting preterm labour. *Cochrane Database Syst Rev.* 2003;1: CD002255.

14. Lamont RF, Khan KS, Beattie B, *et al.* The quality of nifedipine studies used to assess tocolytic efficacy: a systematic review. *J Perinat Med.* 2005;33(4): 287–95.

15. Lamont RF. The development and introduction of anti-oxytocic tocolytics. *BJOG.* 2003;110(suppl. 20): 108–12.

16. Worldwide Atosiban versus Beta-agonists Study Group. Effectiveness and safety of the oxytocin antagonist atosiban versus beta-adrenergic agonists in the treatment of preterm labour. *BJOG.* 2001;108(2): 133–42.

17. Papatsonis D, Flenady V, Cole S, Liley H. Oxytocin receptor antagonists for inhibiting preterm labour. *Cochrane Database Syst Rev.* 2005;3: CD004452.

18. Lyndrup J, Lamont RF. The choice of a tocolytic for the treatment of preterm labor: a critical evaluation of nifedipine versus atosiban. *Expert Opin Investig Drugs.* 2007;16(6): 843–53.

19. de Heus R, Mol BW, Erwich JJ, *et al.* Adverse drug reactions to tocolytic treatment for preterm labour: prospective cohort study. *BMJ.* 2009;338: b744.

20. Scholz H. Pharmacological aspects of calcium channel blockers. *Cardiovasc Drugs Ther.* 1997;10(suppl. 3): 869–72.

21. Khan K, Zamora J, Lamont RF, *et al.* Safety concerns for the use of calcium channel blockers in pregnancy for the treatment of spontaneous preterm labour and hypertension: a systematic review and meta-regression analysis. *J Matern Fetal Neonat Med.* 2010;23(9): 1030–8.

22. Di Renzo GC, Roura LC, Facchinetti F, *et al.* Guidelines for the management of spontaneous preterm labor: identification of spontaneous preterm labor, diagnosis of preterm premature rupture of membranes, and preventive tools for preterm birth. *J Matern Fetal Neonat Med.* 2011;24(5): 659–67.

23. Lamont RF, Dunlop PD, Crowley P, Levene MI, Elder MG. Comparative mortality and morbidity of infants transferred in utero or postnatally. *J Perinat Med.* 1983;11(4): 200–3.

24. Fellman V, Hellstrom-Westas L, Norman M, *et al.* One-year survival of extremely preterm infants after active perinatal care in Sweden. *JAMA.* 2009;301(21): 2225–33.

25. Roberts D, Dalziel S. Antenatal corticosteroids for accelerating fetal lung maturation for women at risk of preterm birth. *Cochrane Database Syst Rev.* 2006;3: CD004454.

26. Afors K, Chandraharan E. Use of continuous electronic fetal monitoring in a preterm fetus: clinical dilemmas and recommendations for practice. *J Pregnancy.* 2011; 848794. doi: 10.1155/2011/848794.

27. Alfirevic Z, Milan SJ, Livio S. Caesarean section versus vaginal delivery for preterm birth in singletons. *Cochrane Database Syst Rev.* 2013;9: CD000078.

28. Bergenhenegouwen LA, Meertens LJ, Schaaf J, *et al.* Vaginal delivery versus caesarean section in preterm breech delivery: a systematic review. *Eur J Obstet Gynecol Reproduct Biol.* 2014;172: 1–6.

29. Hogberg U, Holmgren PA. Infant mortality of very preterm infants by mode of delivery, institutional policies and maternal diagnosis. *Acta Obstet Gynecol Scand.* 2007;86(6): 693–700.

30. Aberg K, Norman M, Ekeus C. Preterm birth by vacuum extraction and neonatal outcome: a population-based cohort study. *BMC Pregnancy Childbirth.* 2014;14: 42.

31. Ingemarsson I. Tocolytic therapy and clinical experience: combination therapy. *BJOG.* 2005;112 (suppl. 1): 89–93.

32. Langhoff-Roos J, Kesmodel U, Jacobsson B, Rasmussen S, Vogel I. Spontaneous preterm delivery in primiparous women at low risk in Denmark: population based study. *BMJ.* 2006;332(7547): 937–9.

33. Conde-Agudelo A, Romero R. Antenatal magnesium sulfate for the prevention of cerebral palsy in preterm infants less than 34 weeks' gestation: a systematic review and metaanalysis. *Am J Obstet Gynecol.* 2009;200(6): 595–609.

34. Doyle LW, Crowther CA, Middleton P, Marret S. Antenatal magnesium sulfate and neurologic outcome in preterm infants: a systematic review. *Obstet Gynecol.* 2009;113(6): 1327–33.

35. ACOG. Committee opinion no. 455: magnesium sulfate before anticipated preterm birth for neuroprotection. *Obstet Gynecol.* 2010;115(3): 669–71.

36. Lamont CD, Jorgensen JS, Lamont RF. The safety of tocolytics used for the inhibition of preterm labour. *Expert Opin Drug Saf.* 2016, May 9.

Chapter 22

Labour in Women with Medical Disorders

Mandish K. Dhanjal and Catherine Nelson-Piercy

Introduction

The process of labour and delivery affects the maternal physiology in a number of ways that are important to consider when managing women with medical disorders. Cardiac output greatly increases and the pain of labour causes extreme stress and increases catecholamine release. Extra energy is required to push in the second stage and the rise in arterial and venous pressure may raise concerns in those with vulnerable coronary and cerebral circulations. Bowel transit time is reduced and this and gastric stasis leads to delayed drug absorption such that many drugs will need to be administered parenterally to be effective.

There are relatively few conditions where caesarean section (CS) is recommended for medical indications. There is an increased tendency for obstetricians to induce labour or to perform a CS in women with medical disorders, often to ensure the availability of suitable personnel or to adjust anticoagulation. However, induction is more likely to lead to prolonged labour, epidural use and an increase in instrumental delivery. Caesarean section carries inherent risks of thrombosis and infection which may compound a pre-existing tendency to these complications in conditions such as previous venothromboembolism and those on immunosuppressive agents or steroids.

Some conditions may deteriorate around labour and delivery, such as sickle cell disease, diabetes, epilepsy, critical heart disease and restrictive lung disease. Others, such as asthma and arrhythmias, are not affected by labour.

Some drugs which are commonly used in labour and delivery such as ergometrine, boluses of Syntocinon and prostaglandin F2α (carboprost) may cause deterioration in certain forms of heart and respiratory disease. Clearly documented plans for suitable alternatives should be made prior to labour in the event of postpartum haemorrhage (PPH).

Clear management plans for delivery and postnatal care should be made and agreed by the multidisciplinary team and the woman in advance and should be placed at the front of the patient's handheld notes, allowing all members of the intrapartum and postnatal team to be fully informed. As the patient may need medical attention as an emergency in a different hospital, contact information for the multidisciplinary team should also be written in the delivery care plan [1].

Key conditions which require multidisciplinary management plans prior to labour and delivery will be discussed in this chapter.

Heart Disease

The intrapartum management of women with heart disease should be supervised by an obstetrician and anaesthetist experienced in the care of women with heart disease. An appropriately experienced cardiologist or obstetric physician should also be readily available.

The key concerns in labour and delivery in a woman with heart disease are [2]:

- reducing the effect of tachycardia and increased cardiac output in labour;
- managing anticoagulation;
- timing and mode of delivery;
- ensuring effective analgesia;
- bacterial endocarditis prophylaxis; and
- management of PPH.

By term the cardiac output will have increased by 25% due mainly to an increase in stroke volume, but also a 10–20 bpm increase in the resting heart rate. In

---

Best Practice in Labour and Delivery, Second Edition, ed. Sir Sabaratnam Arulkumaran. Published by Cambridge University Press. © Cambridge University Press 2016.

labour the cardiac output increases further, by 15% in the first stage and 50% in the second stage to a mean of 10.6 l/min. The sympathetic response to uncontrolled pain in labour is likely to contribute significantly to this increased cardiac output. There are similar, but less marked, increases in cardiac output during CS. Following delivery of the placenta there is up to a 1 l auto-transfusion of blood, necessitating a further rise in cardiac output by 60–80%. This is followed by a rapid decline back to prelabour values within one hour of delivery. These dramatic cardiovascular changes may be poorly tolerated by women with heart disease. Avoidance of tachycardia is possible through effective analgesia, limited exertion in the second stage of labour and cautious use of Syntocinon for the third stage.

Managing Anticoagulation

See the section below on intrapartum management of anticoagulation.

Timing of Delivery

This is usually dependent on the severity of maternal disease and any associated maternal compromise. In women with cyanotic heart disease there may be significant fetal growth restriction which may warrant preterm delivery. A judgement needs to be made as to the gestation of delivery, taking into consideration the neonatal morbidity and mortality associated with preterm birth. If delivery is to occur before 34 weeks' gestation, antenatal steroids should be administered for fetal lung maturity. In a woman at risk of pulmonary oedema, due care and monitoring should occur for 24–48 hours following steroid administration, which can result in fluid retention and cardiac decompensation responsive to diuretics.

Delivery in a tertiary unit is recommended for those with moderate or severe cardiac disease. Induction of labour may be considered in those on therapeutic anticoagulation or those with complex or severe heart disease to allow for adjustment of anticoagulation, insertion of lines for invasive monitoring and availability of relevant senior staff to be present for the delivery. Induction of labour may also be required if maternal cardiac function starts deteriorating near term. Prostaglandin E2 can be used for induction of labour, as can Syntocinon. The doses of Syntocinon used for induction and augmentation of labour are not sufficient to cause concern about maternal

> **Box 22.1** Cardiac Indications for Caesarean Section
>
> - Aortic root dilatation: progressive enlargement or ≥4.5 cm
> - Severe peripartum cardiomyopathy/severe left ventricular dysfunction
> - Aortic dissection

tachycardia; however, prolonged use can result in fluid retention through its antidiuretic effect, which may precipitate pulmonary oedema. To prevent this it is sensible to administer the oxytocin though a syringe driver in a small volume of normal saline, e.g. 50 ml rather than 1 l.

Mode of Delivery

In general, vaginal delivery should be the aim for most women with congenital or acquired heart disease unless there is an obstetric or specific cardiac indication for CS. There are few conditions where CS is recommended (see Box 22.1). Consideration should be given to performing a sterilization at the same time as CS in non-reversible severe conditions such as pulmonary arterial hypertension. This should be fully discussed with the patient antenatally. The CS should be performed in operating theatres that have access to cardiothoracic facilities when it is being performed for cardiac indications.

Lithotomy and supine positions should be avoided during vaginal delivery. Lithotomy results in increased venous return, which may not be tolerated in those with severe stenotic heart lesions or those at risk of heart failure. The supine position reduces venous return and can reduce cardiac output by 25%, resulting in fetal compromise. The delivery position best tolerated is with the woman sitting upright with her legs lower than her abdomen and her feet supported on foot rests or on reversed lithotomy poles.

The active second stage may need to be shortened or avoided in those with severe heart disease who would not tolerate the increased cardiac output associated with pushing, such as those with ischaemic heart disease, critical mitral or aortic stenosis. In such cases the head descends through the pelvis in the passive second stage followed by an instrumental delivery of the baby.

A dilute infusion of 5 units of Syntocinon in 20 ml normal saline over 30 min is recommended for the third stage in women with moderate or severe heart disease. Ergometrine can be used in women with peripartum cardiomyopathy, but should not be used in patients who will decompensate with the resulting peripheral vasoconstriction and coronary vasospasm and tachycardia, i.e. those with stenotic valvular lesions, pulmonary hypertension, ischaemic heart disease or hypertension.

Effective Regional Analgesia

This is an important element in the management of delivery in women with severe heart disease. The advantages are that of minimization of pain and hence a reduced heart rate and blood pressure, peripheral vasodilatation, reducing preload and effective analgesia so that procedures such as assisted vaginal delivery and CS can be performed. Consultant anaesthetic involvement is imperative.

Monitoring

Invasive monitoring in labour is recommended, with arterial and central venous lines for those with severe heart disease. Pulmonary wedge pressure readings are not usually necessary.

Infective Endocarditis

Infective endocarditis (IE) is a rare, potentially fatal condition that may arise following bacteraemia in a patient with a predisposing cardiac lesion. Cardiac conditions at risk of developing infective endocarditis are:

- acquired valvular heart disease with stenosis or regurgitation;
- valve replacement;
- structural congenital heart disease, including surgically corrected or palliated structural conditions;
- previous infective endocarditis; and
- hypertrophic cardiomyopathy.

Cardiac conditions not considered to be at risk of developing infective endocarditis include isolated atrial septal defect, fully repaired ventricular septal defect or fully repaired patent ductus arteriosus, and closure devices that are judged to be endothelialized.

Since 2008 the National Institute of Health and Clinical Excellence (NICE) no longer recommends antibiotic cover to prevent IE in someone at risk of developing it during the process of gynaecological and obstetric procedures and childbirth *unless* they require antibiotics for a suspected infection at the site of the procedure, e.g. chorioamnionitis [3]. In these circumstances, in addition to antibiotics for the infection suspected, they should be given an antibiotic that covers organisms causing IE, e.g. gentamicin or vancomycin. This approach should also be used in a woman with sepsis.

Postpartum Haemorrhage

Syntocinon may be given cautiously in women with severe heart disease, as long as it is given slowly and in low doses. Bolus doses of Syntocinon can cause vasodilatation and severe hypotension. Ergometrine should be avoided in the conditions described previously. Carboprost, a synthetic prostaglandin F2α, causes bronchospasm and is generally avoided in cardiac patients. Misoprostol, a synthetic prostaglandin analogue, given orally, sublingually or rectally, can cause hyperthermia, particularly at higher doses, but is otherwise well tolerated and is an effective agent at stopping PPH due to uterine atony.

Intrauterine tamponade using hydrostatic balloons such as the Rusch balloon can be used in cases of uterine atony. Antibiotic cover should be given while the balloon is *in situ*. At CS, mechanical uterine compression sutures, such as the B-Lynch brace suture, may be effective at controlling uterine haemorrhage due to atony.

Postpartum Care

High vigilance should be employed postnatally, and multidisciplinary maternal surveillance maintained due to the haemodynamic changes that occur postpartum.

Thrombosis

Women with a venous thromboembolism (VTE) in pregnancy will be on treatment doses of low molecular weight heparin (LMWH). Induction of labour and CS should be for obstetric indications. Operative delivery increases the risk of further thrombosis and should be avoided if possible. Low molecular weight

Table 22.1 Therapeutic doses of LMWH

	Early pregnancy weight (kg)	Enoxaparin	Dalteparin	Tinzaparin
Antenatally		1 mg/kg bd	100 units/kg bd	175 units/kg daily for all weights
	<50	40 mg bd	5000 IU bd	
	50–69	60 mg bd	6000 IU bd	
	70–89	80 mg bd	8000 IU bd	
	>90	100 mg bd	10 000 IU bd	
Postnatally		1.5 mg/kg od or 0.75 mg/kg bd	70 units/kg bd	175 units/kg daily

heparin should be stopped as described in the intrapartum management of anticoagulation section below. During labour, graduated elastic compression stockings should be worn. If Flowtron boots are available, these should be used. The woman should be kept well hydrated and remain mobile if possible.

Intrapartum Management of Anticoagulation

Women may present for delivery on prophylactic (e.g. 40 mg enoxaparin) high prophylactic (e.g. 40 mg 12-hourly enoxaparin daily), or full anticoagulant doses of LMWH (see Table 22.1), occasionally fully anticoagulated on warfarin. The approach to the management of anticoagulation for labour and delivery is dependent on the indication for anticoagulation, and therefore the importance of maintaining a given antithrombotic or anticoagulant effect [4,5].

For women receiving prophylactic doses of LMWH, this is usually because of previous thromboembolic events or because of an increased risk of venous thromboembolism in, for example, women admitted with pre-eclampsia. Some women with antiphospholipid syndrome may be receiving prophylactic LMWH for previous adverse pregnancy outcome.

In all the situations described below it is imperative that joint protocols are developed, agreed and documented between obstetricians and obstetric anaesthetists such that women may be informed prior to delivery of the issues and likely plan for discontinuation of anticoagulants, delivery, and analgesia and anaesthesia. In some circumstances, including the fully anticoagulated woman, individual referral to an obstetric anaesthetist is appropriate. Epidural haematoma is a very rare complication of regional anaesthesia in patients receiving LMWH; however,

Table 22.2 Cautionary use of regional analgesia techniques in pregnant women on LMWH

Action	Criteria	Timing to avoid epidural haematoma
Regional analgesia can be given	On prophylactic LMWH	≥12 h after last dose
	On therapeutic LMWH	≥24 h after last dose
Epidural catheter removal	On LMWH	10–12 h after last dose
	Next dose LMWH	≥3 h after removal

caution is recommended. There is international consensus regarding the desired intervals between LMWH doses and insertion or removal of regional analgesia/anaesthesia catheters or needles (see Table 22.2).

If analgesia is required for labour before it is considered safe to administer a regional block, fentanyl patient-controlled analgesia may be used with senior anaesthetic involvement.

Intrapartum Anticoagulation Management in Specific Situations

Women Receiving Prophylactic Low-Dose LMWH for Recurrent Miscarriage or Previous Adverse Pregnancy Outcome

In these circumstances, LMWH can be discontinued at 34–37 weeks unless there are risk factors for VTE, in which case it can be discontinued 12 hours prior to planned induction, CS or at the onset of labour. There is no need to restart LMWH postpartum unless there is a thrombophilia or other identified risk factors for VTE.

Women Receiving Prophylactic Low-Dose LMWH for VTE Prophylaxis Because of Previous VTE or Other Identified Risk Factors for VTE

These women may be advised to discontinue LMWH 12 hours prior to planned induction, CS or at the onset of labour. This ensures that for planned delivery there is at least a 12-hour window to allow siting of regional anaesthesia or analgesia.

There is a possibility that with this strategy, particularly in a multiparous woman in whom the plan is to await the onset of spontaneous labour, that she may request (and be declined) an epidural within 12 hours of her last dose of LMWH. This is also more likely in women receiving high-dose prophylaxis (e.g. enoxaparin 40 mg twice daily). This possibility should be discussed with the individual patient and a risk assessment made of the relative merits of earlier discontinuation of LMWH versus a possible delay in receiving pain relief via an epidural.

If a CS is required less than 12 hours after the last dose of LMWH, this will need to be performed under general anaesthetic. Alternatively, it may be appropriate to request an anti-Xa level and proceed with a regional block if this is very low.

LMWH should be restarted within 4–6 hours postpartum and continued for six weeks in the case of previous VTE, hereditary thrombophilia with a family history, or sickle cell disease.

Women Fully Anticoagulated with LMWH

The main indications for full anticoagulation in pregnancy are:

1. VTE in the current pregnancy; and
2. metal heart valves.

VTE in the Current Pregnancy [4]

The highest risk of further thrombosis or a pulmonary embolus following a deep venous thrombosis is in the first few weeks after the index event. This provides a very strong rationale for delaying delivery if possible in women who develop VTE at or near term. This allows for a longer period of full anticoagulation before the necessary temporary interruption for delivery. These women can be managed in a similar way to women on prophylactic LMWH but with cessation of LMWH 24 hours prior to planned induction, CS or at the onset of labour. For a CS, regional anaesthesia can then be safely employed. For women in labour or undergoing induction of labour, several strategies are possible starting from 24 hours after the last therapeutic dose of LMWH:

1. Withhold heparin until after delivery (facilitating use of regional analgesia if required); not suitable if VTE less than one week before delivery.
2. Give further prophylactic dose of LMWH every 24 hours in labour (considering/offering siting of an epidural prior to each dose).
3. Give doses of subcutaneous prophylactic unfractionated heparin (7500 IU) every 12 hours (allowing siting of an epidural after two hours).
4. Elective placement of an epidural catheter that may be used if required (allowing a further dose of LMWH to be given after three hours).
5. Use intravenous unfractionated heparin (UFH). The dose of intravenous heparin used is designed to provide prophylactic levels (about 1000 units/hour). The infusion is discontinued at onset of the second stage of labour or interrupted 1–2 hours prior to regional anaesthesia or analgesia.

All strategies should include use of grade II elastic compression stockings. Whichever option is employed, the implications should be carefully explained to the woman. Full anticoagulant doses of LMWH should be recommended after delivery, remembering that the correct therapeutic dose for enoxaparin and dalteparin falls to the normal non-pregnant dose, i.e. 1.5 mg/kg daily. This can be divided into a bd regime if there is concern about giving a large bolus dose. If there is concern about PPH, the dose can be kept at high prophylactic levels until this concern passes. It is important to remember that PPH and blood transfusion are independent risk factors for VTE.

Metal Heart Valves

Women with metal heart valves may be on warfarin or full therapeutic doses of LMWH antenatally to prevent valve thrombosis [6]. Warfarin should be stopped ten days to two weeks prior to delivery to allow clearance of warfarin by the fetus. Anticoagulation should then be continued with full anticoagulant doses of LMWH which does not cross the placenta. When LMWH is used, low-dose aspirin (75 mg daily) should be added as an adjunctive antithrombotic therapy.

Many clinicians prefer to plan delivery in women with mechanical heart valves. The risk of valve thrombosis is high in these women and for those maintained on warfarin antenatally, stopping this at 36 weeks, replacing it with full anti-coagulation doses of heparin, and inducing labour or performing a CS (if obstetrically indicated) at 38 weeks minimizes the time spent off warfarin. In women where the risk of thrombosis is lower (large aortic new-generation valves, e.g. Carbomedics) for whom the decision was taken to convert to LMWH for the entire pregnancy, it would seem reasonable to await spontaneous labour unless there is an obstetric reason for earlier delivery.

LMWH should be stopped as soon as contractions start. If labour is to be induced, LMWH should be stopped 24 hours before induction. Regional analgesia can be administered 24 hours after the last dose of therapeutic LMWH.

As a general rule, some form of anticoagulation should be administered within 24 hours of the last dose of therapeutic LMWH. Thus option (1) above is not appropriate for women with metal valves. Options (2)–(4) may be employed, but some clinicians prefer to use option (5). The latter is labour intensive, requires admission to hospital and careful monitoring of APTT levels which can be very problematic, and often leads to under- or overanticoagulation.

For women with VTE in the index pregnancy or those with mechanical valves, full anticoagulant doses of heparin should be resumed after delivery. This can be with subcutaneous LMWH. Conversion back to warfarin should be delayed for at least 5–7 days to minimize the risk of secondary PPH. It is important to continue LMWH until the INR is ≥ 2 for VTE or INR ≥ 2.5 with mechanical valves.

Women Presenting in Labour or Needing Urgent Delivery Fully Anticoagulated on Warfarin or Heparin

In the event of an urgent need to deliver a fully anticoagulated patient, warfarin may be reversed with fresh frozen plasma (FFP) and vitamin K (1 mg intravenously is usually sufficient), and UFH with protamine sulphate. Unfractionated heparin has a short half-life and reversal is not usually required (especially not with doses of 1000 units per hour as suggested above). LMWH is partially reversed with protamine sulphate. However, bleeding complications are uncommon with LMWH. There is a 2% chance of

Table 22.3 Action for treatment and delivery according to platelet count

Platelet count × 10⁹/L	Action
<20	Treat*
>20	Treat if symptomatic*
30	Possibly safe for vaginal delivery
>50	Safe for vaginal delivery and caesarean section
>80#	Considered safe for regional analgesia

Notes
* treatment may be with steroids, intravenous human IgG (IVIG), anti-D or platelet transfusion, depending on aetiology of thrombocytopenia
\# thromboelastography may be helpful

wound haematoma with both LMWH and UFH. If a fully anticoagulated patient requires a CS, this should be performed under general anaesthesia with consideration given to insertion of wound drains and use of staples or interrupted skin sutures.

If vitamin K has been given, anticoagulation with warfarin postpartum becomes very difficult. Both warfarin and LMWH are safe to use in a mother who is or intends to breastfeed.

Thrombocytopenia

The key concerns in labour and delivery in a woman with thrombocytopenia are [7]:

- administering a regional anaesthetic;
- surgical bleeding;
- PPH; and
- fetal intracranial haemorrhage in a thrombocytopenic fetus.

Anaesthetists will usually not site a regional anaesthetic if the platelet count is $<80 \times 10^9/L$ due to concerns around epidural haematoma. Surgical incisions can, however, be made safely with counts of $>50 \times 10^9/L$. The aim of pre-delivery is to keep the platelet count above $50 \times 10^9/L$ (see Table 22.3).

Delivery is the time of maximum concern for the thrombocytopenic mother. The risk of maternal and fetal haemorrhage is not reduced with CS compared with an uncomplicated vaginal delivery. Caesarean section should therefore only be performed for obstetric reasons. Ventouse delivery should be avoided, but the use of traction forceps should be considered if there is a delay in the second stage.

If the third stage is managed actively using oxytocin, there is seldom excessive bleeding from the placental bed. However, there is a risk of bleeding from surgical incisions, soft tissue injuries and tears. A cord platelet count should be performed.

Imminent Delivery with a Platelet Count $<50 \times 10^9/L$

Management of a patient with a platelet count of $<50 \times 10^9/L$ who is soon to deliver will depend on the aetiology of the thrombocytopenia. It is important to increase the platelet count above $50 \times 10^9/L$ to prevent maternal bleeding. Close liaison with the consultant haematologist should occur. If the diagnosis is idiopathic thrombocytopenic purpura (ITP), a condition caused by anti-platelet antibodies, platelet transfusion will only help transiently, as the antibodies will destroy the platelets transfused. Platelets should only be transfused in this instance if delivery is imminent or if an invasive procedure such as central venous line insertion is required. They should be transfused immediately prior to the procedure. If delivery is not imminent, treatment should be with intravenous human IgG (IVIG), which can raise the count within 48–72 hours. Anti-D can be used as an alternative if the woman is Rhesus positive, but may not be available at the high doses required. Steroids take longer to elevate the platelet count.

If the thrombocytopenia is not due to anti-platelet antibodies, then platelets can be transfused to elevate the count. Platelet transfusion will also be beneficial where there are abnormally functioning platelets. In conditions where the patient may require recurrent platelet transfusions in the future, HLA-matched platelets should be ordered if time permits.

Inherited Coagulation Deficiencies

Haemophilia and von Willebrand Disease (VWD)

Haemophilia A and B are sex-linked recessive disorders with a deficiency of coagulation factors VIII (FVIII) and factor IX (FIX) respectively. Heterozygous female carriers usually have FVIII and FIX levels 50% of normal, but are usually asymptomatic. There is a 50% chance that any male offspring will have haemophilia A or B.

> **Box 22.2 Situations in which Prophylactic Treatment will be Required**
>
> - Any clotting factor level of <50 IU/dl prior to insertion of a regional block (which should be performed by a senior anaesthetist) and for all types of delivery.
> - Type 2 VWD for operative delivery or perineal trauma.
> - Type 3 VWD for all types of delivery.
>
> Regional analgesia/anaesthesia is generally not recommended for those with type 2 or 3 VWD.

Von Willebrand disease is a quantitative or qualitative deficiency of von Willebrand factor (VWF). Deficiency of VWF results in FVIII deficiency and abnormal platelet function. Types 1 and 2 are autosomal dominant and type 3 is autosomal recessive.

Treatment

Maternal FVIII levels and VWF increase with gestation and may be normal by the time of labour and delivery. Maternal FIX levels do not rise significantly in pregnancy. A plan for delivery should be made with the haematologist, obstetrician and anaesthetist before delivery [8,9].

Treatment should be given with haematological advice (see Box 22.2). Recombinant factor VIII or IX may be used as well as Desmopressin (DDAVP). DDAVP is a synthetic analogue of vasopressin which increases the levels of endogenous VWF and FVIII in patients with mild haemophilia A, in carriers of haemophilia A and in most patients with VWD. It increases the level of VWF and FVIII 3–5-fold within half-hour. The increased levels are maintained for 6–8 hours. Close monitoring for water retention should accompany DDAVP use. It should be used only with caution in women who also have pre-eclampsia.

Delivery

Women with hereditary coagulation deficiencies who are pregnant with an affected fetus and women with severe VWD should deliver at a unit where the necessary expertise in the management of these disorders and resources for laboratory testing and clotting factor treatments are readily available. Blood should be grouped and saved.

The male fetus of a haemophilia A or B carrier and the male or female fetus of a woman with VWD types

1 and 2 have a 50% chance of being affected. Vaginal delivery carries a small risk of serious fetal or neonatal bleeding in an affected fetus, which may be reduced, but is not eliminated by CS. After discussion with the couple, if vaginal delivery is chosen with an affected or potentially affected fetus, fetal scalp electrodes, scalp fetal blood sampling, ventouse extraction and rotational forceps delivery should not be performed. Lift-out forceps may be used if required. A prolonged second stage should be avoided. The third stage should be actively managed. Cord blood should be sent for clotting factor assay in all male offspring of haemophilia carriers. VWF is elevated in the neonate and testing should be delayed.

Postnatally

The gestation-related rise in FVIII and VWF reverts postnatally. Prophylactic recombinant clotting factor or DDAVP may be required to keep clotting factor levels >50 IU/dl for 3–5 days following delivery. Tranexamic acid may help control prolonged and/or intermittent secondary PPH. The affected neonate should be given oral vitamin K.

Sickle Cell Disease

Women with sickle cell disease should be delivered in hospitals which have the relevant multidisciplinary team available to manage any complications that may arise from sickle cell disease and from high-risk pregnancies [10]. This will usually be a tertiary unit. Preterm birth is common in those with sickle cell disease. This is due to spontaneous preterm labour as well as iatrogenic due to complications including preeclampsia, recurrent crises and placental insufficiency from placental infarcts leading to fetal growth restriction.

Pregnant women with sickle cell disease who have a normally grown fetus should be offered delivery after 38 weeks' gestation, usually by induction of labour. Vaginal birth after CS can be considered. When aiming for a vaginal delivery, consideration should be given to suitable birthing positions in women who have avascular necrosis of the hips, with or without hip replacement(s).

Operative delivery increases the risk of infection, sickle cell crises, acute chest syndrome (ACS) and thromboembolism in women with sickle cell disease and hence CS should only be performed for obstetric reasons.

There should be close involvement with the haematology consultant. Before a planned delivery in a woman with recurrent crises or ACS, it may be necessary to perform an exchange transfusion, particularly if the percentage of sickle cells is high.

Sickle cell crises can be precipitated by dehydration, infection and the increased catecholamine response to pain, all of which may occur in labour. Women should be kept well hydrated and warm, and receive 2 l/min oxygen via nasal prongs or mask. Regional analgesia is recommended for pain control. Pethidine should be avoided, although other opiates can be used if necessary. Blood should be grouped and saved, but if atypical antibodies are present it is recommended that blood should be cross-matched. Broad-spectrum antibiotics should be administered if there is any suspicion of infection and routinely after operative delivery. The fetus is often growth-restricted and hence continuous fetal monitoring should be performed.

Continuous positive airway pressure (CPAP) may be advocated postnatally to reduce the incidence of ACS, particularly in postoperative patients. Acute chest syndrome is the most common cause of postoperative death among patients with sickle cell disease. Women should use graduated elastic compression stockings and be given prophylactic LMWH for six weeks postnatally to prevent thromboses.

Diabetes

Women with diabetes should be delivered in a consultant-led maternity unit with access to senior medical, obstetric and neonatal staff [11].

Pre-Existing Diabetes

The key concerns in labour and delivery in a diabetic pregnancy are:

- timing of delivery to avoid stillbirth and shoulder dystocia;
- mode of delivery to avoid shoulder dystocia; and
- diabetic control in labour to prevent maternal diabetic ketoacidosis and neonatal hypoglycaemia.

Delivery

Women with diabetes should be advised to give birth in hospitals where advanced neonatal resuscitation skills are available 24 hours per day. Delivery of a woman with pre-existing diabetes by 38 completed weeks is recommended in uncomplicated pregnancies

Box 22.3 Setting Up a Sliding Scale of Insulin

Fifty units of short-acting insulin, e.g. actrapid or Humulin S in 50 ml of 0.9% sodium chloride at a rate determined by capillary blood glucose.

Fluid regimen:

- 5% dextrose + 20–40 mmol of KCl infusion 1 l per eight hours if blood glucose <12 mmol/l.
- 0.9% sodium chloride + 20–40 mmol of KCl 1 l in eight hours if blood glucose >12 mmol/l, switch to 5% glucose when blood glucose falls to <12 mmol/l.

Table 22.4 Sliding scale regimen for type 1 diabetes once in established labour

Capillary blood glucose (BM)	Rate of insulin infusion (ml/h)	Comment
<3	0	Treat for hypoglycaemia and recheck in 15 min
3.1–5	1	
5.1–10	2	
10.1–15	3	
15.1–20	4	Check for urinary ketones
>20	5	Check for urinary ketones and call for assistance

If having elective CS, give one-third of the normal dose of long-acting insulin the night before and put first on the list.

with normal growth to avoid the increased risk of stillbirth, reduce the prevalence of macrosomia and reduce the risk of shoulder dystocia. Vaginal delivery is preferable, hence many diabetic women are induced. Vaginal birth after CS can be offered to diabetics. For women who have diabetes and a diagnosis of fetal macrosomia based on ultrasound, there should be a discussion regarding the merits and risks of vaginal birth, induction of labour and CS. In diabetic pregnancies 80% of cases of shoulder dystocia occur above a birth weight of 4.25 kg.

Diabetic Control in Labour and Delivery

Glucose control throughout active labour and delivery should be maintained between 4–7 mmol/l. Often this is best achieved with a sliding scale of short-acting intravenous insulin and dextrose, as the dietary intake in labour is reduced and metabolism is varied (see Box 22.3). This infusion should be considered from the onset of established labour in women with type 1 diabetes.

The sliding scale used will depend on whether they have type 1 or type 2 diabetes and the individual daily insulin requirements. Examples of such scales are shown in Tables 22.4–22.5. The capillary blood glucose (BM) is estimated each hour and the insulin infusion rate adjusted accordingly. The usual insulin dose range is 2–6 units per hour. The aim is to maintain

Table 22.5 Different sliding scale regimens for type 2 diabetes depending on total daily insulin requirement once in established labour

| Capillary blood glucose mmol/l(BM) | Total daily insulin dose | | | If target not achieved with sliding scale C, increase sliding scale each 2 h by following no. of units until target achieved |
| | A <60 units | B 60–120 units | C >120 units | |
	Rate of insulin infusion (ml/h)			
≤ 3.0	0#	0#	0#	0#
3.1–5.0	1	2	3	1
5.1–8.0	2	3	4	2
8.1–11.0	3	4	6	2
11.1–15.0	4	6	8	2
15.1–20.0*	5	8	10	2
>20.0*	6	10	12	2

Notes
* call for assistance from obstetric medicine/diabetic team; check for ketonuria.
# treat for hypoglycaemia and recheck in 20 min.
Select initial sliding scale (A–C) from table depending on final pregnancy total insulin dose. If target not achieved in two hours, move to next sliding scale. If hypoglycaemia occurs, move to previous sliding scale.
If having elective CS, give half of the normal dose of long-acting insulin the night before and put first on the list.

glucose levels of 4–7 mmol/l during labour and delivery, avoiding hypoglycaemia and preventing ketoacidosis. This may be difficult and most centres will aim for 4–8 mmol/l. Separate giving sets should be used for the insulin and dextrose so that in the event of hypoglycaemia, the glucose infusion can be increased and insulin infusion can be stopped. Women with type 1 diabetes are at particular risk of diabetic ketoacidosis which has a high mortality rate. Urinary ketones should be checked each time urine is passed and particularly if the BM is greater than 15.

Insulin drives extracellular potassium into the cells. It is important therefore to include potassium replacement with the intravenous dextrose to avoid hypokalaemia which may otherwise result, especially if glucose levels are high.

Diabetic Control Postpartum

Insulin requirements in women with type 1 diabetes drop significantly following delivery of the placenta. The rate of infusion of insulin should therefore be halved to prevent hypoglycaemia. Postpartum, insulin requirements return rapidly to pre-pregnancy levels. Once women with type 1 diabetes are eating normally, subcutaneous insulin should be recommenced at either the pre-pregnancy dose, or at a 25% lower dose if the woman intends to breastfeed, which is associated with increased energy expenditure. They should monitor their blood glucose levels carefully during this period. Most women with established diabetes are capable of adjusting their own insulin doses and can be advised that tight glycaemic control is not as important during the postpartum period. Indeed, the risk of hypoglycaemia is higher in the postnatal period, especially when breastfeeding, and they should be advised to have a meal or snack available before or during feeds.

Women with type 2 diabetes who were diet controlled pre-pregnancy can discontinue insulin immediately after delivery, even if they were on high doses in pregnancy. Those previously on metformin or glibenclamide can switch back to (or continue on) this treatment immediately postnatally if they are breastfeeding. Other oral hypoglycaemic drugs should be avoided while breastfeeding.

Neonate

Paediatricians do not need to be at the delivery of mothers with diabetes routinely, but should see the baby as soon as possible after birth. The baby should be fed early. Neonatal capillary blood glucose should be checked at 2–4 hours after birth if there are no signs of hypoglycaemia. The mother and baby should be kept together unless there is a clinical complication or clinical signs determining a need for admission into the neonatal unit.

Gestational Diabetes

Delivery

Delivery of a woman with gestational diabetes (GDM) who has an otherwise uncomplicated pregnancy should be at 38 completed weeks. Vaginal delivery is preferable unless there is an obstetric contraindication or if the fetal weight at delivery is estimated to be >4.25 kg.

Diabetic Control

Women with diet-controlled GDM and those on small amounts of insulin (≤40 units/day) do not usually require a sliding scale in active labour due to the reduced oral intake. If taking >40 units/day, they should be started on a sliding scale as described for type 2 diabetes (see Table 22.5).

Following delivery of the placenta, the insulin infusion should be discontinued as insulin resistance falls quickly. Oral hypoglycaemic drugs should also be stopped immediately postpartum. Monitoring of blood glucose should continue for 24 hours following resumption of oral intake as some women diagnosed with GDM will actually have type 2 diabetes.

All women with GDM should have a fasting plasma glucose measured six weeks following delivery and annually thereafter to exclude impaired glucose tolerance or pre-existing diabetes. Women with GDM should be counselled that the risks of future diabetes may be as high as 80%. They should be made aware of diabetic symptoms and should receive lifestyle advice concerning exercise and diet, particularly reduced fat intake. Obese women should be encouraged to lose weight postpartum and all should be advised to avoid obesity.

Addison's Disease

Adrenal insufficiency requires daily hydrocortisone and fludrocortisone (mineralocorticoid) supplementation. Clinical well-being and blood pressure together provide a good index of the adequacy of steroid replacement.

Table 22.6 Steroid support in labour for women on prednisolone ≥7.5mg/day for more than two weeks

Dose of prednisolone per day	Dose of IV hydrocortisone to cover labour (and until drinking)
>7.5 to ≤20 mg	50 mg tds
>20 mg	100 mg tds

In labour and other situations of acute stress, such as infection, there is normally an increased output of endogenous steroids from the adrenal gland. Those with Addison's disease cannot mount such a response and need increased doses of steroid. Labour should be managed with parenteral hydrocortisone 100 mg, intramuscularly, six-hourly.

The physiological diuresis that occurs following delivery may cause profound hypotension in women with Addison's disease. This can be treated with IV saline. Alternatively, the higher dose of steroids to cover labour could be weaned gradually over a number of days rather than over 24 hours to prevent hypotension.

Asthma

Asthma attacks are very rare in labour because of endogenous steroid production. Women should continue to use all their inhalers during labour. There is no evidence that inhaled β_2-agonists delay the onset of labour or impair uterine contractions. Women taking oral steroids (prednisolone ≥7.5 mg/day for more than two weeks prior to delivery) should receive parenteral hydrocortisone to cover the stress of labour, and until oral medication is restarted (Table 22.6) [12].

Caesarean section is only indicated for obstetric reasons. Induction of labour with prostaglandin E2 is safe as this is a bronchodilator. Syntocinon can be used safely for augmentation of labour, the third stage and for treatment of PPH. Misoprostol is preferable to prostaglandin F2α for the treatment of PPH. Prostaglandin F2α (carboprost) can cause bronchospasm and should be avoided if possible. It may be used with caution, and only after informing the anaesthetist, to treat life-threatening PPH. Ergometrine has been reported to cause bronchospasm, in particular in association with general anaesthesia, but this does not seem to be a practical problem when Syntometrine (oxytocin and ergometrine) is used for the prophylaxis of PPH.

All forms of pain relief in labour, including Entonox, opiates and regional analgesia can be used safely by women with controlled asthma. In the unlikely event of an acute severe asthmatic attack, opiates for pain relief should be avoided. Regional, rather than general, anaesthesia is preferable if CS is required because of the decreased risk of chest infection and atelectasis. General anaesthesia should particularly be avoided in those with brittle asthma, and if required, should be supervised by a consultant anaesthetist.

Cystic Fibrosis

Most women with cystic fibrosis (CF) deliver vaginally at term. Some may be inpatients by the end of pregnancy because of a resting hypoxia or fetal growth restriction, necessitating bed rest, oxygen therapy and nutritional supplements. Early delivery may be necessary if there is a significant deterioration in maternal or fetal well-being. Caesarean section is only necessary for obstetric indications and general anaesthesia should be avoided if possible [13].

Patients with CF are particularly prone to pneumothoraces, which may be precipitated by prolonged attempts at pushing and repeated Valsalva manoeuvres in the second stage of labour. Instrumental delivery may be indicated to avoid a prolonged second stage.

Breastfeeding should usually be encouraged, although the mother may continue to require nutritional supplements in the puerperium, especially if she is breastfeeding. Most of the drugs used will be secreted into the breast milk, but this is rarely a contraindication to breastfeeding. Analysis of breast milk of women with CF has shown normal content of sodium and protein.

Epilepsy

Women with major convulsive seizures should deliver in hospital as the risk of seizures increases around the time of delivery. Between 1% and 2% of women with epilepsy will have a seizure during labour and 1–2% will have one in the first 24 hours postpartum [14,15]. This is because seizures are more likely with stress, tiredness and sleep deprivation, all of which occur in labour and postpartum. Additionally there is reduced absorption of antiepileptic medication due to reduced gastric motility. Antiepileptic drugs (AEDs) may be inadvertently omitted.

Box 22.4 Actions when Seizures that are Not Rapidly Self-Limiting Occur in Labour

Give oxygen and either:

- intravenous lorazepam 4 mg over 2 min; or
- diazepam 10–20 mg (rectal gel); or
- diazepam 10–20 mg intravenously at 2 mg/min.

If seizures continue, an intravenous infusion of phenytoin will be required.

Women should not be left unattended in labour or for the first 24 hours postpartum. They should continue their regular AEDs in labour. Consideration should be given to giving AEDs in suppository form or the use of clobazam short term. To limit the risk of precipitating a seizure due to pain and anxiety, early epidural analgesia should be considered.

Most women with epilepsy have normal vaginal deliveries and CS is only required if there are recurrent generalized seizures in late pregnancy or in labour. Women with epilepsy should not use the birth pool to labour or have a water birth.

For women who have had seizures during previous deliveries despite taking their AEDs regularly, clobazam can be started prior to labour in addition to their usual AEDs and discontinued 48 hours after delivery. Another option is to use rectal carbamazepine, which will ensure adequate absorption in labour.

If admitted antenatally or postnatally, women with epilepsy should not be looked after in a side room due to the risk of having a fatal unwitnessed seizure.

All children born to mothers taking enzyme-inducing AEDs should be given 1 mg of vitamin K parenterally at delivery.

Myasthenia Gravis

Myasthenia gravis (MG) is an autoimmune neuromuscular disorder causing fatigable weakness of the skeletal muscles following repetitive activity. It results in ptosis, diplopia, difficulty speaking and occasionally respiratory distress due to fatigue of the intercostal muscles. It does not affect the smooth muscle of the myometrium, therefore contractions and uterine involution are not impaired.

A vaginal delivery should be the aim, although instrumental delivery may be required to prevent maternal exhaustion. Postpartum haemorrhage is not increased in women with myasthenia. Caesarean section should only be performed for obstetric indications [16].

The key concerns in labour and delivery in a woman with MG are:

- drug use and drug interactions;
- neonatal myasthenia gravis; and
- puerperal infection.

Drug Use and Drug Interactions in MG

Treatment of MG includes anticholinesterase inhibitors such as pyridostigmine. These can be administered parenterally in labour. Postnatally, shorter dose intervals should be used as large doses can cause gastrointestinal upset in breastfed newborns.

Pregnant women with myasthenia should see an experienced obstetric anaesthetist, preferably prior to delivery, to make appropriate plans for safe analgesic and anaesthetic use in labour:

- Regional analgesia is safe but if the mother is being treated with anticholinesterases avoid the ester type of local anaesthetics (e.g. chlorprocaine, tetracaine). These depend on maternal plasma cholinesterase for their metabolism. Bupivicaine and lignocaine are the amide type of local anaesthetics and are metabolized by a different pathway and are therefore safe for use in labour and delivery.
- General anaesthesia: if an inhalational anaesthetic is required, ether and halothane should be avoided. Myasthenics are also particularly sensitive to non-depolarizing muscle relaxants such as curare and suxamethonium, which may have an exaggerated or prolonged effect.

Other drugs that may exacerbate or cause muscle fatigue include aminoglycosides (e.g. gentamicin) and β-adrenergics (salbutamol, terbutaline and ritodrine). Narcotics should be used with caution as they can reduce respiratory drive.

Although magnesium sulphate is the drug of choice for seizure prophylaxis in eclampsia and pre-eclampsia (see Chapter 25), it should be avoided in women with MG since it may precipitate a myasthenic crisis. Clinical judgement needs to be used when considering use of magnesium sulphate in a myasthenic woman who has an eclamptic seizure.

Myasthenics on immunosuppression should continue these drugs during labour. If on steroids, they will need IV hydrocortisone in labour (see Table 22.6).

Neonatal Myasthenia Gravis

Transient neonatal myasthenia gravis (TNMG) presents with poor sucking and generalized hypotonia, usually up to four days (and at times up to one week) of life. It is due to transplacental transfer of anticholinesterase receptor (AChR) antibodies. Respiratory distress is usually mild but may be severe and life threatening, requiring ventilation. Neonates of women with MG should be monitored with an apnoea monitor. Treatment is with anticholinesterase inhibitors. The development of TNMG does not mean the child will develop MG in later life.

Puerperal Infection

This is not more common in myasthenics, but if it occurs can result in severe deterioration and should therefore be treated promptly.

Berry Aneurysms and Cerebral Arteriovenous Malformations

There is an increased tendency for untreated cerebral aneurysms and arteriovenous malformations (AVM) to rupture in pregnancy [17]. Berry aneurysms rarely bleed for the first time in labour, although rebleeding can occur if they have not been surgically treated or clipped. Caesarean section is therefore recommended if they have not been treated. The risk of rupture is considered to be related to the increased intracranial pressure that occurs with pushing. Vaginal delivery is possible with a passive second stage and a forceps delivery without maternal effort, but should probably be reserved for the informed multiparous woman who should have an epidural in labour. Elective CS is recommended for those with a large AVM close to term.

If a woman has had a previous AVM which has been treated, or a berry aneurysm which has been clipped, she can be delivered vaginally without any special precautions even if her surgery occurred in pregnancy following an intracerebral bleed.

Infectious Diseases

HIV

The key concerns in labour and delivery in a woman with HIV are:

- prevention of mother-to-child transmission (MTCT); and
- avoidance of maternal infection/sepsis.

Vertical transmission of HIV without any intervention is around 25%. This risk is reduced to around 1% by using antiretroviral treatment (ART) antenatally, during delivery and for the neonate postnatally, performing a CS and avoiding breastfeeding. In women on combination ART (cART) with an undetectable viral load, MTCT of HIV is <0.5% irrespective of mode of delivery [18].

Mode of Delivery

See Table 22.7. The mode of delivery should be discussed by a multidisciplinary team including the HIV physician, the obstetrician and the woman, and a plan made at 36 weeks' gestation. Over 98% of women with HIV in the UK are now on ART in pregnancy.

Those who are on cART with viral loads of <50 copies/ml should aim for vaginal delivery unless there is an obstetric reason for CS. These patients can be managed obstetrically the same as women without HIV. They do not require continuous monitoring in labour as long as they are otherwise low risk. The British HIV Association guidelines state they can deliver in a midwifery-led unit or at home as there is no increase in the incidence of fetal hypoxia. They should continue their cART throughout labour. Evidence shows that this group does not have an increased incidence of MTCT with interventions in labour, including artificial rupture of membranes, use of a fetal scalp electrode, fetal blood sampling, instrumental delivery or episiotomy. If instrumental delivery is required, the most appropriate instrument for the obstetric circumstances which the obstetrician is competent using should be used. Women on cART with undetectable viral loads can be induced and can have a vaginal birth after caesarean (VBAC) if this is not contraindicated for another reason. If they rupture their membranes after 34 weeks' gestation, their labour should be augmented.

A prelabour CS should be offered to HIV-positive women with either a viral load of >400 copies/ml or those on zidovudine monotherapy irrespective of viral load as this will reduce MTCT (to <1% in the latter group). The CS should be performed at 38–39 weeks' gestation in this circumstance as those on retroviral treatment often labour earlier. If an elective CS is being performed for an obstetric indication, rather than to

Table 22.7 Mode of delivery in women with HIV

Obstetric scenario	Vaginal delivery	Consider elective CS*	Recommend elective CS
Term	On cART and VL <50** Elite controllers CD4 ≥350 VL <50	On cART and VL 50–399	On cART and VL ≥400 On zidovudine monotherapy (not elite controllers) irrespective of VL VL >400*** regardless of ART
Term SROM: all cases expedite delivery	VL <50 immediate IOL and low threshold to treat intrapartum pyrexia	VL 50–999	VL ≥1000 regardless of treatment
pPROM ≥ 34/40	VL <50 immediate IOL and low threshold to treat intrapartum pyrexia GBS prophylaxis	VL 50–999 GBS prophylaxis	VL ≥1000 regardless of treatment GBS prophylaxis

Notes
cART = combination antiretroviral treatment
VL = viral load (copies/ml)
* taking into account viral load, trajectory of viral load, length of time on treatment and compliance
** MTCT <0.5% – can have induction of labour, fetal blood sampling, instrumental delivery and vaginal birth after CS
** MTCT <1%

reduce MTCT, then it should be performed at 39–40 weeks' gestation.

Women on cART with a HIV viral load of 50–399 copies/ml have been shown to have a doubling of the MTCT rates with vaginal delivery compared to elective CS. In absolute terms this is around a 0.5% increase. Therefore, in this group CS can be considered, taking into consideration the viral load, the trajectory of the viral load, length of time on treatment and compliance. If a vaginal delivery is agreed in this scenario and instrumental delivery is required, it may be preferable to use forceps as this reduces the likelihood of fetal trauma.

Caesarean section is less effective at reducing transmission when performed in labour or after membrane rupture. Transmission increases with increasing duration of membrane rupture.

A maternal blood sample for CD4 cell count and HIV viral load should be taken at delivery. The umbilical cord should be clamped as quickly as possible after delivery.

Antiretroviral Treatment

Antiretroviral therapy should be continued up to delivery.

Intravenous zidovudine should be given intrapartum to women:

- with viral loads >1000 in labour, with spontaneous ruptured membranes or having a planned CS;

- who are untreated with unknown viral loads who attend in labour or with spontaneous ruptured membranes; and
- on zidovudine monotherapy and planned caesarean section.

This should be started four hours before CS, or at the onset of labour. It should continue until the cord is clamped.

Untreated Women with HIV in Labour

These women should have bloods taken for CD4 cell count, HIV viral load and be given nevirapine 200 mg orally stat. They should be commenced on cART in the form of fixed dose zidovudine (intravenous infusion in labour and delivery and then change to oral), lamivudine and raltegramir. They should have a CS if delivery is not imminent. If in preterm labour, double dose tenofivir should be added to the cART regimen to further load the baby with antiretrovirals before birth in case the neonate cannot tolerate oral ART once born.

Women attending in labour or with spontaneous rupture of the membranes who have not been tested for HIV in pregnancy or who were previously tested as negative but who have remained at risk of contracting HIV, should have a rapid test for HIV. If the result is positive, they should be commenced on treatment before the results of the confirmatory test are received.

All women who are HIV-positive should exclusively bottle feed their babies with infant formula milk.

Table 22.8 Neonatal risks of maternal genital herpes at delivery

Maternal genital herpes	Risk of neonatal herpes	Elective CS recommended
Primary episode >6 weeks before delivery	0%	No
Primary episode <6 weeks before delivery	41%	Yes
Recurrent episode at the onset of labour	1–3%	No

Hepatitis B

Hepatitis B can be vertically transmitted to the fetus if the mother has acute hepatitis B infection in the third trimester or if she is a chronic hepatitis B antigen carrier. Caesarean section is not protective. Neonatal infection is prevented by administering hepatitis B vaccine to all neonates of women who are hepatitis B surface antigen (HBsAg) positive at birth, four weeks and one year. Additional hepatitis B immune globulin is administered in a different site to the vaccine within 12 hours of birth if the mother is Hepatitis B e antigen (HBeAg) positive.

Hepatitis C

Current evidence does not show that elective CS is protective in women with hepatitis C unless they are co-infected with HIV [19].

Genital Herpes

Caesarean section should be recommended to all women who have a primary episode of genital herpes at or within six weeks of delivery to prevent risks of neonatal herpes (Table 22.8) [20]. If the woman opts for a vaginal birth, the membranes should not be artificially ruptured and consideration should be given to treatment with intravenous aciclovir to the mother and subsequently to the neonate. The neonatologist should be informed.

Women with recurrent genital herpes at the onset of labour have a small risk of neonatal herpes (Table 22.8). If their membranes rupture, delivery should be expedited, usually by augmentation of labour. Invasive procedures in labour should be avoided. The neonatologist should be informed during labour.

Renal Disease

Renal function, blood pressure and fluid balance should be monitored during labour and delivery in women with renal disease. Treatment should be continued and parenteral steroids should be administered to those on prednisolone as with any woman on maintenance steroids (see Table 22.6). Those who are immunosuppressed will be at increased risk of infection and should be given prophylactic antibiotics to cover any surgical procedure, including episiotomy.

Caesarean section is only required for obstetric indications, although the overall section rate is increased compared to background rates. The renal allograft in the pelvis does not obstruct vaginal delivery. If a CS is required in a renal transplant patient it should be performed by the most senior obstetrician available.

Obstetric Cholestasis

Labour should be induced at 37–38 weeks' gestation in cases where the bile acids have been greater than 40 μ mol/l in the pregnancy, to avoid the increased risk of stillbirth [21]. There is a higher risk of fetal distress in obstetric cholestasis, therefore continuous fetal monitoring is required throughout induction and labour. Ursodeoxycholic acid can be discontinued postnatally.

The neonate should receive IM vitamin K.

References

1. Knight M, Kenyon S, Brocklehurst P, *et al.* (eds). *Saving Lives, Improving Mothers' Care – Lessons Learned to Inform Future Maternity Care From the UK and Ireland Confidential Enquiries into Maternal Deaths and Morbidity 2009–12.* Oxford: National Perinatal Epidemiology Unit, University of Oxford; 2014.

2. Adamson DL, Dhanjal MK, Nelson-Piercy C. Heart disease and its management in obstetrics. In Greer IA, Nelson-Piercy C, Walters B (eds), *Maternal Medicine: Medical Problems in Pregnancy* (pp. 14–33). New York: Elsevier Ltd; 2007.

3. NICE. Prophylaxis against infective endocarditis: antimicrobial prophylaxis against infective endocarditis in adults and children undergoing interventional procedures: clinical guideline 64; 2008. www.nice.org.uk/guidance/cg64/resources/guidance-prophylaxis-against-infective-endocarditis-pdf (accessed January 2015).

4. RCOG. *Thrombosis and Embolism Disease in Pregnancy and the Puerperium: Acute Management.* London: RCOG Press; 2015.

5. Greer IA, Nelson-Piercy C. Low-molecular-weight heparins for thromboprophylaxis and treatment of venous thromboembolism in pregnancy: a systematic review of safety and efficacy. *Blood.* 2005; 106(2): 401–7.

6. Chan WS, Anand S, Ginsberg JS. Anticoagulation of pregnant women with mechanical heart valves. *Arch Intern Med.* 2000; 160: 191–6.

7. British Committee for Standards in Haematology, General Haematology Task Force. Guidelines for the investigation and management of idiopathic thrombocytopenic purpura in adults, children and in pregnancy. *Br J Haematol.* 2003; 120: 574–96.

8. Lee CA, Chi C, Pavord SR, *et al.* The obstetric and gynaecological management of women with inherited bleeding disorders: review with guidelines produced by a taskforce of UK Haemophilia Centre Doctors' Organization. *Haemophilia.* 2006; 12(4): 301–36.

9. Mumford AD, Ackroyd S, Alikhan R, *et al.* Guideline for the diagnosis and management of the rare coagulation disorders: a United Kingdom Haemophilia Centre Doctors' Organization guideline on behalf of the British Committee for Standards in Haematology. *Br J Haematol.* 2014; 167(3): 304–26.

10. RCOG. *Management of Sickle Cell Disease in Pregnancy.* London: RCOG Press; 2011.

11. NICE. Diabetes in pregnancy: management of diabetes and its complications from pre-conception to the postnatal period: clinical guideline 63; 2014.

12. British Thoracic Society/Scottish Intercollegiate Guidelines Network. British guideline on the management of asthma: a national clinical guideline. *Thorax.* 2014; 69: i1–i192.

13. Geake J, Tay G, Callaway L, Bell SC. Pregnancy and cystic fibrosis: approach to contemporary management. *Obstet Med.* 2014; 7: 147–55.

14. Tomson T, Hiilesmaa V. Epilepsy in pregnancy. *BMJ.* 2007; 335(7623): 769–73.

15. NICE. *Epilepsies: Diagnosis and Management.* Clinical Guideline 137. London: NICE; 2016.

16. Norwood F, Dhanjal M, Hill M, *et al.* Myasthenia in pregnancy: best practice guidelines from a UK multispeciality working group. *JNNP.* 2014; 85: 538–43.

17. Kittner SJ, Stern BJ, Feeser BR, *et al.* Pregnancy and the risk of stroke. *N Engl J Med.* 1996; 335(11): 768–74.

18. British HIV Association. British HIV Association guidelines for the management of HIV infection in pregnant women 2012 (2014 interim review). *HIV Med.* 2014; 15 (suppl. 4): 1–77.

19. Cottrell EB, Chou R, Wasson N, Rahman B, Guise JM. Reducing risk for mother-to-infant transmission of hepatitis C virus: a systematic review for the U.S. Preventive Services Task Force. *Ann Intern Med*; 2013; 158(2): 109–13.

20. RCOG. *Management of Genital Herpes in Pregnancy.* London: RCOG Press; 2007.

21. RCOG. *Obstetric Cholestasis.* London: RCOG Press; 2011.

www.guidance.nice.org.uk/cg63 (accessed 15 May 2016).

Management of Women with Previous Caesarean Section

Tsz Kin Lo and Tak Yeung Leung

The management of pregnant women with a previous caesarean delivery is a unique challenge. The overall success for a trial of labour after caesarean birth (TOLAC) is 60–80%, while the intrapartum uterine rupture risk is 0.5%. Although complications are rare for both TOLAC and elective repeat caesarean delivery (ERCD), the former in general poses slightly higher risk to the baby and the mother. On balance, TOLAC is preferred for most women with one prior lower transverse uterine incision. Although there remains an element of unpredictability in scar rupture, risk stratification helps to fill in the gap between safety in TOLAC, women's preference during childbirth and resource allocation. Labour induction with previous caesarean scar is still feasible in the presence of a good indication. Other special conditions such as preterm and postterm pregnancies, fetal macrosomia, twins and breech-presenting pregnancy are also discussed in detail.

Introduction

Nowadays it is common to encounter women with a previous caesarean scar in obstetric practice. The caesarean birth rate in the developed world varies from 14% in the Netherlands to 20.8% in France, 25% in the UK, 32.3% in the USA, 35% in Korea and 40% in Italy [1–3]. Two important issues stand out in the management for this group of women:

1. exclusion of placenta praevia and accreta by ultrasound; and
2. helping the women to reach a decision on the mode of delivery (MOD), namely TOLAC or ERCD.

Without an adherent placenta overlying a caesarean scar, uterine rupture before labour is exceedingly rare.

The assessment and management of placenta praevia, adherent placenta and uterine rupture is dealt with in other chapters. This chapter focuses on antenatal assessment and counselling on the MOD, and intrapartum management. Special and difficult conditions for TOLAC are also discussed.

Antenatal Management

When a pregnant woman with a previous caesarean section (CS) comes to the antenatal clinic, a detailed history of the previous operation must be reviewed, and should include the indication for CS, the number and type of incision and complication such as uterine tear. This information is relevant for risk assessment and decision making on the mode of subsequent childbirth.

Contraindication to TOLAC

ERCD is recommended with [3]:

1. a history of at least three previous CSs, except in the case of intrauterine death (IUD) or termination of pregnancy (TOP);
2. a T-incision or uterine body incision during a previous CS (rupture risk 4–9% [2]);
3. history of uterine rupture (rupture risk 6–32% [4]);
4. history of dehiscence of a uterine scar discovered during a CS; and
5. medical or obstetric complications that preclude vaginal birth [5].

TOLAC is relatively contraindicated with [3]:

1. uterine malformations;
2. a low vertical incision in the lower segment during a previous CS;

Best Practice in Labour and Delivery, Second Edition, ed. Sir Sabaratnam Arulkumaran. Published by Cambridge University Press. © Cambridge University Press 2016.

Table 23.1 Comparing short-term maternal outcomes between TOLAC and ERCD [7,8]

Maternal outcomes	TOLAC	ERCD	Direction of effect	Grade of evidence
Death	0.004%	0.013%	$p = 0.027$	High
Rupture	0.47%	0.026%	$p < 0.001$	Moderate
Hysterectomy	0.17%	0.28%	$p = 0.50$	Moderate
Bleeding	Insufficient data	Insufficient data	Insufficient data	Low
Transfusion	0.9%	1.2%	$p = 0.25$	Moderate
Infection	4.6%	3.2%	Difference insignificant	Low
Surgical injury	Insufficient data	Insufficient data	Difference insignificant	Low
Hospital stay	Shorter overall	Longer overall	–	Low
DVT	0.04%	0.1%	Reduced by TOLAC	Low

3. unavailability of a surgical report from the preceding CS;
4. two previous CSs;
5. conception under six months from the date of the previous CS;
6. history of postpartum fever; and
7. previous CS <37 weeks.

Benefits and Risks of TOLAC vs ERCD

It is inappropriate to compare outcomes of vaginal birth after caesarean (VBAC) versus ERCD, or of repeat caesarean after failed TOLAC versus ERCD, because VBAC is not guaranteed for TOLAC. Ideally, the appropriate comparison is by intention to deliver (TOLAC vs ERCD). However, these data are not always available, especially for long-term outcomes. Neither are they addressed adequately by randomized trials [6]. Some outcomes may have a low level of evidence. They should, nevertheless, also be shared with the women as they might be important to them [5].

Maternal Benefits and Risks of TOLAC vs ERCD

Short-Term Maternal Outcomes

There are similar short-term risks of concern with TOLAC or ERCD, but the magnitudes are different and should be disclosed to the patient during counselling; these are given in Table 23.1.

Long-Term Maternal Outcomes

There is no high-grade evidence for the long-term benefit or harm of TOLAC vs ERCD. Vaginal birth after caesarean reduces the chance of a woman having *placenta praevia or accrete* in her next pregnancy. On the other hand, CS for the second time significantly increases the chance of a woman having CS in her future pregnancies. The risk of placenta praevia and accreta spectrum disorder increases with the number of caesareans a woman undergoes [8].

Women with multiple repeat caesareans are also at increased risk of hysterectomy, cystotomy, bowel injury, ureteral injury, ileus, blood transfusion of at least four units, need for postoperative ventilation, ICU admission, increased operative time and increased hospital stay. The risk increases with the number of caesareans experienced. The risk is much higher after the fourth CS [9].

After CS, future pregnancies are potentially associated with increased risk for reduced fetal growth, preterm birth and possibly stillbirth. There may also be increased risk of adverse reproductive effects, namely decreased fertility, increased risk of miscarriage and ectopic pregnancy [9].

Therefore, a decision regarding MOD should ideally take future plans for pregnancy into consideration. For women desiring bigger families, VBAC from TOLAC may, in the future, avoid potential maternal complications related to multiple caesarean deliveries [10].

ERCD should not be considered protective against pelvic floor dysfunction (stress incontinence and genital prolapse) because evidence is insufficient and the timing of the original caesarean may influence the risk [8].

Most of the maternal morbidity associated with TOLAC occurs when TOLAC fails, necessitating emergency repeat caesarean. Vaginal birth after caesarean is associated with fewer complications and a failed TOLAC with more complications than ERCD. Therefore, the risk for maternal morbidity is related to

Table 23.2 Comparison of fetal and neonatal outcomes between TOLAC and ERCD [7,8]

Fetal & neonatal outcomes	TOLAC	ERCD	Direction of effect	Grade of evidence
Perinatal death*	0.13%	0.05%	$p = 0.002$	Moderate
Neonatal death**	0.11%	0.06%	$p = 0.001$	Moderate
Fetal mortality***	0.05–0.3%	0–0.04%	Higher in TOLAC****	Low
Respiratory conditions				
1. Bag/mask ventilation	5.4%	2.5%	Insufficient data	Low
2. TTN	3.6%	4.2%	Insufficient data	Low
HIE	Insufficient data	Insufficient data	Insufficient data	Low
Sepsis	Insufficient data	Insufficient data	Insufficient data	Low
Birth trauma	Insufficient data	Insufficient data	Insufficient data	Insufficient
Persistent neurological impairment after brachial plexus injury	Insufficient data	Insufficient data	Not appear to be substantially different	Insufficient
NICU admissions	Insufficient data	Insufficient data	Insufficient data	Low
Neurological outcome	Insufficient data	Insufficient data	Insufficient data	Insufficient
Breastfeeding outcomes	Insufficient data	Insufficient data	Insufficient data	Insufficient

Notes
* Death between 20 weeks of gestation and 28 days of life.
** Death in the first 28 days of life.
*** Deaths in utero at 20 weeks of gestation or greater.
**** ERCD may reduce stillbirth in late third trimester.

the chance of achieving VBAC [10]. Women with at least 60–70% chance of VBAC should have no more maternal morbidity to undergo TOLAC than ERCD [10].

Fetal and Neonatal Benefits and Risks of TOLAC vs ERCD

Only relatively short-term outcome data are available for the baby (Table 23.2).

The neonatal morbidity from ERCD is similar to that from TOLAC, with the best chance of achieving VBAC because failed TOLAC is associated with higher neonatal morbidity than ERCD [8].

Overall

Risks of serious complications are generally low for both mother and baby regardless of TOLAC or ERCD. Except for uterine rupture, risk–benefit ratio for mother both in the short- and long-term favours TOLAC. On the other hand, short-term risk–benefit ratio for baby favours ERCD. On balance, TOLAC is the preferred option in the great majority of cases [3].

Factors Affecting VBAC in TOLAC

In general, success rate of TOLAC is 60–80% and uterine rupture risk 0.5% for women with one prior

low transverse caesarean [2]. The crude success rate of TOLAC is similar to the chance that a nulliparous woman in labour at term has a vaginal birth with today's caesarean rate (76.5%) [5].

Three factors are strongly associated with success of TOLAC [3]:

1. history of vaginal birth (OR 4.2 (3.9–4.6)), especially if vaginal delivery after caesarean (OR 7.4 (4.5–12.2));
2. favourable cervix at entry into labour room (OR 0.39 (0.36–0.42), <4 cm vs ≥4 cm)); and
3. spontaneous labour (OR 1.6 (1.5–1.8)).

VBAC rate after TOLAC is 63% with no prior vaginal deliveries, 83% with a prior vaginal delivery before caesarean and 94% with a prior VBAC [8]. A higher VBAC rate is also observed with greater cervical dilation at admission or at membrane rupture [8].

A number of factors are associated with a reduced TOLAC success [3]:

1. previous caesarean for failure to progress or non-descent at full dilation (OR 0.34 (0.30–0.37)), malpresentation vs dystocia;
2. history of two caesareans (OR for failed TOLAC 1.48 (1.23–1.78));

3. maternal age >35 years (OR for failed TOLAC 1.14 (1.03–1.25), >35 years vs 21–34 years) (but no threshold);
4. body mass index >30 (OR 0.55 (0.51–0.60));
5. pregnancy prolonged past 41 weeks (OR 0.61 (0.55–0.68));
6. birth weight >4000 g (OR 0.55 (0.49–0.61), >4000 g vs 2500–3999 g);
7. induction of labour (OR 0.50 (0.45–0.55));
8. non-White ethnicity [9] (OR 0.69 (0.63–0.75), African vs Caucasian; 0.65 (0.59–0.72), Hispanic vs Caucasian; 0.71 (0.68–0.84), others vs Caucasian);
9. pre-eclampsia [9] (RR for failed TOLAC 1.55 (1.22–2.00)); and
10. short inter-pregnancy interval [10] (OR 0.70 (0.64–0.76), ≤2 years vs >2 years).

Trial of labour after caesarean birth success rate is 65–75% with arrest of dilation between 5 and 9 cm and only 15% with arrest of descent at full dilation [2]. Elective repeat caesarean delivery is preferable to TOLAC with BMI greater than 50 because TOLAC failure rate is 87% and it is difficult to move them rapidly in an emergency. The overall VBAC rate is 63% with labour induction [8]. Labour induction reduces VBAC rate, regardless of the induction method used and whether the cervix is favourable, although unfavourable cervix decreases chance of success to the greatest extent [10]. Rigorous studies have not compared different induction methods. Gestational diabetes successfully managed by diet is not a risk factor for TOLAC failure.

X-ray pelvimetry and scores are largely unhelpful in deciding the MOD [3]. X-ray pelvimetry reduces update of TOLAC [11] and increases repeat caesarean rate without reduction in uterine rupture rate. Scores and nomogram have only limited clinical utility in identifying women at risk of failed TOLAC [11].

There are non-clinical factors potentially affecting uptake and success of TOLAC [12], including national guidelines, local and institutional guidelines, feedback to obstetricians about mode of birth rates, individualized information to women and health insurance policies.

Counselling on Mode of Delivery

Discussion on MOD should be initiated early in pregnancy to allow more time for women to consider options, and to allow for coordination of delivery with another physician and facility if TOLAC is not an option locally [4].

The counselling should be non-judgemental and fact-based, honestly discussing the current issue including facilities, availability of personnel, preparation and protocol for emergency caesarean, chance of successful VBAC, women's understanding of failed TOLAC and the rare possibility of uterine rupture. It is good practice to obtain and review the previous obstetric records and operative notes. Risk assessment should be individualized and based on data that are most personally relevant. Women prefer information that addresses their individual situation, personal values and beliefs that best meet their needs. Women's autonomy should be honoured. Studies specific to TOLAC decision making found that women are more satisfied with their experience, regardless of the type of birth they have, when they believe they were involved in the decision to the degree that was comfortable for them [5].

Presentation of information should be in a way the patient can understand. Framing should be avoided [5]. Following are some techniques for communicating risk that ensure an objective approach and increase patient comprehension [5]:

1. Consistently use absolute numbers in place of relative risks or risk ratios.
2. Avoid using words like 'rare' or 'uncommon'. These are inexact concepts because one individual's interpretation can be different from another's.
3. It is easier to understand smaller denominators and whole numbers. For example, '2 in 100' is more accurately interpreted than '18 to 20 in 1000'. Use the same numeric denominator.
4. Use round numbers and avoid the use of decimals.
5. Use of visual decision aids such as the Paling Perspective Scale helps avoid framing and improve risk communication for most individuals regardless of educational level.

Decision aids are videos, leaflets or computer programs that assist women to make a decision about delivery options wherein both have benefits and harms. Studies have shown that decision aids improve knowledge and accurate understanding of risk, benefits and implications of TOLAC vs ERCD. They reduce anxiety and decisional conflict, increase perceived participation and help women make decisions [5,8].

The counselling should also take into consideration the intended family size and women's plans for future fertility. Risk of multiple caesareans should be considered in all women who are not electing permanent sterilization, as women tend to underestimate their future parity [4].

Women's planned MOD should be validated by the eighth month of pregnancy. There should be documentation in writing of informed consent, the MOD chosen with the reason and an agreed plan in the event that labour begins before an ERCD [3].

Labour Management for TOLAC

Setting

Previous caesarean is among factors indicating increased risk, suggesting planned birth at an obstetric unit [13]. The Royal College of Obstetricians and Gynaecologists (RCOG) in the UK advised that VBAC labours be undertaken in hospitals with facilities for emergency surgery with continuous fetal heart monitoring (CFHM) [14]. The French College of Gynecologists and Obstetricians (CNGOF) stated that TOLAC must not be at home or in a birthing centre, although it can take place at a maternity unit that does not have an obstetrician or anaesthetist on-site 24/7 [3]. It recommended that an obstetrician be present on-site when the obstetric context suggests a higher than normal risk of TOLAC failure or uterine rupture risk.

The American College of Obstetricians and Gynecologists (ACOG) likewise recommended that resources for emergency caesarean be 'immediately available'. In the ACOG and American Society of Anesthesiologists (ASA) joint statement, the definition of 'immediately available' personnel and facilities is a local decision based on each institution's available resources and geographic location [15]. When resources for immediate caesarean are not available, ACOG recommends that the healthcare provider and patients considering TOLAC discuss hospital resources. The process for gathering needed staff when emergency arises should be clear. If the healthcare provider is uncomfortable with a woman's choice, an alternative is to refer the patient to a facility with available resources. Another alternative is to create regional centres where patients interested in TOLAC can be referred and resources more efficiently and economically organized. Transfer of care to facilitate TOLAC is best effected antenatally. Respect for patient

Table 23.3 Dose–response relationship in the last 90 min of labour in women with rupture

One dose	Hazard ratio for rupture	2.8
Two		3.1
Three		6.7
Four or more		8.1

autonomy supports that women be allowed to accept increased levels of risk, and argues that a policy not to offer TOLAC in a centre cannot be used to force women to have ERCD, or to deny care to women in labour who decline to have repeat caesarean. However, the patient should be clearly informed of potential increase in risk and management alternatives. All centres should have a plan for managing uterine rupture. Drills or other simulation may be useful in preparing for rare emergencies [10]. In light of limited physician and nursing resources and low levels of evidence for requirement for 'immediately available' surgical and anaesthesia personnel, there was call for ACOG and ASA to reassess this requirement with reference to other obstetric complications of comparable risk [8].

Analgesia and Anaesthesia

Epidural analgesia is encouraged, as adequate pain relief is helpful in encouraging women to choose TOLAC. The success rate for VBAC is similar to those receiving other types of pain relief [16]. Epidural analgesia does not mask signs and symptoms of uterine rupture; particularly the most common sign of rupture, fetal heart rate (FHR) abnormality [15]. Pain associated with rupture occurs even when epidural is in use. In fact, escalating dosing requirement can be used as an objective clinical sign of impending rupture. There is a dose–response relationship in the last 90 min of labour in women with rupture (Table 23.3).

It is the recommendation of the ASA that neuraxial techniques be offered to patients attempting TOLAC. Early placement of the neuraxial catheter should be considered as it can be used later for labour analgesia, or for anaesthesia in the event of an operative delivery [15].

The anaesthesia team should be notified when a patient is having TOLAC in the labour and delivery room so they can perform pre-anaesthesia evaluation early in labour. If there are medical factors that might complicate her course, the anaesthetist should be consulted before labour in the antepartum period. During labour, the obstetrician updates and clearly communicates any concern to the anaesthetist [15].

Solid foods are best avoided in labour [16]. Clear liquids in labour are acceptable in modest amounts [15]. A randomized controlled trial of a light diet of solid foods versus clear fluids in labour showed no difference in vaginal delivery rate [15]. The ASA states that patients at increased risk of caesarean should remain nothing by mouth [15].

Patients at higher risk of emergency caesarean and those with symptoms of gastro-oesophageal reflux should receive some form of pharmacologic aspiration prophylaxis, such as H_2-receptor antagonist, metoclopramide and/or clear antacid [15].

Women undergoing TOLAC on the labour floor should have intravenous access and blood taken for type and screen [4].

Induction and Augmentation

Nearly one-quarter of women who are candidates for TOLAC may require induction or augmentation of labour [17]. Current guidelines of ACOG, RCOG and the Society of Obstetricians and Gynaecologists of Canada (SOGC) all agree that induction is an option for women undergoing TOLAC [17]. Induction is more likely to result in caesarean than spontaneous labour and roughly doubles the risk of uterine rupture [3]. Therefore, induction should only be considered if medically indicated. Induction is contraindicated with two previous caesareans [3]. The risk of uterine rupture is 0.5% for spontaneous labour [16], 1% with the use of oxytocin, 2% for prostaglandin E2 (PGE2) and 6% for prostaglandin E1 (PGE1) [17]. It is unknown if the increased risk is due to unfavourable cervix or the induction method used, although some showed rupture is no more likely with an unfavourable cervix [10]. There is suggestion for increase in rupture risk only in induction with no prior vaginal deliveries (1.5% vs 0.8%, $p = 0.02$) [10].

Membrane Stripping

Membrane stripping has not been studied in relation to uterine rupture in women with previous caesarean [18]. One report concluded that serial membrane sweeping at term for cervical ripening and labour induction in women with previous caesarean had no significant effect on onset of labour, rate

of induction, repeat caesarean or uterine rupture [17].

Oxytocin

Oxytocin has been used for both labour induction and augmentation. It is associated with minimal to moderate increase in risk of uterine rupture. Should dilation cease, amniotomy is recommended as the first line treatment [3]. The uterine rupture risk associated with oxytocin is dose-dependent. Although there is no established maximum dose of oxytocin for TOLAC, doses exceeding 20 mU/min increase the risk of rupture at least four-fold [16]. ACOG, SOGC and RCOG all support the use of oxytocin for labour augmentation in TOLAC. RCOG states that oxytocin augmentation be titrated to not exceed the maximum rate of four contractions in 10 min. The ideal contraction frequency is 3–4 in 10 min. There should be careful serial cervical assessment, preferably by the same person each time [14].

Prostaglandins E2

PGE2 is associated with increase in risk of uterine rupture. TOLAC success rate falls when PGE2 is used with an unfavourable cervix. It must be used only with great prudence [3]. ACOG agrees to the use of PGE2 in rare circumstances, selecting women most likely to give birth vaginally, and avoiding sequential use of prostaglandins and oxytocin, as one large study found increase in rupture only when oxytocin was used after cervical ripening with prostaglandin [10].

Trans-cervical Balloon Catheter

Current data are insufficient to draw conclusions. A moderate increase in risk of uterine rupture is reported. ACOG, SOGC and CNGOF stated that it may be used for TOLC candidates with unfavourable cervix [3]. RCOG has not provided any recommendations about cervical ripening with mechanical methods.

Misoprostol

Misoprostol should not be used for third trimester cervical priming or induction in women with a history of caesarean birth [10,16]. It substantially increases the risk of uterine rupture (6%) [3,17]. It can be used, however, if gestation is less than 28 weeks [4]. It is the agent of choice for labour induction in early fetal demise even in women with a history of caesarean [4].

Uterine Rupture

Reported prevalence of rupture is 0.2–0.8% of women in TOLAC [3]. For women with one prior low transverse caesarean, the risk of rupture is no different from that of other equivalent serious adverse outcomes faced by all nulliparous women in labour, e.g. risk of abruption 1/100 [5].

Predicting Uterine Rupture

Uterine rupture is a real though unpredictable risk in TOLAC [15]. Clinical factors that increase the risk of uterine rupture during TOLAC include: [19]

1. short inter-delivery interval (≤24mths, OR 2.65 (1.08–5.46) and ≤18mths OR 3.0 (1.2–7.2));
2. short inter-pregnancy interval (<6mths, OR 2.66 (1.21–5.82));
3. birth weight ≥4 kg (OR 1.52 (1.09–2.11)),
4. locked single-layer closure versus double-layer closure (OR 4.96 (2.58–9.52)), locked single layer vs double (OR 0.49 (0.21–1.16)), and unlocked single vs double; and
5. labour induction (OR 2.6 (1.46–3.08)).

During labour induction, uterine rupture is more likely to occur in women:

1. without previous vaginal delivery [4] (OR 1.84 (1.11–3.05), induced vs spontaneous, with no prior vaginal delivery; OR 1.39 (0.62–3.13), induced vs spontaneous, with prior vaginal delivery); or
2. on epidural analgesia [17] (OR 2.12 (1.42–3.08)).

Those experiencing a rupture were significantly more likely to progress more slowly in the active phase of labour [2].

Previous vaginal delivery is the major clinical factor that decreases the risk of uterine rupture during TOLAC [19].

The following clinical factors do not affect the risk of uterine rupture during TOLAC [3]:

1. twins;
2. prolonged pregnancy;
3. maternal diabetes; and
4. maternal obesity.

Imaging is unreliable for forecasting which patient will rupture intrapartum. Neither ultrasound of lower segment at 35–40 weeks of pregnancy nor ultrasound appearance of scar 6–9 months after caesarean delivery is ready for clinical use [19]. They are not recommended to decide MOD [3]. Models and scores have been proposed, but none performed well enough for clinical use [19]. We currently lack a method for reliably estimating risk of rupture during labour [19]. Rupture can occur even in good candidates for VBAC [16].

Consequence of Uterine Rupture

Maternal Risks

Severe maternal morbidity, including hysterectomy, ICU transfer, visceral injuries and blood transfusion, happen in 15% of cases with uterine rupture. Maternal mortality is less than 1% [3].

Perinatal Risks

The risk of neonatal death or neurologic injury is more concerning than maternal morbidity. Perinatal death happens in 6% of cases with uterine rupture [14], asphyxia (umbilical pH <7.0 or neonatal encephalopathy) in 6–15% [3] and hypoxic-ischaemic encephalopathy with long-term disability in 0.5–19% [16]. Neurologic injury is rare if delivery can be accomplished within 18 min, and in many cases outcome has been good when delivered within 30 min [16].

Diagnosis of Uterine Rupture

The most frequently reported sign is non-reassuring FHR tracing, namely prolonged variable decelerations and bradycardia [2]. It is reported in up to 70% of cases with rupture, supporting the recommendation of CFHM. Less frequent symptoms include abdominal pain in the area of prior caesarean incision despite epidural analgesia [4], recession of the presenting vertex and vaginal bleeding. With concealed intraperitoneal bleeding, the woman might present with shoulder pain, restlessness and shock [16]. Persistent abdominal pain, defined as continuously present and specifically noted between contractions, is more strongly correlated with uterine rupture than either bradycardia or late decelerations [2].

Labour Monitoring

For women attempting TOLAC with no previous vaginal birth, the progress of labour is similar to that in normal nulliparas; with history of vaginal delivery, the labour pattern is comparable with that in multigravida. Continuous fetal heart monitoring is used to diagnose early signs of uterine rupture. The use of intrauterine pressure catheter has not been found to be superior to external monitoring or to assist in predicting or detecting uterine rupture [16].

In one small study using partogram for TOLAC, the alert line was 1 cm/h and the uterine rupture rate 2.9%. All uterine rupture occurred 2–6 hours after dilation stopped progressing. If caesarean had been performed at two or three hours after the alert line was crossed rather than later, the rupture rates would have been 0.8% and 1.6% respectively [5]. It is recommended that, in the active phase, the total duration of failure to progress should not exceed three hours; at this point, caesarean should be performed. There are no data to justify a recommendation during latent phase [3].

For augmented labour in a case of TOLAC, progress should be evaluated on a regular basis (ideally every two hours) to titrate oxytocin [4].

Third Stage Management

There is no evidence that an asymptomatic uterine scar should be routinely examined after delivery, or the uterus explored. The clinical relevance of asymptomatic uterine defect/dehiscence diagnosed by manual examination is low. It does not require surgical correction and data are insufficient for a recommendation about MOD in future pregnancies [3]. Only symptomatic rupture might require surgical repair [3].

All obstetric services should have a protocol for management of postpartum haemorrhage [15]. In the case of postpartum haemorrhage or hypovolaemic shock, make sure bleeding is not from a previous uterine incision. Among the differentials, uterine rupture and placenta accreta should be considered [4].

Special Clinical Situations

Breech

Uterine scar does not affect the success rate of external cephalic version (ECV) for breech, nor increase risk of uterine rupture. External cephalic version should be offered to women eligible for TOLAC [3]. After adequate assessment, vaginal breech delivery in a case of TOLAC is considered permissible, although data are insufficient [3].

Table 23.4 Increasing birth weight decreases the chance of VBAC

Birth weight (g)	TOLAC success rate (%)
<4000	68
4000–4249	52
4250–4500	45
>4500	38

Twin

TOLAC success rate for twins is similar to that for singletons with no clinically significant increase in uterine rupture rate and no greater risk of maternal or perinatal morbidity. TOLAC is possible for twins [3,10].

Fetal Macrosomia

Increasing birth weight decreases the chance of VBAC (Table 23.4) [2].

The chance of VBAC is also reduced if the previous caesarean was for dystocia and the current predicted birth weight is greater than that of the previous pregnancy. However, the false-positive rate for predicting estimated fetal weight over 4 kg by ultrasound is approximately 50%. The TOLAC success rate is >60% and increase in risk of uterine rupture, although doubled, is sufficiently minimal even for birth weight >4 kg. It is agreed that suspected macrosomia alone should not preclude TOLAC [3,10]. When the estimated fetal weight is >4.5 kg, particularly in women with no history of vaginal delivery, the TOLAC success rate is <40% and uterine rupture rate is increased three-fold, hence ERCD is recommended [3].

Preterm Pregnancy

The TOLAC success rate <37 weeks is similar to that at term with a lower risk for uterine rupture. The neonatal outcome is similar after TOLAC and ERCD <37 weeks. TOLAC should be encouraged for women in preterm labour [3].

Prolonged Pregnancy

Prolonged pregnancy reduces TOLAC success rate (failure beyond 40 weeks 31% vs 22%, OR 1.36 95% CI 1.24–1.50) [2]. Uterine rupture rate is not increased. TOLAC is possible for prolonged pregnancy >41 weeks [3].

Table 23.5 Comparing the outcomes between TOLAC after two caesareans, after one caesarean and ERCD after two caesareans

	TOLAC after 2 caesarean (%)	TOLAC after 1 caesarean (%)	ERCD after 2 caesarean (%)	P
VBAC	71.1	76.5		<0.001
Uterine rupture	1.36	0.72		<0.001
Hysterectomy	0.56 0.40	0.19	0.63	0.001 0.63
Transfusion	1.68		1.67	0.86
Fever	6.03		6.39	0.27

Previous Low Vertical Incision

Rate of successful TOLAC is similar to that of previous low transverse incision. There has not been consistent evidence of increased risk of rupture. Women with previous low vertical incision may choose to have TOLAC [10].

Unknown Type of Previous Uterine Incision

TOLAC success and uterine rupture rates are similar to those with low transverse incision. TOLAC is not contraindicated unless there is high clinical suspicion of classical scar [10].

Two Previous Caesareans

A recent review concluded that women with two previous caesareans requesting TOLAC had a success rate of 71%, uterine rupture risk of 1.36% and comparable maternal morbidity with ERCD (Table 23.5) [20].

Neonatal morbidity data are too limited to draw conclusions. However, there is no significant difference in the three comparison groups in neonatal unit admission rate, asphyxia injury and neonatal death rate [20].

It is reasonable to consider TOLAC after two previous caesareans. Data regarding risk for TOLAC with more than two prior caesareans are limited [10].

TOP or IUD

Over 28 weeks, cervical ripening with trans-cervical Foley for IUD cases is associated with rupture rate comparable to spontaneous labour [10].

In the second trimester, outcome of induction with prostaglandins (including PGE1) is similar to those with unscarred uterus (e.g. length of time until delivery, failed labour induction and complication rates). The frequency of rupture is <1% in most series [10].

RCOG recommends the use of a lower dose of misoprostol by cutting the tablet or dilution [19]. Mifepristone or hygroscopic dilators are not contraindicated [3]. Mifepristone could increase the chance of labour without PGE2 [21].

For those with two previous caesareans, risk of induction for IUD is only a little higher than with one previous caesarean [21]. With more than two caesareans or an atypical scar, the safety of induction is unknown [21]. Nevertheless, induction is preferable to ERCD in most cases, regardless of the number of past caesareans [3]. TOLAC may even be judged appropriate for prior classical scar after patient and healthcare providers weigh the risks and benefits [10].

TOLAC in Midwifery Practice

The debate regarding the site of birth is steeped over the controversial 'immediately available' standard. There is an argument that TOLAC has been singled out as a high-liability practice although rupture risk is similar to rate of abruption or other adverse events intrapartum with equally adverse outcomes [18]. In fact, most women may safely choose TOLAC under the care of a certified nurse-midwife (CNM) or certified midwife (CM) [18]. Midwifery practice is an attractive alternative to TOLAC candidates who treasure natural birth and, after assessment, are considered to have low uterine rupture risk and good prospect of VBAC.

To select the right candidate requires risk stratification [18]. Low-risk cases could attempt TOLAC in the community, while cases with higher risk should be managed in a hospital setting that has obstetric and anaesthesia services immediately available. One example of risk stratification on the basis of obstetric history and labour characteristics is as shown in Table 23.6 [18].

Common midwifery practice, such as admission only in active labour, continuous labour support, use of non-pharmacologic pain control, freedom of movement and delayed pushing are all evidence-based to promote vaginal birth. Continuous fetal heart monitoring, as routinely practised in obstetrician-led hospital units for women attempting VBAC, usually requires

Table 23.6 Risk stratification [18]

Low risk	One prior low transverse caesarean birth Spontaneous onset of labour No need for augmentation No repetitive FHR abnormalities Previous successful VBAC
Medium risk	Mechanical or oxytocin induction of labour Oxytocin augmentation Two or more previous low transverse caesarean births Fewer than 18 months between prior caesarean birth and current birth
High risk	Repetitive non-reassuring FHR abnormalities Not responsive to clinical intervention Bleeding suggestive of abruption Two hours without cervical change in active phase of labour

Table 23.7 TOLAC in out-of-hospital midwife-led birth centres [18]

	USA [22]	Germany [23]
Sample size	$N = 1453$	$N = 364$
Design	Prospective	Retrospective
One prior caesarean	93%	100%
Two prior caesareans	7%	0%
Postterm (≥42 weeks)	3.2%	0%
Prior vaginal birth	46%	29%
Hospital transfer in labour	24%	41.2%
Median time from decision to transfer to caesarean*	35min	NA
MOD		
Vaginal in birth centre	76%	58.8%
Vaginal in hospital	11%	19.2%
Caesarean	13%	22.3%
Uterine rupture		
One prior caesarean	0.2%	0
More than one prior caesarean	3%	NA
Maternal mortality	0	0
Perinatal mortality		
One prior caesarean	0.3%	0
More than one prior caesarean	2%	NA
Among cases of uterine rupture	33% (2/6)	0

Note
* Among women for whom data were available. NA, not applicable

bed rest, which disallows several labour support measures that have been documented to increase patient satisfaction and that facilitate vaginal birth [5]. The American College of Nurse-Midwives (ACNM) recommended either CFHM or intermittent monitoring as required for high-risk patients (i.e. every 15 min in active labour and every 5 min in the second stage) for women undergoing TOLAC [18]. The use of herbal or homeopathic uterotonics is not well supported by scientific evidence to date, and no data currently exist on the safety of these agents for patients with uterine scar. Their use is discouraged by ACNM for women attempting TOLAC [18].

Hospital-based Midwifery Practice

In a report of TOLAC in a hospital-based midwifery practice, the policy was to await spontaneous onset of labour, admission after active labour was established and intermittent FHR monitoring in labour. Women with more than one previous lower transverse scar or other medical or obstetrical complications were excluded. Of the 303 subjects, 84% had previous vaginal birth. The intrapartum medical transfer rate is 8.7%, similar to that of labouring women with no prior caesarean (10.4%), and VBAC rate is 98.3% with no uterine rupture. Midwifery care of women undergoing TOLAC has been reported safe and is associated with similar success rates, but studies are not big enough to determine incidence of rupture [5].

Out-of-hospital TOLAC

Several studies have looked into TOLAC in out-of-hospital midwife-led birth centres (Table 23.7) [18].

Among women with one prior caesarean, the uterine rupture and perinatal death rate is lower than the national rate for all women. Therefore, when women in medium- or high-risk categories are excluded, an out-of-hospital birthing centre is an option for TOLAC [5].

Unconventional TOLAC

On occasion, there are high-risk cases insisting on TOLAC in a setting with resources that cannot meet their risk level. An example is a 47-year-old woman in her second pregnancy contemplating TOLAC by water birth at home and the pregnancy has now gone beyond 43 weeks. This section outlines some of the principles in managing such difficult situations.

Patient-centred care is the standard in modern medicine, which treasures *patient autonomy* in decision making. Both professional guidelines and the law recognize the right of an adult to refuse medical intervention even if that refusal results in harm, and even death, to the patient. We must respect a woman's decision even if we do not agree with it.

There is no legal obligation for one person to help another through their body as in pregnancy, although some ethicists argue that women have a moral duty to protect the unborn fetus within them. In English law, a fetus is not considered a legal person until it is born. A fetus has no legal rights while in utero. *Our duty of care is to the pregnant women only. There is no legal duty to the unborn child* [1].

For women wishing to embark on non-conventional TOLAC, we should ensure that *they are fully informed to make such a decision.* The decisions made by an adult concerning medical treatment are governed by valid informed consent, which requires that sufficient relevant information must be given to make a decision. Recommended information for women who consider non-conventional TOLAC should include risks and benefits of both the recommended and her non-conventional birth plan. *Alternative and second opinion* should also be offered. We must be content that *she has capacity to make a decision* and she is *making a choice without duress.* Her reason for her choice should be explored in the absence of family and parents. If an interpreter is needed, it should be a professional interpreter rather than a family member. Be alert to the possibility of domestic violence in women who opt for home birth. Regardless of her choice, *we should continue to provide the care and support* that they require in pregnancy. If complications arise from an unconventional birth plan, we will have no legal liability unless there is proven negligence on our part, e.g. failure to give relevant information. However, we must still provide care according to our professional standards. We may be held liable if our care falls below these standards. A clear *birth plan made ahead of delivery* disseminated to relevant staff ensures that all staff are aware of the plan once in labour, and has the legal benefit of ensuring capacity at the time the plan is made. Women in labour are considered to lack capacity with relative ease, e.g. due to pain and emotional stress of labour. Documentation must be legible, meticulous and unambiguous. There should be *explicit documentation of acting contrary to medical advice* [1].

Good communication skills can facilitate collaboration and compromise in proposed risky TOLAC choices, and can reduce the prospects of liability claims. A paternalistic manner is more likely to alienate a woman. Even if we do not agree with a woman's choice, *a collaborative approach* aimed at maximizing fetal and maternal safety is more conducive to a good doctor–patient relationship. It helps to ensure that the woman will continue to seek help if needed rather than as a last resort [1].

ERCD

Timing of ERCD

To reduce respiratory morbidity of the newborn, ERCD should be performed after 39 weeks. For cases at higher risk of intrapartum uterine rupture, e.g. previous uterine rupture, consideration should be given to performing ERCD at 36–37 weeks [4].

Adhesion Prevention in ERCD

Surgical principles in adhesion prevention should be observed, including careful tissue handling, keeping tissue moist, meticulous haemostasis, minimizing ischaemia and desiccation, and using micro- and atraumatic instruments to reduce serosal injury. Foreign bodies, glove powder in particular, are strongly associated with adhesion formation. Powdered gloves should be avoided if possible. Irrigation of the peritoneal cavity and packing the gutters to limit spread of contaminated fluid and the practice of not exteriorizing the uterus has no proven impact on adhesion formation. Data concerning peritoneal closure are conflicting [24].

The Joel-Cohen method for opening the abdomen, suturing the uterus in one layer plus non-closure of visceral and parietal peritoneal layers is associated with significantly lower incidence of adhesion upon repeat caesarean. The type of suture material used during caesarean does not appear to have an effect on adhesion formation. Fibrin glue may be an acceptable alternative to suturing as animal studies showed a reduction in adhesion following its use [24].

Peritoneal lavage with crystalloid has little benefit for adhesion prevention. A 4% icodextrin solution has been approved by the FDA for secondary prevention of adhesion. It was recently introduced in laparoscopic surgery and has not been described for caesarean [24].

Two FDA-approved barrier membranes for adhesion prevention are available. Both have some suggestion of efficacy in reducing adhesion following caesarean. The use of *Interceed* during caesarean may be limited by requirement for complete haemostasis.

Use with incomplete haemostasis may promote adhesion. A case series found reduced incidence and severity of vesico-uterine adhesions at repeat caesarean. The efficacy of *Seprafilm adhesion barrier (HA-CMC)* is unaffected by the presence of blood. However, rare paradoxical inflammatory reaction with peritoneal granuloma formation has been reported. A reduction in the proportion of women with adhesion has been demonstrated during repeat caesarean (7.4% vs 48%, $p = 0.001$) [24].

Conclusion

A previous caesarean delivery presents a unique challenge. With few exceptions, TOLAC is a permissible option with an overall success rate of 60–80% and intrapartum uterine rupture risk of 0.5% for women with one prior lower transverse caesarean. Although complications are rare for both options, TOLAC in general poses slightly higher risk to the baby and ERCD to the mother. On balance, TOLAC is preferred for most women with one prior lower transverse uterine incision. For this group of women, labour induction is feasible in the presence of a solid indication. Although there remains an element of unpredictability in scar rupture, risk stratification helps to fill in the gap between safety in TOLAC, women's preference during childbirth and resource allocation. Occasional unconventional TOLAC birth plans should be treated with respect by a collaborative approach aimed at maximizing fetal and maternal safety. To reduce long-term maternal morbidity, care should be exercised in adhesion prevention during ERCD.

References

1. Dexter SC, Windsor S, Watkinson SJ. Meeting the challenge of maternal choice in mode of delivery with vaginal birth after caesarean section: a medical, legal and ethical commentary. *Br J Obstet Gynaecol*. 2014; 121: 133–40.

2. Holmgren CM. Uterine rupture associated with VBAC. *Clin Obstet Gynecol*. 2012; 55(4): 978–87.

3. Sentilhes L, Vayssière C, Beucher G, *et al.* Delivery for women with a previous cesarean: guidelines for clinical practice from the French College of Gynecologists and Obstetricians (CNGOF). *Eur J Obstet Gynecol Reprod Biol*. 2013; 170: 25–32.

4. Metz T, Scott JR. Contemporary management of VBAC. *Clin Obstet Gynaecol*. 2012; 55(4): 1026–32.

5. King TL. Can a vaginal birth after cesarean delivery be a normal labor and birth? Lessons from midwifery applied to trial of labor after a previous cesarean delivery. *Clin Perinatol*. 2011; 38: 247–63.

6. Dodd JM, Crowther CA, Huertas E, *et al.* Planned elective repeat caesarean section versus planned vaginal birth for women with a previous caesarean birth. *Cochrane Database Syst Rev*. 2013; 12: CD004224.

7. Guise JM, Denman MA, Emeis C, *et al.* Vaginal birth after cesarean: new insights on maternal and neonatal outcomes. *Obstet Gynecol*. 2010; 115(6): 1267–78.

8. National Institutes of Health. NIH Consensus Development Conference Statement vaginal birth after cesarean: new insights March 8–10, 2010. *Semin Perinatol*. 2010; 34(5): 351–65.

9. Clark EA, Silver RM. Long-term maternal morbidity associated with repeat cesarean delivery. *Am J Obstet Gynecol*. 2011; 205(6): s2–10.

10. ACOG. Practice Bulletin no. 115: vaginal birth after previous cesarean delivery. *Obstet Gynecol*. 2010; 116: 450–63.

11. Catling-Paull C, Johnston R, Ryan C, *et al.* Clinical interventions that increase the uptake and success of vaginal birth after caesarean section: a systematic review. *J Adv Nurs*. 2011; 67(8): 1646–61.

12. Catling-Paull C, Johnston R, Ryan C, *et al.* Non-clinical interventions that increase the uptake and success of vaginal birth after caesarean section: a systematic review. *J Adv Nurs*. 2011; 67(8): 1662–76.

13. NICE. Intrapartum care: caring of healthy women and their babies during childbirth: clinical guideline 190; 2014. www.nice.org.uk/guidance/cg190 (accessed 11 December 2014).

14. RCOG. *Birth After Previous Caesarean Birth*. London: RCOG Press; 2007.

15. Hawkins JL. The anesthesiologist's role during attempted VBAC. *Clin Obstet Gynecol*. 2012; 55(4): 1005–13.

16. Scott JR. Intrapartum management of trial of labour after caesarean delivery: evidence and experience. *Br J Obstet Gynaecol*. 2014; 121: 157–62.

17. Ophir E, Odeh M, Hirsch Y, *et al.* Uterine rupture during trial of labor: controversy of induction's methods. *Obstet Gynecol Surv*. 2012; 67(11): 734–45.

18. American College of Nurse-Midwives. Clinical Bulletin no. 12: care for women desiring vaginal birth after cesarean. *J Midwifery Womens Health*. 2011; 56(5): 517–25.

19. Valenti L. Prediction of scar integrity and vaginal birth after caesarean delivery. *Best Pract Res Clin Obstet Gynaecol*. 2013; 27: 285–95.

20. Tahseen S, Griffiths M. Vaginal birth after two caesarean sections (VBAC-2): a systematic review with meta-analysis of success rate and adverse outcomes of VBAC-2 versus VBAC-1 and repeat (third) caesarean sections. *Br J Obstet Gynaecol.* 2010; 117: 5–19.

21. RCOG. *Late Intrauterine Fetal Death and Stillbirth.* London: RCOG Press; 2010.

22. Lieberman E, Ernst EK, Rooks JP, Stapleton S, Flamm B. Results of the national study of vaginal birth after cesarean in birth centers. *Obstet Gynecol.* 2014; 104(5): 933–42.

23. David M, Gross MM, Wiemer A, Pachaly J, Vetter K. Prior cesarean section: an acceptable risk for vaginal delivery at free-standing midwife-led birth center? Results of the analysis of vaginal birth after cesarean section (VBAC) in German birth centers. *Euro J Obstet Gynecol Rep Biol.* 2009: 142(2): 106–10.

24. Bates GW, Shomento S. Adhesion prevention in patients with multiple cesarean deliveries. *Am J Obstet Gynecol.* 2011; 205(6): s19–24.

Chapter 24

Rupture of the Uterus

Ana Pinas Carrillo and Edwin Chandraharan

Introduction

Uterine rupture is an obstetric emergency that arises due to the disruption of the uterine wall, which occurs most frequently during labour and delivery but, rarely, may also occur during pregnancy. It is a catastrophic emergency, associated with high rates of both maternal and neonatal morbidity and mortality. The incidence of uterine rupture in an *unscarred* uterus is 1 in 10 000 deliveries; however, it increases up to 1% in women with previous caesarean section (CS). It can have dramatic consequences from infertility due to irreparable damage to the uterus that may necessitate hysterectomy, to maternal or neonatal death if diagnosis and surgical treatment are delayed.

Although uterine rupture is a rare event in modern obstetric practice, progressively increasing CS rates, especially in Western countries, could potentially increase its incidence. Uterine rupture can happen during the antenatal period, especially in the presence of a previous classical CS scar. However, it occurs most commonly during labour after the onset of uterine contractions. It is also more common in a scarred uterus, but in some parts of the developing world with poor healthcare, it can occur in an unscarred uterus often due to 'grand multiparity' and adverse intrapartum factors such as prolonged or obstructed labour, especially associated with undiagnosed cephalo-pelvic disproportion.

Epidemiology

Uterine rupture is rare in developed countries. The prevalence for women with previous CS is around 1%, while on an unscarred uterus it is extremely rare (<1 per 10 000). The World Health Organization (WHO) undertook a systematic review to obtain data on prevalence/incidence of maternal mortality and morbidity from uterine rupture. They included 86 groups of women and concluded that the prevalence of uterine rupture tended to be lower for countries defined as developed than those classified as less or least developed. For women with a previous CS, the prevalence of uterine rupture was reported to be approximately 1%. Only one group from a developed country reported data for women with an unscarred uterus and the prevalence was extremely low (0.006%) [1].

Classification and Risk Factors

There are two types of uterine rupture. Complete uterine rupture is defined as a full-thickness separation of the uterine muscle and the overlying visceral peritoneum; it can be associated with the extrusion of the fetus, placenta or both into the abdominal cavity. It is a dramatic life-threatening emergency for both the mother and the baby. An incomplete rupture is a disruption of the uterine muscle, but the visceral peritoneum remains intact, which is frequently due to a dehiscence of the CS scar. It is usually uncomplicated. Figure 24.1a shows a complete rupture and Figure 24.1b shows a partial rupture or dehiscence.

The most important risk factor for uterine rupture is the presence of a previous scar. Other causes are shown in Table 24.1.

Previous Caesarean Section

Antepartum rupture is rare and imaging studies of the previous caesarean scar are unreliable to predict the likelihood of intrapartum uterine rupture [2]. A systematic review that analysed 59 full-text articles including one randomized controlled trial (RCT)

Best Practice in Labour and Delivery, Second Edition, ed. Sir Sabaratnam Arulkumaran. Published by Cambridge University Press. © Cambridge University Press 2016.

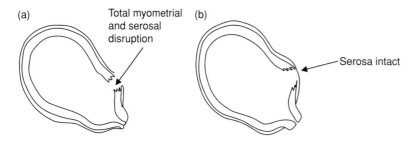

(a) Total myometrial and serosal disruption (b) Serosa intact

Figure 24.1 Types of scar rupture: (a) complete rupture; (b) scar dehiscence.

Table 24.1 Classification of causes of uterine rupture

Uterine injury or anomaly sustained *before* current pregnancy	Uterine injury or abnormality during current pregnancy
1. *Surgery involving the myometrium* Caesarean section or hysterotomy Previously repaired uterine rupture Myomectomy Deep cornual resection Metroplasty	1. *Before delivery* Induction or augmentation of labour External trauma External cephalic version (ECV)
2. *Coincidental uterine trauma* Abortion Sharp or blunt trauma	2. *During delivery* Internal podalic version Difficult forceps Breech extraction
3. *Congenital anomaly* Pregnancy in undeveloped uterine horn	3. *Acquired in pregnancy* Placenta increta or percreta Adenomyosis Sacculation of entrapped retroverted uterus

reported that the prevalence of rupture ranged from 0.5% to 1% [3].

There is no clear evidence on the effectiveness and safety of the agents used for induction of labour in women with a previous uterine scar. A Cochrane review [4] concluded that there was insufficient evidence available on which to base clinical decisions regarding management. It is, however, widely accepted that the use of misoprostol for induction of labour is contraindicated in the presence of a scarred uterus. One large study (20 095 cases) which analysed women who delivered a second singleton following a previous CS reported a uterine rupture rate of 5.2 per 1000 for spontaneous labour and 24.5 per 1000 for labour induced with prostaglandins [5]. Oxytocin used for induction and augmentation remains an option. However, it has been reported that doses exceeding 20 mU/min increase the risk of uterine rupture at least four-fold [3].

Previous Uterine Surgery

Despite the lack of evidence, the vast majority of obstetricians recommend an elective CS after myomectomy if the cavity has been entered into (i.e. 'breached') [6].

The location of the fibroid, the surgical technique and the occurrence of postoperative infection are other factors that can contribute to uterine rupture in subsequent pregnancy [7].

A comparison of the rates of uterine rupture between women with prior myomectomy (176) or prior classical caesarean delivery (455) with women with a prior low transverse caesarean (13 273) showed no statistical difference in the frequency of uterine rupture between the group with a prior myomectomy and the one with low transverse CS [8].

However, this study unfortunately does not state how many patients with a previous myomectomy delivered vaginally.

Laparoscopic myomectomies appear to be safe. A study reviewed 47 pregnancies in 40 patients after laparoscopic myomectomy. Vaginal delivery was attempted in 72% and was achieved in 83% in those who attempted a vaginal delivery with no cases of rupture. The authors advised that vaginal birth can be safely achieved provided they are managed as patients with previous CS [9].

Advances in the subspecialty of fetal medicine have resulted in an increasing number of intrauterine fetal surgeries. Fetoscopic procedures and open procedures such as ex utero intrapartum treatment (EXIT) procedure or mid-gestation open maternal–fetal surgery (OMFS) involve injury to a pregnant uterus and, subsequently, an increased risk of uterine rupture. Wilson *et al.* [10] reviewed the reproductive outcomes of 97 women undergoing maternal–fetal surgery. The number of subsequent pregnancies was 47, with a uterine dehiscence rate of 14% and rupture rate of 14%. These outcomes in a subsequent pregnancy should form part of counselling prior to OMFS.

Obstructed Labour

This represents an important cause of spontaneous rupture in the developing world, especially in women labouring outside hospital. There is a high incidence of cephalo-pelvic disproportion in Black African women. A retrospective review of 82 cases of uterine rupture in a Nigerian hospital (incidence 0.85%) showed that obstructed labour was the third commonest cause (18.7%) and occurred only in unbooked patients [11].

Multiparity is an independent risk factor for uterine rupture and it is considered to be due to the presence of a greater proportion of collagen compared to smooth muscle.

Congenital Uterine Malformations and Connective Tissue Disorders

In the presence of uterine congenital malformations, the walls are likely to be thinner and tend to diminish in thickness as gestation advances. Moreover, additional thinning can occur in the presence of uterine contractions [12]. Overall, uterine malformations complicate 1 in 594 pregnancies and the greatest risk of uterine rupture occurs during labour.

Disorders of connective tissue can also affect the structure and function of the uterus. There are cases described of uterine rupture associated with Ehlers–Danlos syndrome [13].

Induction of Labour and Termination of Pregnancy

There are only a few RCTs of induction of labour in women with a previous CS. Different methods have different incidence of uterine rupture. Ophir *et al.* [14] reviewed the existing evidence and concluded that the lowest rate of uterine rupture occurred with oxytocin (1.1%), then dinoprostone (2%), and the highest rate was with misoprostol (6%).

Trauma

Trauma contributes to only a minority of cases of uterine rupture. It usually occurs in the context of a road traffic accident or a history of assault. It is important to optimize education in trauma prevention in pregnancy and exclude uterine rupture in cases of domestic violence [15].

Mechanisms

It is well known that the risk of uterine rupture increases with the use of prostaglandins for induction of labour. However, the exact pathophysiology is not completely clear. Although one of the contributing factors is increased uterine contractility, it is believed that there may also be some biochemical changes within the collagen component of the scar tissue. This is illustrated by the observation that women treated with prostaglandins are more likely to experience rupture at the site of the old scar, whereas women treated with oxytocin experience uterine rupture on sites remote from the old scar [16]. Prostaglandins may induce changes in the collagen and ground substance (glycosaminoglycans) of the uterine scar, predisposing to an increased incidence of scar dehiscence or rupture.

Clinical Features

Uterine rupture can manifest with a wide spectrum of symptoms and signs depending on the site, extent and timing of rupture. While a scar dehiscence can be asymptomatic, a complete rupture can represent a dramatic emergency with fatal consequences for the mother, the fetus or both. Classical symptoms and signs include sudden onset of abdominal pain which is continuous and persistent between contractions, fresh vaginal bleeding, 'scar tenderness', evidence of fetal compromise (changes in fetal heart rate (FHR)) and alteration in the shape of the abdomen with the presence of easily palpable fetal parts. It is rare to observe all classical features in a single patient and a high index of clinical suspicion is required.

Abnormal FHR patterns can be detected on a cardiotocograph (CTG). These include cessation of uterine contractions often preceded by tachysystole or hypertonia, reduced baseline variability, variable or late decelerations or a single prolonged deceleration. The mechanisms underlying these CTG features include cord prolapse through the ruptured scar showing variable decelerations and abruption leading to late or prolonged decelerations.

Other symptoms include haematuria and bladder tenderness, especially with a previous lower segment uterine scar, as well as maternal tachycardia and signs of hypovolaemic shock and collapse that can lead to fetal demise or even maternal death, if immediate resuscitation and surgical treatment are delayed.

Uterine rupture presents most commonly as an intrapartum event but it can also occur in the antepartum period and very rarely in the immediate postpartum period.

Antepartum Rupture

Antepartum uterine rupture is characterized by abdominal pain as the most important clinical symptom. Vaginal bleeding may be present, but haemorrhage may be intra-abdominal, resulting in irritation of the diaphragm and causing pain referred to chest or to the shoulder. Antepartum rupture can occur in early pregnancy in patients with previous upper segment scars and not associated with contractions [17].

The patient can present with signs of shock, mainly due to hypovolaemia, although it can also have a neurogenic component. There may be abdominal tenderness, especially if associated with haemoperitoneum or presence of fetal parts into the abdominal cavity; however, uterine scar tenderness is not a reliable sign of uterine rupture.

Intrapartum Rupture

This is the most common presentation of uterine rupture. Abdominal pain is also a common symptom, classically presenting as constant acute pain that doesn't subside between contractions. Parallel to this, it is possible to observe a loss of contractions on the CTG, usually preceded by tachysystole or hypertonia. It can be difficult to interpret in the context of labour, but should raise the suspicion of uterine rupture or abruption. 'Scar tenderness', changes in uterine shape and palpation of fetal parts are other signs suggestive of rupture. They have high sensitivity but low specificity and are frequently unreliable. Vaginal bleeding may or may not occur. Haematuria might be present if there is bladder involvement.

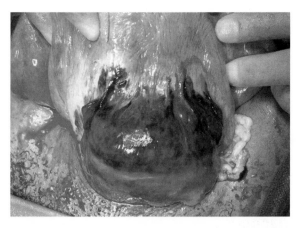

Figure 24.2 Uterine scar dehiscence during second stage of labour with a haematoma under the visceral peritoneum during laparotomy. See the colour plate section for a colour version of this figure.

Continuous FHR monitoring is recommended in all women aiming for vaginal delivery after CS (VBAC). Several studies report the association between FHR changes and uterine rupture. Prolonged deceleration, reduced baseline variability and uterine tachysystole were found to be common patterns with uterine rupture [18,19].

A receding presenting part ('loss of station') may also be a sign of uterine rupture, if the fetal presenting part had already entered the pelvis prior to the rupture. Abdominal and vaginal examination can identify the presenting part rising above the pelvic inlet.

Postpartum Rupture

This is an extremely rare event that usually presents with abdominal pain and postpartum haemorrhage. On vaginal examination, it is sometimes possible to palpate a dehiscence in the uterine wall and if the rupture is complete the fingers can be passed into the peritoneal cavity. However, studies have shown that systematic manual uterine exploration after VBAC does not improve the outcomes. Moreover, it can increase the risk of manual uterine rupture [20], and therefore this practice should be avoided. Figure 24.2 shows uterine scar dehiscence that occurred during active pushing which was followed by maternal collapse in the immediate postpartum period.

Findings on Laparotomy

Low uterine segment (LUS) is the part most commonly involved in rupture, with some studies reporting up to 92% of cases [21]. However, other parts may be involved, especially on previous classical CS, or involvement of the cervix among patients with an unscarred uterus. Rupture of the lower segment can also extend anteriorly towards the bladder, laterally towards the uterine arteries and into the broad ligament. It is important to perform a systematic examination of the uterus and other abdominal organs to ensure appropriate identification of all areas involved. Posterior rupture is rare but it can occur associated with uterine malformations, obstructed labour or instrumental delivery.

Diagnosis

There have been several attempts to predict the risk of uterine rupture in patients with a previous CS using ultrasound antenatally. A recent review included 21 articles that described LUS thickness in relation to the occurrence of a uterine dehiscence or rupture during labour. They found an LUS thickness cut-off of 3.1–5.1 mm and a myometrium thickness cut-off of 2.1–4.0 mm provided a strong negative predictive value for the occurrence of a uterine rupture during VBAC. A myometrial thickness between 0.6 and 2 mm provided a strong positive predictive value for the occurrence of a rupture. However, they could not determine an ideal cut-off to aid clinical practice [22].

The use of magnetic resonance imaging has also been described, but results are still inconclusive [23]. Clinical parameters include extension of uterine incision to the upper segment, uterine tears and very preterm CS.

Management

When uterine rupture is diagnosed, immediate delivery should be expedited to improve maternal and neonatal outcome. Initially, maternal vital signs need to be assessed, if the woman presents with signs of haemorrhagic shock, she needs to be resuscitated and stabilized. Fluid resuscitation and blood transfusion are vital to correct hypovolaemia, hypoxia and acidosis. Complete uterine rupture is an obstetric emergency that can lead to fetal demise and even maternal death if there is delayed intervention. The gravid uterus receives 12% of the cardiac output and thus uterine haemorrhage can lead to rapid hypovolaemic shock, which may pose an anaesthetic challenge. This is because inducing anaesthesia in patients who are hypovolaemic and hypotensive and maintaining

haemodynamic status before haemostasis is achieved could be challenging. Moreover, these patients can frequently develop coagulopathy and require blood products. The presence of an experienced obstetrician as well as an anaesthetist is essential. Senior neonatal input is also needed as the neonate is often born in poor condition.

Immediate laparotomy is essential and delivery of the fetus should be achieved within 15 min (category 1 CS). Occasionally the fetus may be completely extruded in the abdominal cavity and this is associated with worse outcomes.

Once the fetus and placenta are delivered, it is recommended to exteriorize the uterus in order to help arrest the bleeding and give a better view of the posterior aspect, the broad ligament and uterine angles to identify the site(s) of the rupture and associated lacerations. Once this has been done, the surgeon should decide on the most appropriate surgery depending on the patient's general condition, type and extent of the rupture, facilities available, previous obstetric history and own experience.

In case of a simple laceration or scar rupture, repair is appropriate, after ensuring that there are no lateral extensions or involvement of the broad ligament, parametrial vessels, ureters and bladder.

In cases of dehiscence of lower segment CS scars, it is advisable to trim the edges and suture the most viable parts [24].

Tubal sterilization could be considered, provided the circumstances have allowed to discuss this with the patient. However, if the rupture is simple and uninfected and the patient has a strong desire to preserve fertility, this can be omitted.

Hysterectomy should be considered in a lifethreatening situation when the patient is haemodynamically unstable and it is not possible to achieve haemostasis. It may also be considered in cases of extensive laceration. A subtotal hysterectomy is the advisable procedure if the cervix and paracolpos are not involved and if there is no associated sepsis. Uterine artery embolization is generally not feasible due to accompanying haemodynamic instability.

Insertion of a drain should be considered if there is evidence of continuous bleeding due to coagulopathy. Perioperative care includes appropriate administration of prophylactic antibiotics and thromboprophylaxis.

Appropriate documentation of the sequence of events that led to the uterine rupture along with the subsequent management plan is very important. Umbilical cord gases are mandatory.

An adverse incident report should be completed to inform the risk management team. In developed countries, uterine rupture is one of the most common clinical causes of medical litigation in obstetrics and gynaecology. In most cases, it is driven by poor clinical outcomes. Injudicious use of oxytocin is indefensible.

An appropriate debrief to the patient to discuss the sequence of events and consequences is very important. If the uterus has been preserved and no tubal ligation was performed, it is advisable to recommend contraception for a minimum of two years. Any future pregnancy should be closely monitored and an early elective CS should be considered after 37 weeks.

Differential Diagnosis

The main symptoms that present on uterine rupture are abdominal pain, hypovolaemia and fetal compromise. In the presence of these symptoms it is important to exclude placental abruption that may or may not present with vaginal bleeding. The obstetric history and clinical picture can help differentiate these two emergencies. Other less common conditions that can present with similar symptoms include subcapsular liver haematoma with or without rupture, splenic rupture, rupture of the broad ligament uterine vein and uterine torsion. All of these conditions require urgent surgical intervention and immediate laparotomy is generally indicated in patients presenting with these symptoms.

Complications

Maternal

Maternal morbidity and mortality very much depend on the extent of the rupture, the timeliness of diagnosis and intervention, and the availability of resources. Haemoperitoneum, the subsequent haemorrhagic shock and the complications derived from the interventions are responsible for the maternal complications.

In developed countries, maternal death is extremely rare but morbidity is significant. Complications secondary to the emergency intervention including bladder and ureteric injuries are not uncommon, especially during peripartum hysterectomy. Other complications include acute renal failure due to the

hypovolaemia, adverse effects derived from the massive blood transfusion and postoperative complications such as infection and thromboembolism. In more dramatic cases of massive haemorrhage, patients can develop renal, pituitary or liver failure that expedite transfer to the intensive care unit.

Long-term sequelae include renal failure and Sheehan's syndrome and psychological disorders secondary to the permanent loss of fertility in cases of hysterectomy, and post-traumatic stress disorder when there is a poor neonatal outcome.

The rare cases of maternal death in the developed world may be due to haemorrhage, shock, sepsis, disseminated intravascular coagulation and pulmonary embolism [25]. There is also an important human factor; failure to recognize the clinical condition and institute timely and appropriate intervention, failure to seek timely senior help and failure in effective multidisciplinary communication are some of the factors that may increase the likelihood of maternal mortality.

In less developed countries uterine rupture represents an important cause of mortality accounting for as many as 9.3% of maternal deaths as reported by one Indian study [26]. In the *Second Report on Confidential Enquiries into Maternal Deaths in South Africa 1999–2001*, ruptured uterus was responsible for 6.2% of deaths due to direct causes and 3.7% of all deaths (1.9% due to rupture of an unscarred uterus and 1.8% due to a scarred uterus) [1]. This increase is believed to be due to the use of misoprostol in uncontrolled dosages for induction of labour.

Perinatal

Disruption of uteroplacental circulation, secondary to placental abruption, results in fetal hypoxia and metabolic acidosis. This may result in neurological sequelae. If severe and not acted on in time it may result in perinatal death. The median umbilical cord gases reported are 6.80, median base excess −22 and median five minute Apgar score 4 [27]. Approximately 6% of uterine ruptures will result in perinatal death. The risk of hypoxic-ischaemic encephalopathy with long-term disability ranges from 0.5% to 19% [3]. In addition, short-term complications such as neonatal seizures and multiple organ failure requiring intubation and ventilation may ensue. Long-term implications include impaired motor development, learning difficulties and cerebral palsy. Neurological injury is rare if the infant is delivered within 18 min and good outcomes have been reported when delivered within 30 min [3]. Severe complications are more likely to occur in more dramatic cases of uterine rupture with placental or fetal extrusion into the abdominal cavity as the hypoxic insult is more acute in these cases [27].

Reproductive Outcome

Pregnancy after uterine rupture can be successfully managed with good antenatal, intrapartum and post-partum surveillance. There is no clear evidence on the course of action to be taken but there is a general consensus that delivery should be by elective CS as the risk of uterine rupture is too high. The timing of delivery will be assessed individually according to the gestational age of presentation of uterine rupture in the previous pregnancy, type of scar and individual obstetric history.

Recurrent uterine ruptures are associated with a high incidence of maternal and perinatal morbidity. It has been reported that recurrences are frequent, especially after longitudinal ruptures and short intervals between pregnancies.

Conclusion

Uterine rupture can occur at any gestational age. In developed countries uterine rupture is most commonly related to the presence of previous CS. The key steps to improve the outcomes are anticipation of uterine rupture and early diagnosis. Continuous electronic fetal monitoring in high-risk patients such as women undergoing trial of labour with the aim of vaginal delivery with a scarred uterus and recognition of cephalo-pelvic disproportion or malposition prior to augmentation of labour, especially with prolonged second stage of labour, will help to reduce uterine scar rupture.

In low-resource settings, primary precautions are the most important. These include health education such as recommendation of contraception in high-risk women, improving the access to healthcare services and provision of resources to deal with obstetric emergencies.

Although it is not currently possible to predict the occurrence of uterine rupture, early diagnosis and establishment of appropriate interventions are the key to improve the outcome for mothers and their babies.

References

1. Hoffmeyr GJ, Say L, Gulmezoglu AM. WHO systematic review of maternal mortality and morbidity: the prevalence of uterine rupture. *BJOG*. 2005; 112: 1221–8.

2. Varner M. Cesarean scar imaging and prediction of subsequent obstetric complications. *Clin Obstet Gynecol*. 2012; 55: 533–41.

3. Scott JR. Intrapartum management of trial of labour after caesarean delivery: evidence and experience. *BJOG*. 2014; 121: 157–62.

4. Jozwiak M, Dodd JM. Methods of term labour induction for women with a previous caesarean section. *Cochrane Database Syst Rev*. 2013; 3: CD009792.

5. Lydon-Rochelle M, Holt VL, Easterling TR, Martin DP. Risk of uterine rupture during labour in patients with a prior caesarean delivery. *N Engl J Med*. 2001; 345: 3–8.

6. Weibel HS, Jarcevic R, Gagnon R, Tulandi T. Perspectives of obstetricians on labour and delivery after abdominal or laparoscopic myomectomy. *J Obstet Gynaecol Can*. 2014; 36(2): 128–32.

7. Walsh CA, Baxi LV. Rupture of the primigravid uterus: a review of the literature. *Obstet Gynecol Surv*. 2007; 62(5): 327–34.

8. Gyamfi-Bannerman C, Gilbert S, Landon MB, *et al.* Risk of uterine rupture and placenta accreta with prior uterine surgery outside of the lower segment. *Obstet Gynecol*. 2012; 120(6): 1332–7.

9. Hurst BS, Matthews ML, Marshburn PB. Laparoscpic myomectomy for symptomatic uterine myomas. *Fertil Steril*. 2005; 12: 241–6.

10. Wilson RD, Lemerand K, Johnson MP, *et al.* Reproductive outcomes in subsequent pregnancies after a pregnancy complicated by open maternal–fetal surgery (1996–2007). *Am J Obstet Gynecol*. 2010; 203(3): e1–6. doi: 10.1016/j.ajog.2010.03.029.

11. Akaba GO, Onafowokan O, Offiong RA, Omonua K, Ekele BA. Uterine rupture: trends and feto-maternal outcome in a Nigerian teaching hospital. *Niger J Med*. 2013; 22(4): 304–8.

12. Nahum GG. Uterine anomalies, induction of labour and uterine rupture. *Obstet Gynecol*. 2005; 106(5 Pt 2): 1150–2.

13. Murray ML, Pepin M, Peterson S, Byers PH. Pregnancy-related deaths and complications in women with vascular Ehlers–Danlos syndrome. *Genet Med*. 2014; 16(12): 874–80. doi: 10.1038/gim.2014.53.

14. Ophir E, Odeh M, Hirsch Y, Bornstein J. Uterine rupture during trial of labor: controversy of induction's methods. *Obstet Gynecol Surv*. 2012;

67(11): 734–45. doi: 10.1097/OGX.0b013e318273 feeb.

15. El Kady D, Gilbert WM, Xing G, Smith LH. Maternal and neonatal outcomes of assaults during pregnancy. *Obstet Gynecol.* 2005; 105(2): 357–63.

16. Buhimschi CS, Buhimschi IA, Patel S, Malinow AM, Weiner CP. Rupture of the uterine scar during term labour: contractility or biochemistry? *BJOG.* 2005; 112(1): 38–42.

17. Turner MJ. Uterine rupture. *Best Pract Res Clin Obstet Gynaecol.* 2002; 16: 69–79.

18. Ridgeway JR, Weyrich DL, Benedetti TJ. Fetal heart rate changes associated with uterine rupture. *Obstet Gynecol.* 2004; 103: 506–12.

19. Sheiner E, Levy A, Ofir K, *et al.* Changes in fetal heart rate pattern and uterine patterns associated with uterine rupture. *J Reprod Med.* 2004; 49: 373–8.

20. Dinglas C, Rafael TJ, Vintzileos A. Is manual palpation of the uterine scar following vaginal birth after cesarean section (VBAC) helpful? *J Matern Fetal Neonatal Med.* 2015; 28(7): 839–41. doi: 10.3109/14767058.2014.935326

21. Ofir K, Sheiner E, Levy A, Katz M, Mazor M. Uterine rupture: differences between a scarred and an unscarred uterus. *Am J Obstet Gynecol.* 2004; 191(2): 425–9.

22. Kok N, Wiersma IC, Opmeer BC, *et al.* Sonographic measurement of lower uterine segment thickness to predict uterine rupture during a trial of labor in women with previous Cesarean section: a meta-analysis. *Ultrasound Obstet Gynecol.* 2013; 42(2): 132–9. doi: 10.1002/uog.12479.

23. Murphy DJ. Uterine rupture. *Curr Opin Obstet Gynecol.* 2006; 18(2): 135–40.

24. Rameez MFM, Goonewardene M. Uterine rupture. In Chandraharan E, Arulkumaran S (eds), *Obstetric and Intrapartum Emergencies* (pp. 52–8). Cambridge: Cambridge University Press; 2012.

25. Nagarkatti RS, Ambiye VR, Vaidya PR. Rupture uterus: changing trends in etiology and management. *J Postgrad Med.* 1991; 37(3): 136–9.

26. Rajaram P, Agarwal A, Swain S. Determinants of maternal mortality: a hospital based study from South India. *Indian J Matern Child Health.* 1995; 6(1): 7–10.

27. Bujold E, Gauthier RJ. Neonatal morbidity associated with uterine rupture: what are the risk factors? *Am J Obstet Gynecol.* 2002; 186: 311–14.

Management of Severe Pre-Eclampsia/Eclampsia

James J. Walker

Introduction

Although pre-eclampsia is recognized as a placental disease which leads to varied systemic manifestations, it is the systemic signs and symptoms that bring it to the attention of the clinician [1,2]. The placental pathology is responsible for the fetal growth restriction, but is benign to the mother. However, the clinical diseases of severe pre-eclampsia and eclampsia are, along with haemorrhage and sepsis, one of the three major killers of pregnant women worldwide [3]. Within the UK, the incidence of maternal death for both pre-eclampsia and eclampsia has fallen dramatically over the last 50 years [4,5] to the lowest level it has ever been (Figures 25.1, 25.2), but its continuing potential dangers cannot be understated [3,6]. Much of the reduction in death was before the advent of modern methods of care and was due to the increasing health of society, vigilant antenatal care, admission to hospital and expedited delivery. In recent years, the further reductions in death and morbidity have been helped by evidence-based guidelines [1,7], good-quality randomized trials [8–10], reviews [6,11–15] and large case studies [3,6,12,16–19]. Despite this, the Confidential Enquiries into maternal deaths persistently show substandard care in a significant percentage of the deaths that do occur [4]. The aim of this chapter is to give guidance on the diagnosis and management of severe pre-eclampsia and eclampsia in the immediate pre- and postdelivery interval, and is based on established evidence-based guidelines and extensive experience.

Presentation and Diagnosis

The diagnosis of pre-eclampsia has been greatly improved by vigilant antenatal care, but only around 60% of cases are picked up in this way, with many still presenting acutely with varied signs and symptoms. Although the primary diagnosis is based on hypertension and proteinuria (Table 25.1), these are only signs of the underlying disease, and other wide-ranging complications can be present and virtually any organ system may be affected (Table 25.1). Although these complications can be given other labels such as HELLP (haemolysis, elevated liver enzymes and low platelet count) syndrome, they are all variations of the same underlying disease process and point to severity rather than a different diagnosis [2,20]. These variations contribute greatly to the complications found with this condition, with up to 35% of women having significant morbidities [6].

Definitions

See Table 25.1. However, it is high blood pressure that is the biggest immediate risk to the mother, and is the most common presenting sign. Even in women who present with other symptoms, such as headache or abdominal pain, it is the elevation of blood pressure that makes the diagnosis and initiates intervention. There is now general agreement that severe hypertension is present if the systolic blood pressure is over 160 mmHg or the diastolic blood pressure is over 110 mmHg on three occasions within a space of 15 min [1,7,21]. Moderate hypertension is present if the systolic blood pressure is between 140 and 159 mmHg and the diastolic blood pressure between 100 and 109 mmHg on three occasions. This is also classified as severe if it is present with significant proteinuria and/or at least two other significant signs or symptoms (Table 25.1). Eclampsia is defined as the occurrence of one or more convulsions superimposed on

Best Practice in Labour and Delivery, Second Edition, ed. Sir Sabaratnam Arulkumaran. Published by Cambridge University Press. © Cambridge University Press 2016.

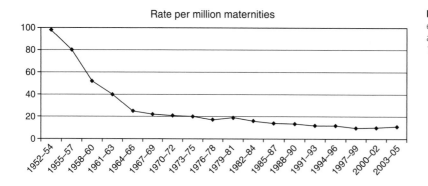

Figure 25.1 Maternal mortality from eclampsia and pre-eclampsia: England and Wales 1952–84; United Kingdom 1985–2005.

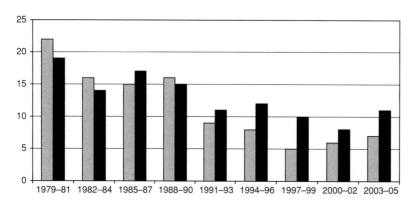

Figure 25.2 Maternal mortality from eclampsia (grey) and pre-eclampsia (black) in the United Kingdom.

pre-eclampsia. Up to 40% of women presenting with eclampsia may have no obvious prodromal signs or symptoms, but have a clear diagnosis of pre-eclampsia after the convulsion has occurred [22].

Table 25.1 Classification of pre-eclampsia/eclampsia

1. Eclampsia	The occurrence of one or more convulsions superimposed on pre-eclampsia
2. Severe pre-eclampsia	Systolic blood pressure over 160 mmHg; or diastolic blood pressure over 110 mmHg (*three blood pressure readings in a 15 min period*) with at least proteinuria of a + + or >0.3 g in 24 hours.
3. Moderate pre-eclampsia	Systolic blood pressure over 140 mmHg; or diastolic blood pressure over 90 mmHg (three blood pressure readings in a 45 min period) with at least proteinuria + + or >0.3 g in 24 hours.
And any of the following	Symptoms of headache; visual disturbance; epigastric pain; signs of clonus; papilloedema; liver tenderness; platelet count falling to below 100 × 10⁹/L; alanine amino transferase (ALT) above 50 IU/l

The Problem

Although the classification of pre-eclampsia and its severity is primarily based on the level of blood pressure and the presence of proteinuria, clinicians should be aware of the potential involvement of other organs when assessing maternal risk and the degree of placental disease causing fetal manifestations. It is important that any presenting woman is managed on clinical grounds and not on any perceived presence or absence of a given diagnosis. Many of the maternal deaths and severe morbidity that occur are in women who do not fit the strict criteria of pre-eclampsia. Therefore, clinical signs should not be ignored simply because the precise diagnosis is in doubt.

In the UK, the majority of deaths have been due to cerebral causes, with cardiorespiratory complications being the next most common (Table 25.2). Renal failure, a commonly perceived risk in pre-eclampsia, is a rare event, occurring in around 1/200 cases [6]. It is also a rare cause of death, largely due to the fact that it is not that common, is generally due to acute tubular necrosis which is recoverable, and can be relatively easily managed with dialysis support if required. There has been no maternal death from renal failure

Table 25.2 The causes of maternal death from pre-eclampsia/eclampsia in the UK over the last 40 years. The breakdown of causes is not yet available for the last triennium

Year	Cerebral	Pulmonary	Hepatic	Renal	Other	Total
1970–72	25	8	5	3	6	47
1973–75	23	7	14	1	4	49
1976–78	21	4	5	0	3	33
1979–81	17	8	8	0	3	36
1982–84	21	3	0	0	1	25
1985–87	11	11	1	1	2	26
1988–90	14	10	1	0	2	27
1991–93	5	11	0	1	3	20
1994–96	7	8	3	0	2	20
1997–99	7	2	2	0	5	16
2000–02	9	1	0	0	4	14
2003–05	12	0	2	0	4	18
2006–08	12	0	6	0	2	19
2009–11	?	?	?	?	?	9
Total	184	73	46	6	41	359

in the UK for over 20 years (Table 25.2). This has led to the establishment of guidelines that concentrate on the control of hypertension and the management of fluid balance [7]. Using this form of standardized care package for pre-eclampsia, the Yorkshire series had no maternal deaths in over 1000 cases of severe pre-eclampsia and eclampsia with reduced maternal and neonatal morbidity [6].

Although the main disease morbidity for the baby is placental insufficiency and its consequences, the main cause of death is iatrogenic prematurity due to the need to end the pregnancy because of disease severity. The fact that growth restriction is more common in early onset disease means that these problems are additive.

Therefore, the approach on admission should be to assess the severity of the disease and the risk to both the mother and the baby. Blood pressure control should be the first line of management, as it is easy and life-saving. Convulsions, if present, need to be controlled, but the use of prophylactic anticonvulsive therapy is more controversial. Fluid management is more of a problem for intra- and postpartum care, but antenatally, judicious fluid replacement is necessary if delivery is planned. As far as the baby is concerned, emergency delivery on admission is rarely necessary in the absence of placental abruption, but careful assessment of fetal well-being and the likelihood of prolonging the

pregnancy needs to be assessed as part of the decision-making process.

How Should Women be Assessed at Initial Presentation?

Many women with severe disease may have few, if any, symptoms and the high blood pressure is discovered as part of routine antenatal care. Others will present with convulsions, abdominal pain or general malaise. As in all medical situations, a clear history and examination should be carried out, and pre-eclampsia should always be considered as a potential diagnosis. The presence or absence of symptoms, particularly headache and abdominal pain, is important, as their presence implies systemic involvement, worsening disease and the increased risk of morbidity. Increasing oedema is a common presenting feature, but is not in itself a sign that should determine management. Enquiry about fetal movement should not be forgotten as an immediate assessment of fetal well-being and as their presence is reassuring.

Examination should start with the diagnostic signs of blood pressure measurement and urine analysis. Abdominal examination should be carried out to assess uterine size and liquor volume, presence of uterine tenderness suggestive of concomitant placental abruption or upper abdominal tenderness suggestive of liver tenderness and HELLP syndrome. Maternal tendon reflexes, although useful to assess magnesium toxicity, are not of value in assessing the risk of convulsion, although the presence of clonus may be. If the woman is extremely unwell, particularly in the postpartum period, she should be assessed for signs of pulmonary oedema, and continuous oxygen saturation monitoring with a pulse oximeter can be invaluable. Auscultation of the fetal heart and commencing of electronic fetal heart monitoring allows further fetal assessment.

An important consideration is the early involvement of senior obstetric and anaesthetic staff and experienced midwives in the assessment and management of women with severe pre-eclampsia and eclampsia. Repeatedly, the Confidential Enquiry into maternal deaths associates the absence of senior involvement with the occurrence of substandard care [4].

How Should the Blood Pressure be Taken?

It is important to take the blood pressure with a cuff of the appropriate size. If in doubt, it is better to use a larger cuff as this will result in less error in a normal size arm than a smaller cuff in overweight women. At least three readings should be carried out and averaged to confirm the diagnosis because of natural variation (see Table 25.1). Korotkoff phase 5 is the appropriate measurement of diastolic blood pressure [23]. Whatever method is used, it should be consistent and documented. Automated methods need to be used with caution, as they systematically underestimate blood pressure readings in pre-eclampsia, especially at higher blood pressure levels [24]. Validation using a mercury sphygmomanometer or other validated device should be carried out if there is concern.

The blood pressure should be checked every 15 min in the acute phase until the woman is stabilized, and then less often depending on the clinical situation.

High blood pressure is the main maternal risk and commencement of antihypertensive therapy if the blood pressure is above 160/100 mmHg is recommended without requiring further assessment. Using the recommended drugs and doses has been shown to be beneficial to the mother and carries no increased risk to the baby [7,25].

How Should the Woman be Monitored?

The presence of proteinuria confirms the diagnosis of pre-eclampsia and systemic involvement, but the level does not differentiate severity and therefore does not need to be repeated once its presence is established [7,26]. Its presence is particularly associated with increased risk to the baby.

The usual screening test for proteinuria is visual dipstick assessment. While it is accepted that there is a poor predictive value from urine dipstick testing [16,27], an approximate equivalence is 1+ = 0.3 g/l, 2+ = 1 g/l and 3+ = 3 g/l. Therefore, generally, a 2+ dipstick measurement can be taken as evidence of proteinuria for clinical management. If a more accurate test is required, this should be a 24-hour urine collection, the 'gold standard', or a spot protein creatinine ratio where a level of 0.03 g/mmol appears to be equivalent to 0.3 g/24 hours, the accepted threshold diagnostic level [7].

Therefore, the immediate presumptive diagnosis and presumed severity can be assessed at the bedside: blood pressure and proteinuria measurement along with clinical history and examination. Initial treatment can be instigated without waiting for biochemical, haematological and ultrasound examination.

What Further Tests are Required?

Once a woman has been assessed clinically and any high blood pressure or convulsion managed, a fuller assessment of her and her disease and her baby can be made. This requires a full blood count, liver and renal function tests. These should be repeated as required to assess clinical stability or deterioration. Generally, clotting studies are not required if the platelet count is over 100×10^6/l.

Uric Acid

In pre-eclampsia, there is a rise in uric acid in most cases which helps to confirm the diagnosis of pre-eclampsia and confers an increased risk to the mother and baby, but the absolute levels should not be used for clinical decision making. It is no longer recommended as part of the routine assessment of pre-eclampsia [7].

Urea and Creatinine

Renal function is generally maintained in pre-eclampsia until the late stage. If urea or creatinine is elevated early in the disease process, underlying renal disease should be suspected. There tends to be a rise postpartum, which is of little significance as renal failure is uncommon in pre-eclampsia in the absence of haemorrhage, HELLP syndrome or sepsis.

Platelets

A falling platelet count is associated with worsening disease and is in itself a risk to the mother. However, it is not until the count is less than $100 \times 10^6/l$ that there may be an associated coagulation abnormality. A count of less than 100 should be a consideration for delivery, as this will tend to fall further, particularly postpartum.

Liver Function Tests

An AST level of above 75 IU/l is seen as significant and a level above 150 IU/l is associated with increased morbidity to the mother. A diagnosis of HELLP syndrome needs confirmation of haemolysis, either by LDH levels or by blood film. These tests are not generally done in the UK, and the diagnosis of HELLP is usually based on platelets and liver function tests (LFTs) alone (ELLP).

Fluid Management

If delivery is planned, close fluid balance with charting of input and output is essential. A catheter with a urometer is helpful during delivery and in the immediate postpartum period. The use of continuous oxygen saturation monitoring with a pulse oximeter can demonstrate early signs of pulmonary oedema [6], the best sign of fluid overload.

How Should the Fetus be Assessed?

After an initial clinical assessment, a cardiotocograph should be carried out. This gives immediate information about fetal well-being and a reactive reassuring tracing suggests that the fetus is not in any immediate danger. Women in labour with severe pre-eclampsia should have continuous electronic fetal monitoring.

The main pathology affecting the fetus is placental insufficiency leading to intrauterine growth restriction (IUGR) in around 30% of pre-eclamptic pregnancies. If conservative management is planned, then further assessment of the fetus using ultrasound should be carried out. Ultrasound assessment of fetal size at presentation is a valuable one-off measurement to assess fetal growth, and can be informative for the decision to deliver, assessment of survival chance and to inform the neonatal unit. Liquor volume should be assessed at the same time, along with umbilical artery Doppler waveform, using absent or reversed-end diastolic flow as a diagnostic criterion [28]. In the presence of normal liquor volume and umbilical Doppler waveforms, continuation of the pregnancy for an average of 15 days is possible if the mother is stable [25]. If abnormalities of fetal assessment are found, prolongation for more than a few days is unlikely, although a course of antenatal steroids should still be attempted if required. Repeat assessment of liquor volume and umbilical artery Doppler waveform can be used along with cardiotocography to assess fetal well-being and optimize delivery. Daily assessment of the changes in umbilical artery and the mid-cerebral artery Doppler waveforms and their ratio can give a more accurate estimate of fetal well-being and decompensation [29].

Pre-delivery Care

General Measures

Initially, the woman should be managed in a high-dependency area, ideally with one-to-one midwifery care. After initial assessment, a decision has to be made about continued management, particularly the need for antihypertensive therapy, magnesium sulphate and antenatal steroids. If delivery is planned, the need for transfer because of fetal and/or maternal care should be considered. This management should be led by the most senior obstetrician present and the consultant should be called to attend. Close liaison with neonatal and anaesthetic colleagues is necessary, again at senior level.

An intravenous cannula should always be inserted, but fluid given with care. A urinary catheter is not always necessary, but may be helpful to monitor urine output over delivery and postpartum.

Antihypertensive Therapy

A blood pressure greater than 160/110 mmHg requires treatment in the maternal interest and many authorities, including the author, recommend that a threshold diastolic blood pressure of over 100 mmHg should be used. Similarly, if the blood pressure is below 160/100 mmHg, there is no immediate need for antihypertensive therapy unless it is associated with other markers of severe disease, such as heavy proteinuria or disordered liver or haematological test results. In these situations, antihypertensive treatment can be used to prevent a hypertensive crisis. Most women can be managed with oral therapy alone [6], with the preferred therapeutic agents being labetalol, nifedipine, hydralazine or methyldopa (Table 25.3) [1,7].

Table 25.3 Antihypertensive therapy

Labetalol

Oral dose of 200 mg repeated hourly as required.

Daily dose range from 200 mg bd to a maximum of 400 mg qid.

IV bolus dose 50 mg (= 10 ml of labetalol 5 mg/ml) given over at least 1 min. Can be repeated every 10 min if required to a maximum dose of 200 mg.

The pulse rate should be monitored and remain over 60 beats per minute.

IV infusion of neat labetalol at a rate of 4 ml/h via a syringe pump. The infusion rate should be doubled every half-hour to a maximum of 32 ml (160 mg)/h until the blood pressure has reduced and stabilized at an acceptable level.

Nifedipine

Oral dose of 10 mg repeated six-hourly.

After delivery initially this may be changed to the slow-release preparation given 12-hourly.

Hydralazine

IV bolus dose of 5 mg with repeating 5–10 mg IV every 30 min until control is achieved to a maximum of 20 mg.

IV infusion of 0.5–10 mg/h IV to a maximum of 20 mg.

IM dose – intermittent doses of 5–10 mg up to a maximum of 30 mg.

Methyldopa

Oral dose of 250 mg orally usually given three times a day. This can be increased to a 500 mg dose up to four times a day with a maximum daily dose of 2 g.

Labetalol

Labetalol has the advantage that it can be given initially by mouth and then, if needed, intravenously by bolus or infusion. Most women will respond to an initial 200 mg oral dose, which should lead to a reduction in blood pressure in about half an hour. A second oral dose can be given if needed an hour later. Regular daily medication can then be commenced. If there is no response to oral therapy, or if it cannot be tolerated, control should be by repeated IV bolus of labetalol followed by a labetalol infusion if required (Table 25.3). Labetalol should be avoided, if possible, in women with known asthma.

Nifedipine

If labetalol is contraindicated or fails to control the blood pressure, then nifedipine is an alternative or additive agent. This should be given as a 10 mg oral tablet. If it controls blood pressure, it should be repeated six-hourly initially, although it may be changed after delivery to a slow-release preparation

which lasts 12 hours. Blood pressure should be measured every 10 min in the first half-hour after treatment, as often there can be a very marked drop in pressure. The previous voiced concern over interaction between magnesium sulphate and nifedipine does not appear to be a clinical problem.

Hydralazine

Hydralazine has traditionally been the drug of choice in the acute situation, but a review has suggested that hydralazine may be less preferable compared with labetalol [9]. Although the evidence is not strong enough to preclude its use, it has largely been superseded by labetalol, which has the advantages of the oral as well as intravenous route. When using hydralazine there is an increased risk of hypotension, so the starting dose should be 5 mg IV and repeated as required. An infusion can also be used, as can the intramuscular route (Table 25.3).

Methyldopa

Methyldopa is still commonly used in the UK and throughout the world, and has been proven safe in long-term follow-up of the delivered babies. However, studies have suggested superior benefits of labetalol. Methyldopa is less effective in the acute situation, but may be the only drug available if others are contraindicated or fail. If used, the starting dose is 250 mg orally, usually given three times a day. This can be increased to a 500 mg dose up to four times a day, with a maximum daily dose of 2 g.

Hospitals should have a guideline available outlining their drug of choice. It is important that attendant staff know how to give the drug and what effect to expect. Too often, too little drug is given, with the resulting lack of benefit.

If the mother is easily stabilized and the fetus appears well, a prolongation of pregnancy of an average of 15 days is possible, as long as there is no other reason to deliver [25]. In most cases a delay of 48 hours is possible to allow the use of antenatal steroids in pregnancies under 34 weeks' gestation.

Management of Seizures

See Table 25.4. Usually, women will present after the convulsion has occurred, and sometimes it is diagnosed by history alone. However, if attending during the convulsion, this is a medical emergency and

Table 25.4 Magnesium sulphate intravenous protocol

Magnesium sulphate is given as a loading dose followed by a continuous infusion for 24 hours or until 24 hours after delivery, whichever is later. The actual dosage used varies around the world, but that used in the Collaborative Eclampsia Trial is recommended in the UK [8].

Loading dose Loading dose of 4 g should be given intravenously over 5 min, equating to 20 ml magnesium sulphate 20% IV over 5 min.

Maintenance dose An infusion of 1 g/h maintained for 24 hours equating to 50 ml magnesium sulphate 20% IV via a syringe pump at an infusion rate of 5 ml/hr. Each syringe should last ten hours.

There is no need to measure magnesium levels with the above protocol.

Important observations

The following observations should be performed:
1. continuous pulse oximetry;
2. hourly urine output (should be greater than 100 ml in four hours);
3. hourly respiratory rate (should be >12/min); and
4. deep tendon reflexes (should be present).

The antidote is 10 ml 10% calcium gluconate given slowly intravenously over 10 min.

Table 25.5 Causes of death in women in the MAGPIE study [9]

	Magnesium group	Placebo	Total
Cardiorespiratory failure	5	7	12
Stroke	3	2	5
Other	3	3	6
Renal failure	0	3	3
PE	0	3	3
Infection	0	2	2
Total	11	20	31

its management should be subject to regular multidisciplinary training drills. The woman should be protected from injury during the convulsion and not left alone. Help should be summoned, including the anaesthetist and senior obstetrician. The usual assessment of airway, breathing and circulation (ABC) is the primary approach, with the woman in the left lateral position and oxygen administered by facemask. The respiratory rate, pulse and blood pressure should be checked.

Magnesium sulphate is the therapy of choice, even in the acute situation, and diazepam and phenytoin should not be first line drugs. This should be given by standard regime (Table 25.4). Since 97% of magnesium is excreted in the urine, the presence of oliguria can lead to toxic levels. If oliguria is present, further magnesium sulphate infusion should be withheld. Since magnesium is not being excreted, no other anticonvulsant is needed. Magnesium can then be re-introduced if urine output improves.

Recurrent seizures can be treated with either a further bolus of 2 g magnesium sulphate or an increase in the infusion rate to 1.5 or 2.0 g/h. If seizures persist, then alternative agents such as diazepam or thiopentone can be used, but prolonged use of diazepam is associated with an increase in maternal death and neonatal respiratory depression. If all therapy fails and convulsions persist, intubation and transfer to intensive care facilities for intermittent positive pressure ventilation may be needed.

The main side-effects of magnesium are motor paralysis demonstrated by absent tendon reflexes and respiratory depression as well as cardiac arrhythmia, but these are unusual with the 1 g/h dosage. If there is any concern, the antidote calcium gluconate should be given (Table 25.4).

Once stabilized, delivery should be planned, but a delay of several hours is allowable to allow full preparation, assuming that there is no acute fetal concern, such as a fetal bradycardia.

How Should Seizures be Prevented?

Although it is clear that, in the presence of convulsions, magnesium sulphate is the drug of choice, its role in prevention of convulsions in severe pre-eclampsia is less clear. The MAGPIE trial has demonstrated that administration of magnesium sulphate to women with pre-eclampsia reduces the risk of an eclamptic seizure by 58% compared to placebo [9]. Although the relative risk reduction was similar regardless of the severity of pre-eclampsia, the number needed to treat depended on the absolute risk of convulsion. Therefore, its benefit is less clear in low-risk countries and premature presentations where the background incidence of eclampsia is low. In the trial, there was also a reduction in the rate of complications independent of the convulsions. The cases of death were similar in both groups except for the more unusual causes, for the developed world, of thrombosis and sepsis (Table 25.5).

Therefore, it would seem that its benefit to women in the developed world is less definite. In the last 12 years there has been a rise in the number of women

307

dying of pre-eclampsia/eclampsia in the UK, despite the use of magnesium. These have been mostly due to cerebral vascular accident. Therefore, in the UK, where the incidence of eclampsia is low, lowering blood pressure in severe pre-eclampsia should be the first line therapy, not magnesium sulphate, as this is the main risk of death. Magnesium sulphate should be limited to those women who are being delivered, the blood pressure is poorly controlled or there are other concerning signs, particularly persistent headache. If used, the infusion should be continued for 24 hours following delivery or 24 hours after the last seizure, whichever is the later, unless there is a clinical reason to continue.

How Should Fluid Balance be Managed?

Pulmonary oedema is the second most common cause of maternal death (Table 25.2), often associated with inappropriate fluid management, but this was also seen in the MAGPIE trial. Since the main risk of pulmonary oedema is in the first 48 hours postpartum, fluid replacement should be managed carefully throughout the intrapartum/postnatal period. There is no evidence for the benefit of fluid expansion and it should not be used [30], since fluid restriction is associated with a good maternal outcome [6]. Total fluids should be limited to 80 ml/h or 1 ml/kg/h. Urine output should be measured as part of the input/output assessment, but there is no need to maintain a particular output volume to prevent renal failure, as oliguria occurs in around 30% of women with severe pre-eclampsia and renal failure is rare. Fluid restriction should be maintained until there is a postpartum diuresis. If there is associated maternal haemorrhage, fluid restriction is inappropriate, but replacement should be given using some form of invasive monitoring. This is usually by central venous pressure (CVP) monitoring, which needs to be used with care, as pulmonary oedema can occur even in the presence of a 'normal' CVP.

Thrombo-prophylaxis

Women with severe pre-eclampsia are at risk of venous thrombosis. Antenatally, in labour and postnatally, all patients should have thrombo-prophylaxis in the form of antiembolic stockings and/or heparin until they are mobile. Heparin administration is not a contraindication to the insertion of an epidural catheter. However, low molecular weight heparin should not

Table 25.6 Preparation for transfer

Prior to transfer the condition must be stabilized. The following is required:

1. Transfer should be discussed with appropriate consultant medical staff and all the relevant people at the receiving unit, e.g. the neonatal unit and neonatal medical staff, the resident obstetrician, the midwife in charge of the delivery suite, intensive care and the intensive care anaesthetist (where appropriate).
2. All basic investigations should have been performed and the results clearly recorded in the accompanying notes or telephoned through as soon as available.
3. Blood pressure should be stabilized at an acceptable level and maintained.
4. If the woman is ventilated, it is important to ensure ventilatory requirements are stable and oxygen saturations are being maintained.
5. Fetal well-being has been assessed to be certain that transfer is in the fetal interest before delivery. Steroids should be given if the woman is preterm.
6. Appropriate personnel are available to transfer the woman. This will normally mean at least a senior midwife, but may require an obstetrician or anaesthetist.

be given until two hours after spinal anaesthesia and an epidural catheter should not be removed until ten hours after the last dose because of the risk of an epidural haematoma.

Delivery Guidelines

The timing, place and mode of delivery is the most important decision in the care of the pre-eclamptic woman. Delivery should be 'on the best day in the best way'. Delay in delivery can help with stabilizing the mother, transferring the woman to another unit, use of corticosteroids to mature fetal lungs or even prolongation of the pregnancy for a period of time. However, delaying delivery could also increase the risk to the mother and her baby and close monitoring is essential.

Gestation Before 34 Weeks

If the gestation is less than 34 weeks and delivery can be deferred, corticosteroids should be given, although this decision needs to be constantly reassessed for any change in maternal or fetal condition. However, even 24 hours of steroid therapy helps to reduce fetal respiratory morbidity and mortality. Conservative management at very early gestations may improve the perinatal outcome, but must be carefully balanced with maternal well-being. If the delivery decision involves transfer to another unit, it is important that the woman is stable prior to transfer (Table 25.6) and, if she is not, it is better to deliver in the base unit and transfer the baby postnatally, if required.

Gestation Between 34 and 37 Weeks

If the gestation is between 34 and 37 weeks, delivery after stabilization should be considered. If the mother is stable and the fetus is well, prolongation of the pregnancy for the benefit of the fetus can be considered.

Gestation After 37 Weeks

After 37 weeks, delivery, once stabilized and the appropriate measures are in place, is recommended as no benefit for mother or baby will be gained from delay except for transfer to a more appropriate unit [31].

The Delivery

The timing, place and mode of delivery need to be carefully planned, involving all appropriate professionals. The aim should be to deliver, particularly premature infants, during normal working hours. The mode of delivery should be influenced by the presentation of the fetus, the fetal condition and the likelihood of success of induction of labour after assessment of the cervix. Although a vaginal delivery is generally preferable, below 32 weeks' gestation caesarean section (CS) is superior, as the success of induction is reduced. After 34 weeks with a cephalic presentation, vaginal delivery should be considered with the likelihood of a successful vaginal delivery being increased by the use of vaginal prostaglandins.

Antihypertensive treatment should be continued throughout, preferably orally; intravenous infusion should be used only if oral therapy fails. Epidural anaesthesia should be used for obstetric need and not as a method of controlling blood pressure. The third stage should be managed with 5 units Syntocinon given intramuscularly or slowly intravenously, and not ergometrine or Syntometrine, as these can cause a sharp rise in both arterial blood pressure and cardiac return, increasing the risk of cardiac failure or cerebrovascular accident.

These women should receive high-dependency care and charts should be commenced to record all physiological monitoring and investigation results. To aid monitoring, an indwelling urinary catheter should be inserted and oxygen saturation should be measured by pulse oximeter and, if a CVP line is present, this should be measured continuously. All results should be charted as outlined.

Units should be moving to using Modified Early Obstetric Warning Scores (MEOWS) and these can be used in conjunction with these charts (see Chapter 29).

Anaesthesia and Fluids

Generally, women with pre-eclampsia tend to maintain their blood pressure during regional blockade, and routine fluid loading is unnecessary and may add to fluid overload. If hypotension occurs, small doses of a vasoconstrictor can be used. Even at CS, fluid replacement of greater than 500 ml of fluid, unless matched against blood loss, is not usually necessary. General anaesthesia should be avoided if possible, as intubation and extubation can lead to increases in systolic and diastolic blood pressure, as well as heart rate, bringing increased risk to the mother. This can be attenuated using either labetalol, alfentanil or remifentanil [32].

How Should the Woman be Managed Following Delivery?

Most women that die do so after delivery. Therefore, although delivery is the start of the reversal process, the first 24–48 hours are critical in care management. Around 60% of women worsen within 24 hours of delivery and the improvement in the maternal condition may not be seen until 48 hours. Therefore, continued vigilance is required. Also, both eclampsia and severe pre-eclampsia can present for the first time postnatally, so women with signs or symptoms compatible with pre-eclampsia should be carefully assessed and managed accordingly.

Women should continue high-dependency care, and all results should be charted. Again, there should be some form of MEOWS chart in place. Blood pressure and pulse should be measured regularly until stable, and then with lengthening intervals depending on the clinical condition. Although initially blood pressure may fall postpartum, it often rises again at around 24 hours. Therefore, a reduction in antihypertensive therapy should be made in a stepwise fashion and titrated against measurements. Temperature should be measured four-hourly or whenever the patient complains of feeling hot. The respiratory rate should be measured hourly, especially if the woman is on magnesium sulphate.

Postpartum Fluid Management

Pulmonary oedema is mostly a postpartum risk. Therefore, fluid restriction should continue until the natural diuresis occurs, which is sometime between 24 and 48 hours postdelivery. If oxygen saturation falls below 95% on air, then medical review is essential to assess fluid overload. If the fluid balance is in positive excess of more than 750 ml since delivery, then 20 mg of IV furosemide should be given. If there is no diuresis in response to this and the oxygen saturation does not rise, then renal referral should be considered.

Cases requiring large volumes of replacement fluid such as fresh frozen plasma, blood or platelets can be problematical and need management by those experienced in these cases. It is never difficult putting more fluid in, but getting it out can be a real problem.

Once the woman is well enough to tolerate free oral fluids, IV fluids can be stopped and the restrictions lifted.

HELLP Syndrome

HELLP syndrome may occur for the first time postpartum and is a reflection of the severity of the underlying disease. It requires no particular treatment apart from the normal supportive measures. Corticosteroids have been used in HELLP syndrome, but although they lead to a more rapid resolution of the biochemical and haematological abnormalities, there is no evidence that they reduce overall morbidity [20].

Ongoing Care and Discharge

Although late eclampsia has been reported up to four weeks postnatally, the incidence of eclampsia and severe pre-eclampsia falls after the fourth postpartum day. Therefore, most severe cases will need inpatient care for at least four days following delivery. Careful review to ensure improving clinical signs is needed before discharge by a senior doctor. However, if all else is well, there is no reason why the woman cannot go home on antihypertensive treatment and be weaned off therapy as an outpatient. Sometimes, blood pressure can take up to three months to return to normal. However, evidence suggests that up to 13% of women with pre-eclampsia will have underlying renal problems or essential hypertension that was not suspected

antenatally. Women with persisting hypertension and proteinuria at six weeks should be considered for further investigation.

References

1. Magee LA, Pels A, Helewa M, *et al.* Diagnosis, evaluation, and management of the hypertensive disorders of pregnancy: executive summary. *J Obstet Gynaecol Can.* 2014;36(7): 575–6.

2. Walker JJ. Pre-eclampsia. *Lancet.* 2000;356(9237): 1260–5.

3. Souza JP, Gulmezoglu AM, Vogel J, *et al.* Moving beyond essential interventions for reduction of maternal mortality (the WHO Multicountry Survey on Maternal and Newborn Health): a cross-sectional study. *Lancet.* 2013;381(9879): 1747–55.

4. CMACE. Saving Mothers' Lives: Reviewing Maternal Deaths to Make Motherhood Safer – 2006–08. *BJOG.* 2011;118(suppl. 1): 1–203.

5. Knight M, Kenyon S, Brocklehurst P, *et al. Saving Lives, Improving Mothers' Care – Lessons Learned to Inform Future Maternity Care from the UK and Ireland Confidential Enquiries into Maternal Deaths and Morbidity 2009–12.* Oxford: National Perinatal Epidemiology Unit, University of Oxford; 2014.

6. Tuffnell DJ, Jankowicz D, Lindow SW, *et al.* Outcomes of severe pre-eclampsia/eclampsia in Yorkshire 1999/2003. *BJOG.* 2005;112(7): 875–80.

7. RCOG. *Hypertension in Pregnancy: The Management of Hypertensive Disorders During Pregnancy.* London: RCOG Press; 2010.

8. The Eclampsia Trial Collaborative Group. Which anticonvulsant for women with eclampsia? Evidence from the Collaborative Eclampsia Trial. *Lancet.* 1995;345(8963): 1455–63.

9. The Magpie Trial Collaboration Group. Do women with pre-eclampsia, and their babies, benefit from magnesium sulphate? The Magpie Trial: a randomised placebo-controlled trial. *Lancet.* 2002;359(9321): 1877–90.

10. Magee LA, von Dadelszen P, Rey E, *et al.* Less-tight versus tight control of hypertension in pregnancy. *N Eng J Med.* 2015;372(5): 407–17.

11. Churchill D, Duley L, Thornton JG, Jones L. Interventionist versus expectant care for severe pre-eclampsia between 24 and 34 weeks' gestation. *Cochrane Database Syst Rev.* 2013;7: CD003106.

12. Dodd JM, McLeod A, Windrim RC, Kingdom J. Antithrombotic therapy for improving maternal or infant health outcomes in women considered at risk of placental dysfunction. *Cochrane Database Syst Rev.* 2013;7: CD006780.

13. Firoz T, Magee LA, MacDonell K, *et al*. Oral antihypertensive therapy for severe hypertension in pregnancy and postpartum: a systematic review. *BJOG*. 2014;121(10): 1210–18.

14. Hofmeyr GJ, Belizan JM, von Dadelszen P, Calcium and Pre-eclampsia Study Group: Low-dose calcium supplementation for preventing pre-eclampsia – a systematic review and commentary. *BJOG*. 2014;121(8): 951–7.

15. Magee LA, Namouz-Haddad S, Cao V, Koren G, von Dadelszen P. Labetalol for hypertension in pregnancy. *Exp Opin on Drug Safety*. 2015;14(3): 453–61.

16. Ebeigbe PN. Inadequacy of dipstick proteinuria in hypertensive pregnancy: evidence for a change to alternatives. *Niger Postgrad Med J*. 2009;16(1): 46–9.

17. Singh S, McGlennan A, England A, Simons R. A validation study of the CEMACH recommended modified early obstetric warning system (MEOWS). *Anaesthesia*. 2012;67(1): 12–18.

18. Chappell LC, Duckworth S, Seed PT, *et al*. Diagnostic accuracy of placental growth factor in women with suspected preeclampsia: a prospective multicenter study. *Circulation*. 2013;128(19): 2121–31.

19. von Beckerath AK, Kollmann M, Rotky-Fast C, *et al*. Perinatal complications and long-term neurodevelopmental outcome of infants with intrauterine growth restriction. *Am J Obstet Gynecol*. 2013;208(2): e1–6.

20. Martin JN Jr, Rinehart BK, May WL, *et al*. The spectrum of severe preeclampsia: comparative analysis by HELLP (hemolysis, elevated liver enzyme levels, and low platelet count) syndrome classification. *Am J Obstet Gynecol*. 1999;180(6 Pt 1): 1373–84.

21. Martin JN Jr, Thigpen BD, Moore RC, *et al*. Stroke and severe preeclampsia and eclampsia: a paradigm shift focusing on systolic blood pressure. *Obstet Gynecol*. 2005;105(2): 246–54.

22. Douglas KA, Redman CW. Eclampsia in the United Kingdom. *BMJ*. 1994;309(6966): 1395–400.

23. Brown MA, Buddle ML, Farrell T, Davis G, Jones M. Randomised trial of management of hypertensive pregnancies by Korotkoff phase IV or phase V. *Lancet*. 1998;352(9130): 777–81.

24. de Greeff A, Shennan A. Blood pressure measuring devices: ubiquitous, essential but imprecise. *Expert Rev Med Devices*. 2008;5(5): 573–9.

25. Magee LA, Ornstein MP, von Dadelszen P. Fortnightly review: management of hypertension in pregnancy. *BMJ*. 1999;318(7194): 1332–6.

26. Ferrazzani S, Caruso A, De Carolis S, Martino IV, Mancuso S. Proteinuria and outcome of 444 pregnancies complicated by hypertension. *Am J Obstet Gynecol*. 1990;162(2): 366–71.

27. Brown MA, Buddle ML. Inadequacy of dipstick proteinuria in hypertensive pregnancy. *Aust N Z J Obstet Gynaecol*. 1995;35(4): 366–9.

28. Neilson JP, Alfirevic Z. Doppler ultrasound for fetal assessment in high risk pregnancies. *Cochrane Database Syst Rev*. 2000;2: CD000073.

29. RCOG. *The Investigation and Management of the Small-for-Gestational-Age Fetus*. London: RCOG Press; 2014.

30. Duley L, Williams J, Henderson-Smart DJ. Plasma volume expansion for treatment of women with pre-eclampsia. *Cochrane Database Syst Rev*. 2000;2: CD001805.

31. Koopmans CM, Bijlenga D, Groen H, *et al*. Induction of labour versus expectant monitoring for gestational hypertension or mild pre-eclampsia after 36 weeks' gestation (HYPITAT): a multicentre, open-label randomised controlled trial. *Lancet*. 2009;374(9694): 979–88.

32. Yoo KY, Kang DH, Jeong H, *et al*. A dose–response study of remifentanil for attenuation of the hypertensive response to laryngoscopy and tracheal intubation in severely preeclamptic women undergoing caesarean delivery under general anaesthesia. *Int J Obstet Anesth*. 2013;22(1): 10–18.

Chapter 26

Neonatal Resuscitation and the Management of Immediate Neonatal Problems

Paul Mannix

Introduction

The vast majority of newborn babies require no help in adapting to their new extrauterine life. They rapidly clear lung fluid, create a functional residual capacity and breathe on their own within seconds of their birth. However, it is very difficult to predict the baby who will struggle with this transition and hence need resuscitation, and so I start this chapter with the comment that any person involved in the delivery of care to the pregnant woman should have an understanding of the principles of newborn resuscitation. This includes medical students on their obstetric attachment, student midwives in training, midwives, obstetricians and obstetric anaesthetists, as well as neonatologists and paediatricians.

De Lee stated in 1897 that 'there are three grand principles governing the treatment of asphyxia neonatorum: first, maintain the body heat; second, free the air passages from obstructions; third, stimulate respiration, or supply air to the lungs for oxygenation of the blood' [1]. Over 100 years later, these principles remain largely unchanged.

In this chapter, the principles and physiology of neonatal resuscitation are discussed using the animal models of Dawes and Cross from the 1960s and 1970s. The UK Resuscitation Council uses this physiology for the basis of its teaching for newborn life support. It uses a step-by-step approach to the assessment and onward management of the baby who has not achieved normal breathing in the moments immediately after birth. Special cases in which resuscitation is required, such as preterm babies, babies born in the presence of meconium-stained liquor, babies born at home and babies with congenital anomalies, the use of continu-

ous positive airway pressure (CPAP) and the management of some of the more difficult neonatal issues, such as persistent pulmonary hypertension of the newborn and the baby born with shock, are also described. I will also touch on the controversy relating to the timing of cord clamping

Prior to the 1950s, numerous techniques for the resuscitation of the newborn were advocated and employed, all with some degree of apparent success. These included insufflation of the stomach with oxygen [2], hyperbaric oxygen [3], rapid hypothermia [4] and the use of respiratory stimulants on the tongue [5,6].

In the 1960s and 1970s, physiologists such as Kenneth Cross in London, Geoffrey Dawes in Oxford and other neonatal physiologists undertook major studies to assess the effect of a hypoxic insult on the fetus [7–9]. Their seminal work allows a great understanding of what is happening in utero to a baby, and helps to guide our actions in the process of resuscitation.

They used pregnant animals and externalized the fetus. After they had inserted arterial and venous lines for monitoring the physiological parameters, they placed a saline-filled bag over the head of the fetus. They then rendered the fetus hypoxic by occluding the umbilical cord and made recordings until the fetus died or it had responded to resuscitation. Their findings were extrapolated to the human fetus and are represented on the figures used in this chapter to explain their findings.

Consider the graph in Figure 26.1. If a fetus is rendered hypoxic (time 0 on Figure 26.1), it responds by increasing the rate and depth of its breathing pattern, as shown in the lines at the top of the graph – each

Best Practice in Labour and Delivery, Second Edition, ed. Sir Sabaratnam Arulkumaran. Published by Cambridge University Press. © Cambridge University Press 2016.

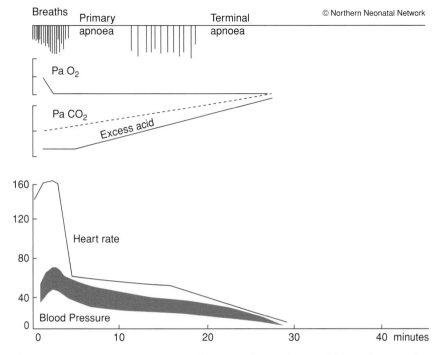

Figure 26.1 Diagrammatic representation of primary and terminal apnoea following the onset of acute total asphyxia at time 0.

vertical line representing a breath. After a period of time, the fetus loses consciousness owing to hypoxia of the cerebral tissues, and this results in a loss of control from higher breathing centres. The period of apnoea which follows is termed 'primary apnoea'. After a period of time, the spinal reflex centres come into play, because they are no longer being inhibited by the higher cerebral centres. This results in intermittent deep gasping respirations – each gasp occurring about every 6–10 s [8]. In the presence of continued hypoxia, this gasping will finally stop, and the fetus enters the phase of 'terminal apnoea'. Some like to call this phase 'secondary apnoea', but it deflects from the reality of the situation. This fetus *will* die unless someone in attendance at this delivery inflates the chest. As such, the more descriptive term 'terminal apnoea' should be used.

The next section in the graph relates to the oxygen, carbon dioxide and pH levels of the fetus. Clearly in this model, the animal has been rendered hypoxic. As such, the oxygen levels fall to a minimum and fail to respond to the rapid and increasing respiratory rate and fail to respond to the gasping. In the same way, the carbon dioxide levels begin to rise as the fetus is unable

to dispose of the carbon dioxide produced. This carbon dioxide is converted to carbonic acid, which along with the increasing lactic acidosis from the hypoxia results in an excess of acid and a fall in the fetal pH. This fact is well known to those practising on a labour ward, and is the physiological basis behind the use of fetal scalp pH assessment to monitor fetal well-being during labour.

Turning to the cardiovascular responses in the hypoxic fetus, we see one of the ways in which the fetus differs from the adult. An adult rendered hypoxic for short periods would quickly develop cardiac failure and suffer a cardiac arrest. The fetus, on the other hand, is designed to cope with the hypoxia associated with birth. Each time the uterus contracts, the flow of oxygenated blood from placenta to fetus is interrupted with the well-recognized consequence of a fetal bradycardia on the CTG. The same is seen in our animal model. The initial response to the hypoxia is an increase in the heart rate, but this is followed by a fall in the heart rate, not to zero as in the adult but to a rate of around 80 beats per minute (bpm). The heart relies on its stores of glycogen for an energy source during the hypoxic episodes, and only after a prolonged period of

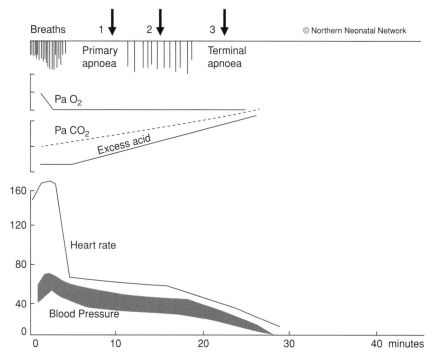

Figure 26.2 Diagrammatic representation of primary and terminal apnoea following the onset of acute total asphyxia at time 0 with three time points marked.

asphyxia does the fetal heart rate (FHR) drop to very low levels and finally stop altogether.

By using other cardiovascular responses, the asphyxiated fetus aims to maintain its blood pressure. It diverts (redistributes) its blood flow away from non-essential organs (skin and splanchnic circulation) and sends it to vital organs (brain, heart, adrenals). As such, the baby who has experienced the longest period of intrauterine asphyxia will appear white and pale owing to this redistribution, the baby having vasoconstricted its peripheral circulation.

Finally, the heart can no longer continue without oxygen, and as the heart fails the blood pressure drops and the fetal heart stops.

That explains the background physiology to intrapartum asphyxia. The difficulty facing the person needing to resuscitate the baby is that they have no idea how far along this asphyxial timescale the baby has travelled in utero.

The baby born at each of the three arrows marked in Figure 26.2 presents the same clinical findings – apnoeic, bradycardic and probably pale. The basis for the resuscitation of these babies is to start by performing the actions needed to resuscitate the baby at point 1 and if there is no response, move on to those actions

needed for the baby at point 2, and so on in a stepwise manner, always assessing any change in colour, tone, respiratory effort and heart rate to the particular manoeuvre that was tried.

The first action in any resuscitation in the newborn, no matter how unwell the baby appears, is to get the baby wiped and dried and wrapped in warmed towels. It is far more difficult to resuscitate a cold, wet baby than it is to resuscitate a warm, dry baby.

Let us consider these babies born at different points along this asphyxial pathway and what they will need for resuscitation.

Let us consider the baby born in the primary apnoeic phase of asphyxia (Figure 26.3 – arrow 1 on Figure 26.2).

We know from the physiology we have just looked at that primary apnoea is always followed by gasping respiration. Therefore we know that this baby will gasp. If, at the point of gasping, this baby has a patent airway, it will be successful in getting oxygen into its lungs. This will quickly pass into the bloodstream and as soon as it passes into the coronary arteries the heart will respond with an increase in rate and the baby will turn pink. To all intents and purposes, the baby has resuscitated itself. We will have dried and wrapped the baby.

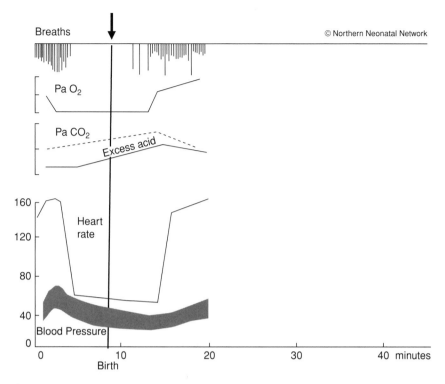

Figure 26.3 Diagrammatic representation of response to birth in primary apnoea.

We might have needed to open or clear the airway, but the rest was down to the baby.

Second, let us consider a baby who has been hypoxic for a little longer than the first baby who has now reached the gasping phase (Figure 26.4 – arrow 2 in Figure 26.2).

As with the previous baby, so long as the baby continues to take gasps and has an open and patent airway, it will resuscitate itself. The gasping will draw air into the lungs which, once absorbed into the bloodstream, will pass to the coronary arteries, resulting in an increase in the heart rate and the baby turning pink. Again, we will have dried and wrapped the baby before anything else, but this baby may take a little while to re-establish a normal respiratory pattern and may need some supportive ventilation breaths but, as with the previous baby, it has to all intents and purposes resuscitated itself.

Let us thirdly consider the baby who has taken its last gasp in utero and has been delivered in the terminal apnoeic phase (Figure 26.5 – arrow 3 in Figure 26.2).

This baby has now taken its last breath. If no action is taken, this baby *will* die. Owing to the fact that the baby has never made an extrauterine breath, its lungs will still be full of fluid. When we start to resuscitate the baby we need to remember this. Having dried and wrapped the baby, the breaths we give need to be long and sustained in order to empty the alveoli of all of the lung fluid and allow the formation of a functional residual capacity.

The initial breaths are called inflation breaths and are normally given at 30 cm of water each for 2–3 s duration. We give five such breaths and are watching to assess if we achieve chest wall movement. It is not uncommon that adequate chest wall movement is only seen on the fourth and fifth breaths, as the first three breaths simply have been effective in pushing that lung fluid out of the alveoli into the interstitial tissues and pulmonary lymphatics for drainage.

Inflating the chest using a bag and mask or a T-piece and mask is a skill which requires some learning, and it would be useful to practise this in your own delivery unit. We recommend the use of the soft-edged laerdal masks. The mask chosen needs to be the correct size – fitting over the nose and mouth but not extending below the chin or onto the orbits. The mask needs to be held in place by a downward pressure on the stem, usually by holding the stem between the thumb and the forefinger. The middle finger can sit on the

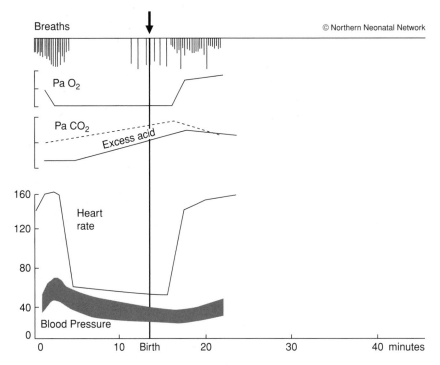

Figure 26.4 Diagrammatic representation of response to birth in gasping phase of intrapartum asphyxia.

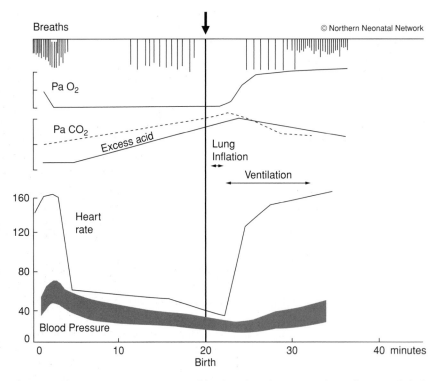

Figure 26.5 Diagrammatic representation of the physiological response to lung inflation in a baby born in early terminal apnoea.

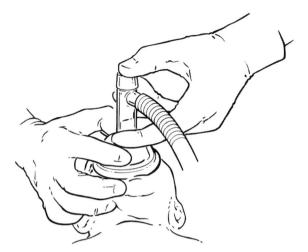

Figure 26.6 Neutral head position and correct hand position for use of T-piece and mask.

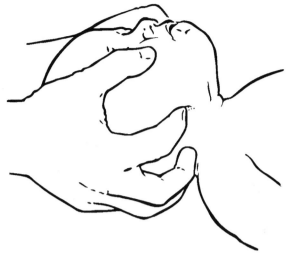

Figure 26.7 Double-handed jaw thrust with head in neutral position.

chin to allow support and to hold the head in a neutral position. The fourth and fifth fingers should rest on the jaw, making sure they are in contact with bone and not with the submandibular soft tissues. Pressure in the latter area will simply push the tongue up into the airway and make effective chest wall inflation more difficult by occluding the airway. The correct hand position for using a T-piece is shown in Figure 26.6.

If still unable to get the chest wall to move, ensure you are not overextending the neck. Once certain you are in the neutral position (Figures 26.6, 26.7 and 26.10), it may be appropriate to inspect the oropharynx by direct vision using a laryngoscope. When doing this one should be prepared to suction out any particulate material that may be occluding the airway (e.g. vernix, blood, meconium). It might also be useful at this point to insert an oropharyngeal (Guedel) airway, remembering that in the baby these are inserted in the same alignment as it will sit, unlike in the adult in which it is inserted and then rotated. The Guedal airway is sized by measuring from the mid-point of the chin to the angle of the jaw.

If you are still unable to effect chest wall movements, you will need to enlist the help of another. In such circumstances, you can use two hands to achieve adequate airway control and hold the mask while your colleague provides the inflation from the bag or T-piece. With two people, it allows you to provide a forward movement of the jaw, pushing the angle of the jaw anteriorly to increase the pharyngeal space by moving the tongue forward, which is known as a jaw thrust. This is shown in Figure 26.7.

How do we know if the baby has responded to our inflation breaths? Well, consider the baby who gasped in the first two scenarios. If you remember, the measure of the baby responding was by finding an increase in the heart rate. There is no difference in this baby. Yes, it is further along the asphyxial pathway of our animal model, but adequate inflation breaths should result in an increase in the heart rate, as that air gets oxygen into the bloodstream and into the coronary arteries. You will see from Figure 26.5 that the lung inflation results in an increase in the heart rate although the baby has not yet established its own respiratory pattern. We need to provide shorter ventilation breaths for a short period of time, after which we will see the baby begin to gasp. This gasping will then be interspersed with normal respiratory effort, just like we had seen in the two previous scenarios.

Finally, let us consider another baby who has also reached the terminal apnoeic phase (Figure 26.8 – arrow 3 in Figure 26.2).

This baby will not breathe for itself, and requires us to give five inflation breaths in order to oxygenate it and then allow an improvement in the heart rate. Let us consider that we have given the baby five inflation breaths and we are certain that we have seen good chest wall movement. Our assessment of effectiveness of the resuscitation thus far is to assess the heart rate, but in this case there has been no increase. The heart rate is still at 40 bpm, for example. Why is this, and what do we need to do?

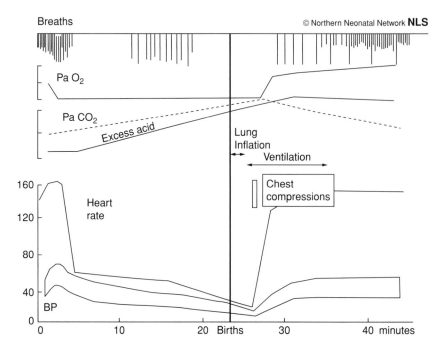

Figure 26.8 Diagrammatic representation of the physiological response to cardiac compressions in a baby born in early terminal apnoea who has not responded to lung inflation.

What we can assume is that this heart has been too compromised by the episode of intrapartum asphyxia. It has failed to respond to the effective inflation breaths. This tells us that this baby requires a short (30 s) period of cardiac compressions in order to try to move blood from the pulmonary vasculature into the coronaries so that the oxygen given with successful inflation breaths can get into the coronaries and give the heart the bump-start it needs.

Chest compressions are best given with two hands encircling the chest wall. Fingers at the back, thumbs at the front. The thumbs should be on the lower third of the xiphisternum on a point one finger's breadth below an imaginary line drawn between the baby's nipples. The compressions should be about one-third of the depth of the chest to the baby's spine (Figure 26.9).

The compressions should be given in a ratio of 3:1 with short ventilation breaths. A total of 120 events in a minute should be the aim – but the quality of the compression and ventilation is probably more important than the quantity [10]. They should be continued for 30 s and then the baby reassessed. Hopefully, there will have been an increase in the heart rate and the baby will be becoming pink and active. If not, and one is happy that chest wall movement is effective and

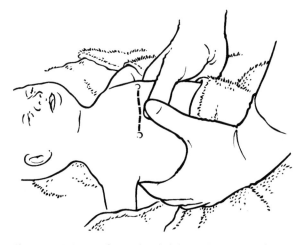

Figure 26.9 Position for two-handed chest compressions when standing at the side or foot of the baby.

compressions are adequate, one should consider the use of drugs after gaining venous access via the insertion of an umbilical venous catheter (UVC). Such action would almost certainly be the domain of the neonatal team, but with more trainees spending some time in neonatal training posts or attending Newborn Life Support courses, it would not be inappropriate for an obstetrician, midwife or anaesthetist with some

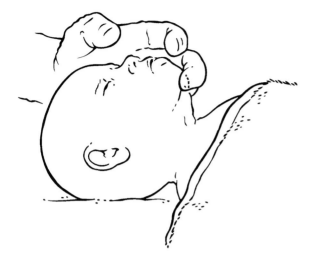

Figure 26.10 Placing the head in the neutral position using chin lift.

UVC experience to insert the line. One would consider using sodium bicarbonate, adrenaline and dextrose as part of the resuscitation. In babies remaining pale and bradycardic, one should always consider blood loss, and in such cases volume (O negative blood) can be life-saving.

All this can be summarized in the algorithm shown in Figure 26.11. This is the 2010 UK Resuscitation Council newborn life support algorithm for the resuscitation of the newborn baby.

Opening the Airway

The neonate has a relatively large occiput and if the infant is floppy this often results in the neck flexing the chin onto the chest wall, leading to obstruction of the airway. In such cases, one needs to be able to open the airway using simple manoeuvres. The simplest manoeuvre is the 'chin lift', which simply puts the newborn baby's head into a neutral position, opening the airway and allowing the baby to take in air if it is making any sort of respiratory effort (Figure 26.10). Note that in opening the airway, the baby's face should be parallel to the surface on which it is being resuscitated, with the eyes looking straight upwards. This is different from the adult position, where the neck is extended with the patient 'sniffing the morning air'. Figure 26.10 illustrates the correct position of the newborn baby's head to achieve the neutral position.

If this fails to allow air entry, one can consider the jaw thrust manoeuvres described above.

Whatever the condition of the baby at birth, it is vital to remember that the baby will be wet and have a large surface area to body mass ratio. These two issues mean that the baby will lose heat very quickly. A cold, wet baby is much more difficult to resuscitate than a warm, dry baby.

For the newborn term baby, it is important that the baby is wiped and dried and wrapped in warm towels as quickly as possible after birth, particularly if it has not established a normal breathing pattern. Remember particularly to dry the head and, if need be, place a hat on the baby's head. Premature infants are now placed into warming bags undried, which has shown to be an effective method of conserving heat for the baby. The use of a warmer bag is only advocated if the baby will remain under an overhead radiant heater which would allow the child to maintain warmth or they were able to go into contact with their mother for warmth. If a radiant heater is not available, then even the premature baby should be towelled dry and wrapped in warm, dry towels using a hat in the same way as the term baby.

Resuscitation of the Premature Baby

The resuscitation of the premature baby should be performed along exactly the same lines as that for the term baby. The differences are the two highlighted earlier. First, the baby tends to be placed in a warming bag directly and left under a radiant heater for maximum temperature control; and second, the initial inflation breaths given may be at a lower pressure to effect the chest wall movements than in the term baby. Data from the EPICure study showed that temperature on admission to the neonatal unit was directly related to outcome and that too many babies born at less than 25 weeks' completed gestation were too cold [11]. Following these results, much work was done to try to improve the temperature of these fragile babies, and the use of warmer bags and overhead radiant heaters is now commonplace and has been shown to be highly effective [12]. One needs to remember that the premature infant is more fragile than the term baby, is more prone to hypotension and hypoglycaemia than the term infant, and has far less energy stores for the resuscitation. As a consequence, it will get colder quicker, take longer to rewarm and, due to the probable lack of surfactant, have less-compliant lungs and need more help in establishing their respiration. Most of the premature babies who are being resuscitated are

Resuscitation Council (UK) GUIDELINES 2015   **Newborn Life Support**

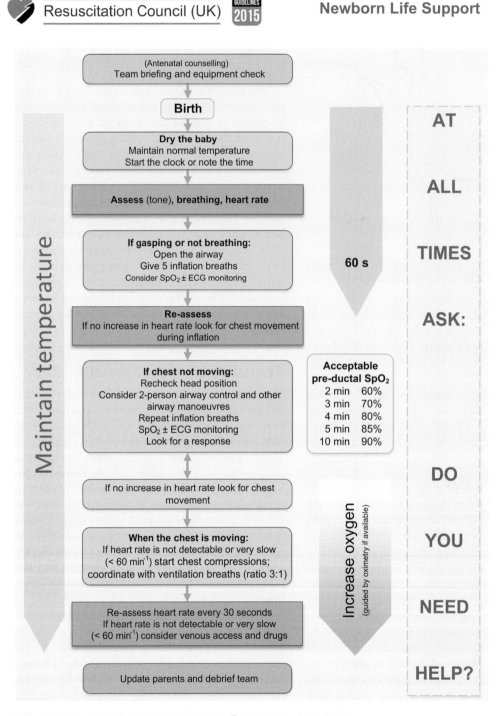

Figure 26.11 Newborn Life Support Algorithm 2015 © Resuscitation Council (UK).

babies who require stabilization rather than resuscitation [13]. The preterm baby who has undergone the same asphyxial events as the term babies described earlier is not likely to survive, and most of the babies where the neonatal team are involved in the resuscitation are those preterm babies who are born and show signs not only of vitality but also of viability.

This whole question may be considered in other parts of this book, but the recent publication by the Nuffield Bioethics Council does give some sensible guidance on which babies should or should not be resuscitated [14].

Continuous Positive Airway Pressure (CPAP)

As mentioned above, most of the preterm babies requiring help at birth are really requiring stabilization in this transition period rather than full resuscitation as in the term babies described. One aspect of their management is related to their poor compliance and the tendency for their alveoli to empty at end expiration rather than retaining some functional residual capacity. Their lungs and alveoli could be likened to a party balloon – difficult to get the first breath into but each subsequent breath then becoming easier. For some of these babies who exhibit a good respiratory drive it is possible to maintain a low but continuous positive pressure at the end of expiration which prevents the alveolar collapse and makes it easier for the baby to maintain their own lung aeration without resorting to full ventilation. It is known that babies who receive CPAP as compared to controls not receiving CPAP have higher lung volumes and less histological inflammation [15].

Cord Clamping

The question of how soon to clamp the umbilical cord has been debated for many years and comes and goes as a 'hot topic' for discussion. At present credence is given to the views taken in the 1970s relating to the active management of the third stage of labour to prevent postpartum haemorrhage. This led to an almost immediate clamping of the cord with the delivery of the head of the baby; recent views wanting to allow a longer period between delivery and cord clamping have met with some resistance, not least owing to the use of the term 'delayed cord clamping'. In a sphere of medicine in which every moment counts, the suggestion of a 'delay' can for some be seen as a cause for concern.

However, there are good physiological reasons on the fetal side why the immediate clamping of the cord may not be in the best interests of the newborn baby. The baby who has their cord clamped prior to their first breath is found to have a drop in their heart rate that is not seen in those babies who have their cords clamped after their first breath [16]. Recent animal studies have shown improved circulatory stability in preterm infants with delayed cord clamping and that ventilation prior to cord clamping has a marked effect on stabilizing cerebral blood flow. This is adding to the view that a delay in clamping of the cord until the baby has established its own ventilation or has had this done for it provides a smoother transition to newborn life [17]. Many units are now beginning to introduce a delay.

Later clamping of the cord results in improved iron stores in infancy for term babies, and for preterm babies later clamping of the cord if possible allows greater stability during their transition, with less hypotension and need for inotropic support – but one has to be able to provide this delay without allowing the baby to become cold. Studies are underway looking at the ability to resuscitate the baby at the maternal bedside with an unclamped cord to assess both the feasibility and the benefits of such actions.

In 2010 the International Liaison Committee on Resuscitation (ILCOR) suggested that a delay of up to 1 min would be recommended for newborn babies not requiring resuscitation, but there was insufficient evidence to support or refute a delay for those requiring resuscitation or for the preterm babies. We await the result of clinical trials and at present most teams will want some delay to the cord clamping based on how vigorous the baby looks at birth if there is no maternal contraindication [18,19].

Meconium-stained Liquor

The newborn baby is born with its bowels containing meconium. This is a mixture of sloughed-off cells and bowel secretions formed over the time that the fetus has been developing in utero. Babies who are nearing term may, in the presence of an asphyxial insult, evacuate their bowels and hence the liquor will appear meconium-stained. From the earlier physiology which we have described (Figure 26.1), it will be understood that if the baby reaches the gasping phase of asphyxia and the liquor contains meconium, then that fetus is very likely to aspirate the meconium into their lungs. There is little that anyone can do about this meconium even at the time of the delivery, and the job of the resuscitator under such circumstances is to try to prevent any further aspiration of meconium which may be in the nose and the mouth of the newborn infant.

The guidance about what to do for a baby born with meconium-stained liquor has become simpler since the advent of the newborn life support algorithms (Figure 26.11). The baby born in the presence of meconium who is active, pink and crying should be wiped and wrapped in the same way as we have already described, and should be watched for any signs of respiratory distress owing to the meconium which may have been aspirated prior to the delivery. For the baby who is born floppy and not breathing, once the baby has been gently dried and covered with a warmed towel, direct inspection of the oropharynx would be advocated with the use of a laryngoscope and any particulate material present in the mouth should be aspirated using a Yankauer sucker. Once this has been done, the resuscitation can proceed in the ways already outlined, with manoeuvring of the airway to make it patent and, if necessary, giving the sustained inflation breaths in order to effect chest wall movement and allow oxygenation of the blood passing into the coronary arteries. The practice of suction of the nose and mouth with the child's head on the perineum, or of splinting the chest at birth, are no longer advocated in the UK, nor is there any need to be suctioning from the nose and mouth thin meconium-stained liquor once the child has established its own respiratory effort, as these have been shown to provide no benefit [20].

Babies Born Outside Hospital

Some women choose electively to give birth in the comfort of their own home. When such a decision has been made, a plan is put in place with the midwifery teams caring for that mother and her unborn child so that the child can be delivered safely in the home. Occasionally, some of these babies may not establish normal respiratory effort, or the child may be born without the midwife being present. Furthermore, some women may deliver outside hospital unplanned, and therefore it is important that people working in the field of obstetrics, maternity and paediatrics, as well as other highlighted specialities, should understand the basic principles of the resuscitation. In a hospital setting nowadays, we have developed resuscitaires that carry all of the equipment necessary for us to perform an effective resuscitation of the newborn baby but, in essence, all that is really required is a flat surface, some warmed towels and some light. We must remember that the baby born out of hospital, particularly if unexpected, is more likely to get cold and therefore attention to drying the baby with something that is available and getting them wrapped and kept warm is of vital importance. The airway manoeuvres described can be done very simply, and if the child does not establish their own respiration then mouth to nose-and-mouth resuscitation can be given by someone who is present at the time of the delivery. This may be life-saving. One needs to pay particular attention to temperature control. Cold rooms need warming and draughts from windows need to be minimized in order to allow the maximum warmth to the baby. Instruction can be reasonably easily given to any other helper as to how to perform cardiac massage if it were indicated, and if one is calling for an emergency ambulance one ought to be clear that the ambulance is required for a newborn baby so that paramedics with the correct skills can be sent to assist whoever else is involved in the onward resuscitation. Remember to cover the head, that a baby can be placed in direct contact with the mother in order to maintain warmth and that hot water bottles can be useful, but should not be in direct contact with the child's skin and would be better wrapped in a towel. It is also helpful to look at your watch to have an accurate assessment of the time of the birth of the child and how long any attempts at resuscitation have been continuing.

Babies with Congenital Abnormalities

With the improvements in fetal medicine scanning, it is unusual now to be presented with a baby with a major unexpected congenital anomaly. Babies born with Pierre Robin sequence are a particular risk, owing to the small mouth due to their mandibular hypoplasia. The insertion of a nasopharyngeal or oropharyngeal airway in these cases can be of great benefit, as it allows better passage of air into the pharynx.

In babies known to have a diaphragmatic hernia it is always preferable not to provide mask inflation of the lungs if it can be avoided. Inevitably some of that masked gas will pass into the intestines and can compromise the aeration of the lungs. It would always be preferable to intubate such a baby if it was showing signs of respiratory compromise, but one must do what they are capable of doing and in the absence of someone trained in neonatal intubation it would be entirely sensible to offer inflation breath and onward resuscitation in the same manner as outlined earlier in the chapter.

Persistent Pulmonary Hypertension of the Newborn (PPHN)

At birth the baby needs to change the flows of blood through its circulation. The first breath leads to a massive fall in the pulmonary vascular resistance, and that coupled with the clamping of the cord and the relative increase in the systemic vascular resistance are the major factors that cause the change from the fetal to the neonatal/adult circulation. Failure for this to occur results in an inappropriately high pulmonary vascular resistance, a reduction in effective pulmonary blood flow, shunting of blood from the right to the left side through both the *foramen ovale* and the *ductus arteriosus* and a baby who remains blue. There are many conditions that can result in PPHN, some of which can be anticipated from a knowledge of the pregnancy and the labour. Such causes would include perinatal asphyxia, meconium aspiration syndrome, congenital pneumonia, pulmonary hypoplasia secondary to oligohydramnios, and congenital lung abnormalities. The presence of such a shunt can often be easily demonstrated by assessing the saturations on the right hand (preductal) and either foot (postductal). A difference of more than 10% would be considered as significant [21]. Persistent pulmonary hypertension has a quoted incidence of about 1–5 per 1000 births [22].

The immediate management of the baby at birth is the same and is in line with what has been outlined in the earlier pages of this chapter: wipe and dry the baby to keep it warm, open the airway and assess the response. If there is no respiratory effort, then you need to give inflation breaths and follow the NLS algorithm appropriately. Unfortunately, in some of these babies they need more intensive resuscitation and onward care. The mainstay of the management is to try to reduce the effective pulmonary vascular resistance or to increase the systemic vascular resistance by artificial means to allow a reversal of the right-to-left shunts. The manoeuvres needed include sedation and paralysis of the baby, ventilation with 100% oxygen

(FiO_2 1.0), alkalinization of the pH either by hyperventilation to reduce the $PaCO_2$ or by the use of $NaHCO_3$ and the use of pulmonary vasodilator agents such as prostacyclin or tolazoline. More recently, inhaled nitric oxide has become more widely available, and is a very useful addition to the pharmacopoeia for this difficult condition.

Shock

We have stated that the baby who has undergone a significant period of asphyxia will appear pale owing to the vasoconstriction of their peripheral circulation in order to maintain their blood pressure. It is also important to remember that the baby who has lost blood will also appear pale. A history of antepartum haemorrhage or the presence of a retro-placental clot can be the important clue to the failure of a baby to respond to a well-performed resuscitation. If the baby has (1) good chest wall movements with mask ventilation; (2) is having adequate cardiac massage; and (3) has failed to respond to drugs, it is important to consider a loss of circulating volume as a possible cause. The baby should be given 20 ml/kg of packed red blood cells as a bolus. This can have a dramatic effect by providing the red cells to deliver the oxygen to the coronaries, allowing the baby to respond to the resuscitation being carried out.

Summary

It is often difficult to predict which babies will require resuscitation at birth. As a consequence, it is of great importance that all staff involved in the management of pregnant women should have the basic skills required for basic neonatal resuscitation. The pathway follows a logical system based on an understanding of the physiology of intrapartum asphyxia.

The baby needs to be wiped and dried and kept warm. The airway needs to be opened by placing the head in a neutral position, and if breathing is not established then resuscitation with inflation breaths needs to be given. The success of the inflation breaths is determined by the response in the heart rate. Cardiac compressions may be needed if the chest wall has inflated but the heart rate has not responded. Drugs may be needed if the heart rate does not respond. In a small number of cases, the baby will need blood because they are hypovolaemic following a fetal–maternal bleed, massive APH or a retro-placental clot.

The vast majority of babies born need no resuscitation and of those who do require help, about 95% will have responded with an increase in heart rate within 1–2 min of effective resuscitation.

References

1. De Lee JB. Asphyxia neonatorum: causation and treatment. *Medicine (Detroit)*. 1897; 3: 643–60.

2. Akerren Y, Furstenberg N. Gastrointestinal administration of oxygen in the treatment of asphyxia in the newborn. *J Obstet Gynaecol Br Emp*. 1950; 57: 705–13.

3. Hutchinson J, Kerr M, Williams K, Hopkinson W. Hyperbaric oxygen in the resuscitation of the newborn. *Lancet*. 1963; 2: 1019–22.

4. Cordey R, Chiolero R, Miller J. Resuscitation of neonates by hypothermia: report of 20 cases with acid–base determination on 10 cases and long-term development of 33 cases. *Resuscitation*. 1973; 2: 169–87.

5. Daniel SS, Dawes GS, James LS, Ross BB. Analeptics and resuscitation of asphyxiated monkeys. *Br Med J*. 1966; 2: 562–3.

6. Barrie H, Cottom DG, Wilson BDR. Respiratory stimulants in the newborn. *Lancet*. 1962; 2: 742–6.

7. Cross KW. Resuscitation of the asphyxiated infant. *Br Med Bull*. 1966; 22: 73–8.

8. Dawes G. *Fetal and Neonatal Physiology*. Chicago, IL: Year Book Publisher, 1968.

9. Godfrey S. Respiratory and cardiovascular changes during asphyxia and resuscitation of foetal newborn rabbits. *Quart J Exper Physiol*. 1968; 53: 97–118.

10. Whyte SD, Sinha AK, Wyllie JP. Neonatal resuscitation: a practical assessment. *Resuscitation*. 1999; 40: 21–5.

11. Costeloe K, Hennessy E, Gibson AT, Marlow N, Wilkinson AR. The EPICure study: outcomes to discharge from hospital for infants born at the threshold of viability. *Paediatrics*. 2000; 106(4): 659–71.

12. Vohra S, Frent G, Campbell V, Abbott M, Whyte R. Effect of polyethylene occlusive skin wrapping on heat loss in very low birthweight infants at delivery: a randomized trial. *J Pediatr*. 1999; 134(5): 547–51.

13. O'Donnell C, Davis PG, Morley CJ. Resuscitation of premature infants: what are we doing wrong and can do better? *Biol Neonate*. 2003; 84: 76–82.

14. Nuffield Council on Bioethics. Critical care decisions in fetal and neonatal medicine: ethical issues; 2006. http://nuffieldbioethics.org/wp-content/uploads/2014/07/CCD-web-version-22-June-07-updated.pdf (accessed 10 May 2016).

15. Probyn ME, Hooper SB, Dargaville PA, *et al*. Positive end expiratory pressure during resuscitation of premature lambs rapidly improves blood gases without adversely affecting arterial pressures. *Peditr Res*. 2004; 56: 198–204.

16. Brady JP, James LS, Baker MA. Heart rate changes in the fetus and newborn infant during labor, delivery and the immediate neonatal period. *Am J Obstet Gynecol*. 1962; 84: 1–12.

17. Bhatt S, Alison BJ, Wallace EM, *et al*. Delayed cord clamping until ventilation onset improves cardiovascular function at birth in preterm lambs. *J Physiol*. 2013; 591(8): 2113–26.

18. Wylie J, Perlman J, Kattwinkel J, *et al*. 2010 international consensus on cardiopulmonary resuscitation and emergency cardiovascular care science with treatment recommendations: neonatal resuscitation. *Resuscitation*. 2010; 81S: e260–87.

19. Perlman JM, Wylie J, Kattwinkel J, *et al*. Part 11: neonatal resuscitation: 2010 international consensus on cardiopulmonary resuscitation and emergency cardiovascular care science with treatment recommendations. *Circulation*. 2010; 122(suppl. 2): S516–38.

20. Vain NE, Szyld EG, Prudent LM, *et al*. Oropharyngeal and nasopharyngeal suctioning of meconium-stained neonates before delivery of their shoulders: multicentre, randomised controlled trial. *Lancet*. 2004; 364: 597–602.

21. Pearlman SA, Maisels J. Preductal and postductal transcutaneous oxygen tension measurements in premature newborns with hyaline membrane disease. *Pediatrics*. 1989; 83: 98–100.

22. Weigel TJ, Hageman JR. National survey of diagnosis and management of persistent pulmonary hypertension of the newborn. *J Perinatol*. 1990; 10: 369–75.

Chapter 27

The Immediate Puerperium

Shankari Arulkumaran

The first models of postnatal care were established at the start of the twentieth century, in response to high maternal mortality rates. Despite a dramatic reduction in the mortality rates since then, there has been little alteration in the timing or the content of care [1]. It is estimated that up to 47% of women have reported at least one health problem within the first six weeks of giving birth [2] and as many as 76% of women have at least one health problem within two months of giving birth [3]. The puerperium is usually taken to describe the six weeks in which a woman's anatomy and physiology return to their pre-pregnancy states following childbirth. There is no specific definition for the immediate puerperium, but here it is taken to address the issues a woman may face in at least the first two weeks following delivery.

One of the challenges in postnatal care is that it crosses both the acute and primary healthcare sectors. A solution is to ensure that there is a system in place to provide women and their babies with an individualized postnatal care plan, which is reviewed and documented at each postnatal contact [4]. This should include relevant factors from the antenatal, intrapartum and immediate postnatal period. There should be details of a named midwife or health visitor, including a 24-hour telephone number to enable the woman to contact her named healthcare practitioner or an alternative practitioner should he or she not be available.

Specific plans for the postnatal period include managing medically related conditions when they occur, such as hypertension, thromboembolism, blood loss, infection, urinary tract- and bowel-related symptoms, postnatal wound care, pain, fatigue and mental health conditions. Other details such as adjustment to motherhood, emotional well-being and family support structures should be covered. Plans for feeding, including specific advice about either breastfeeding support or formula feeding, need to be included, as well as plans for contraceptive care [4]. Relevant adjustments will need to be in place for anyone who has communication difficulties, and for those who do not speak or read English [5].

The Postnatal Check

Women should be advised, within 24 hours of the birth, of the symptoms and signs of conditions that may threaten their lives and require them to access emergency treatment. Table 27.1 summarizes the signs and symptoms that are suggestive of potentially life-threatening physical and mental health conditions in the woman [4].

Maternal Observations

The importance of routine measurements such as pulse, temperature, respiratory rate and blood pressure in any ill postnatal women cannot be over-emphasized. The results should be documented and acted upon; normality cannot be presumed without measurement [5]. The uterus should be examined and any deviation from normal noted. In addition, attention should be paid to the amount and nature of lochia passed, any caesarean section (CS) scars or perineal trauma, bladder and bowel function, as well as thrombosis risk.

Infant Care

Women should also be warned about a major change in the baby's behaviour, as highlighted in Table 27.2 [4].

There are specific behaviours that increase a baby's risk of sudden infant death syndrome. Providing the

Best Practice in Labour and Delivery, Second Edition, ed. Sir Sabaratnam Arulkumaran. Published by Cambridge University Press. © Cambridge University Press 2016.

Table 27.1 Signs and symptoms of potentially life-threatening physical and mental health conditions [4]

Physical signs	Mental health signs
Sudden and profuse blood loss or persistent, increased blood loss	Severe depression, such as feeling extreme unnecessary worry
Faintness, dizziness, palpitations or tachycardia	Being unable to concentrate due to distraction from depressive feelings
Fever, shivering, abdominal pain, especially if combined with offensive vaginal loss or a slow- healing perineal wound	Severe anxiety, such as uncontrollable feelings of panic
Headaches accompanied by visual disturbances or nausea or vomiting within 72 hours of birth	Being unable to cope or becoming obsessive
Leg pain, associated with redness or swelling	The desire to hurt others or oneself
Shortness of breath or chest pain	Thoughts about taking one's own life
Widespread rash	Confused and disturbed thoughts, including hallucinations and delusions

Table 27.2 Major changes in the baby's behaviour [4]

Less active/responsive than usual, or more irritable than usual.
Breathing faster than usual or grunting when breathing.
Feeding less than usual or nappies much less wet than usual.
Has blue lips or, with the exception of hands and feet, feels cold when dressed appropriately for the environment temperature.
Has a fit or is floppy.
Vomits green fluid or has blood in their stools.
Has a rash that does not fade when pressed with a glass or has a temperature higher than 38 °C.
Has a bulging or very depressed fontanelle.
Within the first 24 hours after the birth, has not passed urine, faeces (meconium) or develops a yellow skin colour (jaundice).

woman, her partner or the main carer with the opportunity to regularly discuss infant sleeping practices can help to identify and support them and the wider family to establish safer infant sleeping habits, and to reduce the baby's risk of sudden infant death syndrome [4].

Infant Feeding

Women should receive breastfeeding support through an integrated service that uses an evaluated, structured programme [4]. Babies who are fully or partially formula fed can develop infections and illnesses if their formula milk is not prepared safely. In a small number of babies these cause serious harm which may be life threatening, and require the baby to be admitted to hospital. The mother or main carer of the baby needs consistent, evidence-based advice about how to sterilize feeding equipment and safely prepare formula milk.

The baby's relationship with the mother has a significant impact on the baby's social and emotional development. In turn, the woman's ability to provide a nurturing relationship is partly dependent on her own emotional well-being. Regular assessment of the woman's emotional well-being and the impact of this on her attachment to her baby may lead to earlier detection of problems.

Mental State

Women experience emotional changes in the immediate postnatal period, which usually resolves within 10–14 days after the birth. Women who are still feeling low in mood, anxious, experiencing negative thoughts or lacking interest in their baby at 10–14 days after the birth may be at increased risk of mental health problems. These women should receive an assessment of their mental well-being [4].

General Health

The woman's eating habits and physical activity levels could influence the health behaviour of the wider family, including children who are developing habits that may remain with them for life [4]. Supporting the woman in the postnatal period to change her eating habits and physical activity levels may improve her health, her infant's health and the health of the wider family. It may also improve the outcomes of future pregnancies.

Advice on healthy eating and physical exercise (advising them to take a brisk walk or other moderate exercise for at least 30 min at least five days of the week) should be tailored to each individual woman [4]. Ongoing support over a sufficient period of time will allow for sustained lifestyle changes.

All non-sensitized Rhesus negative women should be offered an appropriate dose of anti-D immunoglobulin within 72 hours of delivery of a Rhesus positive baby. This should be based on the postdelivery Kleihauer Betke test. Similarly, the MMR (measles, mumps, rubella) vaccine should be offered to any woman found to be seronegative on antenatal screening for rubella. She should be advised not to get pregnant in the next three months.

Puerperal Complications

Postpartum Haemorrhage

Figures from the latest *Confidential Enquiry into Maternal Deaths* in the UK estimate that 13% of all maternities in England in 2011–12 were affected by a blood loss ≥500 ml. These figures have doubled since 2005 [5]. There are a number of preventive measures to reduce the complications caused by a postpartum haemorrhage. In the antenatal period, low haemoglobin levels should be investigated and optimized prior to delivery.

Physiological observations including the respiratory rate recorded within a trigger system such as the Modified Early Obstetric Warning Score (MEOWS) chart should be used to monitor all postnatal admissions. Concerns should be escalated to a senior doctor or midwife if a woman's health deteriorates, and there should be a named senior doctor in charge of ongoing care [5]. Fluid resuscitation and blood transfusion should not be delayed because of false reassurance from a single haemoglobin result; the whole clinical picture should be considered.

While significant haemorrhage may be apparent from observed physiological disturbances, young, fit, pregnant women compensate remarkably well. While a tachycardia commonly develops, there can be a paradoxical bradycardia, and hypotension is always a very late sign; therefore, ongoing bleeding should be acted on without delay [5].

In a woman who is bleeding and is likely to develop a coagulopathy or has evidence of a coagulopathy, it is prudent to give blood components before coagulation indices deteriorate and worsen the bleeding. If pharmacological measures fail to control the haemorrhage, initiate surgical haemostasis sooner rather than later. Early recourse to hysterectomy is recommended if simpler medical and surgical interventions prove ineffective [5].

Postpartum Haematomas

Postpartum haematomas can present as vulval, paravaginal, intra-ligamentous (broad ligament) and retroperitoneal. Vulval haematomas can be further subdivided into perineal, ischiorectal and labial [6]. Vulvovaginal haematomas are an uncommon complication postpartum and the incidence can vary from 1 in 500 to 1 in over 12 000 [6].

In most cases, normal rather than abnormal labour and delivery are associated with their occurrence. Factors such as primiparity, a fetus over 4 kg, delayed second stage of labour, instrumental deliveries, episiotomies and genital tract varicosities are poor predictors of vulval haematomas [6].

Paravaginal haematomas can occur with trauma to the pudendal vessels because of their arterial component and lack of counter pressure; expansion within the vaginal, subvaginal and retroperitoneal tissues of the pelvis can occur. Vulval veins have no valves and therefore continued bleeding from trauma can cause gross distention of the soft tissues of the vagina and vulva [6].

The aim of surgical management is to alleviate the pain caused by the haematoma, prevent further bleeding and damage to tissue as well as to reduce the risk of subsequent infection. The clots should be evacuated to start with and if any bleeding vessels are identified, they should be clamped and ligated. Some authors have advised that the haematoma cavity be tightly packed with gauze and drained, with subsequent removal of the packs and healing by secondary intention [6]. Others advocate draining of the haematoma and primary repair. Angiographic embolization of the bleeding internal iliac artery tributaries and internal iliac artery ligation may be required in more severe cases [6].

What is crucial in the management of such cases is early recourse to treatment, as prolonged delay may result in increased pain and discomfort for the patient as well as further bleeding, tissue distortion, damage and necrosis. On diagnosing a vulvovaginal haematoma, aggressive fluid replacement, blood transfusion, antibiotics, indwelling urinary catheter and surgery are mandatory unless the haematoma is small, self-limiting and presents with minimal symptoms. In other cases, prompt treatment will result in reduced scarring, postpartum pain and dyspareunia.

Sepsis

Pregnant women are uniquely at risk from sepsis. Their immune system is modulated to accept foreign proteins from the feto-placental unit and usually they are young and fit, and able to withstand the physiological insults of widespread inflammation for long periods of time. Pregnant or postpartum women can appear well until the point of collapse, which can occur with little warning. However, more often than not a woman's physiological vital signs, the pulse, blood pressure, temperature and respiratory rate, will give an indication of the early stages of sepsis [5]. In the majority of cases, the organism group A *Streptococcus* (GAS) is responsible for women who die from genital tract sepsis following term births. Most are following vaginal deliveries; in the few that are CS, this occurred despite the administration of antibiotics [5].

'Severe sepsis' is sepsis associated with organ dysfunction, for example acute renal failure or hypotension. 'Septic shock' is a vasodilatory form of shock and is defined as persisting hypotension despite adequate fluid resuscitation in the presence of sepsis [5]. Lactic acid is an important marker of tissue hypoxia and a strong indicator of the potential for multi-organ failure and mortality. A serum lactate measurement of >2 mmol/l indicates severe sepsis and >4 mmol/l indicates septic shock [5].

Antibiotic administration is crucial to the immediate management. From the recognition of signs of septic shock, each hour's delay in administering antibiotic therapy increases the chance of mortality by 8% [5]. The choice of antibiotic is as important as timely administration. In most women with sepsis, antibiotics will be started prior to culture of the infecting organism. Antibiotic choice should therefore be based on the suspected site of infection, with the antibiotics chosen to have an appropriate spectrum of activity based on local prescribing guidelines. If the source of sepsis is unknown then antibiotics covering a broad range of possible organisms should be used and later the spectrum can be narrowed or targeted based on the culture results, radiological imaging or the development of specific signs or symptoms [5].

A woman with sepsis must receive the level of care she needs and critical care should be provided on the delivery unit if this is the most appropriate setting. Alternatively, maternity care should be provided on the critical care unit if this is the most appropriate setting [5].

Influenza A and B are highly infectious acute viral infections of the respiratory tract and should also be considered as a source of maternal sepsis. It usually occurs in a seasonal pattern, with epidemics in the winter months. Vaccination is the main public health response to influenza in general. Influenza vaccination in pregnancy reduces maternal morbidity and mortality, reduces the likelihood of perinatal death, prematurity and low birth weight and prevents influenza in the infant up to six months of age through transfer of maternal antibodies [5].

Ogilvie's Syndrome

Ogilvie's syndrome can occur after CS and result in caecal perforation. This is an extremely rare phenomenon following normal vaginal delivery, especially the progression to caecal perforation [7]. The exact aetiology of Ogilvie's syndrome is unknown, but it has been associated with severe trauma, abdominal and/or pelvic surgery, and sepsis. Bed rest and abnormal electrolytes are listed as factors associated with the development of the syndrome. The mechanism of the condition is thought to involve loss of tone in the parasympathetic nerves S2 to S4. This, in turn, results in an atonic distal colon and pseudo obstruction [7].

A cut-off sign relating to an area of dilated and collapsed bowel around the splenic flexure corresponds to the transition zone between the vagal and sacral parasympathetic nerve supply. The cut-off sign is used to support the hypothesis of parasympathetic inhibition causing Ogilvie's syndrome [7]. The diagnosis of Ogilvie's syndrome can be difficult due to the non-specific clinical features. Abdominal distension is considered to be the most common symptom. As with any case of suspected ileus or obstruction, electrolyte levels are an essential investigation, with hypocalcaemia being the most common [7]. Abdominal radiography is the standard first line investigation, and a caecal diameter of 9 cm or more is the only definitive sign of imminent perforation [7]. Several sources have discussed non-surgical management options, which include decompression of the bowel and intravenous fluid support, unless signs of peritonism are evident. The use of prokinetic, parasympathomimetic drugs such as neostigmine can be successful in the management of Ogilvie's syndrome, although the benefit in cases of idiopathic Ogilvie's syndrome is not certain [7]. The importance of early diagnosis cannot be underestimated.

Venous Thromboembolism and Pulmonary Embolus

The prothrombotic changes of pregnancy do not revert completely to normal until several weeks after delivery.

Indeed the time of greatest risk for venous thromboembolism (VTE) associated with pregnancy is the early puerperium and, although most VTE occurs antenatally, the risk per day is greatest in the weeks immediately after delivery. For women at high risk of postpartum VTE, the recommended duration of thrombo-prophylaxis is six weeks [8]. All women with a body mass index greater than 40 kg/m^2 should be considered for prophylactic low molecular weight heparin for seven days after delivery [8]. Additional risk factors relevant for postpartum thrombo-prophylaxis after delivery include prolonged labour, immobility, infection, haemorrhage and blood transfusion.

The first thrombo-prophylactic dose of low molecular weight heparin should be given as soon as possible after delivery, provided that there is no postpartum haemorrhage. If there has been regional analgesia, low molecular weight heparin should be given by four hours after delivery or four hours after removal of the epidural catheter [8]. If the epidural catheter is left in place after delivery, it should be removed 12 hours after a dose or four hours before the next dose of low molecular weight heparin [8]. Women delivered by emergency CS have a roughly four-fold increased risk of postpartum VTE compared with women delivered vaginally and should be considered for low molecular weight heparin for seven days after delivery [8].

Low molecular weight heparin is appropriate for postpartum thrombo-prophylaxis although, if women are receiving long-term anticoagulation with warfarin, this can be started when the risk of haemorrhage is low, usually 5–7 days after delivery [8]. Both warfarin and low molecular weight heparin are safe when breastfeeding. Low molecular weight heparin has the advantage of not requiring monitoring.

Warfarin requires close monitoring and carries an increased risk of postpartum haemorrhage and perineal haematoma compared with low molecular weight heparin [8]. It is not appropriate for those women requiring seven days of postpartum prophylaxis. However, it is appropriate for those on maintenance warfarin outside pregnancy.

The incidence of pulmonary embolism is reported to be about 13/10 000 pregnancies, about half occurring in the puerperium; the risk of pulmonary embolism is highest in the immediate postpartum period [9]. In massive life-threatening pulmonary embolism with haemodynamic compromise, both the Royal College of Obstetricians and Gynaecologists (RCOG) and the American College of Chest Physicians (ACCP) recommend the use of fibrinolysis in selected cases. Furthermore, to minimize the risk of bleeding, fibrinolytic agents with short infusion times or bolus therapy and adjunctive anticoagulant therapy more than four hours postpartum is recommended [9]. Postpartum massive pulmonary embolism represents a significant management dilemma, as the possible benefit from fibrinolysis needs to be weighed against the risk of inducing postpartum haemorrhage. The risk of death in pulmonary embolism with sustained hypotension and cardiogenic shock is high (15.3% at three months), whereas the risk of non-fatal bleeding from fibrinolytic therapy in pregnant women is only 2.9%, with no recorded maternal deaths [9].

Postnatal Hypertension

Blood pressure rises progressively over the first five postnatal days, peaking on days three to six after delivery. This pattern of blood pressure is thought to result from mobilization, from the extravascular to the intravascular space, of the six to eight litres of total body water and the 950 mEq of total body sodium accumulated during pregnancy [10].

Postpartum hypertension may represent a continuation of an antenatal hypertensive disorder (regardless of aetiology), or the appearance of a new hypertensive disorder after delivery. Hypertension is defined as a blood pressure of 140/90 mmHg or more; mild to moderate hypertension is usually defined as a blood pressure of 140/90 to 169/109 mmHg, and severe hypertension as 170/110 mmHg or more. Compared with women with pre-eclampsia, fewer women with gestational hypertension appear to have postpartum hypertension. Also, the duration of this hypertension appears to be shorter than in women with pre-eclampsia [10].

It is generally understood that severe hypertension should be treated (to prevent acute maternal vascular complications such as stroke), but no such consensus exists for mild to moderate postpartum hypertension, regardless of type. Several drugs are commonly prescribed in the postpartum period: methyldopa, beta-blockers, angiotensin-converting enzyme inhibitors and some calcium channel blockers. They have minimal milk to maternal plasma ratios to make breastfeeding acceptable [10]. Methyldopa, however, is associated with an increased risk of maternal depression and is therefore not advised.

Anaesthetic Complications

Postpartum women recovering from anaesthesia require the same standard of postoperative monitoring, including documentation, as non-obstetric patients [5]. The association between post-dural puncture headache and subdural haematoma is well described, even after an intentional dural puncture. Cerebral venous sinus thrombosis occurring postpartum is also well described [5]. In both instances, women often complain of a persistent headache. Prompt and appropriate imaging and transfer to a neurosurgical unit is key to the management unless it is postural that follows an epidural analgesia, the treatment of which is described in Chapter 3. Outpatient follow-up and notification of the woman's GP, in case subsequent complications occur, are also crucial.

Pelvic Girdle Pain

One in five women report pelvic girdle pain during pregnancy and the majority experience regression of the pain postpartum. Nevertheless, 2–3% of all women report significant symptoms up to one year after delivery [11]. Some women with severe pelvic girdle pain fear the consequences of labour and delivery and therefore lack the confidence to deliver vaginally. Therefore, more evidence is needed on the impact of the mode of delivery on the prognosis of pelvic girdle pain. It appears that women with a high body mass index have higher incidences of pelvic girdle pain following delivery. There appears to be an association with increased pain following an instrumental delivery over a spontaneous vaginal delivery. However, women who have had an elective CS appear to have a two-fold increase in severe pelvic girdle pain up to six months following delivery [11].

Urine Infection

Urine is bacteriostatic to most local commensal bacteria and this is thought to result from its relatively acidic pH, high osmolality and high urea concentration. In an anatomically normal urinary tract, sterility is maintained by free antegrade flow through the ureteral and urethral valves [12].

In pregnancy, significant physiological changes occur in the urogenital tract, increasing the potential for pathogenic colonization. Bladder volume increases and detrusor tone decreases. Additionally, 90% of pregnant women develop ureteric dilatation as the result of a combination of progestogenic relaxation of ureteric smooth muscle and pressure from the expanding uterus [12]. There is relative sparing of the left ureter because of protection from the sigmoid colon and upper rectum. The net effect, however, is increased urinary stasis, compromised ureteric valves and vesicoureteric reflux, which facilitate bacterial colonization and ascending infection [12]. Early recognition and treatment can reduce maternal morbidity, but while antibiotic treatment is effective at curing urinary tract infections, there are insufficient data with which to recommend any specific treatment regimen or duration [13].

Lower Urinary Tract Dysfunction

The incidence of urinary incontinence in pregnancy varies between 32% and 64% and is higher in parous than in nulliparous women. However, the prevalence of persistent urinary incontinence in the postpartum period is considered to be around 24% [13]. Stress urinary incontinence, which is common during pregnancy, generally resolves in the postpartum period. On the other hand, symptoms of overactive bladder syndrome symptoms appear to increase with greater gestation but decrease rapidly after childbirth [13].

Vaginal delivery has been thought to cause postpartum stress urinary incontinence. Several reports show an increased risk of stress urinary incontinence following vaginal delivery compared with CS; however, CS appears to be only partially protective against the development of stress urinary incontinence six years after delivery [13]. The development of stress urinary incontinence after vaginal delivery is thought to be due to a consequence of muscular and neuromuscular injuries of the pelvic floor as well as damage to the suburethral fascia. Damage to the levator ani has been well documented following vaginal delivery and is thought to be associated with the subsequent development of lower urinary tract symptoms [13].

Management in the early postpartum period is mainly conservative and includes lifestyle interventions, physical therapies and the use of anti-incontinence devices, pads and catheters: these are considered to have a low risk of adverse effects and do not affect subsequent treatments. There is evidence that pelvic floor muscle training during a first pregnancy reduces the likelihood of postnatal urinary incontinence. Pelvic floor muscle training should also be offered as first line therapy to women with persistent urinary incontinence three months after delivery [13].

Poor response to pelvic floor muscle training in the early postpartum period may be caused by neurogenic injury, which may resolve over time. This may take several months to recover and may interfere with women's ability to isolate and contract the pelvic floor muscles in the early postpartum period [13].

Continence pessaries are used in the management of stress urinary incontinence and can be considered as an alternative to other conservative treatment. They are believed to increase urethral resistance by augmenting urethral closure during episodes of increased intra-abdominal pressure. They may be offered to women who do not respond well to pelvic floor muscle training [13].

There appears to be little evidence available on the treatment of overactive bladder symptoms in puerperium; neither are there any studies that assess the effect of bladder and pelvic floor muscle training. The mainstay of treatment is conservative and includes lifestyle modifications, fluid manipulation, avoiding caffeine, bladder and pelvic floor muscle training, and alternative therapies such as acupuncture. The use of antimuscarinics during breastfeeding is recommended only when the medication is of clear benefit to the mother [13].

Pelvic Organ Prolapse

The severity of pelvic organ prolapse as measured by the Pelvic Organ Prolapse Quantification (POP-Q) staging system appears to increase during pregnancy in nulliparous women. However, the stage does not change significantly postpartum. The POP-Q stage may be higher in women delivered vaginally than in women delivered by CS, with the most frequent site of prolapse being the anterior compartment [13].

Pelvic organ prolapse in the immediate puerperium should be managed conservatively. These include lifestyle interventions such as stopping smoking, and reducing exacerbating or predisposing factors that include: avoidance of heavy lifting, treating chronic cough and constipation, and pelvic floor muscle training [13].

Vaginal rings and pessaries can also be offered as a conservative treatment option. The aim is to manage pelvic organ prolapse by mechanically supporting the pelvic viscera. Modern pessaries are made from a variety of materials, including rubber, plastic and silicone.

While there are no studies about the use of rings and pessaries during pregnancy and the postpartum, there is good evidence that they provide symptomatic relief and may prevent worsening of pelvic organ prolapse in the non-pregnant population; this evidence has been adopted for use in pregnancy and the immediate puerperium [13].

Wound Breakdown

The incidence of perianal wound breakdown is generally considered to be between 0.1% and 2.1%. There is little evidence in the literature with regards to risk factors, but infection is a common cause in over 40% of cases [14]. Dehiscence may range in severity from simple separation of the skin or mucosa to more severe separations that involve the anal sphincter or mucosa. The consequence of these include pain, infection, loss of perineal body mass, loss of tone to the vaginal introitus and loss of continence [14].

Some of studies have shown that perineal laceration repair breakdown is associated with instrumental deliveries in conjunction with mediolateral episiotomy, third- or fourth-degree tears, the presence of meconium-stained amniotic fluid and a prolonged second stage [14]. Delayed closures of perineal laceration repair breakdown may be related to the integrity of the tissue and high rates of infections. This results in pain and discomfort for the patient as well as loss of sexual function and embarrassment. Alternative management options that provide good results and high patient satisfaction include wound preparation with irrigation, debridement and early surgical repair. Attention to these details and appropriate use of antibiotics is often successful [14].

Breast Pain

Up to 16% of breastfeeding women complain of mastitis [15]. However, not all breast pain is mastitis. Engorgement due to the accumulation of milk causes mild bilateral breast pain and tenderness. This tends to re-occur at regular intervals as the milk is being produced. If the breast is not completely emptied during feeding, stasis can cause milk extravasation into adjacent tissue, increasing the likelihood of mastitis [15]. Nipple pain is common in breastfeeding women and is an independent risk factor for mastitis [15]. The normal discomfort subsides within one minute of commencing feeding. Pain that worsens during feeding is, however, due to cracks and sores on the nipples that may occur. The treatment involves proper positioning and consistent topical nipple care.

Anaemia

The occurrence of postpartum anaemia is not unusual. Around 15% of women may lose over 500 ml of blood during delivery, with the risk of anaemia and the subsequent depletion of iron stores. Oral iron therapy is regularly used to treat iron deficiency in these women, achieving a mean increase in haemoglobin values of approximately 2.83 g/dl at 30 days [16]. Postpartum anaemia may increase the risk of depression, anxiety, asthenia, lethargy, lactation failure and other morbidities, resulting in a longer hospital stay and reinforcing the need to seek appropriate therapy [16]. Oral iron seems to be a valid, simple and effective treatment approach in women with severe postpartum anaemia. The low cost of oral iron tablets supports the fact that this therapy is used as the first choice in women with severe postpartum anaemia without clinical indication for blood transfusion; however, intravenous therapy may be a good option in cases of oral iron intolerance or presumed poor adherence to oral therapy.

Mental Health

In pregnancy and the postnatal period, many mental health problems have a similar nature, course and potential for relapse as at other times. However, there can be differences; for example, bipolar disorder shows an increased rate of relapse and first presentation in the postnatal period [17]. Some changes in mental health state and functioning (such as appetite) may represent normal pregnancy changes, but they may be a symptom of a mental health problem.

The management of mental health problems during pregnancy and the postnatal period differs from at other times because of the nature of this life stage and the potential impact of any difficulties and treatments on the woman and the baby. There are risks associated with taking psychotropic medication in pregnancy and during breastfeeding and risks of stopping medication taken for an existing mental health problem. There is also an increased risk of postpartum psychosis [17].

Depression and anxiety affect 15–20% of women in the first year after childbirth. During pregnancy and the postnatal period, anxiety disorders, including panic disorder, generalized anxiety disorder, obsessive-compulsive disorder and post-traumatic stress disorder can occur on their own or can co-exist with depression [17]. Psychosis can re-emerge or be exacerbated during pregnancy and the postnatal period. Postpartum psychosis affects between 1 and 2 in 1000 women who have given birth. Women with bipolar disorder are at particular risk, but postpartum psychosis can occur in women with no previous psychiatric history [17].

Changes to body shape, including weight gain, in pregnancy and after childbirth may be a concern for women with an eating disorder. Although the prevalence of anorexia nervosa and bulimia nervosa is lower in pregnant women, the prevalence of binge eating disorder is higher [17].

Mental health professionals providing detailed advice about the possible risks of mental health problems or the benefits and harms of treatment in the postnatal period should include in the discussion the uncertainty about the benefits, risks and harms of treatments for mental health problems in the postnatal period, as well as the likely benefits of each treatment, taking into account the severity of the mental health problem [17]. In addition, the woman's response to any previous treatment should be taken into account. A risk assessment should be made as to whether there is more risk to the mother and baby associated with the background mental health problem or parenting associated with no treatment in a mother with symptoms [17]. There will be risks to the woman and the baby associated with each treatment option, but there is also a need for prompt treatment because of the potential effect of an untreated mental health problem on the baby. Ultimately, managers and senior healthcare professionals responsible for perinatal mental health services should ensure that there are clearly specified care pathways so that all primary and secondary healthcare professionals involved in the care of women during the postnatal period know how to access assessment and treatment [17].

Stillbirth

The WHO defines stillbirth as a fetal death late in pregnancy and individual countries define the gestational age at which a miscarriage becomes a stillbirth. Stillbirth accounts for 60% of all perinatal deaths and 75% of all potentially preventable losses [18]. For women and their families who experience stillbirths, the loss can be devastating. In high-income countries, maternal age, smoking and obesity are the new contributors to risk, in addition to infections, congenital anomalies, diabetes and postdate pregnancies [19].

Induction of labour 24 hours following a stillbirth is usual practice and delayed induction carries with it the potential risk of disseminated intravascular coagulation. The infant should be carefully inspected following the delivery and the findings documented in detail [18]. Parents are given the option of holding their baby following the delivery and some may find this of some comfort, whereas others may suffer psychological sequalae. A postmortem examination should be discussed, with specific consent relating to the retention of tissue [18]. Other investigations should be discussed, including maternal blood for direct causes and risk factors, karyotyping, examination of the placenta and membranes, external examination of the fetus (if a postmortem is declined) and a radiographical examination of the infant, where possible [18]. A dedicated bereavement midwife should be made available, in addition to religious leaders from different faith groups.

Mother should be cared for in a different bereavement suite or room with no immediate connection to the delivery or postnatal unit, i.e. away from the sounds of other newborns crying or mothers feeding their babies. The husband or partner should be able to stay with the mother until the time of discharge from the hospital. Counselling services are essential, and in the UK a consultant normally sees the woman and her partner or family member four to six weeks later to go through the results of any investigations, discuss any questions they may have regarding their loss and to make plans for any future pregnancy [18].

Conclusion

The immediate postpartum period is normal or is associated with minor symptoms or anxiety in the vast majority of women. In some mothers complications of labour and delivery may be associated with physical or mental ill health. Midwives and doctors should pay attention to details while talking to the mother and methodically inquire for symptoms and check for early signs of illness. Early recognition and prompt treatment is the key to limiting or avoiding complications in the postnatal period.

References

1. Demott K, Bick D, Norman R, *et al. Clinical Guidelines and Evidence Review for Post Natal Care: Routine Post Natal Care of Recently Delivered Women and Their Babies.* London: National Collaborating Centre for Primary Care and Royal College of General Practitioners; 2006.

2. MacArthur C, Lewis M, Knox EG. Comparison of long-term health-problems following childbirth among Asian and caucasian mothers. *Br J Gen Pract.* 1993;43(377): 519–22.

3. Glazener CM, Abdalla M, Stroud P, *et al.* Postnatal maternal morbidity: extent, causes, prevention and treatment. *Br J Obstet Gynaecol.* 1995;102(4): 282–7.

4. NICE. *Postnatal Care.* London: NICE; 2013.

5. Knight M, Kenyon S, Brocklehurst P, *et al.* (eds). *Saving Lives, Improving Mothers' Care – Lessons Learned to Inform Future Maternity Care from the UK and Ireland Confidential Enquiries into Maternal Deaths and Morbidity 2009–12.* Oxford: National Perinatal Epidemiology Unit, University of Oxford; 2014.

6. Morgans D, Chan N, Clark CA. Vulval perineal haematomas in the immediate postpartum period and their management. *Aust N Z J Obstet Gynaecol.* 1999;39(2): 223–7.

7. Harish E, Sundeep VK, Sivasi KK, Dharma Kumar KG. Spontaneous caecal perforation associated with Ogilvie's syndrome following vaginal delivery – a case report. *J Clin Diagn Res.* 2014;8(6): ND8–9.

8. Nelson-Piercy C, MacCallum P, Mackillop L. *Thrombosis and Embolism during Pregnancy and the Puerperium, Reducing the Risk.* London: RCOG Press; 2009.

9. Azarisman SM, Liza RA, Radhiana H, *et al.* Immediate postpartum cardiorespiratory collapse: a management quandary. *Blood Coagul Fibrinolysis.* 2010;21(6): 601–4.

10. Magee L, von Dadelszen P. Prevention and treatment of postpartum hypertension. *Cochrane Database Syst Rev.* 2013;4: CD004351.

11. Bjelland EK, Stuge B, Vangen S, Stray-Pedersen B, Eberhard-Gran M. Mode of delivery and persistence of pelvic girdle syndrome 6 months postpartum. *Am J Obstet Gynecol.* 2013;208(4): 298.

12. McCormick T, Ashe RG, Kearney P. Urinary tract infection in pregnancy. *TOG.* 2008;10: 156–62.

13. Asali F, Mahfouz I, Phillips C. The management of urogynaecological problems in pregnancy and the early postpartum period. *TOG.* 2012;14: 153–8.

14. Williams MK, Chames MC. Risk factors for the breakdown of perineal laceration repair after vaginal delivery. *Am J Obstet Gynecol.* 2006;195(3): 755–9.

15. Schoenfeld EM, McKay MP. Mastitis and methicillin-resistant *Staphylococcus aureus* (MRSA):

the calm before the storm? *J Emerg Med*. 2010;38(4): e31–4.

16. Perello MF, Coloma JL, Masoller N, Esteve J, Palacio M. Intravenous ferrous sucrose versus placebo in addition to oral iron therapy for the treatment of severe postpartum anaemia: a randomised controlled trial. *BJOG*. 2014;121(6): 706–13.

17. NICE. *Antenatal and Postnatal Mental Health: Clinical Management and Service Guidance:* Clinical Guideline 192. London: NICE; 2014.

18. Smith G, Fretts R. Stillbirth. *Lancet*. 2007;370: 1715–25.

19. Goldenberg R, McClure E, Bhutta Z, *et al*. Stillbirths: the vision for 2020. *Lancet*. 2011;377: 1798–805.

Chapter 28

Triage and Prioritization in a Busy Labour Ward

Nina Johns

Introduction and Definition

The term 'triage' originates from the French language, meaning 'to sort' or 'sift'. Within medical practice, the term has come to describe a system used to rapidly assess the clinical needs of large numbers of casualties and assign management priorities. Although initially introduced within military settings to deal with huge casualties in wartime, triage has become a daily management tool in certain healthcare settings. It is a procedure for standardized clinical assessment, prioritization and delivery of emergency care when workload exceeds capacity. It is particularly useful in areas of high-flow patient care with diverse clinical needs, such as accident and emergency and obstetrics.

The primary aim of triage is to deliver the appropriate care to each patient with the correct urgency required, in the right order, with the resources available at that time, in the most efficient way – 'do the most for the most, in the right order'. Four categories exist within the basic triage structure; these indicate the need for clinical intervention rather than the severity of injury, and are described in Table 28.1. Those requiring immediate intervention need further prioritization, using the well-recognized ABC systems assessment: airway, breathing and circulation [1].

A = Airway An airway problem will result in death if not dealt with rapidly.

B = Breathing If the airway is clear but there is a problem with breathing this must be addressed before C.

C = Circulation This covers cardiac output, control of haemorrhage and volume, and red cell replacement.

Table 28.1 Trauma triage prioritization [1]

Priority	Category	
1	Immediate	Requires immediate resuscitation or emergency treatment, or may die.
2	Urgent	Treatment may be delayed for a few hours.
3	Expectant	Can tolerate a significant delay.
4	Dead	Condition so severe unlikely to survive.

The end point of triage is the allocation of a priority to each case and a mechanical resource to carry out care to each individual. The optimal care is received when the most appropriate priority is set and resources are used most efficiently. It is essential that all cases are assessed before treatment is carried out, as resources may be allocated to one when another still awaiting assessment is in greater need.

The key to successful triage is to be able to assess patients rapidly and accurately, and thus allocate them to intervention correctly.

Triage and Prioritization in Obstetrics

While triage is an effective tool throughout medical practice, there are a number of specific difficulties within obstetrics that need to be considered. Prioritization on the labour ward must reflect constantly changing events. Not only do the numbers of patients within the department change, but also the clinical needs of those patients vary with time. Labour is a dynamic process, which results in changes in both the maternal and fetal condition. As such, the urgency of treatment required will also change with time. Those with seemingly less urgent concerns will continue to

Best Practice in Labour and Delivery, Second Edition, ed. Sir Sabaratnam Arulkumaran. Published by Cambridge University Press. © Cambridge University Press 2016.

labour and will need ongoing care. These individuals may then develop concerns requiring immediate priority over others, with unpredictable and unpreventable complications arising in normal labour. Regular reassessment of individual and departmental priorities is therefore essential.

The labour ward not only provides support for women in normal labour, it must be equipped to manage abnormal labour, life-threatening emergencies, severe maternal medical conditions and acute surgical events. In addition to this, elective work on any labour ward, such as induction of labour and elective caesarean sections (CSs), also requires allocation of appropriate resources. The routine midwifery and obstetric care provided by the labour ward is coupled with high-dependency care, the management of surgical theatres, postoperative recovery and assessment of unscheduled antenatal 'drop-ins' and admissions.

The majority of admissions to the labour ward are unplanned, with women attending from home, general practice, hospital antenatal clinics, community midwifery clinics and other departments within the hospital. These admissions present with a spectrum of conditions, ranging from physiological labour to minor complaints unrelated to pregnancy, to acute emergencies. Following recommendations from a number of national enquiries (CEMACE, *Safer Childbirth*), separate departments or areas adjacent to the labour ward have been developed for women presenting with unscheduled pregnancy-related conditions who are not in labour. Many of these departments are themselves named triage, but this does not necessarily represent a standardized assessment and process of clinical prioritization for these women and many of these departments share clinical space with elective day assessment admissions and women attending for induction of labour. Local pathways are beginning to emerge that have developed from the current systems available in emergency medicine, such as the Birmingham Symptom Specific Obstetric Triage System [2–4]. This novel pathway includes a standardized assessment of all women and their babies within 15 min of arrival and the use of symptom-specific algorithms to determine the clinical urgency of further investigations and seniority of review. Such systems allow standard initial assessment, facilitates clinical prioritization and the patient receives the level and quality of care appropriate to their clinical needs. Effective triage systems maximize effective use of available resources

and allow midwives and medical staff to know exactly who is in the department and their level of clinical need, and enable more effective communication and handover.

For those admissions that are planned, such as elective CS and induction of labour, their progress of care will also depend on the resources available and the emergency workload of the department.

The workload on the labour ward is concurrently linked to that of other departments, such as the neonatal intensive care unit and the postnatal wards. The inability of the neonatal unit to accept an admission of a preterm infant may necessitate an in utero transfer to another unit, taking time to organize and using valuable midwifery staff time to escort, while a lack of beds on the postnatal ward means that delivery rooms are blocked with postnatal women, and labour ward midwifery resources are used for their care. Therefore, the entire maternity and neonatal services must work together and communicate effectively to maintain continued flow and safe care throughout.

Staffing

Coordination of the diverse clinical events on the labour ward requires appropriate numbers of medical, midwifery and support staff, with the relevant clinical skills and experience. There is clear evidence that one-to-one midwifery care in labour reduces intervention and improves women's satisfaction [5], but many units struggle to provide this. In the UK, almost three-quarters of heads of midwifery feel that their funded establishment is inadequate to cope with the workload [6]. The number of midwives required to provide one-to-one care in labour depends on the case mix, with more midwives being required to provide care for women with complex pregnancies and those requiring emergency intervention. Appropriate midwifery staffing levels and the means to calculate the numbers required have been summarized recently in the national NICE guidance on *Safe Midwifery Staffing for Maternity Settings* [7]. This guidance has used evidence from numerous national reports to provide regulated targets for midwifery staffing which includes the core standard of one-to-one care for women in labour, but allows local skill mix to reflect complexity and workload, with the ability to uplift to cover leave and sickness absence and enable fluctuations in workload to be dealt with. The guidance has also outlined

Box 28.1 Red Flag Events [7]

A midwifery red flag event is a warning sign that something may be wrong with midwifery staffing. If a midwifery red flag event occurs, the midwife in charge of the service should be notified. The midwife in charge should determine whether midwifery staffing is the cause, and the action that is needed.

- Delayed or cancelled time-critical activity.
- Missed or delayed care (for example, delay of 60 min or more in washing and suturing).
- Missed medication during an admission to hospital or midwifery-led unit (for example, diabetes medication).
- Delay of more than 30 min in providing pain relief.
- Delay of 30 min or more between presentation and triage.
- Full clinical examination not carried out when presenting in labour.
- Delay of two hours or more between admission for induction and beginning of process.
- Delayed recognition of and action on abnormal vital signs (for example, sepsis or urine output).
- Any occasion when one midwife is not able to provide continuous one-to-one care and support to a woman during established labour.
- Other midwifery red flags may be agreed locally.

organizational and clinical indicators – red flag events (see Box 28.1), which can be used to assess whether the midwifery staffing levels are safe for an individual unit [7].

As with midwifery staffing, the number of medical staff that should be allocated to the labour ward depends on the size of the unit and the complexity of the case mix. Again, *Safer Childbirth* [8] has addressed this in detail, looking at obstetric, anaesthetic and paediatric requirements with regard to UK practice. Table 28.2 summarizes the recommendations of this document with regard to obstetric staffing, but recognizes the financial implications of providing this.

Consultant input is essential for leadership, experience and teaching. Emergency workload varies little over the 24-hour period in the labour ward [10], and there is evidence that morbidity and mortality are increased overnight, when consultants are not routinely present [11,12]. Although it has always been presumed, evidence is emerging that demonstrates that consultant input reduces intervention [13] and

improves outcomes [14]. Junior medical staff should be allocated to clinical tasks appropriate for their level of training and demonstrated competencies while learning new clinical and management skills with proper supervision. The use of competency-based training in the UK means that junior obstetric staff need to be directly supervised and observed when performing clinical interventions to allow assessment of their competencies, and this can only be carried out if the consultant is present at the time.

As most medical staff in the UK now work in a shift pattern on the labour ward, there is loss of continuity of care and an increased tendency to defer decision making and intervention across shift boundaries. This increases the risk of a number of problems likely to occur at the same time, having to be dealt with by the on-coming shift who are unfamiliar with the patients. Changes in shift are ideally handled with effective handovers and regular ward rounds. In addition to medical staff, midwifery staff allocations should also be based on the midwives' experience and the woman's needs.

During each shift a single senior midwife is needed to allocate midwifery staff appropriately, coordinate and supervise their practice. The 'shift leader' will provide all staff with a central and easily accessible person for advice and help, and is the essential point of contact and communication with medical staff. When workload demand exceeds the staff available, it is paramount that this is identified early. Each unit should have an 'escalation policy' which can be implemented when demand exceeds resource, to allow mobilization of staff from other areas to manage the workload safely and to allow redistribution of cases, such as cancelling elective work and discharging appropriate women home.

Space

Despite adequate staffing levels, physical resources such as delivery rooms, high-dependency beds and operating theatres are limited to a finite number. Once workload exceeds these resources, meticulous reassessment is required to organize which women can be transferred to antenatal or postnatal wards or discharged. Regular ward rounds by senior medical staff on both the antenatal and postnatal wards are also required to identify women and babies who can be discharged, allowing rapid transfer from the labour

Table 28.2 Proposed obstetric staffing targets 2007–10, reproduced with kind permission from *Safer Childbirth* [8], adapted from *The Future Role of the Consultant* [9]

Category	Definition (births/year)	Consultant presence (year of adoption)			Specialist trainees (n)
		60-hour	98-hour	168-hour	
A	<2500	Units to continually review staffing to ensure adequate based on local needs			1
B	2500–4000	2009	–	–	2
C1	4000–5000	2008	2009	–	3
C2	5000–6000	Immediate	2008	2010	
C3	>6000	Immediate	Immediate if possible	2008	

ward. It is essential to ensure that the service provided is safe, and the escalation policy should also address what happens when there are physically no beds in the department. Some units will choose to deliver appropriate women on the antenatal ward, whereas others will have arrangements with neighbouring units who will then take women for delivery when their own unit closes.

Surgical cases must be prioritized for the most efficient use of theatre time and personnel. Many units now perform elective operative obstetrics as a planned list, with dedicated staff that are separate from those covering the labour ward, using a theatre that is not the emergency labour ward theatre. This clearly has cost implications, but has the huge benefit of ensuring that the management of obstetric emergencies is not being compromised by lack of staff or theatre space because of elective work. With regard to emergency work, simultaneous high-risk interventions should be avoided if possible. For example, a controlled amniotomy should not be carried out at the same time as fetal blood sampling on the department, as both may subsequently require immediate transfer to theatre for delivery by emergency CS. Despite all this, there will be, on occasion, instances where emergency intervention is delayed because of theatre being blocked by another case, or staff not being immediately available. With meticulous planning and risk assessment to ensure that staffing and physical resources such as theatres are appropriate to the annual workload, and taking measures such as minimizing annual leave when high numbers of deliveries are predicted, or allocating extra staff to particularly high-risk elective cases, these incidences should be kept to a minimum, and we need to accept that very occasionally these things will happen. As part of serious untoward incident reporting, review of such cases should ensure that nothing different could have been done to avoid the event.

Workload

Obstetrics and midwifery is a speciality of peaks and troughs. All of us that work on the labour ward are aware of this, and resources must be in place to deal with these often-unpredictable variations in workload. Staffing and space, and the role of an effective, accepted escalation policy have been discussed above. It is, however, essential to recognize that workload can be managed in the longer term. The number of deliveries expected in the future can be estimated by the number of women booked to deliver each month. Capacity can be calculated, and if the workload is predicted to exceed capacity, bookings can be capped. The effect of other influences should be assessed carefully, as one of the contributors to the problems experienced at Northwick Park, as described by the Healthcare Commission [15], was the impact of extra workload generated by the closure of a neighbouring unit.

Routine elective work on the labour ward, such as elective caesarean sections and routine induction of labour, continues to occur in parallel with the unscheduled workload. However, for the labour ward to be managed effectively, the routine work must be limited, with finite numbers of cases each day. A central booking system or diary is essential to coordinate this. Ideally this should be held on the labour ward, but should coordinate with the antenatal wards and the central theatre office. This communication allows the wards and theatres to anticipate their workload and alter their staffing levels appropriately. Regular reports from the antenatal wards, with regard to the inductions in progress and potential transfers to the labour ward, also assist the shift leader to calculate

Table 28.3 Obstetric triage guide [17]

Category of obstetric priorities	Pathology	Examples
1. Immediately life threatening	Airway obstruction (1A)	Laryngeal oedema (anaphylaxis/severe PET) Trauma Eclampsia (during/post fit)
	Breathing problem (1B)	Respiratory or cardiac arrest Pulmonary oedema (severe PET) Bronchospasm (asthma/anaphylaxis/AFE)
	Circulatory collapse (1C)	Massive haemorrhage (can be concealed) Uterine rupture Severe sepsis
	Fetal problems (1F)	Shoulder dystocia Terminal bradycardia (abruption/cord prolapse/uterine rupture)
2. Urgent (can deteriorate rapidly)	Maternal (2M)	Severe hypertension Unstable or ill diabetic Chest pain
	Fetal (2F)	Pathological CTG Chorioamnionitis
3. Semi-urgent, attention needed (to prevent future disaster)	Maternal (3M) Fetal (3F)	Postpartum 'trickling' Prolonged second stage of labour with a normal CTG
4. Can wait until other emergencies are under control	Maternal (4M) Fetal (4F)	Rupture of membranes with no contractions and normal CTG Meconium staining of liquor in the presence of a normal CTG
5. Delay/postpone until things quieten down	Elective deliveries (5)	Elective CS/induction of labour with no maternal or fetal problem

changes in the workload on their department. This information can also be used to stagger clinical activities and interventions to avoid simultaneous problems occurring as a result – for example, delaying the commencement of an oxytocin infusion or administration of prostaglandins until another problem has been resolved. Furthermore, it must also be recognized that elective work can be postponed when there is excessive emergency work. While it is disappointing for a woman to have her elective CS postponed or her induction delayed, all women would want us to ensure safe conditions within the department.

General Principles of Triage and Prioritization in Obstetrics

As previously stated, the primary aim of triage is to deliver the appropriate care to each patient with the correct urgency required, with the resources available at that time, in the most efficient way and order. In pregnant women, assessment of the fetus immediately follows assessment of the mother. This may result in further conflicts in obstetric triage, as the fetal condition also needs to be considered. While the fetus is best served by the resuscitation of its own mother, other mothers should take priority over unborn babies [16]. For example, assessment and resuscitation of an antenatal woman with an eclamptic seizure would take immediate priority over a fetal bradycardia in the same department. Difficulties on the labour ward, however, more commonly involve the management of multiple urgent problems rather than immediately life-threatening emergencies. The obstetric triage system therefore needs to provide a framework to prioritize several urgent problems, while maintaining the traditional structure for life-threatening emergencies. Sen and Paterson-Brown have outlined a comprehensive obstetric triage guide, which provides such a framework [17] (Table 28.3). The categorization is slightly different in that there are five categories (Table 28.3), and in the category 1 cases, instead of the traditional A, B, C, D approach used for trauma, the D is replaced by F for fetal. In categories 2–5 they should be identified as a maternal problem (M) or a fetal problem (F) or both. By using this system, it becomes clear which problems need to be dealt with first, remembering that within the same category, a mother takes precedence over a fetus.

Additional to the skill of prioritization is the ability to allocate the most appropriately skilled member of staff to the individual patients. To achieve the most efficient use of the resources available, initial assessment of the labour ward requires detailed handover of the workload, together with knowledge of skills and experience of the staff on duty. Once the initial priorities have been defined and staff distributed appropriately, good communication, regular reviews and comprehensive ward rounds are needed to summarize and reassess the workload and changing priorities. Regular ward rounds also provide an opportunity to identify potential future problems and encourage positive decision making, with clear plans outlined for each individual, including timing of examinations and stepwise decisions based on their findings, documented in the case notes. Problems tend to accumulate if decisions are deferred, resulting in simultaneous emergencies. Multidisciplinary ward rounds, including obstetric and anaesthetic medical staff and the midwifery shift leader, promote good communication between members of the team and enable planning of interventions which may require regional anaesthesia or analgesia, matched against the ongoing workload of the labour ward.

Within the systems of prioritization and triage in obstetrics there must always be the ability to deal with unexpected and unpredictable emergencies. Some obstetric emergencies can be anticipated, such as a large postpartum haemorrhage following a prolonged dysfunctional labour with oxytocin augmentation. If anticipated, these emergencies may be averted or, at least, planned for. For example, additional intravenous access prior to delivery and active management of the third stage with additional uterotonic agents can prevent or minimize postpartum haemorrhage. The outcome from other obstetric emergencies can be altered with swift identification of the problem and rapid intervention. For example, the use of continuous electronic fetal monitoring in women labouring after a previous CS can identify scar complications early and allow rapid intervention and emergency delivery. For emergencies that are often unpredictable, regular rehearsal drills and detailed departmental guidelines enable all staff to be familiar with the actions needed and their individual role.

Good communication on the labour ward is paramount, between patients, relatives and staff, and between members of staff. It is not possible to antici-pate and recognize problems within individual delivery rooms without being fully aware of what is going on in that room. Ward rounds by the shift leader and medical staff should review each room occupied, although not all women need to be reviewed personally unless clinically indicated. An update from the midwife looking after the woman is enough, as long as there is good ongoing communication with the shift leader. Following ward rounds, the labour ward board, detailing all the women on the department, should be revisited and the cases summarized. Potential problems should be communicated to the anaesthetic staff, theatre staff and the neonatal unit, as they also form part of the team needed to coordinate safe practice. If this communication and teamwork is not well established it will lead to errors and conflicts between members of staff. For example, if the correct category of urgency for an emergency CS is not communicated to the anaesthetist and theatre team, they may not attend quickly and will delay the time to delivery. Both national and local enquiries looking at poor obstetric outcomes frequently highlight problems with communication being prominent in the series of events leading to the outcome. Multidisciplinary ward rounds, rehearsal drills and teaching sessions will help to improve teamwork and communication and should be encouraged. Clear lines of communication are required in emergencies, with calm and precise coordination from a single leading individual. These lines of communication can be established and practised during drills.

Clinical Scenarios

The following clinical scenarios (Tables 28.4, 28.5) have been designed to represent the workload of a busy labour ward. Read through the tables as if you were receiving handover for your shift. Consider how you would prioritize the cases and how you would allocate the staff you have available, which are described at the bottom of the table. Initially the workload may seem impossible to manage, but use the obstetric triage system outlined in Table 28.3 then check your ideas with those suggested below.

Clinical Scenario A

Having allocated a priority to all cases, staffing needs to be reviewed to allow staff allocation. The first priority when faced with a number of complex problems

Table 28.4 Clinical scenario A, according to room numbers

1	24 years, 28/40, nulliparous, chest pain and cough O$_2$ saturation 93% on air	7	32 years, G2P1 previous stillbirth at 38/40 36/40; decreased fetal movements
2	28 years, 41/40, nulliparous; Cx 2 cm dilated at 02:30; Cx 3 cm dilated at 06:30; ARM	8	36 years, nulliparous insulin-dependent diabetic; prostin induction at 38/40; last BM 4.1, 90 min ago
3	18 years, 40/40, nulliparous, transferred from birth centre, APH 150 ml	9	31 years, G3P2; previous LSCS; followed by SVD; Cx fully dilated at 06:30
4	27 years, para 1 SVD at 06:30; awaiting suturing of second-degree tear	10	28 years, nulliparous, 31/40 dichorionic twins; IVF; painless PV bleeding
5	No case	11	33 years, nulliparous; Cx 7 cm dilated at 04:30; Cx 9 cm dilated at 07:30
6	22 years, G2P1; Cx 4 cm dilated at 05:30; meconium-stained liquor; variable decelerations of FHR	12	34 years, G2P1; maternal lupus BP 160/90, 1+ proteinuria; abdominal pain; no fetal movement
HDU1	37 years, nulliparous, 34/40, BP 175/112 3+ proteinuria, headache	HDU2	No case
Rec 1	33 years, para 1 emergency LSCS at 9 cm dilated; vaginal bleeding; estimated blood loss 1100 ml	Rec 2	35 years, para 3; manual removal of placenta; oxytocin infusion, PR misoprostol; tachycardia HR 128 bpm

Notes:
08:30 handover
Two elective LSCS – first case: maternal congenital heart disease, needs HDU
Three prostin inductions
Staff available:
Two ST1/2 (SHO)
Eight midwives – three senior who suture and cannulate
One shift leader midwife
One recovery nurse
One ST 3–7 – obstetrics (registrar)
One ST 3–7 – anaesthetics (registrar)
Anaesthetic and obstetric consultants available at 10 a.m. after risk management meeting.

Table 28.5 Clinical scenario B, according to room numbers

1	22 years, nulliparous, transferred from birth centre; Cx 9 cm dilated since 03:30	7	29 years, G2P1; hepatitis B; Cx 3 cm dilated at 06:30
2	38 years, nulliparous; undiagnosed breech; contracting 2:10; Cx 1 cm dilated 07:30	8	36 years, G10P8; Cx 6 cm dilated at 07:30; thick meconium; fetal bradycardia of 90 bpm for 4 min
3	32 years, G3P2; previous LSCS; followed by SVD; Cx 5 cm dilated at 06:30; meconium-stained liquor	9	No case
4	31 years, nulliparous; prostin induction at 40+12/40; Cx 3 cm dilated at 04:00; variable decelerations of FHR	10	24 years, nulliparous, 40+4/40; APH 200 ml
5	28 years, G4P2+1 33/40; abdominal pain	11	33 years, G3P0+2; previous stillbirth at 40/40; prostin induction at 38/40; awaiting ARM
6	34 years, nulliparous, 40/40; spontaneous labour; Cx 4 cm dilated at 00:00; Cx 4 cm dilated at 04:00; ARM Cx 5 cm dilated at 08:00	12	41 years, G2P1; dichorionic twins, 34/40; backache; small PV bleed
HDU1	35 years, para 1; epileptic 2 seizures following spontaneous vaginal delivery	HDU2	No case
Rec 1	32 years, para 1; forceps, third-degree tear PPH 1800 ml	Rec 2	29 years, para 2; emergency LSCS for fetal tachycardia; prolonged SROM pyrexial; HR 112; O$_2$ saturation 93%

Notes:
In theatre with LSCS + hysterectomy, massive PPH 3500 ml
08:30 handover – two elective LSCS, two prostin inductions
Staff available:
Two ST 1/2 (SHO)
Eight midwives – four senior who suture and cannulate
One shift leader midwife
One recovery nurse
One ST 3–7 – obstetrics (registrar)
One ST 3–7 – anaesthetics (registrar)
Anaesthetic and obstetric consultants available if requested.

requiring intervention simultaneously is to ask available staff to attend. The consultant obstetrician and consultant anaesthetist should be contacted and asked to attend immediately (patient care has to take priority, so the meeting can continue without them or be postponed).

1. The immediate priority is the woman in room 1 (priority 1B), who is hypoxic and needs full assessment and investigation for pulmonary embolus. She should be seen by the obstetric ST 1/2, as this is primarily a medical problem rather than an obstetric problem. She needs oxygen and anticoagulation with subcutaneous low molecular weight heparin, and investigations instituted to confirm the diagnosis. Midwife 1 should stay with her once medical staff have left.

2. The women in Recovery 1 and 2 are also an immediate priority (1C) as they may be haemodynamically unstable. The anaesthetic ST 3–7 should review the woman in Recovery 2 to try to determine the cause of the tachycardia, which is most likely to be hypovolaemia secondary to blood loss. He can institute initial resuscitation while midwife 2 assesses the degree of blood loss and uterine tone, and sends off appropriate bloods. The obstetric consultant should see the woman in Recovery 1, who is being cared for by the recovery nurse, as she is still bleeding and may need to return to theatre for further examination, with or without a laparotomy.

3. The urgent maternal priority is in high-dependency bed 1 (priority 2M). The obstetric ST 3–7 can see her, assess the degree of severity of her pre-eclampsia and proceed to treatment of her hypertension. The anaesthetic consultant should see this woman and institute invasive monitoring. Assessment of the fetal condition should follow stabilization of the mother, and initially midwife 3 can carry this out.

4. The urgent fetal priorities are in rooms 12 and 6 (priority 2F). The second obstetric ST 1/2 can review room 6, who is being cared for by midwife 4, and assess the potential fetal distress and carry out a fetal blood sample. The concern in room 12 is both fetal and maternal. This woman is at high risk of a placental abruption and intrauterine fetal demise. Initially the shift leader can attend to

auscultate the fetal heart. If it is present, the fetal priority changes, but the concern remains. She will need urgent obstetric review as soon as an obstetrician is free. If the women in recovery are stable and able to both be cared for by the recovery nurse, or returning to theatre, midwife 2 can attend to this woman, otherwise midwife 5 can attend.

5. The semi-urgent maternal priorities are in rooms 9, 10 and 3 (priority 3M). Midwife 6 can assess the woman in room 9 initially to confirm full dilatation, review the continuous fetal heart rate monitoring and assess the progress in second stage. The midwife can then discuss her findings with the shift leader and obstetric registrar, to plan her further management. Midwife 7 can initially carry out review of the woman in room 3. Assessment of blood loss, blood pressure, pulse and fetal condition can be established, as well as intravenous cannulation. One of the obstetricians can then subsequently examine the woman and diagnose the cause of antepartum haemorrhage when they are free. During this time, midwife 8 can review the woman in room 10, assess the quantity of blood loss, the maternal and fetal conditions and establish intravenous access. If all is stable, the woman can then await review by obstetric staff once they are free, or be sent for a departmental ultrasound scan for placental localization.

6. The semi-urgent fetal priorities are in rooms 7 and 11 (priority 3F). The shift leader can see room 7, auscultate the fetal heart and commence electronic fetal monitoring. Once she has seen to room 10, midwife 8 can assess the woman in room 11 in terms of uterine activity and assess the need for a further vaginal examination (VE). If required, she can discuss the need for augmentation of labour with the shift leader. In many units, augmentation with an oxytocin infusion in a nulliparous labourer can be started by the shift leader, without the immediate need for medical staff review. This can, however, be delayed if other women still need to be seen.

7. The other rooms, 2, 4 and 8, can now wait until the other emergencies are under control (priority 4M and 4F). The woman in room 8 can be reviewed by the shift leader, who can carry out BM monitoring and then ensure that the woman in room 2 is

alright until a midwife is free to provide one-to-one care. The first available midwife or ST 1/2 can then suture the woman in room 4.

8. The elective work (priority 5) can be delayed until the labour ward is more composed.

It is clear from this that optimal care is not being delivered, as women in labour are not receiving one-to-one care, and resources are being utilized based on a priority of need. This principle is fundamental to triage. If staff are available elsewhere they should be asked to come and help out until the crisis is over (implement the escalation policy), and all elective work should be deferred until it is safe to continue.

Clinical Scenario B

1. The immediate priorities are in theatre and recovery bed 2 (priority 1C). The case in theatre is already being managed by the night shift; however, they should be contacted to confirm that the situation is controlled and that any additional help is not required. If further help is needed, the consultant obstetrician and anaesthetist should be asked to attend. This patient will need a high-dependency bed once she is out of theatre. The woman in recovery bed 2, who is being cared for by the recovery nurse, appears to be septic; she should be assessed by the daytime anaesthetic ST 3–7 and transferred to a high-dependency bed for further treatment and invasive monitoring.

2. The immediate fetal priority is room 8 (priority 1F). The obstetric ST 3–7 should review this case. A fetal bradycardia in a multiparous patient in established labour may be due to rapid progress to full dilation. If this patient is in the second stage she may need an instrumental delivery. Midwife 1 is present to deliver if she progresses rapidly, or to assist the obstetrician if required.

3. The urgent maternal priorities are recovery bed 1 and room 10 (priority 2M). The obstetric ST 1/2 should assess the woman in recovery bed 1 with midwife 2, as she has had a significant postpartum haemorrhage. Review of her blood pressure, pulse, repeat haemoglobin level and any ongoing blood loss will ascertain whether she is stable or requires further treatment. Midwife 3 should initially assess room 10. Assessment of blood loss, blood pressure, pulse and fetal condition can be established, as well as intravenous cannulation.

The obstetric ST 1/2 can then subsequently examine the woman and diagnose the cause of antepartum haemorrhage.

4. The urgent fetal priority is in room 4 (priority 2F). The pattern of the electronic fetal heart rate monitoring needs to be identified and the woman needs to be examined to determine progress in labour. Midwife 4 should perform a VE to assess the stage of labour, and ask the obstetric ST 1/2 to review whether there is suspected fetal compromise, with a view to fetal blood sampling.

5. It is difficult to prioritize the woman in room 5 based on the information available. The shift leader should quickly see this lady and prioritize her further after a rapid assessment. The abdominal pain may be something as simple as indigestion, in which case resources do not need to be allocated, or may be a massive abruption or preterm labour.

6. The semi-urgent maternal priorities are in HDU 1 and room 1 (priority 3M). The obstetric ST 3–7 should review the woman in high-dependency when he has finished in room 8. If this postnatal woman is stable with no further seizures, she can be transferred to the ward, as high-dependency will be needed by the case currently in theatre. Midwife 5 can assess the maternal and fetal condition in room 1. The obstetric ST 3–7 can then examine the woman when he has completed his assessment in HDU 1, and determine whether oxytocin or delivery is indicated.

7. The semi-urgent fetal priority is room 12 (3F). Midwife 6 needs to assess the maternal and fetal conditions and the degree of bleeding. If appropriate, she should gain IV access and send the appropriate bloods and commence fetal monitoring. The obstetric ST 1/2 should then assess to determine the cause of the bleeding and rule out preterm labour when one is free.

8. Room 3 (priority 4F) and room 6 (priority 4 F/M) can now wait until the other emergencies are resolved. Midwife 7 can provide care and review the fetal condition in room 3. Midwife 8 can insert an intravenous cannula in room 6 and commence an oxytocin infusion after discussion with the shift leader, although this can be delayed until other priorities have been addressed.

9. Room 11 does not require care at the moment, and could be moved to the antenatal ward until

the workload has settled. Similarly, room 2 does not require one-to-one care, as she is not in established labour. Although she needs to be seen to discuss her options for delivery, this can be deferred and, again, she could be transferred to the antenatal ward in the meantime. Room 7 may need care. With the information available it is again difficult to allocate a priority as she may still be in the latent phase of labour, or may be contracting well and established. The shift leader should assess her further so she can be triaged properly.

As discussed above in relation to clinical scenario A, the escalation policy should be implemented to draft staff in when appropriate. All elective work should be deferred until it is safe to proceed, and if possible moved out of the labour ward area. Even if consultant input is not immediately required, both the consultant obstetrician and the consultant anaesthetist can provide extra pairs of hands as well as support and guidance, and should be called to attend immediately. It is also clear that doing this as a paper exercise is somewhat artificial, as the labour ward is dynamic and the clinical situation changes all the time. What may be prioritized as requiring immediate intervention using up skilled staff can resolve quickly (e.g. the woman in room 8 delivers before the obstetric ST 3–7 attends), and cases that seem to be low priority may suddenly require immediate attention (e.g. the woman in room 3 ruptures her uterus with massive haemorrhage and a profound bradycardia).

In both the above scenarios there are a number of ways to prioritize the workload presented, and you may not agree with the suggestions given, but a systematic approach using a logical framework enables you to anticipate a likely series of events and allocate staff appropriately. Rapid and logical decision making is a key skill in prioritization on a busy labour ward. As with most other skills in obstetrics, it can be taught, but there is also a degree of art and style that can only be improved by experience. We are all familiar with those we like to be on call with, as things always seem calm and under control even when busy; and there are others who never seem to quite know what is going on even when relatively quiet. Triage is something we all practise every day on the labour ward, although this has rarely been taught formally. With the structures and approaches in this chapter, the art of triage can be formalized to a degree, with the aim of optimizing

outcomes for both our patients – the mother and the baby.

References

1. Cox C, Grady K, Howell C. *Managing Obstetric Emergencies and Trauma: The MOET Course Manual*, 2nd edition. Oxford: RCOG Press; 2007.

2. Kenyon S, Dann S, Jeffery J, Johns N. Evaluation of the implementation of the Birmingham Symptom Specific Obstetric Triage System. *Arch Dis Child Fetal Neonatal Ed*. 2014;99(suppl. 1): A19–A20. doi: 10.1136/archdischild-2014-306576.54.

3. Beckmann A, Hamilton-Giachritsis C, Johns N, Kenyon S. Inter-rater reliability of the Birmingham Symptom specific Obstetric Triage System. *Arch Dis Child Fetal Neonatal Ed*. 2014;99(suppl. 1): A24–A25. doi: 10.1136/archdischild-2014-306576.68.

4. Easterbrook J, Hewison A, Johns N, Kenyon S. Midwives' views of the implementation of the Birmingham Symptom Specific Obstetric Triage System. *Arch Dis Child Fetal Neonatal Ed*. 2014;99(suppl. 1): A26–A27. doi: 10.1136/archdischild-2014-306576.74.

5. Hodnett ED, Gates S, Hofmeyr GJ, Sakala C. Continuous support for women during childbirth. *Cochrane Database of Syst Rev*. 2007; 3: CD003766. doi: 10.1002/14651858.CD003766.pub2.

6. Royal College of Midwives. *RCM Annual Survey of Heads of Midwifery Service*. London: RCM; 2005.

7. NICE. Safe midwifery staffing for maternity settings; 2015. www.nice.org.uk/guidance/ng4/evidence (accessed 15 May 2016).

8. RCOG. *Safer Childbirth: Minimum Standards for the Organisation and Delivery of Care in Labour*. London: RCOG Press; 2007.

9. RCOG. *The Future Role of the Consultant: A Working Party Report*. London: RCOG Press; 2005.

10. NHS ModernisationAgency. *Findings and Recommendations from the Hospital at Night Project*. London: NHSMA; 2005.

11. NHS Litigation Authority. *Ten Years of Maternity Claims: An Analysis of NHS Litigation Authority Data*. London: NHS Litigation Authority; 2012.

12. Luo ZC, Karlberg J. Timing of birth and infant and early neonatal mortality in Sweden 1973–95: longitudinal birth register study. *Br Med J*. 2001;323: 1327–34.

13. Olah KS. Reversal of the decision for caesarean section second in the vaginal stage of labour on the basis of a consultant assessment. *J Obstet Gynaecol*. 2005;25: 115–16.

14. Murphy DJ, Liebling RE, Patel R, Verity L, Swingler R. Cohort study of operative delivery in the second stage of labour and standard of obstetric care. *Br J Obstet Gynaecol.* 2003;110: 610–15.

15. Healthcare Commision. *Investigation into 10 Maternal Deaths at, or Following Delivery at, Northwick Park Hospital, North West London Hospitals NHS Trust,* *Between April 2002 and April 2005.* London: Healthcare Commission; 2006.

16. Macdonald C, Redondo V, Baetz L, Boyle M. Obstetrical triage. *Canadian Nurse.* 1993;89(7): 17–20.

17. Sen R, Paterson-Brown S. Prioritisation on the delivery suite. *Curr Obstet Gynaecol.* 2005;15(4): 228–36.

Chapter 29

Risk Management in Intrapartum Care

Leroy C. Edozien

Intrapartum care is a high-risk activity. Even when there is no obvious imminent threat to mother and baby, care providers have to be vigilant as the transition from low risk to high risk could be swift and occur with little or no forewarning. When patient safety incidents occur in intrapartum care, the financial and emotional cost could be high. The spending on maternity clinical negligence cover in the UK equates to nearly one-fifth of the spending on maternity services. Human error cannot be eliminated but the risk of harm could be managed. Risk management comprises the concepts, processes and behaviours that are applied to facilitate delivery of safer care, mitigate the effects of any errors and learn from incidents. This chapter discusses the application of risk management in intrapartum care, using the RADICAL framework (Raise Awareness, Design for safety, Involve users, Collect and Analyse data, Learn from incidents) as its basis.

Introduction

Health professionals seek the best clinical and psychological outcomes for their patients, but sometimes patients get harmed rather than healed by the care we deliver. Such harm may be the unanticipated consequence of an intended action or omission, or the result of what is commonly referred to as 'human error'. Historically, a linear relationship between competency and clinical outcome was assumed: all competent healthcare practitioners were expected to deliver their expertise flawlessly, and practically all adverse incidents were taken as indicative of less-than-competent practice. The delivery of healthcare, however, is not fundamentally different from other aspects of day-to-day life, as far as safety is concerned. A parallel can be drawn, for example, with road safety. Road

safety cannot be secured solely by ensuring that all drivers are skilled in the mechanical processes of moving a vehicle. Roads have to be designed in such a way that opportunities for accidents to occur are minimized. Additional measures are required in areas of high risk, such as near schools. Environmental factors, such as weather conditions or difficult terrain, are important. Driver behaviour is also important: road rage is eschewed, drink-driving is outlawed and seat belts must be worn. The same principles apply to the protection of patient safety in the delivery suite. Doctors and midwives must be knowledgeable in the management of maternal and fetal conditions in labour, but the physical and cultural environment in which they work is also important; so too is their behaviour.

Risk management integrates these systemic and individual practitioner factors in order to minimize accidents, mitigate the effects of any errors and promote patient safety. It comprises the framework, principles and processes that are applied to achieve the cardinal objective of ensuring that the care we provide is safe. When applied appropriately, risk management is more of a clinical activity than an administrative one; it should be intrinsic to clinical care. For example, clinical competence in the management of pre-eclampsia will be incomplete without awareness of the risk that the locally used monitoring device may underestimate systolic blood pressure, or without a culture in which obstetricians, anaesthetists and midwives work in harmony.

Implementing Risk Management in the Delivery Suite

There should be a designated lead consultant for risk management in the delivery suite, and a risk manager

---

Best Practice in Labour and Delivery, Second Edition, ed. Sir Sabaratnam Arulkumaran. Published by Cambridge University Press. © Cambridge University Press 2016.

Box 29.1 Attributes of Good Risk Management in a Delivery Suite

- Comprehensive (includes all domains of the RADICAL framework)
- Evidence-supported (incorporates best practice, user experience and available resources)
- Takes account of human factors
- Intrinsic to clinical practice (not a standalone activity but applied as part of clinical care)
- Applies across professional and disciplinary boundaries
- Visibly fair to all and promotes a just culture
- Tailored to local requirements
- Responsive to evolving challenges (such as structural or staff changes; new threats to patient safety)
- Integrated with clinical audit and other quality initiatives

(usually a midwife, but nothing stops a unit from designating a doctor, psychologist or other professional as risk manager), but these persons should not be seen as the sole custodians of risk management – their role is to facilitate and coordinate the management of risk, not to manage risk in the day-to-day practice of every doctor or midwife. Individual practitioners should be encouraged and trained to deliver risk management in their own clinical practice.

The lead consultant and the risk manager should be supported by a committee (or similar forum) where risk management policies, strategy and operational issues are discussed and agreed. The nature of this forum will vary from one unit to another. It may be limited to risk management in some units but have a wider clinical governance remit in other units. Whichever form it takes, the lines of communication and accountability in relation to the shop-floor and other elements of the departmental/directorate management should be clearly outlined. It is the responsibility of this committee and its members to implement a risk management programme that meets the criteria outlined in Box 29.1.

For many years, risk management in UK maternity units focused on fulfilling standards set by the Clinical Negligence Scheme for Trusts (CNST) sponsored by the National Health Service Litigation Authority. This resulted in transactional change (policies, processes and rules were standardized) but there was only limited transformational change (little or no fundamental change in the thinking or behaviour of

clinicians and managers occurred). Using the road safety analogy introduced at the beginning of this chapter, this approach was akin to concentrating on the Highway Code and driver training, without commensurate attention to driver behaviour and environmental correlates of road safety. There is now more emphasis on safety culture in maternity units, with risk management being intrinsic to clinical practice.

Transformational change through *integrated* risk management is the key to reducing the huge and expanding burden of clinical negligence litigation. In 2012–13 there were 1146 clinical negligence claims relating to maternity care in the UK, equivalent to around one claim for every 600 births; the number of claims increased by 80% in the five years from 2007–08 to 2012–13 [1].

Designing and implementing a system for protecting patient safety in the delivery suite could be challenging, given the vast range of activities that could positively or negatively have an impact on safety. It is, therefore, helpful to have a framework that covers the various domains of risk management and facilitates both implementation and monitoring of risk management initiatives. In this regard, the RADICAL framework simultaneously offers both comprehensiveness and simplicity. It comprises the following domains in an integrated grid: Raise Awareness, Design for safety, Involve users, Collect and Analyse safety data, and Learn from patient safety incidents [2,3]. The RADICAL framework could be used not only for setting out plans and projects, but also to provide standing agenda for meetings of the risk management/clinical governance committee.

Raising Awareness

What Patient Safety Incidents Occur in Intrapartum Care?

Avoidable maternal death still occurs in delivery suites in both developed and resource-poor countries. In the UK there has been a drop in overall maternal mortality rate but avoidable deaths still occur, with substandard care featuring in nearly three-quarters of direct deaths [4,5]. Clearly, there is an unmet need for focused risk management interventions addressing this challenge.

Avoidable intrapartum-related stillbirth and neonatal death also occurs. The UK Chief Medical Officer, in his annual report 2006, expressed concern that

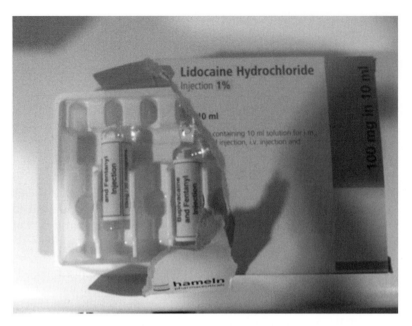

Figure 29.1 Bupivacaine and fentanyl returned to lidocaine box in error. See the colour plate section for a colour version of this figure.

the rate of intrapartum-related deaths (nearly 500 each year) was not decreasing [6]. This relates to babies that are apparently healthy at the onset of labour, but die during or soon after birth. Using a well-established confidential case review methodology, the West Midlands Perinatal Institute investigated 25 such cases (16 stillbirths and 9 early neonatal deaths) that occurred at 15 different maternity units during 2008/9 [7]. The review showed that there was substandard care in all cases. In 16 cases (64%), panels concluded that different management *would have* avoided the outcome. In another five cases, different management *might have* resulted in a different outcome, suggesting that 21 of 25 (or 84%) of the deaths were potentially avoidable.

In a study of 51 countries [8], intrapartum stillbirth rates averaged 0.9/1000 births for developed countries and 7.3/1000 for developing countries, and the intrapartum stillbirth rate was more closely related to measures of obstetric care than the antepartum stillbirth rate.

Intrapartum-related fetal or neonatal deaths are only the tip of the iceberg. Other babies survive but are brain-damaged, and this is also often preventable. In a case control study of 28 486 deliveries, of which 161 neonates ≥34 weeks of gestational age were born with metabolic acidosis, suboptimal care was noted in 49.1% of cases versus 13.0% of controls ($p < 0.001$) [9].

Other patient safety incidents that may occur in intrapartum care include retained swabs, deficiencies in the management of obstetric haemorrhage, fetal or maternal trauma resulting from errors in operative vaginal delivery, medication errors, delays in medical intervention, failure to recognize or to respond appropriately to maternal deterioration, and anaesthetic incidents.

In a near-miss incident, an obstetrician who was about to repair a perineal tear under local anaesthetic was presented with an ampoule of what was thought to be lidocaine. It was actually an ampoule of bupivacaine and fentanyl (used for epidural analgesia), which had previously been returned to the wrong box (Figure 29.1). Fortunately this was recognized during the process of double witnessing, a check routinely performed before a drug is administered. In a similar incident at another hospital, the mix-up was not detected and a midwife mistakenly administered an epidural anaesthetic (bupivacaine) via an intravenous drip. This resulted in the death of a newly delivered mother. The Health and Safety Executive successfully brought a prosecution under the Health and Safety at Work Act 1974, and the hospital was ordered to pay £100 000 for failing to manage the risk of drug errors [10]. The judge blamed 'systematic and individual fault'. The substances had been mixed up as, despite being completely different, the two drugs had near-identical packaging and were stored side-by-side in the same unlocked cupboard. The trial concluded that avoiding any one of a number of errors would probably have averted the woman's death. Significantly, the court noted that a similar mistake made sometime earlier in the same hospital was not fatal but should have served as sufficient warning.

What are the Underlying Causes of Patient Safety Incidents in Intrapartum Care?

In 16 of the 25 cases of intrapartum-related stillbirth reviewed by the Perinatal Institute, there was poor interpretation of the fetal heart rate [7]. In six cases, there was no appropriate management plan for labour. Other factors implicated in the review include failure to escalate a problem and obtain senior input (18 cases); delay in management/expediting delivery (12 cases); inappropriate use of oxytocics, causing hyperstimulation (5 cases); and substandard neonatal resuscitation (7 of the 9 neonatal deaths). There was concern about the quality of record keeping in 21 of the 25 cases.

In the study of term or near-term babies born with metabolic acidosis, suboptimal care included failure to respond within the specified time limit in response to a pathological cardiotocograph (CTG) pattern of ≥40 min duration (with the exception of bradycardia), and failure to perform a CTG despite indications [9]. Care was considered suboptimal in relation to administration of oxytocin if this drug was administered without a valid indication, started or increased despite a pathological CTG pattern or uterine hyperactivity or short increment intervals were applied (less than 15 min), or there was uterine hyper-stimulation (six or more uterine contractions per 10 min interval, for more than 20 min), or a CTG tracing was not used continuously.

These deficiencies in clinical care are commonly manifestations of generic deficiencies relating to teamwork. The King's Fund inquiry into the safety of maternity units in the UK identified inter-professional relationships between doctors and midwives, difficulties with leadership and management, and difficulties with communication between clinicians, 'particularly at crunch points such as referrals between health professionals, shift changes and in emergencies', as key problems [11].

These findings from clinical studies and national inquiry indicate that intrapartum risk management could save many mothers and babies from death, neurodevelopmental handicap and other physical or psychological trauma.

Design for Safety

Error in clinical practice cannot be completely eradicated, and risk management should focus more on prevention of harm. In the delivery suite, the vast majority of preventable harm to mothers and babies can be minimized by adopting the following strategies and tactics: (a) standardization of care; (b) good handover practice; (c) maintaining situational awareness; (d) appropriately interpreting and responding to CTGs; (d) judicious use of oxytocin; and (e) early detection of deterioration in maternal condition and responding appropriately to any such deterioration.

Standardization of Care

Variance in clinical care, particularly where such variance is arbitrary, provides fertile ground for unsafe practice. Standardization helps to reduce variance, minimize confusion and promote patient safety. All maternity units should have evidence-supported protocols and guidelines covering various conditions and treatments, including high-risk situations such as vaginal birth after caesarean delivery, medical disorders such as pre-eclampsia, obstetric emergencies such as postpartum haemorrhage and shoulder dystocia, and operative interventions such as instrumental delivery and repair of perineal tears. Although these guidelines are in place in many units, they are often lengthy and unwieldy.

Good Handover Practice

Patient safety requires effective communication and shared mental models with respect to evolving clinical and logistic challenges. The points in the patient's journey at which there is a transfer of care from one clinician or team to another are 'hot spots' of vulnerability: pathogens that threaten patient safety could creep in as a result of communication defects and poor execution of care plans. There is also the risk of the patient's care falling into the virtual space between professionals. On the delivery suite, the key to avoiding these risks is the inter-shift handover, which affords an opportunity for the team to undertake a baseline assessment of the current clinical situation, assess the resources available (staff, beds, cots, etc.), anticipate developments ('feed-forward'), plan contingencies and disseminate lessons learned from safety incidents. Each delivery suite should have a structured multi-disciplinary inter-shift handover (SMITH) protocol which encompasses pre-handover, handover and post-handover behaviour [12]. This will also help address the inter-professional communication problem identified by the King's Fund inquiry, as mentioned above. Clarity of purpose and goals is fostered when structured communication (such as the SBAR – Situation, Background, Assessment, Recommendation – framework) is used to report assessments.

Maintaining Situational Awareness

The King's Fund inquiry recommended that safety awareness training should be introduced into mainstream professional education. Situational awareness is a skill that should be a major part of such training. It is the cognitive state of being aware of what is happening around oneself and understanding how evolving events could affect one's goals and objectives; it is the ability to maintain the 'big picture' and think ahead. It is essential for patient safety on the delivery suite, and without it there can be no effective leadership, appropriate decision making or coherent teamwork [13]. Strategies for maintaining situational awareness include proactively seeking and managing information on unfolding events (e.g. by undertaking periodic ward rounds), implementing a buddy system (periodically the CTG is assessed by a fresh pair of eyes) and use of checklists [14–16]. The World Health Organization (WHO) Surgical Safety checklist has been shown in a random-allocation trial to be effective in reducing perioperative complications, and has been adapted for use in maternity units. In addition to the checks stipulated in the WHO checklist, the maternity checklist requires staff to: check that the resuscitaire is in working order and the neonatal team have been called, if required; ensure that the urinary catheter is draining; check that the baby/babies have been identified with ID bands; and check that cord bloods have been taken, if required.

Checklists have also been used for reporting vaginal examinations, electronic fetal monitoring, fetal scalp blood sampling and operative vaginal deliveries, and for documenting the management of a range of conditions such as shoulder dystocia and postpartum haemorrhage. They help to standardize care and to avoid the deleterious effects of fatigue and cognitive overload, but clinicians using checklists should beware of involuntary automaticity, the phenomenon where an operator drifts into an 'autopilot' mode without being aware, devotes minimal attention to the task

in hand and becomes at risk of perpetrating an error [17].

Team situational awareness can easily be compromised when staff are working in conditions of high cognitive load and psychological stress due to workforce pressures. A UK national audit showed that there was a shortfall of 2300 in midwives in 2012 (calculated using a benchmark of 29.5 births per midwife per year) and 28 per cent of maternity units reported that they closed to admissions for half a day or more between April and September 2012 [1].

Appropriately Interpreting and Responding to CTGs

Despite the widespread use of electronic fetal monitoring in intrapartum care in resource-rich countries for over three decades, misinterpretation of CTGs in labour and failure to respond appropriately to abnormal traces remain frequent and are major causes of harm to babies. In this author's opinion, there are two reasons for this. First, the teaching of CTG interpretation has traditionally been based on pattern recognition, with a tendency to bypass the underlying physiology. Such an approach confers the advantage of expediency, but encourages 'superficial' rather than deep learning (in educational theory, the 'superficial' approach limits learning to isolated facts that are subsequently reproduced, whereas 'deep learning' promotes understanding that can be applied in unfamiliar as well as familiar contexts). Second, there is a tacit assumption that failures of interpretation are always due to knowledge deficits, whereas in many cases the problem is not *lack of knowledge* but *perception deficit* associated with fatigue, cognitive overload or other factors associated with loss of situational awareness. Risk management interventions aimed at improving CTG interpretation should take account of these two underlying causes of poor interpretation and/or response [18]. The use of a buddy system ('a fresh pair of eyes'), for example, attempts to pick up perception defects before they result in harm [14].

Judicious Use of Oxytocin

Oxytocin is the most commonly used but also the most dangerous drug in routine obstetric practice. When used judiciously, it is generally safe. Injudicious use is associated with uterine tachysystole, uterine rupture, fetal heart rate abnormalities and concomitant problems, including fetal demise. This risk of serious harm if the drug is administered incorrectly warrants an oxytocin administration protocol based on the best available evidence. In high-risk situations, particularly in the presence of a uterine scar, intrapartum oxytocin should not be administered without the prior approval of a senior obstetrician and without discussing the risk with the woman.

A practical problem is that care providers do not always find the right balance between 'pushing' the oxytocin infusion in order to achieve optimal strength and frequency of contractions, and ensuring the safety of mother and baby. Attempts to reduce the incidence of harm and litigation associated with oxytocin have focused on implementation of conservative protocols, with mixed results. In one study, the protocol led to lower oxytocin maximal dosing and lower intensive care nursery admission rates, but greater postpartum blood loss, wound infection and a trend towards higher caesarean delivery rates [19]. In another study, low-dose oxytocin protocols resulted in fewer caesarean deliveries performed for fetal distress (32.52% vs. 38.67%; $p = 0.02$), but there were significantly higher rates of chorioamnionitis, longer median time from admission to delivery and more caesarean deliveries performed for lack of progress in labour [20].

A meta-analysis did not resolve the question, partly because the definition of high- and low-dose protocols and the outcomes that were measured varied considerably across the nine trials that were included in the analysis [21].

From a practical rather than academic standpoint, perhaps the key issue is not necessarily the oxytocin regime, but the superficial learning of the attending staff (akin to that discussed above in relation to CTGs). The training of staff who are involved in the administration of intrapartum oxytocin should include information about the uterine response rate to oxytocin, the half-life of oxytocin and down-regulation of oxytocin receptors [22]. Knowledge of these facts and concepts should inform clinical practice.

Early Detection of Deterioration in Maternal Condition and Responding Appropriately

With the uptake of scenario training ('skills drills'), maternity units have progressively become better at managing acute emergencies such as massive haemorrhage and shoulder dystocia. There has, however,

been slower progress in the recognition and management of situations where there is a gradual, rather than acute or precipitate, deterioration in the condition of the woman or her baby. Sadly, many women suffer serious morbidity or mortality because their deterioration has not been recognized or has not been managed appropriately [5]. To address the problem of recognition, a Modified Early Obstetric Warning Score (MEOWS) chart was introduced for routine use in the care of all pregnant or postpartum women who become unwell (Figure 29.2) [4,5]. The UK Confidential Enquiry report recommends that care providers should use the charted observations in order to 'ensure confirmation of normality rather than presumption' [5]. In other words, use of the chart should change behaviour such that clinicians constantly seek objective confirmation of normality, rather than presume normality and passively await any development that challenges this presumption. The report also states that 'it is the response to the abnormal score that will affect outcome, not simply its documentation' – another pointer to the importance of clinician behaviour in the management of risk.

Maternity units in tertiary centres where there is a relatively heavy caseload of high-risk cases should have a dedicated high-dependency room or bay for women who need closer monitoring. Local protocols should specify thresholds for escalation of clinical concerns so that critically ill women are seen by staff with appropriate experience and expertise. With increased consultant presence in the delivery suite, the recurring problem of failure to escalate concerns should be less frequent.

Involve Users

In the last two decades there has been a gradual retreat from the paternalistic approach to clinical practice ('the doctor knows best'), with concomitantly increasing recognition of the patient's right to be involved in decisions about her care. 'Nothing about me without me' has become the mantra for champions of patient involvement in healthcare delivery. There are, however, two conceptual problems in the current movement.

One is that patient involvement in health services delivery has largely been conceived in terms of patient representation on committees (exemplified by the recruitment of patients into Maternity Services Liaison Committees) – but this is only one dimension of patient involvement. Involvement of pregnant,

Please complete or affix label		Date	Observation pathway	Signature	Name
Surname					
Forename					
Date of birth					
Hospital No					

		Date Time																Date Time
Looks Well		Yes																Yes
		No																No
Respiration	Write rate in box	>25																>25
		21 - 24																21 - 24
		14 - 20																14 - 20
		11 - 13																11 - 13
		<10																<10
SpO₂		≥96																≥96
		<96																<96
Temperature °C	Write rate in box	39																>38
		38																37.5 - 38.0
		37																
		36																35.1 - 37.4
		35																<35.0
Heart Rate	Mark as X & Write rate in	130																>110
		120																
		110																
		100																91 - 110
		90																
		80																61 - 90
		70																
		60																
		50																41 - 50
		40																<40
Systolic Blood Pressure	Mark as V & Write rate in	200																>160
		190																
		180																
		170																
		160																140 - 159
		150																
		140																
		130																90 - 139
		120																
		110																
		100																
		90																80 - 89
		80																
		70																<79
		60																
		50																
MAP mmHhg																		
Diastolic Blood Pressure	Mark as A & Write rate in	130																>110
		120																
		110																
		100																90 - 109
		90																
		80																
		70																60 - 89
		60																
		50																50 - 59
		40																<49
Neuro response		Alert/Verbal																Alert/Verbal
		Confusion/ Unrousable																Confusion/ Unrousable
Pain score		7																7
		>4 - 6																>4 - 6
		0 - 4																0 - 4
Urine		Protein																Protein
		No protein																No protein
PV Loss		Heavy/Offensive																Heavy/Offensive
		Normal																Normal
Total Red																		Total Red
Total Yellow																		Total Yellow

Escalate if : One RED or TWO Yellow or Any changes concerns

Ref. 100368

Figure 29.2 Modified Early Obstetric Warning Score Chart. The reference to the colour red in the footnote corresponds to the darker shade of grey in the chart. Reproduced with permission from St George's University Hospitals NHS.

recently pregnant and non-pregnant women as committee members in policy making and in the design and organization of maternity services is important, but their involvement as front line individuals at the point of healthcare delivery is also important.

The other is that this domain of the RADICAL framework encompasses all users of health services, not just the woman/patient. 'Users' of maternity services include not only the woman but also her family and birth partner (who may be a friend or other associate). The engagement of partners is particularly important. Often, partners are witnesses as an error chain develops, and if they are engaged, informed and empowered, they will be in a better position to break the error chain – by asking questions, expressing concerns, alerting midwives and doctors, and supporting the woman in decision making.

The Scottish Health Council has published a document to guide boards and managers in promoting service user involvement in maternity services [23]. The recommendations in this guidance include the use of tools (such as questionnaires, comments cards, graffiti boards, kiosks and handheld patient devices) which encourage women to provide feedback *during* their hospital treatment, and the use of new technologies (such as Skype, Twitter and social networking sites) to promote user involvement. Community groups, employment networks and education networks could be used to engage maternity service users and to disseminate safety information.

Data collected using the tools and networks listed above also fall under the 'Collect and Analyse data' domain of the RADICAL framework, and should be applied in other domains such as raising awareness, design of services and organizational learning. This way, the essence of the framework – that all risk management domains should be integrated – is achieved.

Engagement of users at the front line of intrapartum care should start with antenatal education. A contentious and challenging issue in intrapartum care is how to obtain a valid consent for interventions such as caesarean delivery and operative vaginal delivery when a woman is in the throes of labour. While it is usually an institutional requirement for a consent form to be signed for an emergency caesarean delivery, such 'consent' is of questionable (and in many cases, no) legal standing. In the Western world, at least two in every ten deliveries is caesarean, and one in ten deliveries is an operative vaginal delivery. This means that at least three of every ten women will have an operative

delivery. All women and their birth partners should be made aware of this chance antenatally, and be provided with appropriate quantity and quality of information. This would help make consent discussions in an emergency intrapartum situation easier and more meaningful.

Involving users also entails finding out how they perceive and respond to safety concerns. Constructive engagement of users during intrapartum care promotes not only clinical safety but also psychological safety. A qualitative study funded by the King's Fund found that the woman was far more likely to feel unsafe in cases where she and her midwife failed to form this bond; when asked to consider the most important elements of a safe birth, all women talked about having enough experienced staff available [24].

It is also essential to communicate risk in an appropriate and clear manner to women and their families, in order to facilitate safe health behaviour and compliance with medical advice. The UK Confidential Enquiry found that 'it was not clear that women were made aware of the gravity of the risks they may encounter when refusing to take the advised course of action recommended by their doctor or midwife' [5].

Collect and Analyse Data

Obstetricians are familiar with, and mostly operate within the ambit of, the positivist tradition, with its emphasis on empirical data and scientific methods. The collection and analysis of data constitutes a bedrock in risk management. This data collection and analysis includes proactive and prospective risk analysis, incident reporting, case note reviews, clinical audit and safety culture measurement. The data are used to establish baseline parameters, to benchmark local performance against agreed standards and to set targets for quality improvement. The findings of this exercise should inform other RADICAL domains – such as raising awareness, designing services to optimize safety and involving service users in quality improvement.

The data collected from surveys, risk assessments, interviews, systems analyses ('root-cause analysis') and clinical audit could be used to populate risk registers and score cards. The Maternity Dashboard is a score card akin to the dashboard of a motor vehicle, providing real-time indicators of the quality and safety of care (Figure 29.3) [25]. Four categories of activity are covered in the dashboard: clinical activity;

Performance and Governance Scorecard: Always Aiming for Excellence

St George's Maternity Unit
The 'Maternity Dashboard' 2013

Category	Metric	Goal	Red Flag	Comment	Data Source	2008 Nov	2009 Nov	2010 Nov	2011 Nov	2012 Nov	JAN	FEB	MAR	APR	MAY	JUN	JUL	AUG	SEP	OCT	NOV	DEC	COMMENTS / ACTION THIS MONTH
Clinical Activity	Births — Benchmarked to 5000 per annum	5000 (425)	>433 (5200)	Review 3 monthly	Maternity System	498	447	459	431	452	458	380	359	421	402	405	434	413	445	415	402		
	Scheduled Bookings — Bookings (1st visit) scheduled	5680 (500)	>525 (6300)		Maternity System	442	512	541	516	407	481	338	457	504	458	477	516	481	469	476	520		
	Bookings <12Wks6	>90%	<90%		Maternity System	NA	NA	86	92.8	85	79	83	81	81	81	80	76	75	73	76	75		
	Carmen Suite — Benchmarked 500 /year	>60/Month	<50/month	Review 6 monthly	Maternity System	NA	NA	58	49	59	68	47	43	48	48	52	56	54	56	54	57		
	Transfers to D/Suite for reasons other than — Calculated based on National Data	<40	>41%		Lead Midwife Carmen Suite	NA	39	20.5	44	32	24	24	27	23.8	31%	35	31	38	41	38	25		Epid (32%), Mec (29%), Failure to progress (24%), Fetal cpompromise 9%.
	Normal Vaginal Births — 50 % (based on National Average of 46%)	>60%	<45% (<60%)	Review 6 monthly	Maternity System	NA	34.4	69.3	57.6	60.1	60	54.1	59.1	59.7	60.7	60	61.3	57.4	60.7	59.8	64.1		
	Home Births	>3%	<1%		Maternity System	Not monitored during this Period				2.2	0.9	3	1.1	1.9	1.5	1.7	0.2	1.4	2	1.2	1.2		
	Instr. Vag Del — Ventouse & Forceps	10-18%	<5%or >20%		Maternity System	NA	13.1	15	15.1	12	18.8	18.9	14	15.8	17.5	15.3	15	18.2	14.6	15.1	16.1		
	Induction of Labour — Percentage of total birth / month	<28%	>30.5 %	According to NICE, IOL	Maternity System	10.7	17.5	16.9	23	22	22.9	21.9	30	25.9	26.6	26.2	29	23.6	24.3	27.5	32.6		
	Postponed IOL due to overcapacity — Planned induction rebooked due to staffing/activity issues	<4/month	>5/month		D/Suite Escalation	NA	N/A	NA	1	1	4	4	4	4	4	3	4	3	4	2	2		
	C-Section — Total rate (planned & unscheduled)	<28%	>30%	Rate based on other	Maternity System	25.2	24.4	24.0	23.4	22.1	22.2	26.9	25.6	24.2	20.6	22.7	20.7	21.9	21.5	25	18.9		Maternal Request C Section - 18% of all elective C sections and 44 % inclding declining VBAC
	Emergency C-Sections — Excluding 'No Labour Emergency LSCS')	<16%	>16%		Maternity System	NA	NA	10.3	11.6	10	6.1	9.6	7.5	8.2	8.7	8.6	8.5	7.2	8.3	8.2	6.2		
	Maternal Request C. Section — No medical or obstetric indication	14 (aspirational goal 12)	5%	% of total number of	Electronic Diary	Not monitored during this Period				9.1	8	18	8.6	9.2	8.4	9	8.6	8.8	9.1	10.8	9		
	Vaginal Birth After Caesarean Section — UK Sentinel Audit 33%	>33%	< 30 %		Labour Ward Book	Not monitored during this Period				66.7	66.7	60.5	60.7	63.6	65.7	53.6	68	71.4	43.3	61.3	78.5		
	Refusal of NNU Transfers — Awaiting guidance from NNU Team	<4	>6		Maternity System	Not monitored during this Period				6	5	0	4	17	13	5	3	2	3	2	0		
	GA C.Sections	<7%	>10%		Maternity System	NA	NA	NA	6	1.3	0.4	1.3	0.6	1.4	1.5	2.7	0.7	1.3	1.3	2.4	1.2		
Workforce	Locally Agreed Weekly hours of Labour Ward consultant cover	> 98 hours/wk	<92 hours/wk	Per week	Delivery Suite Consultant Rota	NA	58	73	86	86	90	98	98	98	98	98	98	98	98	98	98		
	Safer Childbirth Requirement Weekly hours of labour ward	>168	<168	Per week	Consultant & SR Rota	NA	66	129	104	102	104	116	118	122	124	128	124	116	118	118	116		
	Midwife/birth ratio	<1:30	>1:40		Head of Midwifery	1.36	1.33	1.33	1.3	1.31		1.26			1.26			1.27		Quarterly			Being monitored quarterly - Q4 11/12
	Supernumerary Midwife in Labour Ward	>90%	<75%		Practice Educator							95			97.7			98.7		Quarterly			
	Mandatory Training for CNST Midwives	>75%	<70%	CNST Training	Practice Educator	NA	NA	89	89	88	88	88	90	88	88	92	68	88	88	88	87		
	Mandatory Training for CNST Doctors	>75%	<70%	CNST Training	Practice Educator	NA	92	92	94	94	92	90	90	92	92	92	92	90	90	92	90		

Figure 29.3 Maternity Dashboard: a clinical governance monitoring tool. See the colour plate section for a colour version of this figure.

Figure 29.3 (cont.)

	Indicator	Target (good)	Target (alert)	Review / Notes	Source	Prior period	Monthly data	Comments
Clinical Indicators — Maternal morbidity	All Readmissions	<1%	>3%	Review 6 monthly	Maternity System	N/A	2.7 0.5 0.8 0.4 0.5 0.8 0.7 0.6 0.5 0.5	
	Retained Products / Sepsis			Review 6 monthly	Maternity System	New for 2013		
	Life Threatening PPH >2.0L	<2%	>3%	Review 6 monthly	Maternity System	3 3 0.3 0.7 1.1	0.9 0.6 0.8 1.9 0.7 1.7 2.4 0.6 1.7 1.2	Home birth – admitted with cerebellar infarction to Neuro-ITU
	Unexpected Admission to ITU			ITU, Medical, Surgery,	Maternity System	Not monitored during this Period 0	2 1 0 0 1 1 1 0.6 1 1	
	BMI > 30 Kg/m2			% from Database	Maternity System	New for 2013	16.8 13.1 18.4 12.5 14.7 16 15.6 11.4 16.5 14.6	
	Severe Pre-Eclampsia / eclampsia (MgSO4)	Severe Pre-Eclampsia < 6 cases in 6 months			Maternity System	N/A 0 1 2 0	1 1 0 1 0 0 0 0 1 0	
	Number of cases of meconium aspiration	'Meconium Aspiration' our aspirations Goal is to have < 4			Neonatal Team	NA 1 0 1 0	0 0 0 1 1 0 1 0 0 0	
	Number of cases of hypoxic encephalopathy (Grade 2/3)	Unexpected Admissions < ITU cases 6 months / cases every 6 months		Review 6 monthly	Neonatal Team	NA 3 0 0 1	1 0 0 1 1 0 0 0 1 0	
Peri-natal morbidity & Mortality	Term Stillbirths	<2	>3	Review 6 monthly	Maternity System	1 1 0 1 1	0 1 1 0 0 0 0 0 0 0	
	Preterm Stillbirths 28-36	<3	>3	Review 3 monthly	Maternity System	0 NA NA 2 1	0 2 0 1 5 1 1 1 1 2	Fetal abnormalities & severe growth restriction
	Preterm Stillbirths <28	<2	3	Review 6 monthly	Maternity System	NA NA NA NA 1	0 1 1 0 0 0 2 0 0 1	
	Early Neonatal Deaths	<2	>3	Review 6 monthly	Maternity System	NA NA NA NA 1	0 0 0 3 1 0 0 0 0 0	
	Risk Incidents involving Fetal Monitoring / Syntocinon	<3	>4 (2)	Review 6 monthly	Risk Management	NA NA NA 0 2	0 0 0 0 1 0 0 0 0 1	
	Failed Instrumental Delivery	<1%	>3%	Erb's palsy 14%, #	Maternity System	0.7 0.1 0.6 0.5 0.4	0.4 0 0 1.2 1 0.5 0.7 0.5 0.2 0.2	
	Morbidity Shoulder dystocia	< 2 / month	> 3 / month		Physio Department	NA NA 0 0.4 0.4	0 0 0 0 1 1 1 0 0 0	
Risk Management	Total number of SUIs			Total Number as per revised	Risk Management	NA NA 0 0 0	2 3 1 1 0 2 2 2 2 4	
	SUIs where Clinical Care / Organisational issues identified	<2/month	>4/month		Risk Management	Not monitored during this Period 1 0	0 1 0 1 1 0 0 0 1 1	
	3rd degree tear	<5%	>7%	1.5% of deliveries	Maternity System	4.1 2.7 6 4.2 2.8	2.6 3.6 3.4 3.1 3.5 4.2 3.6 2.7 2.2 2.8 2.7	
Responsive Care — Formal Complaints	Attitude	0	>0			4 4 3 5 5	5 3 4 2 3 4 3 6 4 3	
	Clinical Care					1 1 1 1 1	3 3 3 0 0 2 2 1 3 1 0	Requesting the patient to book after miscarriage, poor environment in pre-op area
	Organisational					2 2 1 2 3	2 0 1 0 1 1 1 3 2 2	
	Commendations					1 3 2 3 2	5 11 2 3 6 6 7 6 2 3 7	

workforce; clinical outcomes; and risk incidents/complaints or patient satisfaction surveys. Individual maternity units set local goals for each of the parameters monitored, and categorize their scores using a traffic-light system: green (the goal is met); amber (the goals is not met, but the score is within a pre-defined threshold and action is needed in order to avoid entering the red zone); red (the threshold is breached and immediate action is needed to maintain safety).

The dashboard is tailored to the identified needs of the local maternity unit, but national-level aggregation of locally collected data could help paint a bigger picture and identify common themes. This is what the Maternity Safety Thermometer seeks to achieve [26]. It is a point of care survey that records rates of the following: maternal infection; perineal trauma; postpartum haemorrhage; mother and baby separation; term babies with an Apgar score of 6 or less at five minutes; and psychosocial harm. Data collected locally (on a chosen day, monthly) are uploaded to a national online database and aggregated data are analysed and published.

The *Each Baby Counts* project is a good example of how locally collected in-depth data on a specific risk management concern could be aggregated to see the bigger picture and share the lessons learned [27]. From January 2015, each Trust/Health Board in the UK has been asked to complete an online data collection form for each case of intrapartum-related stillbirth or neonatal death that occurs under their care. The data collection includes results of local investigations and root-cause analyses, and common themes will be identified.

To set national standards, promote benchmarking and monitor trends, it is important to have standardized data collection – but maternity units generally do not have common systems. One of the findings of the Healthcare Foundation's programme on *Improving the Safety of Maternity Services* was that participating maternity units took different approaches to the collection and management of data on clinical processes and outcomes [28]. Also, the King's Fund inquiry found that clinicians complain of multiple data collection systems taking up large amounts of time at the expense of time for patient care, and that IT systems in many hospitals do not permit integrated data collection and handling.

The non-uniformity and deficiencies in data collection and management also make it more difficult to explain the wide variations in clinical practice (e.g. caesarean delivery rates) and complications (e.g. third- and fourth-degree perineal tears) between hospitals, variations which persist even after adjustments are made for some (but not all) maternal factors.

Learn from Patient Safety Incidents

For investment in risk management to be worthwhile, the organization and its staff have to learn from patient safety incidents. This learning is not something that should happen simply by chance; it has to be planned, nurtured and reinforced. Learning is shaped by qualitative and quantitative patient safety data (Collecting and Analysing data). Lessons learned have to be shared with staff (Raising Awareness) and with patients (Involving Users), and should inform service development (Designing for safety) – the domains of the RADICAL framework inform each other.

One of the best tools for learning from patient safety incidents in the delivery suite is the Systems Analysis conducted after a major incident. This tool is often called 'root-cause analysis', but the term could be a misnomer since there is often not a single root cause, and the purpose of the exercise is not just to find the cause(s) of the incident but to improve the system and make it more resilient. The term 'High-Level Investigation (HLI)' is also used to describe this exercise, but this too is less than satisfactory as it sounds rather inquisitorial.

Regardless of the term used to describe it, the structured analysis of major patient safety incidents in UK maternity units (and secondary care, generally) does not appear to have had an optimum effect on organizational learning. There are a number of reasons for this. First, what was originally intended to be a quality improvement exercise has been coalesced with medico-legal imperatives, and the 'investigation' is taken by hospitals as the first step in preparations for anticipated litigation. Second, the exercise is often conducted by staff who have not been adequately trained to undertake this role, and the quality of the analysis often does not facilitate learning. Third, the analyses conducted in a unit over time need to be meta-analysed to unearth recurring and cross-cutting themes, but this rarely happens.

For a 'root-cause analysis' to serve its purpose of consolidating individual and organizational learning, it has to meet quality standards. There are standards for conducting incident investigation. The process of investigation/analysis should be open and transparent, those involved in the incident should be kept appropriately informed and the focus should be on opportunities for improvement, not fault-finding or apportioning of blame. Hindsight and outcome bias should be avoided.

The UK Confidential Enquiry report made the following observations:

> Serious incident reviews or root cause analyses were not carried out to review the care received by all women who died. Even fewer of the morbidity cases of women who recovered from septic shock underwent a local review. In other instances, where a review was carried out, the quality was poor. This is a lost opportunity, reducing the capability of the host organisation and the wider NHS to learn from these tragic and serious events. When a thorough serious incident review was carried out, it was clear that maternity units learned valuable lessons and in turn that enabled them to improve their systems and processes [5].

Another route to optimizing learning is the integration of risk management with clinical audit. Safety incident reports and risk assessments should inform the clinical audit agenda, and clinical audit findings should inform the risk register. Clinical audit is a good way of ascertaining whether lessons have been learned from some incidents.

Some nuggets of learning extracted from the UK Confidential Enquiries are reproduced in Box 29.2.

Conclusion

The spending on maternity clinical negligence cover in the UK equates to nearly one-fifth of the spending on maternity services [1]. Most claims and huge payments relate to intrapartum events (particularly, management of labour, caesarean delivery and fetal brain injury) [29]. This highlights the importance of risk management in intrapartum care. By reducing the number of claims, financial and other resources can be freed for the further improvement of maternity care and for improvements elsewhere in the health economy. Beyond avoidance of litigation, there are other ethical ('first, do no harm') and professional reasons for employing risk management, as discussed above.

Box 29.2 Some Risk Management Nuggets from the UK Confidential Enquiries into Maternal Mortality and Morbidity (*Saving Lives, Improving Mothers' Care, 2014*)

- Do not hesitate to escalate concerns to senior colleagues. Failure to escalate led to deaths from sepsis and haemorrhage.
- Do not be complacent about 'routine' observations. Inadequate observation suggesting systemic failures in either staffing or routine tasks featured in a number of deaths. In one case, failure to record routine observations during induction of labour led to maternal death (uterine rupture).
- Someone needs to fly the aircraft. Poor coordination and documentation following multidisciplinary specialist review was implicated in maternal deaths.
- Beware of ruptured uterus when using a tamponade balloon to treat postpartum haemorrhage. In two maternal deaths from haemorrhage the problem was uterine rupture but balloons had been inserted.
- Use a blood warmer. There was one death due to cardiac arrest which followed the rapid transfusion of five units of blood with no indication that a rapid warmer infusion device was used.
- Be fastidious in estimating blood loss. There were many deaths where there were inconsistencies in documented loss between different care givers, suggesting lack of both teamwork and communication and resulting in delayed recognition and treatment of massive haemorrhage.
- Persistent headache after dural puncture? Consider the possibility of subdural haematoma and cerebral venous sinus thrombosis

---

For risk management to address this challenge effectively, all domains of risk management should command attention and the domains should be integrated. The RADICAL framework facilitates this, and its application to intrapartum care has been described in this chapter. The framework is both a management tool and a way of thinking. Its implementation has the potential to bring about the transformational change that is essential for optimizing the safety of intrapartum care. The realization of this potential calls for inspired leadership and teamwork [30].

References

1. The National Audit Office. *Maternity Services in England: Report by the Comptroller and Auditor General.* London; The Stationery Office; 2013.

2. Edozien LC. Mapping the patient safety footprint: the RADICAL framework. *Best Pract Res Clin Obstet Gynaecol.* 2013;27: 481–8 doi: 10.1016/j.bpobgyn. 2013.05.001.

3. Edozien LC. The RADICAL framework for implementing and monitoring healthcare risk management. *CGIJ.* 2013;18: 165–75. doi: 10.1108/14777271311317945.

4. Centre for Maternal and Child Enquiries (CMACE). Saving Mothers' Lives: reviewing maternal deaths to make motherhood safer: 2006–08. The Eighth Report on Confidential Enquiries into Maternal Deaths in the United Kingdom. *BJOG.* 2011;118(suppl. 1): 1–203.

5. Knight M, Kenyon S, Brocklehurst P, *et al.* (eds). *Saving Lives, Improving Mothers' Care – Lessons Learned to Inform Future Maternity Care from the UK and Ireland Confidential Enquiries into Maternal Deaths and Morbidity 2009–12.* Oxford: National Perinatal Epidemiology Unit, University of Oxford; 2014.

6. Department of Health. *On the State of Public Health: Annual Report of the Chief Medical Officer 2006.* London: Department of Health; 2007.

7. West Midlands Perinatal Institute. *Confidential Enquiry into Intrapartum Related Deaths.* NHS West Midlands; October 2010.

8. Goldenberg RL, McClure EM, Bann CM. The relationship of intrapartum and antepartum stillbirth rates to measures of obstetric care in developed and developing countries. *Acta Obstet Gynecol Scand.* 2007;86: 1303–9. doi: 10.1080/00016340701644876.

9. Jonsson M, Nordén-Lindeberg S, Ostlund I, Hanson U. Metabolic acidosis at birth and suboptimal care: illustration of the gap between knowledge and clinical practice. *BJOG.* 2009;116: 1453–60. doi: 10.1111/j.1471–0528.2009.02269.x.

10. Morris S. Hospital fined £100,000 after wrong drug killed new mother. *Guardian.* 17 May 2010. www.theguardian.com/society/2010/may/17/mother-killed-myra-cabrera-bupivacaine (accessed 9 February 2016).

11. King's Fund. *Safe Births, Everybody's Business: An Independent Inquiry into the Safety of Maternity Services in England.* London: King's Fund; 2008.

12. Edozien LC. Structured multidisciplinary intershift handover (SMITH): a tool for promoting safer intrapartum care. *J Obstet Gynaecol.* 2011;31: 683–6.

13. Edozien LC. Situational awareness and its application in the delivery suite. *Obstet Gynecol.* 2015;125: 65–9. doi: 10.1097/AOG.0000000000000597.

14. Fitzpatrick T, Holt L. A 'buddy' approach to CTG. *Midwives.* 2008;11: 40–1.

15. Fausett MB, Propst A, Van Doren K, Clark BT. How to develop an effective obstetric checklist. *Am J Obstet Gynecol.* 2011;205: 165–70.

16. Kearns RJ, Uppal V, Bonner J, *et al.* The introduction of a surgical safety checklist in a tertiary referral obstetric centre. *BMJ Qual Saf.* 2011;20: 818–22.

17. Toft B, Mascie-Taylor H. Involuntary automaticity: a work-system induced risk to safe health care. *Health Serv Manage Res.* 2005;18: 211–16.

18. MacEachin SR, Lopez CM, Powell KJ, Corbett NL. The fetal heart rate collaborative practice project: situational awareness in electronic fetal monitoring – a Kaiser Permanente perinatal patient safety program initiative. *J Perinatal Neonatal Nurs.* 2009;23: 314–23.

19. Lewis LS, Pan HY, Heine RP, *et al.* Labor and pregnancy outcomes after adoption of a more conservative oxytocin labor protocol. *Obstet Gynecol.* 2014;123(suppl. 1): 66S. doi: 10.1097/01.AOG. 0000447374.37308.4c.

20. Rohn AE, Bastek JA, Sammel MD, Wang E, Srinivas SK. Unintended clinical consequences of the implementation of a checklist-based, low-dose oxytocin protocol. *Am J Perinatol.* 2014;32: 371–8. doi: 10.1055/s-0034-1387932.

21. Budden A, Chen LJ, Henry A. High-dose versus low-dose oxytocin infusion regimens for induction of labour at term. *Cochrane Database Syst Rev.* 2014;10: CD009701. doi: 10.1002/14651858.CD009701.pub2.

22. Mahlmeister L. Best practices in perinatal care: evidence-based management of oxytocin induction and augmentation of labor. *J Perinat Neonat Nurs.* 2008;22(4): 259–63. doi: 10.1097/01.JPN.0000341354. 99703.b2.

23. Scottish Health Council. *Good Practice in Service User Involvement in Maternity Services: Involving Women to Improve their Care.* Glasgow Scottish Health Council; 2011.

24. Magee H, Askham J. *Women's Views About Safety in Maternity Care: A Qualitative Study.* London: King's Fund and Picker Institute; 2008.

25. Royal College of Obstetricians and Gynaecologists. *Maternity Dashboard: Clinical Performance and Governance Score Card.* London: RCOG Press; 2008.

26. www.safetythermometer.nhs.uk (accessed 9 February 2016).

27. www.rcog.org.uk/eachbabycounts (accessed 9 February 2016).

28. www.health.org.uk (accessed 15 May 2016).

29. National Health Service Litigation Authority. *Ten Years of Maternity Claims: An Analysis of NHS Litigation Authority Data*. London: NHSLA; 2012.

30. Cornthwaite K, Edwards S, Siassakos D. Reducing risk in maternity by optimising teamwork and leadership: an evidence-based approach to save mothers and babies. *Best Pract Res Clin Obstet Gynaecol*. 2013;27: 571–81

Chapter 30

Team Working, Skills and Drills on the Labour Ward

Katie Cornthwaite and Dimitrios M. Siassakos

Effective multi-professional team working is essential for the management of obstetric emergencies. The success of a team is multi-factorial, but simple teamwork behaviours can make a significant difference. Training should focus on improving clinical outcomes and patient safety, while being a fun and beneficial experience for members of staff. 'In-house' programmes are cost-effective and inclusive, and training in teamwork can be seamlessly integrated into skills and drills. This should be mandated for all members of the multi-professional team in order to improve patient outcomes.

Background

In the developed world, labour is usually very safe, but a variety of emergencies can occur (Table 30.1), with, on average, one in six women facing a potentially lethal emergency [1]. These can develop quickly and unexpectedly, and require a rapid and coordinated response from a number of multi-professional team members.

Although some emergencies are common, many occur rarely, and it is therefore difficult to learn by experience alone. The mandatory reduction in doctors' working hours has compounded the problem. Indeed, an Israeli study, in which 60 obstetric trainees and 84 midwives were video-recorded managing obstetric emergencies, showed that while 82% of participants regarded their theoretical knowledge as satisfactory, 68% were not trained to take independent action in any of the four selected obstetric emergencies [2]. Furthermore, in a multi-centre survey of 614 multi-professional staff in the USA, less than two-thirds of the participants replied that there was clear leadership in obstetric emergencies [3].

We need to empower clinicians to feel confident in their practical skills and in leading the manage-

Table 30.1 Obstetric emergencies suitable for rehearsals

Emergency	UK incidence (approximate, per maternities)
Maternal collapse and peri-mortem caesarean section	0.03 per 1000
Seizures/eclampsia	0.5 per 1000
Cardiotocogram (CTG) interpretation	High rate of false-positives
Cord prolapse	1–6 per 1000
Breech delivery	30 per 1000
Shoulder dystocia	2–20 per 1000
Postpartum haemorrhage	Massive in 13 per 1000
Neonatal resuscitation	Common need

ment of these emergencies, despite possibly having less experience.

Furthermore, the stakes are high – at least 50% of maternal deaths are avoidable, and poor or non-existent teamwork has been repeatedly identified as a factor contributing to poor outcomes in national confidential enquiries and medico-legal cases [4,5].

Pregnant women are often younger and fitter than the general medical population and the changes associated with pregnancy can make it difficult to recognize potentially serious complications. One review of the management of critical obstetric emergencies highlighted that poor recognition of concealed complications resulted in suboptimal care for one in three cases [6]. Notably, this was attributed to poor teamwork and deficient interpersonal skills.

However, it is not only mothers who are affected by poor team working. Suboptimal team communication and deficient team training have been identified as the most common root causes for infant death

Best Practice in Labour and Delivery, Second Edition, ed. Sir Sabaratnam Arulkumaran. Published by Cambridge University Press. © Cambridge University Press 2016.

in developed countries [5,7]. Inadequate management from front line teams can result in cerebral palsy [8] and brachial plexus injury [9]. While the management of shoulder dystocia typically focuses on the individual skills of the accoucheur, effective team working remains essential. Importantly, the multi-centre SaFE study revealed that participants training as individuals for shoulder dystocia were less likely to have performed actions requiring a team effort to relieve the shoulder dystocia, such as McRoberts or applying suprapubic pressure [9,10,11].

Consequently, for a number of years, there have been calls across the board for effective teamwork training. In 2008, a report by the House of Commons on Patient Safety recommended that 'those that work together should train together'; focusing on skills such as leadership, teamwork and situational awareness [12]. The recent Keogh report, which reviewed the quality of care provided by hospital trusts with persistently high mortality rates, highlighted the need for customized training in teamwork for all NHS staff [13].

In maternity, the 2004 King's Fund report *Safe Births: Everybody's Business* underlined the need for clarity about team objectives, effective leadership and improved communication. Accordingly it advocated teamwork training for all maternity staff [7]. Further to this, a recent report published by the Royal College of Obstetricians and Gynaecologists (RCOG), *Becoming Tomorrow's Specialist*, promotes team working and reiterates that a clinician who works in isolation is undesirable. The report emphasizes that the attainment of professional skills and attributes such as teamwork and leadership are just as important as clinical competencies. It underlines the need for effective teaching in multi-professional team working from the outset of training [14].

Evidently, there has been a cultural shift from striving for individual technical perfection to better team coordination and communication, which requires integrated teamwork training with multi-professional simulation. Lessons from the aviation industry have traditionally been applied to medicine. However, while their Crew Resource Management (CRM) programmes have been found to improve attitudes towards team working in accident and emergency, the same methods have failed to achieve improvement on the labour ward [1,15]. As a result, there has been a move to developing specific training tools applicable to obstetrics, typically focusing on

'skills and drills' simulation rather than the wholesale adoption of potentially inappropriate models from other disciplines.

It is crucial that teamwork training interventions are simple and relevant to the specific healthcare setting – only then can they truly impact on patient care and safety [16,17].

In this chapter we summarize the current evidence relating to the key characteristics of a good team, and how best to deliver effective teamwork training in obstetrics.

Team Working

Team working is defined as the combined effective action of a group working towards a common goal. It requires individuals with different roles to communicate effectively and work together in a coordinated manner to achieve a successful outcome [18]. Obstetric emergencies can develop rapidly and unpredictably, necessitating hasty formation of an ad hoc team. Often these emergencies occur consecutively or even simultaneously, with little opportunity for teaching or debriefing. So what characteristics are needed for the team to function well?

Knowledge, Skills and Attitude (KSA)

Healthcare professionals involved in obstetric care are inclined to report high levels of competence in dealing with obstetric emergencies [19]. However, important knowledge gaps have been identified [20], which can impact on team performance and patient care. Obstetric emergency training can help to address these deficiencies; in the SaFE study, a definitive improvement in both knowledge and skills occurred after training [2], and was sustained for 6 and 12 months after training [21].

Interestingly, cross-sectional analysis of the pre-training data for 19 randomly selected multi-professional teams who participated in SaFE showed no relation between conventional KSA measures of individual ability and variation in team efficiency [22]. So, what accounts for the variation in team performance, besides KSA? Further analysis of the SaFE study revealed a strong correlation between generic teamwork scores and clinical efficiency [23]. Clearly, team performance is not merely reliant on individual members having the knowledge and skills to pass an assessment, but how those multi-professionals interact to apply that knowledge and skill.

Communication

Clear communication is essential for healthcare teams. Obstetric emergencies frequently involve different professions with varying levels of seniority, which may provide an obstacle to effective communication. Therefore, strategies must be in place to overcome this. Analysis of simulated emergencies and focus groups confirmed the usefulness of structured handover, such as SBAR (clearly states situation (S) and background (B), gives an accurate assessment (A), requests recommended actions (R)), for any team member who may need to handover or lead the team until more experienced staff arrive. Closed-loop communication should also be used. This refers to the sender initiating a message, the receiver receiving the message, interpreting it and acknowledging its receipt, and the sender following up to ensure the intended message was received and acted upon [24,25]. It is also vital that the patient and family are appropriately communicated with to avoid undue psychological distress. Indeed, the recent NICE intrapartum care guideline recommends allocation of a member of the healthcare team to talk with the woman and her birth partner(s) to explain what is happening and offer support throughout the emergency [26].

Leadership

Team leadership is a complex skill. The leader is the figurehead of the team, who is expected to set team objectives and establish behavioural expectations, thereby providing direction and structure. Team leadership also involves supporting and monitoring team members [27]. Leaders require a certain amount of competence but may vary in their level of expertise and also their profession. While knowledge is necessary, good communication and situational awareness are vital.

A deficiency in leadership is associated with poor outcomes [28]; however, until recently there has been no evidence to show how to establish leadership. Findings from recent research on teamwork, leadership and team training are shown in Table 30.2.

Situational Awareness

Situational awareness is defined as 'the perception of the elements in the environment, the comprehension of the meaning, and the projection of their status in the near future'. More simply, it refers to knowing what is

Table 30.2 Findings from recent research on leadership on the labour ward

Leadership Issue	Summary of findings
Who should be the leader?	*Experience* – the person with experience of the emergency who knows team members and their roles/responsibilities, not necessarily the most senior
Who is the leader?	*Verbal declaration* – declare being a leader verbally or allocate leadership verbally
How to lead	*Know the team* (before the emergency, otherwise stop and ask who they are and what they can do) – this will help with task allocation and determination of leadership *SBAR* – clarify the situation and background, then make an assessment and a recommendation loudly for everyone to hear; including patient and companions who can then be informed in the same simple step even without communication directed specifically at them at that point (if not enough staff) *Closed-loop communication* – use closed-loop communication to allocate critical tasks to team members, including communication with the patient and companions (if enough staff); follow simple algorithms that determine the order and/or importance of tasks *Avoid distraction* – it might be useful to focus on leadership and avoid performing tasks that can be done by other members of the team. This allows the leader to take a step back and maintain a broader, 'helicopter' view.

going on, and is frequently found to be deficient in simulation [29–31] or by observation of labour wards [32]. It is a concept that was first defined in aviation, and it has been consistently difficult to define and measure in obstetrics [33–35], where situations are often complex. However, focus groups have identified three teachable components: find out the clinical situation; find out the team abilities; and keep aware of patient and companion needs for communication and information.

Shared Mental Methods

This concept refers to having a shared objective and a plan of work to achieve it. Shared mental models emerge through the interactions of team members. However, in healthcare, teams are often created there and then for an emergency, and individuals may never have worked within the same team, or even met before.

Table 30.3 Teachable teamwork behaviours

1	Find out clinical situation (and maintain regular update).
2	Know or find out what the team members can do for the emergency at hand.
3	Declare or allocate leadership verbally based on relevant experience of emergency at hand.
4	Use closed-loop communication for allocation of critical tasks.
5	Keep patients and companions informed.
6	Team leader should focus on leadership to ensure effective teamwork unless the task is simple or there is no one else who can do it.

Clear and early verbalization of the situation or diagnosis (for example, saying 'this is eclampsia') can help focus team members, improve performance and keep patients and their companions informed [28]. Certain teamwork behaviours can be taught, as shown in Table 30.3.

Teamwork Training: Why Bother?

Acquisition of Knowledge and Skills

As discussed, the SaFE study demonstrated a definitive and sustained improvement in both knowledge and skills following training [21]. Another study revealed that clinical performance for drills requiring multi-professional team effort (postpartum haemorrhage, eclampsia) was poorer than that for drills focusing on skills of the individual accoucheur (breech vaginal delivery, shoulder dystocia) prior to training. Team-based simulation training improved performance in subsequent drills, even when scenarios were changed [2].

Satisfaction of Learners

Evidence shows that clinicians enjoy obstetric emergency training [36]. Multi-professional team training using simulation not only improves knowledge and clinical management of obstetric emergencies, but also confers confidence and enhances communication skills [37].

Change in Attitude

A study using a validated tool (Sexton safety attitude and climate questionnaire) to assess staff attitudes in a maternity unit showed that the introduction of team training enhances teamwork climate and promotes a positive safety culture [38].

Clinical Behaviours

Behavioural changes are difficult to assess, with most evaluation tools relying extensively on self-reporting and subjective assessments by observers [39].

However, clinical and social science methods have been used to describe specific teachable behaviours of effective teams and leaders [24,40]. Better teams are likely to vocalize the nature of the emergency earlier, use closed-loop communication to allocate critical tasks and use more structured handovers.

Patient and Organizational Outcomes

Obstetric emergency training can improve knowledge, skills, satisfaction and team behaviours, but do these changes translate into better outcomes for patients and healthcare organizations?

Patient Safety

A retrospective observational study demonstrated improved perinatal outcomes in a large UK maternity unit after the introduction of 'in-house' obstetric emergency training: low Apgar scores (<7 at five minutes) and moderate, severe or total hypoxic-ischaemic encephalopathy were all reduced by about 50% [41], and brachial plexus injuries by 70% [42].

Notably, the units that demonstrated improved outcomes all made use of department-level incentives to train and 'in-house' training programmes were attended by 100% of staff.

Patient Satisfaction

Obstetric lawsuits repeatedly cite deficient interpersonal skills and communication problems, which adversely affect patients' and relatives' satisfaction and raise concerns about their safety [43].

Training in obstetric emergencies can improve these communication shortages and subsequent patient satisfaction, and reduce litigation [44].

Teams trained 'in-house' with patient-actors demonstrate significantly higher safety and communication scores compared with teams trained at simulation centres using computerized patient mannequins. Accordingly, obstetric training should be designed to closely imitate the demands of a real-life labour ward in order to enhance psychological fidelity [45].

Simulation studies have shown significant improvements in patient-actors' perception of care following training [46]. Furthermore, patient-actor perception was better when the leader had a directive style of communication, which included certain items of information such as condition of the baby, cause of the emergency and aims of treatment [40].

Cost-Effectiveness

'In-house' simulation training is cost-effective and is likely to be less than attendance at external courses [42,46]. Moreover, there is a potential for huge savings from litigation costs and insurance premiums by improving outcomes [47,48].

Teamwork Training: How Should We Organize It?

Lessons for Training

A good clinical outcome should be the decisive factor for the success of a team. Our understanding regarding characteristics of effective teams and how best to organize team training has been enhanced through the study of teams in simulation, in conjunction with inter-professional focus group analysis [25]. In this multi-centre study, team performance during simulation was assessed by measuring the time to administer an essential drug (magnesium for eclampsia), which is a clinically relevant surrogate of team performance and safety [49]. Front line staff participating in focus groups recounted real-life emergencies and enriched our knowledge further. Participants identified a need for teamwork training, which incorporates several methods suited to different learning styles and levels of seniority.

There continues to be evidence of poor inter-professional working in maternity. Training together in realistic settings, via attendance at local skills and drills training, can improve this and provide an opportunity for team bonding. 'In-house' training allows new staff to familiarize themselves with their specific role and environment in emergencies, while maintaining competence for permanent staff. This helps to prepare teams on the 'shop-floor' to rapidly come together as a team and manage any emergency.

Accordingly, the UK NHS Litigation Authority mandate annual multidisciplinary skills drills through its Clinical Negligence Scheme for Trust (CNST) standards [48]. Despite this, in 2003 only 51% of UK centres surveyed were conducting such training. Common causes for not undertaking skills drills were concerns about the impact on service provision and a perception of the training process as threatening or stressful [50].

The following highlights ways to alleviate such fears and maximize the benefit from drills.

Organizing Effective Skills and Drills Training

Course Planning and Administration

The course programme should be finalized by a local training team who can allocate individual modules to specific trainers, who can then practise scenarios prior to running the courses so as to identify any problems.

A practice midwife can be invaluable in administering the course. All presentations, handouts and equipment may be stored centrally, and it is useful if trainers are familiar with each other's workstations and lectures, so that both trainers and workstations are interchangeable when necessary. The programme should ideally change annually to maintain interest. Course manuals should be sent out to all participants prior to the course.

To ensure that staff are released to attend the training day, several dates may be arranged well in advance. A database should be kept of all attendees for clinical negligence scheme assessments. Appraisals of consultants and trainee doctors, and supervision schemes for midwives, should identify non-attendees and a mandatory session can be arranged at the end of the year. Certificates of attendance should be provided and logbooks of training can be signed to increase motivation.

Access

Locally organized emergency training days should be available to both hospital and community staff. In view of the increasing numbers of births outside consultant-led units, it is important to advertise and actively promote in the community [18].

Location

The emergency drills are best undertaken in a delivery room or another clinical area, as it provides the highest environmental fidelity. A suitable seminar room nearby should be used for lectures.

Delivery rooms may not always be available for use, but training in the true clinical environment enables local protocols and procedures to be tested and, if necessary, revised, thereby improving the system and creating a sense of general ownership.

The workload can be reduced in advance, for example by limiting the number of elective caesarean sections. It may be best to leave the decision of which rooms will be used for each drill until the latest possible time, and remain flexible.

Scenarios

The scenarios should be simple and outline the immediate emergency action required. The participation in role-play is a new experience for many healthcare professionals and this is often the first obstacle to be encountered. Given time, participants overcome their initial embarrassment and appreciate the opportunity to actively take part in the scenario as part of 'the team'.

It can be helpful to conduct a drill briefing prior to the first drill, in which the actions the participants are required to undertake can be highlighted. This can then be reinforced between drills if necessary. During each scenario, it works well to take one member of the team into the room first for a handover, while the rest of the team waits outside. Individuals then get an opportunity to practise their handover skills when other team members enter the room.

Facilitation

Between six and ten 'in-house' trainers should be enlisted to facilitate the day. Participants should feel welcome and relaxed, and encouraged to participate in the planning and evaluation of their learning. This is vital to the success of drills.

Patient-Actors

Drills tend to be more successful if the setting is as near to reality as possible [44]. Obstetric emergencies are unique in that there is significant audience participation; good communication with both the woman and their family or friends is essential.

Using a patient-actor, or integrating a patient-actor with a mannequin, is cheap, easy and effective [18]. It can also increase the realism of the situation, enhance communication between team members and women, and lead to improvement in communication scores as assessed by patient-actors [44]. Hence, it can be useful

for the patient-actors to give the team feedback after each drill.

A member of staff with experience of the emergencies portrayed can make an excellent patient. Alternatively, using a healthcare assistant as the patient-actor may be advantageous in giving them an insight into their role as part of the multi-professional team when attending obstetric emergencies.

Equipment

The correct equipment must be available. If mannequins are used, a pregnant abdomen, bra and female wig add realism to the simulated scenario. In the PROMPT (PRactical Obstetric Multi-Professional Training) course, props are used to increase the realism of the scenarios: blood-stained incontinence sheets, trousers that bleed, a pregnant uterus, life-size copy of O Rhesus negative blood bags, a perineum with a prolapsed cord [18].

The level of fidelity of simulations is not as important as designing the drills to suit task demands in real life, and in many cases low-technology props may be as effective as more sophisticated equipment.

Pictorial guidelines can be used to facilitate visual estimation of blood loss [51], otherwise underestimation might occur in as many as 95% of obstetric haemorrhage cases [2].

Record Keeping

A 'made-up' set of patient notes and partogram can be used at the handover in the delivery room as an aide-memoir of the patient's history, and also to document the care given during the scenario.

Structured documentation proforma can be developed and used for both training and real-life emergencies. The team should allocate the role of scribe to one person during the drill. If necessary this can be prompted by the trainer. Documentation, including completion of clinical incident forms, should be discussed following the drill.

Objectives, Feedback and Assessment

Workshops should remain focused, and outcome-based training can achieve this. At the beginning of training sessions, the learning objectives or the most common challenges should be identified. It may be useful to discuss difficulties and omissions identified from past learners, and aim to avoid the same mistakes. Specific checklists can help structure observation

Table 30.4 Pendleton's feedback rules

1 The team members say what they did well.
2 The team members say what can be improved.
3 The facilitator acknowledges what they did well.
4 The facilitator states where they could improve.

of clinical actions, and provide a useful starting point in the discussion and evaluation of management of the scenario [18].

Appropriate feedback to learners is as important as objectives. Learning is about having an experience, reviewing it, concluding and planning the future. Consequently, drills need to incorporate both practical and reflective elements through constructive feedback that is directly linked to the outcome-based objectives. Pendleton's rules are useful but several other feedback models exist (Table 30.4).

So as to avoid intimidating authority gradients, a member of the group can provide feedback to the rest of the team, using the drill-specific checklist(s). Subsequently, the drill leader together with the patient-actor can facilitate group discussion with suggestions about what could be improved, altered or added.

Learners often perceive that they have performed very badly, so it is vital that positive actions are emphasized. We do not use formal assessment. It removes the threat of testing, may promote team ethos and has led to both 100% staff participation and improved outcomes.

Evaluation sheets should be given to all participants as their feedback can lead to both training and infrastructural improvements.

Frequency of Training

Training should take place at least annually in accordance with CNST requirements. While it has been established that improvement in both knowledge and skills is sustained for 12 months after training [21], more frequent training may be beneficial. Focus groups have identified that often members of ad hoc teams do not even know each other's names, professions or responsibilities as a result of staff rotations or turnover [25]. A potential solution to this would be regular training several times per year. Of course, introductions at the start of each shift would enable senior doctors to know their staff so as to determine and allocate tasks appropriately in the case of an emergency.

Additional In-House Training

Other in-house training methods can be used alongside skills drills training in order to suit different learning styles and maximize the benefits of teamwork training.

Focus groups identified three potentially useful additional approaches:

1. debriefing staff after real-life emergencies to learn lessons;
2. video-recorded role-play to identify personal training needs and stimulate self-reflection; and
3. case-based discussions for those who might initially feel intimidated by role-play.

All professions, not just doctors and midwives, can use these concurrent training methods. This will help to foster good collaboration, positive teamwork climate and a sound safety culture [38].

While training in the same team as senior staff can improve learning, the focus groups suggested that junior doctors and midwives may benefit from additional group teaching sessions, without senior staff, in order to develop leadership skills. This is useful experience for occasions when juniors may need to lead emergencies initially while awaiting the arrival of a senior. Nonetheless, focus groups and staff attitude surveys agree that senior (consultant) presence is useful.

Summary

- Obstetric emergencies require a rapid and coordinated response from a multi-professional team.
- Successful team working is multi-factorial, requiring knowledge and skills, clear communication, experienced leadership and a shared objective.
- Effective teamwork training for all maternity staff is high on the agenda.
- Simple teamwork behaviours make a marked difference to team effectiveness during obstetric emergencies.
- Training should first and foremost improve clinical outcomes and patient experience.
- 'In-house' training is effective and inclusive, and reduces costs.
- Multi-professional groups should be encouraged to participate in developing and running courses.

- Mandate and confirm annual attendance by all hospital and community, midwifery, obstetric and managerial staff.
- Patient-actors are cost-effective and improve communication skills.
- Teamwork training should be context-specific and integrated.
- Training should be fun and enjoyable.
- Formal assessment is not necessary and may be detrimental to staff morale.
- Monitor clinical results and feedback to staff.

Conclusion

Effective teamwork training is undoubtedly key to a successful obstetric unit, fostering a positive working environment and improving patient safety outcomes. Studies on teamwork and team training have helped establish the characteristics of effective maternity teams, and teachable behaviours have been identified. We have moved away from theoretical, aviation models of training to high-fidelity methods specific to obstetrics. Local, 'in-house' training has been proven to be cost-effective, while consolidating behaviour changes and improving patient safety and satisfaction.

References

1. Nielsen PE, Goldman MB, Mann S, *et al*. Effects of teamwork training on adverse outcomes and process of care in labor and delivery: a randomized controlled trial. *Obstet Gynecol*. 2007;109(1): 48–55.

2. Maslovitz S, Barkai G, Lessing JB, Ziv A, Many A. Recurrent obstetric management mistakes identified by simulation. *Obstet Gynecol*. 2007;109(6): 1295–300.

3. Guise JM, Segel SY, Larison K, *et al*. STORC safety initiative: a multicentre survey on preparedness & confidence in obstetric emergencies. *Qual Saf Health Care*. 2010;19(6) doi: 10.1136/qshc.2008.030890.

4. Risser DT, Rice MM, Salisbury ML, *et al*. The potential for improved teamwork to reduce medical errors in the emergency department. *Ann Emerg Med*. 1999;34(3): 373–83.

5. Centre for Maternal and Child Enquiries (CMACE). Saving Mothers' Lives: reviewing maternal deaths to make motherhood safer: 2006–08. The Eighth Report on Confidential Enquiries into Maternal Deaths in the United Kingdom. *BJOG*. 2011;118(suppl. 1): 1–203.

6. Maternal and Child Health Consortium. *Antepartum Term Stillbirths. Confidential Enquiries into Stillbirths and Deaths in Infancy. 5th Annual Report*. London: Maternal and Child Health Consortium; 1998.

7. King's Fund. *Safe Births: Everybody's Business. An Independent Enquiry into the Safety of Maternity Services in England*. London: King's Fund; 2008.

8. Department of Health Expert Group. *An Organisation with a Memory: Report of an Expert Group on Learning from Adverse Events in the NHS*. London: The Stationary Office; 2000.

9. Draycott T, Crofts JF, Ash JP, *et al*. Improving neonatal outcome through practical shoulder dystocia training. *Obstet Gynecol*. 2008;112(1): 14–20.

10. Crofts JF, Bartlett C, Ellis D, *et al*. Training for shoulder dystocia: a trial of simulation using low fidelity and high fidelity mannequins. *Obstet Gynecol*. 2006;108(6): 1477–85.

11. Crofts JF, Ellis D, Draycott TJ, *et al*. Change in knowledge of midwives and obstetricians following obstetric emergency training: a randomised controlled trial of local hospital, simulation centre and teamwork training. *BJOG*. 2007;114(12): 1534–41.

12. Health Committee, House of Commons. *Patient Safety, Sixth Report of Session 2008–09*. London: The Stationery Office; 2009.

13. Keogh B. *Review into the Quality of Care and Treatment Provided by 14 Hospital Trusts in England: Overview Report*. London: NHS England; 2013.

14. RCOG. *Becoming Tomorrow's Specialist: Lifelong Professional Development for Specialist in Women's Health Working Party Report*: London: RCOG Press; 2014.

15. Morey JC, Simon R, Jay GD, *et al*. Error reduction and performance improvement in the emergency department through formal teamwork training: evaluation results of the MedTeams project. *Health Serv Res*. 2002;37(6): 1553–81.

16. Baker DP, Day R, Salas E. Teamwork as an essential component of high-reliability organisations. *Health Serv Res*. 2006;41: 1576–98.

17. Lyndon A. Communication and teamwork in patient care: how much can we learn from aviation? *J Obstet Gynecol Neonatal Nurs*. 2006;35: 538–46.

18. Draycott T, Winter C, Crofts J, Barnfield S. *PRactical Obstetric Multiprofessional Training (PROMPT) Trainer's Manual*. Bristol: PROMPT Foundation; 2008.

19. Tucker J, Hundley V, Kiger A, *et al*. Sustainable maternity services in remote and rural Scotland? A qualitative survey of staff views on required skills, competencies and training. *Qual Saf Health Care*. 2005;14(1): 34–40.

20. Thompson S, Neal S, Clark V. Clinical risk management in obstetrics: eclampsia drills. *Qual Saf Health Care.* 2004;13(2): 127–9.

21. Crofts JF, Bartlett C, Ellis D, *et al.* Management of shoulder dystocia: skill retention 6 and 12 months after training. *Obstet Gynecol.* 2007;110(5): 1069–74.

22. Siassakos D, Draycott TJ, Crofts JF, *et al.* More to teamwork than knowledge, skill and attitude. *BJOG.* 2010;117: 1262–9.

23. Siassakos D, Fox R, Crofts JF, *et al.* The management of a simulated emergency: better teamwork, better performance. *Resuscitation.* 2011;82: 203–6.

24. Siassakos D, Bristowe K, Draycott TJ, *et al.* Clinical efficiency in a simulated emergency and relationship to team behaviours: a multisite cross-sectional study. *BJOG.* 2011;118: 596–607.

25. Bristowe K, Siassakos D, Hambly H, *et al.* Teamwork for clinical emergencies: interprofessional focus group analysis and triangulation with simulation. *Qual Health Res.* 2012;22: 1383–94.

26. NICE. *Intrapartum Care: Care of Healthy Women and their Babies during Childbirth*: NICE Clinical Guideline 190. London: NICE; 2014.

27. Salas E, Sims D, Burke S. Is there a big five in teamwork? *Small Group Res.* 2005;36(5): 555–99.

28. Cullinane M, Findlay G, Hargraves C, Lucas S. *An Acute Problem? A Report of the National Confidential Enquiry into Patient Outcome and Death.* London: NCEPOD; 2005.

29. Miller K, Riley W, Davis S. Identifying key nursing and team behaviours to achieve high reliability. *J Nurs Manag.* 2009;17(2): 247–55.

30. Muller MP, Hansel M, Stehr SN, *et al.* Six steps from head to hand: a simulator based transfer oriented psychological training to improve patient safety. *Resuscitation.* 2007;73(1): 137–43.

31. Cooper S, Kinsman L, Buykx P, *et al.* Managing the deteriorating patient in a simulated environment: nursing students' knowledge, skill and situation awareness. *J Clin Nurs.* 2010;19(15–16): 2309–18.

32. Mackintosh N, Berridge EJ, Freeth D. Supporting structures for team situation awareness and decision making: insights from four delivery suites. *J Eval Clin Pract.* 2009;15(1): 46–54.

33. Fletcher G, Flin R, McGeorge P, *et al.* Anaesthetists' non-technical skills (ANTS): evaluation of a behavioural marker system. *Br J Anaesth.* 2003;90: 580–8.

34. Yule S, Flin R, Maran N, *et al.* Surgeons' non-technical skills in the operating room: reliability testing of the NOTSS behavior rating system. *World J Surg.* 2008;32: 548–56.

35. Proctor MD, Panko M, Donovan SJ. Considerations for training team situation awareness and task performance through PC-gamer simulated multiship helicopter operations. *Int J Aviat Psychol.* 2004;14: 191–205.

36. Bower DJ, Wolkomir MS, Schubot DB. The effects of the ALSO course as an educational intervention for residents: Advanced Life Support in Obstetrics. *Family Med.* 1997;29(3): 187–93.

37. Birch L, Jones N, Doyle PM, *et al.* Obstetric skills drills: evaluation of teaching methods. *Nurse Educ Today.* 2007;27(8): 915–22.

38. Siassakos D, Fox R, Hunt L, *et al.* Attitudes toward safety and teamwork in a maternity unit with embedded team training. *Am J Med Qual.* 2011;26: 132–7.

39. Morgan PJ, Pittini R, Regehr G, Marrs C, Haley MF. Evaluating teamwork in a simulated obstetric environment. *Anesthesiology.* 2007;106(5): 907–15.

40. Siassakos D, Bristowe K, Hambly H, *et al.* Team communication with patient actors: findings from a multisite simulation study. *Simul Healthc.* 2011;6: 143–9.

41. Draycott T, Sibanda T, Owen L, *et al.* Does training in obstetric emergencies improve neonatal outcome? *BJOG.* 2006;113(2): 177–82.

42. Draycott T. Litigation, risk management and patient safety; a new approach to old problems. Forum on Maternity and the Newborn of the Royal Society of Medicine, 2005.

43. White AA, Pichert JW, Bledsoe SH, Irwin C, Entman SS. Cause and effect analysis of closed claims in obstetrics and gynecology. *Obstet Gynecol.* 2005; 105(5): 1031–8.

44. Crofts JF, Bartlett C, Ellis D, *et al.* Patient-actor perception of care: a comparison of obstetric emergency training using manikins and patient-actors. *Qual Health Care.* 2008;17(1): 20–4.

45. Beaubien JM, Baker DP. The use of simulation for training teamwork skills in health care: how low can you go? *Qual Saf Health Care.* 2004;13: I51–I56.

46. Weinstock PH, Kappus LJ, Kleinman ME, *et al.* Toward a new paradigm in hospital-based pediatric education: the development of an onsite simulator program. *Pediatr Crit Care Med.* 2005;6(6): 635–41.

47. Mann S, Marcus R, Sachs BP. Lessons from the cockpit: how team training can reduce errors on L&D. *Contemporary Ob/Gyn.* 2006;51(1): 34.

48. NHS Litigation Authority. Clinical Negligence Scheme for Trusts: maternity standards. Criterion 4.1.1; 2006. www.nhsla.com (accessed 29 May 2006).

49. Eppich W, Howard V, Vozenilek J, Curran I. Simulation-based team training in healthcare. *Simul Healthc*. 2011;6(suppl): S14–S19.

50. Anderson ER, Black R, Brocklehurst P. Acute obstetric emergency drill in England and Wales: a survey of practice. *BJOG*. 2005;112(3): 372–5.

51. Bose P, Regan F, Paterson-Brown S. Improving the accuracy of estimated blood loss at obstetric haemorrhage using clinical reconstructions. *BJOG*. 2006;113(8): 919–24.

Chapter 31

Cerebral Palsy Arising from Events in Labour

Mariana Rei and Diogo Ayres-de-Campos

Cerebral palsy (CP) consists of a heterogeneous group of non-progressive movement and posture disorders, which may also include cognitive and sensory components. The spastic quadriplegic and dyskinetic forms are significantly associated with fetal hypoxia, but there is strong evidence indicating that intrapartum events account for only 10–20% of all CP cases, and a number of criteria need to be present to establish a possible causal relationship. The pathways leading to brain injury are very diverse and have only recently become clearer, due to advances in neuroimaging and diagnostic laboratory techniques. Further research is required to determine the effect of intrapartum fetal monitoring and obstetric interventions on the incidence of CP.

Introduction

Cerebral palsy is the most common physical disability of childhood, and consists of a heterogeneous group of non-progressive movement and posture disorders, frequently accompanied by cognitive and sensory impairments, epilepsy, nutritional deficiencies and secondary musculoskeletal lesions. It has a substantial impact on the life of the child and of family members, as well as on healthcare costs [1]. These disorders differ according to the extent and region of the brain that is affected, and consequently the clinical presentation and the severity of impairments will vary.

The earliest description of CP and related musculoskeletal disorders is attributed to the English orthopaedic surgeon William Little, who also first proposed the association between perinatal asphyxia and adverse neurological outcome [2]. The concept that intrapartum events were the leading cause of CP became widely accepted by the medical and scientific communities until, nearly a century later, large population-based studies revealed that only a minor-

ity of cases result from intrapartum fetal hypoxia/acidosis [3].

The worldwide prevalence of CP has remained stable at 2–3 per 1000 live births for more than four decades, despite remarkable improvements in obstetric and neonatal care [4]. In developing countries, approximately half of cases occur in premature infants. In industrialized countries, the prevalence of CP appears to be decreasing in premature births, but has remained stable in full-term infants. The latter account for 50–65% of cases, and tend to be more severely impaired [2].

Definition of Cerebral Palsy

Several efforts were conducted in the past to define the syndrome of motor disorders that constitutes CP. Recently, the International Executive Committee for the Definition of Cerebral Palsy proposed the following: 'Cerebral palsy describes a group of permanent disorders of the development of movement and posture, causing activity limitation, that are attributed to non-progressive disturbances that occurred in the developing fetal or infant brain. The motor disorders of CP are often accompanied by disturbances of sensation, perception, cognition, communication and behaviour, by epilepsy, and by secondary musculoskeletal problems' [5]. While the underlying abnormality of the brain is presumed to be permanent and non-progressive, there is a growing body of evidence to suggest that clinical manifestations and the severity of functional impairment can change over time.

Classification of Cerebral Palsy

Both for clinical and research purposes, CP has been classified according to different criteria: the anatomical

---

Best Practice in Labour and Delivery, Second Edition, ed. Sir Sabaratnam Arulkumaran. Published by Cambridge University Press. © Cambridge University Press 2016.

site of the brain lesion (cerebral cortex, pyramidal tract, extrapyramidal system or cerebellum); the nature of the movement disorder (spasticity, dyskinesia or ataxia); the topographical involvement of the extremities (diplegia, quadriplegia or hemiplegia); the timing of the presumed insult (prepartum, intrapartum or postnatal); and the degree of muscle tone (isotonic, hypotonic or hypertonic). Spasticity refers to the inability to relax the muscles of the extremities, with resulting limb tightness, abnormal posture and difficulty in initiating movement. Dyskinesia is divided into two categories: dystonia and choreoathetosis. In dystonia, the dominant abnormality is generalized hypertonia and extreme difficulty in coordinating movement, while in choreoathetosis, irregular, spasmodic, involuntary movements of the limbs or facial muscles are seen. Ataxia is a disorder of motor function defined by the occurrence of movements with abnormal force, rhythm and accuracy.

Clinically, the nature of the movement disorder (spasticity, dyskinesia or ataxia) and the topographical involvement of the extremities (diplegia, quadriplegia or hemiplegia) are the two most relevant aspects for classification. The traditional classification of 'spastic CP' takes into account the topographical involvement of the motor disorder, and includes spastic diplegia (bilateral spasticity with lower limbs more affected than the upper limbs), hemiplegia (unilateral spasticity of the body) or quadriplegia (bilateral spasticity with arm involvement equal to or greater than the leg). However, the inter-rater reliability of this topographic classification is poor, and a simpler version was proposed by the European Surveillance of Cerebral Palsy network, which became widely adopted. This classification divides CP into the categories: unilateral spastic, bilateral spastic, dystonic, choreoathetoid and ataxic [6].

The 'spastic quadriplegic' and 'dyskinetic' forms of CP are the most strongly associated with fetal hypoxia/acidosis occurring during labour. 'Spastic quadriplegic' (Figure 31.1) is one of the most severe forms of CP, affecting the ability to relax the muscles of all the limbs. Described in ~90% of cases in very low birth weight children, it is associated with parasagittal brain injury to the periventricular and subcortical white matter – periventricular leukomalacia (Figures 31.2, 31.3), arising from intermittent reductions in fetal oxygenation occurring over a period of at least one hour (as occurs with excessive uterine activity, cord compression or recurrent reductions in mater-

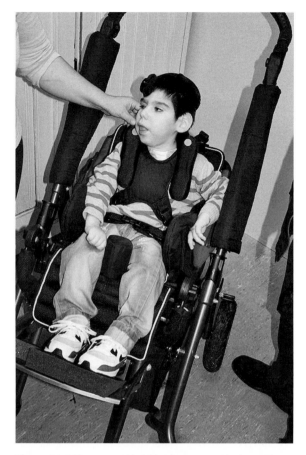

Figure 31.1 Three-year-old child with spastic quadriplegic CP (with kind permission from the parents).

nal oxygenation). 'Dyskinetic CP' typically affects term infants and arises from an acute and severe reduction in fetal oxygenation (as occurs with umbilical cord prolapse, major placental abruption, maternal cardiovascular collapse or uterine rupture). This disorder is consequent to selective neuronal necrosis of the hippocampus, thalamus, basal ganglia, reticular formation, and Purkinje cells of the cerebellum, leading to marble-like lesions, known as 'status marmoratus', on neonatal brain magnetic resonance imaging (MRI) (Figure 31.4).

Individuals with CP, particularly in its most severe forms, frequently have associated neurological abnormalities, namely intellectual disabilities in ~50% of cases, epilepsy in 25–45%, speech and language disorders in 40%, visual deficits in 40% and hearing impairments in 10–20% [7]. Neurodevelopmental disorders are also common, and features of the autism spectrum disorder may appear in up to 7% of

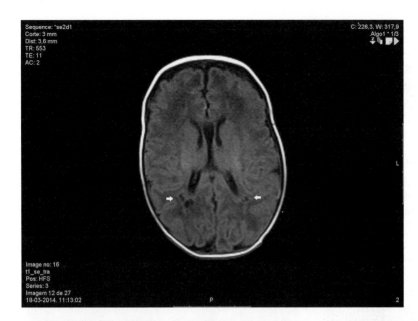

Figure 31.2 MRI showing cystic periventricular leukomalacia (arrows) (courtesy of Dr Carina Reis, Neuroradiology Department, S. Joao Hospital, Porto, Portugal).

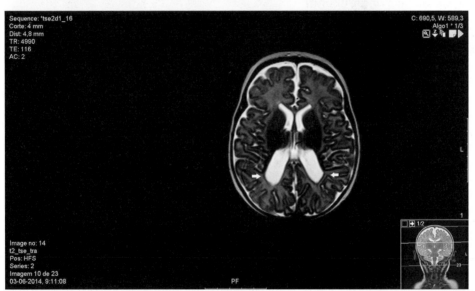

Figure 31.3 MRI showing subcortical white matter injury, enlargement and irregularity of the ventricular walls (arrows), suggesting periventricular leukomalacia (courtesy of Dr Carina Reis, Neuroradiology Department, S. Joao Hospital, Porto, Portugal).

children. Other organs and systems that may be affected are the somatosensory (stereognosis and proprioception impairments), genitourinary (dysfunctional voiding and a high rate of urinary infections), gastrointestinal (dysphagia, oesophageal and bowel dismotility), endocrine (growth failure and osteopenia) and musculoskeletal (subluxation, progressive dysplasia of the hip, foot deformities and scoliosis). Chronic pulmonary disease is a leading cause of

death, due to recurrent pneumonia caused by gastro-oesophageal reflux, palatopharyngeal in-coordination and aspiration of gastric content, as well as to restrictive lung disease related to scoliosis.

In an attempt to establish an accurate, reliable and standardized classification of the severity of CP, Palisano *et al.* developed the Gross Motor Function Classification System, based on the child's gross motor and functional disabilities established by the International

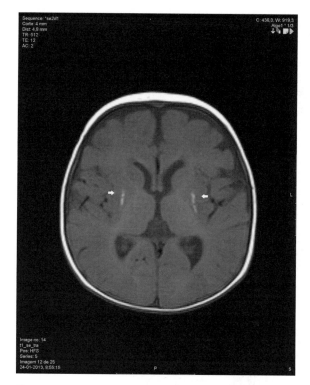

Figure 31.4 MRI showing lesions of the basal ganglia – lenticular nucleous (arrows), (courtesy of Dr Carina Reis, Neuroradiology Department, S. Joao Hospital, Porto, Portugal).

Classification of Impairments, Disabilities and Handicaps [8]. It comprises five levels of dysfunction, according to four different age groups. This classification presents a high inter-rater reliability (particularly after the age of two years) and has been successfully implemented in a variety of settings, including clinical care, research and healthcare administration [9]. Several complementary tools have also been developed to assess fine motor function, such as the ABILHAND-Kids, the Bimanual Fine Motor Function classification and the Manual Ability Classification System [2].

Diagnosis of Cerebral Palsy

Although CP is a static, non-progressive disorder, its clinical expression may evolve as the nervous system matures [10]. Due to the transitory nature of some abnormalities and the low inter-observer agreement associated with their evaluation, a definitive diagnosis usually requires repeated observations and should be deferred until later infancy, particularly in preterm infants. Isolated abnormalities may resolve progressively after nine months of age, spasticity may not

be apparent until six months of age and dyskinetic patterns are typically identified only after 18 months. Despite some disagreement as to the age required for an accurate diagnosis, 36 months usually allows a reliable assessment of motor capacity, in contrast to the false-positive diagnoses that may occur before 18 months of age [11].

CP is a diagnosis of exclusion, so atypical neurological signs should raise the possibility of alternative conditions, including neurodegenerative diseases, inborn errors of metabolism, congenital brain and spinal cord malformations, traumatic lesions, neuromuscular/movement disorders and neoplasms.

Neuroimaging methods do not establish a definite diagnosis of CP, but have been used for early prediction of the disease and for excluding other entities (see below). Neurological, neuromotor and neurophysiological tests have also been used with the same purpose. Among the neuromotor assessment tools assisting in the early diagnosis of CP are the General Movement Assessment, with an estimated sensitivity of 98% (95% CI 74–100%) and specificity of 91% (95% CI 83–93%), the standardized Lacey Assessment of Preterm Infants and the Hammersmith Infant Neurologic Examination.

Pathogenesis and Risk Factors

Cerebral palsy has been linked to a wide range of antenatal, intrapartum and postnatal factors that most likely act along the common pathogenic pathways of hypoxia/acidosis, inflammation and neurodevelopmental abnormalities.

The most commonly reported risk factors for CP are prematurity, low birth weight, intrapartum hypoxia/acidosis, chorioamnionitis, central nervous system malformations, intrapartum fever, multiple gestations, coagulation disorders, ischaemic stroke, maternal thyroid disease, obesity and placental pathology [3,12–14].

Prematurity arises as the single most important risk factor for CP, with a magnitude of risk that is inversely correlated with gestational age and birth weight. The prevalence of CP varies from 90 cases per 1000 neonatal survivors of less than 1000 g, to 1.5 cases per 1000 neonatal survivors weighing more than 2500 g [1]. A recent systematic review of 49 studies reported the highest prevalence in neonates weighing 1000–1499 g (59.2 per 1000 live births; 95% CI 53.06–66.01) and in those born before 28 weeks' gestation

(111.8 per 1000 live births; 95% CI 69.53–179.78) [15]. A strong association was also found between multiple gestation and CP, and although birth weight and gestational age are obvious confounders, an independent four-fold increase in risk was reported in a large study evaluating different populations [16].

A substantial body of evidence indicates that a hostile inflammatory environment is another pathogenic pathway leading to CP. Funisitis, increased cytokine levels in amniotic fluid and in fetal blood have all been associated with white matter injury [17]. Maternal bacteriuria (OR 4.7, 95% CI 1.5–15.2) and antibiotic treatment during pregnancy (OR 6.3, 95% CI 3.0–15.2) are independently associated with an increased risk of spastic hemiplegia, and less pronouncedly with diplegia and tetraplegia [18]. A recent systematic review reported a significant association between clinical and histological chorioamnionitis and CP, with pooled odds ratios of 2.42 (95% CI 1.52–3.84) and 1.83 (95% CI 1.17–2.89) respectively. However, there is no robust evidence to suggest that identification and treatment of these infections will alter the course of the disease [19].

Recent data also support the contribution of multiple genetic factors to the aetiology of CP. The prevalence of congenital anomalies in individuals with CP (11–32%) is significantly higher than in the general population (2–3%). Several single-gene Mendelian disorders, inherited as autosomal dominant, autosomal recessive or X-linked, often present with clinical features similar to CP. Many of these gene disorders appear to be responsible for other neurodevelopmental disorders such as autism, attention deficit disorder, intellectual impairment and epilepsy. Despite the growing body of evidence for the genomic causes of CP, in many countries comprehensive genetic testing is still not offered as part of the diagnostic investigation in affected individuals.

Intrapartum hypoxia/acidosis is perhaps the most studied risk factor for CP, with the clear limitation that an agreed set of criteria to define the former entity has not existed. Nevertheless, even with previously existing markers, several large population-based studies, conducted over different time frames and in different populations, have led to the widely accepted conclusion that intrapartum hypoxia/acidosis accounts for only 10–20% of CP cases [1,20–22]. Many intrapartum events have been associated with CP, including instrumental vaginal delivery, caesarean section (CS) and breech delivery [14]. Other related factors are meconium-stained amniotic fluid, meconium aspiration, severe placental vascular lesions, placental abruption and cord prolapse. On the other hand, a recent meta-analysis including a total of 3810 participants found no association between the use of elective caesarean delivery and CP. An increased risk of CP (OR 2.17, 95% CI 1.58–2.98) was found in emergency CSs, although the indication leading to surgery is a likely confounder [23]. Low five minute Apgar scores, seizures, respiratory distress syndrome, hypoglycaemia, jaundice, hyperbilirubinaemia, neonatal sepsis and meningitis have all been reported as neonatal risk factors for CP [13,14]. Perinatal stroke has been the focus of many studies and is correlated with other antenatal and perinatal risk factors for CP, such as intrauterine growth restriction, pre-eclampsia, infection and thrombophilia, although the evidence regarding the latter remains controversial [13].

Consaguinity, rhesus isoimmunization, iodine deficiency and maternal infections due to rubella and cytomegalovirus have also been associated with neurodevelopment abnormalities and CP [1].

Cerebral Palsy Arising from Events in Labour

The multidisciplinary International Cerebral Palsy Task Force published a consensus statement in 1999 defining the criteria necessary to establish a link between intrapartum hypoxia/acidosis and CP [24]. The subject was also analysed in 2003 by the American College of Obstetricians and Gynecologists (ACOG) together with the American Academy of Pediatricians (AAP). More recently, FIGO published its revised consensus on intrapartum fetal monitoring where the causal relationship between hypoxia/acidosis and CP is also evaluated [22,24,25]. There is a general agreement that a number of findings are necessary to implicate intrapartum hypoxia/acidosis as the possible cause of CP in term infants (Table 31.1).

The application of the ACOG/AAP 2003 criteria was retrospectively evaluated by Phelan and coworkers in 39 neonates with permanent neurologic impairment. Three or more of the essential criteria were met in 94% of cases. Umbilical artery pH below 7.00 was found in 97% of cases, base deficit equal or above 12 mmol/l in 100%, moderate or severe encephalopathy in 97%, spastic quadriplegic or dyskinetic cerebral

Table 31.1 Criteria needed to implicate intrapartum hypoxia/acidosis as a possible cause of CP in term infants, FIGO 2015 [22,24,25]

1. *Metabolic acidosis* in umbilical artery blood or in newborn circulation during the first minutes of life (pH <7.00 and base deficit ≥12 mmol/l or lactate ≥10 mmol/l)
2. *Low Apgar scores* at one and five minutes
3. *Early onset hypoxic-ischaemic encephalopathy* grade 2 or 3
4. *Early imaging studies suggestive* of an acute and non-focal cerebral anomaly
5. *Spastic quadriplegic or dyskinetic* cerebral palsy
6. *Exclusion of other identifiable aetiologies* such as birth trauma, coagulation disorders, infection and genetic disorders

palsy or death attributable to brain injury in 94%. None of these neonates had any other identifiable aetiologies for their CP [26].

No currently available clinical procedure, including continuous cardiotocographic (CTG) monitoring during labour or increased CS rates, has been shown to reduce the risk of CP in term infants. Continuous intrapartum CTG was compared with intermittent auscultation in several randomized trials carried out before 1993 [27]. While it was associated with a 50% reduction in neonatal seizures, no effect was evident in the incidence of CP or perinatal mortality, but the studies were clearly underpowered to show a difference in these rare outcomes. Moreover, the technology has evolved since that time, so the existing evidence comparing continuous CTG with intermittent auscultation regarding the incidence of CP is scientifically inconclusive.

Hypoxic-ischaemic Encephalopathy

Although there is no universally accepted definition, neonatal encephalopathy is a clinical syndrome of near-term neonates that manifests with an abnormal level of consciousness, or seizures, difficulty with initiating and maintaining breathing and a depression of tone and reflexes [28]. It occurs in about 3 per 1000 term live births [29] and is considered the strongest clinical predictor for the occurrence of CP.

Hypoxic-ischaemic encephalopathy (HIE) is a form of neonatal encephalopathy that is caused by intrapartum hypoxia/acidosis, and has an estimated incidence of 1.5 per 1000 live births [29]. Since there are multiple non-hypoxic causes for neonatal encephalopathy, in order to establish the diagnosis of HIE it is necessary to document the occurrence of metabolic acidosis in umbilical cord blood or in the newborn circulation during the first minutes of life [30], together with low Apgar scores and early imag-

ing evidence of cerebral oedema. It is not infrequent for there to be some uncertainty as to the exact cause of neonatal encephalopathy.

According to the Sarnat & Sarnat classification, three grades of HIE are distinguished: grade 1 is characterized by hyperalertness, irritability, jitteriness and a normal electroencephalogram; grade 2 is characterized by obtundation, hypotonia, strong distal flexion, occasional multifocal seizures and has a 20–30% risk of death or major neurological sequelae such as CP; grade 3 is associated with coma, and in the majority of cases there is neonatal death or long-term neurological sequelae such as CP [31]. In a recent systematic review, 14.5% of HIE cases were reported to develop CP [21]. The co-existence of multisystem organ failure, including renal, hepatic, haematologic, cardiac, metabolic and gastrointestinal functions, is frequent in HIE, but the severity of neurological injury does not necessarily correlate with the involvement of other systems.

Similarly to CP, an estimated 70% of cases of neonatal encephalopathy is thought to be consequent to events arising before the onset of labour [22], and less than 10% due to postnatal complications such as severe respiratory distress, sepsis and shock [32]. Most of the remaining cases are due to intrapartum hypoxia/acidosis, but their incidence varies according to the healthcare setting. Hypoxia/acidosis can also occur during pregnancy and in the postnatal period and cause neonatal encephalopathy, but these situations will not display metabolic acidosis at birth. The occurrence of clinical 'sentinel events' may help to differentiate between a prenatal and an intrapartum event, namely when there is documentation of prolonged maternal hypotension, maternal cardiovascular collapse, ruptured vasa praevia, massive feto-maternal haemorrhage, uterine rupture, major placental abruption, umbilical cord prolapse, shoulder dystocia and retention of the after-coming head.

A CTG tracing acquired in the beginning of labour may also help to determine the timing of damage. Reduced variability and absence of accelerations lasting 50 min or more suggests the possibility of a previously damaged fetus, while a normal tracing that later on becomes pathological is more likely to be associated with an intrapartum event [25].

Neuroimaging

Neonatal cranial ultrasound can identify some of the brain lesions associated with subsequent development of CP, including intraventricular haemorrhage, periventricular leukomalacia and haemorrhagic infarction, but more recent methods, such as MRI, magnetic resonance spectroscopy (MRS) and diffusion-weighted MRI, are more helpful in establishing the cause of neonatal encephalopathy and identifying patterns that are strongly predictive of CP [32].

MRI obtained between 24 and 96 hours of life appears to be more sensitive in defining the timing of hypoxic injury, whereas MRI undertaken between 7 days and 21 days (ideally at 10 days) will be more accurate in delineating the full extent of brain injury [28]. Early cerebral oedema, with or without intracerebral haemorrhage, suggests an event that occurred in the last 6–12 hours and usually clears by four days [24]. Diffusion-weighted MRI identifies early injury due to its ability to detect subtle changes in water content [32]. With respect to the prediction of CP, a recent meta-analysis reported that MRI in the late perinatal period has a sensitivity ranging from 86% to 100% and a specificity ranging from 89% to 97% [11]. Two typical patterns of brain lesion have been documented in association with fetal hypoxia/acidosis:

1. Parasagittal brain injury to the periventricular and subcortical white matter – periventricular leukomalacia (Figures 31.2, 31.3) occurs mainly in premature children exposed to intermittent reductions in fetal oxygenation over a period of at least one hour. Moderate and severe cases are associated with a high risk of 'spastic quadriplegic' CP (Figure 31.1), as well as cognitive, psychomotor and neurosensory impairment.
2. Grey matter lesions of the basal ganglia, thalamus, hippocampus, reticular formation and cerebellum (Figure 31.4) occur in full-term infants undergoing acute and severe hypoxia [33]. 'Dyskinetic CP' typically affects these infants.

Multicystic encephalopathy is observed in a minority of newborns, and is frequently followed by an unexpectedly severe encephalopathy, but the hypoxia/acidosis aetiology is uncertain in these cases, as it may be affected by underlying fetal infections or metabolic disorders. Other patterns of brain injury, such as focal arterial or venous infarction, and focal intraparenchymal or intraventricular haemorrhage, are unlikely to be related to peripartum hypoxia/acidosis, and genetic, coagulation and/or metabolic screening tests should be considered in their presence. Neuroimaging findings of unilateral infarction suggest a prothrombotic coagulation disorder and should prompt a screen for coagulation abnormalities. It is important to realize that, despite recent advances in neuroimaging, the ability to correctly predict the occurrence of CP is still limited, as positive and negative predictive values are still modest.

Antenatal Approaches to the Prevention of Cerebral Palsy

Potentially modifiable antenatal risk factors for CP include the management of maternal thyroid disease, prevention of preterm birth (see below), prevention of rubella and cytomegalovirus infection, prevention of Rhesus isoimmunization, diagnosis and treatment of intrauterine infections, prenatal diagnosis of fetal malformations and genetic disorders, avoidance of consanguinity, limiting multiple gestations by reducing the number of embryos transferred in assisted reproduction techniques and control of obesity. In some countries improvements in nutrition also play an important role.

A high level of evidence supports the preventive strategies for preterm birth, which includes smoking cessation and reducing alcohol consumption, screening and treating asymptomatic bacteriuria, aspirin to reduce the incidence of pre-eclampsia in high-risk cases, progesterone and/or cervical cerclage for women with previous preterm labour and short cervix [34]. Prophylactic use of antibiotics for women with preterm rupture of membranes has been shown to reduce the incidence of chorioamnionitis, neonatal infection and abnormal cerebral ultrasound on discharge [35]. There are, however, insufficient data regarding an effect on perinatal mortality and CP.

More recently, there is increasing evidence that antenatal administration of magnesium sulphate to women at risk of preterm labour reduces the incidence and severity of CP and protects gross motor function, particularly in early gestational ages, without adverse long-term fetal or maternal outcome [36].

As previously mentioned, the effect of intrapartum fetal monitoring or any other intrapartum procedure on the rates of CP is inconclusive. Further research is needed to determine the effect of CTG as currently performed, as well as new technologies such as computerized CTG analysis and fetal eletrocardiography. It is possible that, because intrapartum hypoxia/acidosis accounts for such a low percentage of CP cases, even the most accurate technologies may not have a major impact on overall incidence. On the other hand, the acute nature of certain intrapartum events, such as placental abruption, uterine rupture, cord prolapse, shoulder dystocia and retention of the after-coming head, should lead to the emphasis being placed more on adequate management of these situations. Simulation-based training of healthcare teams in management of these rare phenomena has been shown to reduce adverse obstetric outcomes, such as low Apgar scores and HIE [37], but its effect on perinatal mortality and CP needs to be evaluated in adequately sized studies.

Acknowledgements

The authors would like to thank Dr Ana Vilan from the Department of Neonatology at the S. Joao Hospital in Porto for her review of the manuscript.

References

1. Colver A, Fairhurst C, Pharoah PO. Cerebral palsy. *Lancet.* 2014;383(9924): 1240–9.

2. O'Shea M. Cerebral palsy. *Semin Perinatol.* 2008;32(1): 35–41.

3. Moreno-De-Luca A, Ledbetter DH, Martin CL. Genetic [corrected] insights into the causes and classification of [corrected] cerebral palsies. *Lancet Neurol.* 2012;11(3): 283–92.

4. Clark SL, Hankins GD. Temporal and demographic trends in cerebral palsy: fact and fiction. *Am J Obstet Gynecol.* 2003;188(3): 628–33.

5. Rosenbaum P, Paneth N, Leviton A, et al. A report: the definition and classification of cerebral palsy April 2006. *Dev Med Child Neurol.* 2007;109(suppl.): 8–14.

6. Surveillance of Cerebral Palsy in Europe. Surveillance of cerebral palsy in Europe: a collaboration of cerebral palsy surveys and registers. *Dev Med Child Neurol.* 2000;42(12): 816–24.

7. Novak I, Hines M, Goldsmith S, Barclay R. Clinical prognostic messages from a systematic review on cerebral palsy. *Pediatrics.* 2012;130(5):e1285–312.

8. Palisano R, Rosenbaum P, Walter S, et al. Development and reliability of a system to classify gross motor function in children with cerebral palsy. *Dev Med Child Neurol.* 1997;39(4): 214–23.

9. O'Shea TM. Diagnosis, treatment, and prevention of cerebral palsy. *Clinical Obstet Gynecol.* 2008;51(4): 816–28.

10. Hadders-Algra M. Early diagnosis and early intervention in cerebral palsy. *Front Neurol.* 2014;5: 185.

11. Bosanquet M, Copeland L, Ware R, Boyd R. A systematic review of tests to predict cerebral palsy in young children. *Dev Med Child Neurol.* 2013;55(5): 418–26.

12. Nelson KB. Causative factors in cerebral palsy. *Clinical Obstet Gynecol.* 2008;51(4): 749–62.

13. Himmelmann K, Ahlin K, Jacobsson B, Cans C, Thorsen P. Risk factors for cerebral palsy in children born at term. *Acta Obstet Gynecol Scand.* 2011;90(10): 1070–81.

14. McIntyre S, Taitz D, Keogh J, et al. A systematic review of risk factors for cerebral palsy in children born at term in developed countries. *Dev Med Child Neurol.* 2013;55(6): 499–508.

15. Oskoui M, Coutinho F, Dykeman J, Jette N, Pringsheim T. An update on the prevalence of cerebral palsy: a systematic review and meta-analysis. *Dev Med Child Neurol.* 2013;55(6): 509–19.

16. Scher AI, Petterson B, Blair E, et al. The risk of mortality or cerebral palsy in twins: a collaborative population-based study. *Pediatr Res.* 2002;52(5): 671–81.

17. Yoon BH, Jun JK, Romero R, et al. Amniotic fluid inflammatory cytokines (interleukin-6, interleukin-1beta, and tumor necrosis factor-alpha), neonatal brain white matter lesions, and cerebral palsy. *Am J Obstet Gynecol.* 1997;177(1): 19–26.

18. Ahlin K, Himmelmann K, Hagberg G, et al. Cerebral palsy and perinatal infection in children born at term. *Obstet Gynecol.* 2013;122(1): 41–9.

19. Shatrov JG, Birch SC, Lam LT, et al. Chorioamnionitis and cerebral palsy: a meta-analysis. *Obstet Gynecol.* 2010;116(2 Pt 1): 387–92.

20. Nelson KB, Ellenberg JH. Antecedents of cerebral palsy: multivariate analysis of risk. *N Eng J Med.* 1986;315(2): 81–6.

21. Graham EM, Ruis KA, Hartman AL, Northington FJ, Fox HE. A systematic review of the role of intrapartum hypoxia-ischemia in the causation of neonatal encephalopathy. *Am J Obstet Gynecol.* 2008;199(6): 587–95.

22. American College of Gynecologists. Neonatal encephalopathy and cerebral palsy: executive summary. *Obstet Gynecol.* 2004;103(4): 780–1.

23. O'Callaghan M, MacLennan A. Cesarean delivery and cerebral palsy: a systematic review and meta-analysis. *Obstet Gynecol.* 2013;122(6): 1169–75.

24. MacLennan A. A template for defining a causal relation between acute intrapartum events and cerebral palsy: international consensus statement. *BMJ.* 1999;319(7216): 1054–9.

25. Ayres-de-Campos D, Spong KY, Chandraharan E, *et al.* FIGO consensus guidelines on intrapartum fetal monitoring: cardiotocography. *IJGO.* 2015;131(1): 13–24.

26. Phelan JP, Korst LM, Martin GI. Application of criteria developed by the Task Force on Neonatal Encephalopathy and Cerebral Palsy to acutely asphyxiated neonates. *Obstet Gynecol.* 2011;118(4): 824–30.

27. Alfirevic Z, Devane D, Gyte GM. Continuous cardiotocography (CTG) as a form of electronic fetal monitoring (EFM) for fetal assessment during labour. *Cochrane Database Syst Rev.* 2013;5: CD006066.

28. American College of Obstetricians and Gynecologists. Executive summary: neonatal encephalopathy and neurologic outcome, second edition. Report of the American College of Obstetricians and Gynecologists' Task Force on Neonatal Encephalopathy. *Obstet Gynecol.* 2014;123(4): 896–901.

29. Kurinczuk JJ, White-Koning M, Badawi N. Epidemiology of neonatal encephalopathy and hypoxic-ischaemic encephalopathy. *Early Hum Dev.* 2010;86(6): 329–38.

30. Hankins GD, Speer M. Defining the pathogenesis and pathophysiology of neonatal encephalopathy and cerebral palsy. *Obstet Gynecol.* 2003;102(3): 628–36.

31. Sarnat HB, Sarnat MS. Neonatal encephalopathy following fetal distress: a clinical and electroencephalographic study. *Arch Neurol.* 1976;33(10): 696–705.

32. Ferriero DM. Neonatal brain injury. *N Eng J Med.* 2004;351(19): 1985–95.

33. Woodward LJ, Anderson PJ, Austin NC, Howard K, Inder TE. Neonatal MRI to predict neurodevelopmental outcomes in preterm infants. *N Eng J Med.* 2006;355(7): 685–94.

34. Iams JD, Romero R, Culhane JF, Goldenberg RL. Primary, secondary, and tertiary interventions to reduce the morbidity and mortality of preterm birth. *Lancet.* 2008;371(9607): 164–75.

35. Kenyon S, Boulvain M, Neilson JP. Antibiotics for preterm rupture of membranes. *Cochrane Database Syst Rev.* 2013;12: CD001058.

36. Doyle LW, Crowther CA, Middleton P, Marret S, Rouse D. Magnesium sulphate for women at risk of preterm birth for neuroprotection of the fetus. *Cochrane Database Syst Rev.* 2009;1: CD004661.

37. Draycott T, Sibanda T, Owen L, *et al.* Does training in obstetric emergencies improve neonatal outcome? *BJOG.* 2006;113(2): 177–82.

Chapter 32

Objective Structured Assessment of Technical Skills (OSATS) in Obstetrics

Melissa Whitten

Background

The use of the Objective Structured Assessment of Technical Skills (OSATS) tool within obstetrics and gynaecology training has become established since the early 1990s, when Winckel *et al.* demonstrated a form of objective structured assessment which could be developed for use in the operating theatre environment, with good construct validity and inter-rater reliability [1]. Within the UK, introduction of shift working patterns as part of the implementation strategies for the reduction of junior doctor working hours as part of the European Working Time Directive meant that a change in the format of assessment of surgical competence was needed to enable junior doctors to have their competency assessed by a large number of different assessors [2].

The Royal College of Obstetricians and Gynaecologists (RCOG) introduced the widespread use of OSATS within UK training in August 2007, as part of their competency-based Specialty Training Curriculum, developed as part of implementation of the Modernising Medical Careers programme [3,4]. The curriculum is competency-based, with an anticipated training time of seven years to achieve competency as a fully independent practitioner. Training is divided into three phases: basic, intermediate and advanced, with indicative targets regarding the expected acquisition of skills at each stage of training framed within a modular curriculum (Figure 32.1). Each module of the curriculum has specific training targets, and the final level of competence is reached in stages (levels 1–3) [5].

Basic training incorporates the first two years of specialty training, and requires the trainee to develop and demonstrate, among other targets of training, technical competence in a number of surgical procedures, before being able to progress to the next stage of training. Trainees will usually spend a year in two different training units during basic training, within a defined region of training, and once competency is achieved for these key surgical procedures, would be expected to demonstrate continued competency alongside development of more complex technical and clinical skills as their training progresses across other units in the region. OSATS are one of a number of workplace-based assessment (WPBA) formats used to evaluate progression throughout specialty training, aiming to link teaching, learning and assessment in a structured way.

How do OSATS Fit into the RCOG Training Curriculum?

There are three types of WPBA used in O&G training:

1. OSATS (objective structured assessment of technical skills);
2. Mini-CEX (mini-clinical evaluation exercise); and
3. CBD (case-based discussion).

Within the core curriculum, OSATS are expected to be carried out on a number of surgical procedures felt to be fundamental to the practice of O&G:

- diagnostic laparoscopy;
- diagnostic hysteroscopy;
- fetal blood sampling;
- manual removal of placenta;
- opening and closing the abdomen;
- operative laparoscopy;
- operative vaginal delivery;
- caesarean section;
- perineal repair; and
- uterine evacuation.

Best Practice in Labour and Delivery, Second Edition, ed. Sir Sabaratnam Arulkumaran. Published by Cambridge University Press. © Cambridge University Press 2016.

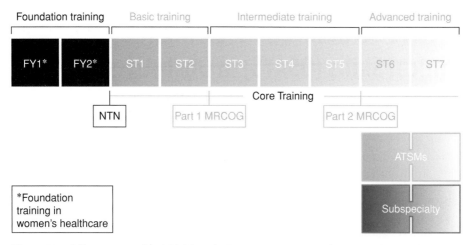

Figure 32.1 Different stages of the RCOG Specialty Training Programme in obstetrics and gynaecology. Reproduced with permission from the RCOG.

For all procedures, trainees are expected to gain competence during their first two years of basic training, and then to continue providing evidence of competence and progression onto more complex cases as they progress through their intermediate and advanced training years. A Matrix of Educational Progression provides guidance to trainees about how many of each procedure are expected to be completed each year [6] to demonstrate development and acquisition of competence and evidence of progression for their trainers and training programme leads. Although it is recognized that within a competency-based curriculum trainees will progress at different rates, the competency levels are the minimum that trainees must achieve before moving to the next stage of training.

In addition to the set requirements outlined above, a generic OSATS form exists to enable trainees to collate evidence of experience and competence for other surgical procedures which they undertake during their training, e.g. cervical cerclage, caesarean hysterectomy.

OSATS Requirements

In order for the OSATS process to be formalized further within the curriculum, several key requirements have been determined by the Specialty Education and Assessment Committee of the RCOG to guide trainees undertaking specialty training, and their trainers:

- The trainee must declare in advance whether an OSATS is summative or formative and there must always be a distinction between the two.

- At least two different assessors must be used for each type of OSATS procedure. The same assessor must not be used for all OSATS and a consultant must do at least one of the assessments for any one procedure.
- The trainee must retain all OSATS forms in their e-Portfolio, whether they were completed satisfactorily or not – in order to enable their educational supervisor to review progress effectively.
- Before a competence can be signed off as 'fully competent for independent practice' in the logbook, each OSATS must have been successfully completed (i.e. every box ticked for independent practice) on at least *three* separate occasions.
- Once the trainee is signed off as fully competent for independent practice for a particular skill, they should undergo an annual OSATS assessment (one per procedure) to demonstrate continued competence until they achieve their Certification of Completion of Training (CCT).
- Trainees must also keep count of the number of each procedure they perform annually until they achieve CCT.

Undertaking an OSATS

When a trainee feels ready to undertake an OSATS, they will be expected to discuss and agree being assessed with a clinical supervisor, who will:

- assess the procedure; and
- complete the OSATS form on the e-Portfolio.

The trainee will need to declare whether they wish the assessment to be a formative or summative process before the start of the procedure in order that the clinical supervisor is able to determine their expectations for performance. Clinical supervisors can be any health professional who is able to carry out the procedure independently themselves. Typically, clinical supervisors will be consultants or trainees at a more senior level than the trainee being assessed, but can include midwives (for example, for assessment of perineal repair competence) and clinical nurse specialists (for some gynaecological procedures). Most trainees will have a wide number of clinical supervisors taking part in their assessment of competence during their training, with the overall assessment of competence during the year being overseen by their dedicated educational supervisor. On completion of the required number of summative OSATS needed to be 'signed off' for that competence in the logbook, the trainee can request that a clinical supervisor, or their educational supervisor, records the date that each OSATS is signed off.

Formative vs. Summative Assessment

OSATS can be carried out as either a formative or summative form of assessment:

- Formative (assessments for learning) are used as an opportunity to practise a skill and to provide feedback for further development of skills.
- Summative (assessments of learning) are used to enable the trainee to demonstrate competence in a given clinical situation.

Trainees are required to undertake both formative and summative OSATS in order to provide evidence of progression of skills acquisition. This model was reinforced in the RCOG curriculum update of August 2014 with the introduction of specific and separate formative and summative completion forms. Trainees are advised to take as many formative OSATS as they feel they need in order to feel sufficiently competent in a procedure *before* requesting a summative OSATS. Before competences can be signed off in the trainee logbook, each OSATS must be completed as a summative process, in full, on at least *three* separate occasions.

The Formative Assessment

Before starting the procedure, the trainee and assessor determine what the procedure is, establish the clinical details of the case and the level of complexity which is expected to exist. The assessor then observes the trainee undertaking the procedure, considering a number of technical and non-technical skills (not an exhaustive list) during the observation:

- checking of equipment/environment;
- communication with patients and/or relatives;
- perioperative planning, e.g. positioning;
- use of assistants;
- technical ability;
- communication with staff;
- selection of instruments and equipment;
- forward planning;
- economy of movement;
- dealing with problems and/or difficulties;
- tissue handling;
- documentation;
- completion of task as appropriate; and
- safety considerations.

The assessor then provides specific, constructive verbal and written feedback to the trainee around their performance, focusing upon:

- what went well;
- what could have gone better; and
- a learning plan for the future.

The trainee is expected to complete a reflection about their learning from the event in order to reinforce a process of reflective learning for future development. For formative assessments, there is no overall judgement on competence – this is assessed summatively once the trainee feels ready to be assessed for competence acquisition.

Written feedback is entered by the assessor into the trainee's e-Portfolio, the online training portfolio onto which all training and assessment evidence is collated for trainees registered in a Specialty Training Programme. The trainee, their educational supervisor, college tutor and the regional training programme directors, will be able to view individual assessment forms and collation of evidence gathered on the e-Portfolio. This is used to assess the trainee against the Matrix of Training as he or she progresses through each year of training. For doctors who are not part of the Specialty Training Programme within a region, it is still recommended to register with the RCOG for online e-Portfolio access to enable coordinated collation of competence progression and acquisition for appraisal and revalidation purposes. For doctors who are not registered on e-Portfolio, the OSATS forms may be downloaded and inserted into a hard-copy portfolio.

The discussion between assessor and trainee about the formative OSATS procedure should take place as quickly as possible after the event, with written feedback being carried out as soon as is feasible, in order that the contemporaneous nature of the discussion is captured effectively.

The Summative Assessment

The summative OSATS is an assessment of performance (AoP) and is a *mandatory*, *summative* tool designed to:

1. enable judgement of surgical competency in the procedure being assessed; and
2. provide specific, constructive feedback to the trainee about their performance.

There is a judgement to be made in each assessment relating to the overall performance observed: *competent* or *working towards competence*. Trainees require a minimum of three procedures deemed competent per core procedure, by more than one assessor, including a consultant or post-CCT holder. For an assessor, the judgement of competence which they make as part of a summative OSATS is specific to that assessment only.

As for formative assessments, the trainee should agree with the assessor beforehand that they are willing and able to carry out an assessment for the procedure, and should specify that the assessment is to be summative in nature. The clinical details and complexity of the procedure need to be detailed in the assessment form, and the assessor needs to indicate whether the procedure falls into the basic, intermediate or advanced section of the curriculum.

The summative OSATS template provides a number of anchor statements to guide assessors in their determination of competence for a particular procedure [7]:

- For the trainee considered *competent* in the observed procedure it would generally be expected that the trainee was able to perform all aspects of the procedure safely and competently with no or minimal need for help, or in the context of an unexpectedly difficult case, may have needed more assistance for the more difficult aspects of the procedure.

- For the trainee considered to be *working towards competence* it would generally be expected that the trainee required significant help throughout or with the majority of steps, or that the trainee was unable to perform any of the necessary procedures to be safe and competent at this stage.

The assessor is directed to consider technical and non-technical skills in determining their assessment of the trainee (using the same list as for formative OSATS). The assessor is then asked to specify which of the following statements apply in their assessment of the procedure completed:

- This trainee performed this observed procedure competently;

or

- This trainee is working towards competence in this procedure.

As with the formative OSATS, the assessor is expected to provide verbal and subsequent written feedback to the trainee about what went well and what could have gone better, and a formulated learning plan. Even for the trainee who is determined to be competent at the procedure, or who is reaching the end of training, the concept of lifelong learning still applies, such that there should always be a learning plan for the future.

OSATS in Practice

Do OSATS work and are they practical in today's clinical learning environment? Both questions were subject to intense scrutiny as part of the original development of appropriate and fit-for-purpose workplace-based assessment tools for the Specialty Training Curriculum. Trainees and trainers who were part of the consultation groups for development of the curriculum highlighted that any new assessment method would have to be fit for purpose and practicable in a busy working environment. Little research on OSATS in the clinical environment existed prior to their development for use within obstetrics and gynaecology; however, early evidence from 'dry' clinical skills laboratory settings of formalized assessment of specific surgical techniques including hysteroscopy, episiotomy repair, laparoscopic suturing and open bladder neck suspension indicated good construct validity and inter-rater reliability [8–12], and Winckel *et al.*'s feedback from development of OSATS-like assessments in the surgical operating environment was encouraging [1].

Prior to the 2007 introduction of the RCOG Specialty Training Curriculum, Bodle *et al.* undertook a detailed investigation of trainee and trainer perceptions of the value and validity of OSATS for the assessment of surgical skills in the theatre environment as part of an RCOG-commissioned study during the development of the postgraduate training portfolio [13]. During a six-month period from October 2005 to March 2006 (during the development of plans for postgraduate training within the new curriculum), Yorkshire and Bristol deaneries piloted OSATS use for obstetrics and gynaecology. Eight-five per cent of trainee and 76% of trainer responses within this relatively small study agreed or strongly agreed that OSATS would improve trainees' surgical skills. Stronger agreement was associated with the more junior grades, perhaps reflecting these trainees' familiarity with objective methods of assessment which now feature in many medical school assessment processes. Face validity was deemed to be good, with 80% of trainee and 76% of trainer responses agreeing or strongly agreeing with the ability of OSATS to assess surgical skills. Trainees differed from trainers in their perception of the practical application of OSATS, with 26% of trainee and 46% of trainer responses agreeing or strongly agreeing that it would be time-consuming and add to the burden of administrative work. However, in terms of the potential for OSATS to be applied as part of training on a formal basis, 76% of trainee and trainer responses agreed or strongly agreed that OSATS should become part of the annual assessment process for trainees.

Following implementation of the training curriculum in late 2007, an RCOG-funded study evaluating the utility of WPBAs in obstetrics and gynaecology was undertaken [14]. Within a related piece of work carried out among 74 trainees in 2008–09 to determine the reliability of WPBAs, Homer *et al.* identified wide variations in the estimates of reliability across the forms being used at the time, and that trainees often required a higher number of assessments completed than the indicative number within the curriculum guide in order to achieve competency sign-off. In six out of nine OSATS studied within this work, at least ten forms were required by the trainee to achieve a G-coefficient of 0.8, the reliability value which, although arbitrary, is usually considered to be an acceptable cut-off value within medical education literature [15,16].

Perineal repair was found to be the procedure requiring the least number of assessments to be 'signed off', while manual removal of the placenta was found to be challenging in terms of numbers of procedures available for trainees to undertake.

An RCOG-led review of trainee feedback carried out by Landau *et al.* in 2013 suggested that the effectiveness of the OSATS as an assessment tool for caesarean section diminished as the seniority of the trainee increased, with technical competence assessed less effectively in more complex procedures. It was thought that this finding was a result of both the generic design of the tool and insufficient training on the part of assessors. This and other work led to the 2014 division of all OSATS into either formative or summative assessments, and the development of additional training resources and guidance for assessors and trainees [17,18]. The impact of the implementation of formative and summative assessments is yet to be formally assessed.

The Future

The use of OSATS as an assessment tool within obstetrics and gynaecology continues to be a developing area of work. Feedback from trainees and assessors is sought on a regular basis by means of direct enquiry at the time of Annual Review of Competence Progression (ARCP), within trainee and trainer evaluation surveys, via e-Portfolio communications and through direct feedback and discussion within and between Local Education Training Boards and the RCOG. The detailed separation of formative and summative assessment, introduced in 2014, will hopefully help to reinforce the importance of both aspects of assessment in determining skills acquisition and learning needs. The RCOG has developed dedicated teaching tools for both trainees and trainers to help reinforce the concepts of best practice in carrying out WPBAs [18,19], and there is guidance from the GMC on the implementation of WPBAs to help support both specialty leads, assessors and trainees [20]. Recent work on the development of a Non-Technical Skills for Surgeons-style assessment format appears promising and may widen the scope for multi-professional assessors in relation to this important area of practice in relation to patient safety [21].

As trainees and assessors become used to the most recent changes to the model for OSATS, one of the remaining challenges will be the ability to complete both the verbal and written feedback aspects of assessment in a timely fashion. In a busy labour ward environment this can be challenging, but developments such as smartphone apps for downloading online forms will surely help in this regard, alongside incorporation of e-Portfolio links on inbuilt IT systems within units. Trainees who have started their specialty training in the years since 2007, many of whom have now progressed through to completion of training, and the trainers who have taken part in OSATS assessment during their 'initial' phase of implementation, will be very well placed to lead on the future development of OSATS to ensure that they remain an appropriate and pertinent format for assessment of training.

Appendices[1]

Appendix 32.1: Example of Formative Assessment

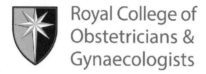

Royal College of
Obstetricians &
Gynaecologists

OSATS Supervised Learning Event

Trainee name: Simon Brown	StR Year: 1	Date: 1/9/2015
Trainer name: Joanne Smith	Grade: Consultant obstetrician	
Procedure: Caesarean section		
Clinical details and complexity: Elective primip caesarean section for breech presentation following unsuccessful ECV		

This is a **formative** tool designed to give feedback to the trainee about their performance in **this** procedure. Please provide specific, constructive **feedback** to the trainee in verbal and written forms in the box below that you feel will enhance training. There is **NO** overall judgement relating to competence for this event.

The following areas are suggestions to consider about the **overall** observed performance. This includes both the technical and non-technical skills necessary for the procedure and is not an exhaustive list.

Checking equipment/environment	Communication with patients and/or relatives
Peri-operative planning e.g. positioning	Use of assistants
Technical ability	Communication with staff
Selection of instruments and equipment	Forward planning
Economy of movement	Dealing with problems and/or difficulties
Tissue handling	Documentation
Completion of task as appropriate	Safety considerations

Feedback (continued overleaf):

What went well?
This was Simon's ninth CS and his second doing a breech delivery. Led the WHO timeout process effectively. Careful and methodical approach on entering the abdomen and making the uterine incision. Was able to deliver the baby with some assistance. Remained calm throughout. Good communication with scrub assistant in terms of instruments and sharps.

---

[1] OSATS templates reproduced with the kind permission from the RCOG.

What could have gone better?

You needed some help in delivering the baby (extended breech) which is to be expected on this first occasion. There was an extension to the left angle for which you needed some assistance in order to secure haemostasis.

Learning Plan:

Practice assisted breech delivery manoeuvres using manikins where possible so that you build up your confidence and competence in getting the baby delivered safely, especially in respect to delivery of the arms and head. Think about what instructions you need to give to your assistant (for example, if you were being assisted by a more junior colleague) in order to help you manage the delivery more effectively. Remember to keep your delivering hand in the midline to minimise surgical trauma such as angle extensions. Remember to communicate with your anaesthetic colleagues if the surgical blood loss is becoming greater than expected so that they can be proactive in managing fluid balance.

Trainee signature: S. Brown   **Trainer signature:** J. Smith

Trainee Reflection:

I was pleased to have been able to start and finish this Caesarean section as it was the first one where I 'led' the procedure from start to finish. However, it was difficult to get the baby delivered as the arms were extended and I hadn't seen that happening before. Having a consultant there to help me made a big difference, as otherwise this could have been very stressful. I will practise doing assisted breech deliveries using the simulation models and in future I would spend more time before the operation starts thinking through my troubleshooting plans for situations where the baby does not come as easily as anticipated. The angle extension was a result of my difficulty in getting the baby delivered and a good lesson in retaining my core surgical principles in order to avoid undue additional complications.

Appendix 32.2: Example of Summative Assessment

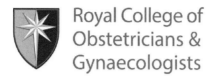

Royal College of
Obstetricians &
Gynaecologists

OSATS Assessment of Performance

Trainee name: Jenny Steele   **StR Year:** 5   **Date:** 1/9/2015

Trainer name: Joanne Smith   **Grade:** Consultant obstetrician

Procedure: Caesarean section

Clinical details and complexity: Emergency repeat Caesarean section at 9cm dilatation. Prolonged rupture of membranes. Meconium-stained liquor and pathological CTG

Degree of difficulty: Basic/Intermediate/Advanced   **Encounter requested in advance:** Yes / No

This assessment is a **mandatory, summative** tool designed to:

1. Enable judgement of surgical competency in **this** procedure and
2. To provide specific, constructive **feedback** to the trainee about their performance.

There is a judgement to be made in this assessment relating to the overall performance observed: **competent** or **working towards competence**.

Trainees require a minimum of three procedures deemed competent per core procedure, by more than one assessor, including a consultant or post-CCT holder. This judgement is **specific** to **this assessment only.**

The following anchor statements are for general guidance about the overall observed level of performance. Suggestions for areas to consider during the assessment are listed overleaf.

For the trainee considered **competent** in the observed procedure it would generally be expected that:

•   The trainee was able to perform all aspects of the procedure safely and competently with no or minimal need for help, or in the context of an unexpectedly difficult case, may have needed more assistance for the more difficult aspects of the procedure.

For the trainee considered to be **working towards competence** it would generally be expected that:

•   The trainee required significant help throughout or with the majority of steps
•   The trainee was unable to perform any of the necessary procedures to be safe and competent at this stage

This trainee performed this observed procedure competently*

This trainee is working towards competence in this procedure*

*Delete as appropriate

Please provide written feedback for the trainee regarding their performance in the box provided overleaf in addition to your direct verbal feedback.

The following areas are suggestions to consider about the overall observed performance. This includes both the technical and non-technical skills necessary for the procedure and is not an exhaustive list.

Checking equipment/environment	Communication with patients and/or relatives
Peri-operative planning e.g. positioning	Use of assistants
Technical ability	Communication with staff
Selection of instruments and equipment	Forward planning
Economy of movement	Dealing with problems and/or difficulties
Tissue handling	Documentation
Completion of task as appropriate	Safety considerations

Feedback:

What went well?

This was a complex situation where the woman was very keen on VBAC but where there was significant concern about fetal wellbeing. You led the team effectively by ensuring clear communication with the anaesthetist and theatre team as to the urgency of the situation, and maintained good situational awareness in this respect when regional blockade was being established. You explained the situation clearly to the woman and her partner and gained consent effectively during this rapidly developing clinical scenario. Good surgical competence displayed in terms of delivery of the deeply engaged head with anticipation for the need for assistance from below (not required).

What could have gone better?

There was a degree of uterine atony which took a while to manage and the eventual blood loss was nearly a litre as a result.

Learning plan:

Remember to anticipate the need for additional uterotonics and communicate this proactively with your anaesthetist and wider theatre team (could discuss in the 'time out'). Think about how you would supervise and support a more junior colleague undertaking this type of delivery in the future, and how you would judge when to 'step in' to assist.

Trainee signature: *Jenny Steele*   **Trainer signature:** *J. Smith*

References

1. Winckel CP, Reznick RK, Cohen R, Taylor B. Reliability and construct validity of a structured technical skills assessment form. *Am J Surg*. 1994; 167: 423–7.

2. Department of Health. *A Compendium of Solutions to Implementing the European Working Time Directive for Doctors in Training from August 2004*. London: HMSO; 2004.

3. RCOG. *Report of the Basic Specialty Training Working Party in Obstetrics and Gynaecology*. London: RCOG Press; 2006.

4. Department of Health. *Modernising Medical Careers: Operational Framework for Foundation Training*. London: HMSO; 2005.

5. www.rcog.org.uk/en/careers-training/about-specialty-training-in-og/assessment-and-progression-through-training/Sign-off-of-competency-acquisition (accessed 15 May 2016).

6. www.rcog.org.uk/en/careers-training/about-specialty-training-in-og/assessment-and-progression-through-training (accessed 15 May 2016).

7. www.rcog.org.uk/globalassets/documents/careers-and-training/assessment-and-progression-through-training/osats_summative_1_august_2014.pdf (accessed 15 May 2016).

8. Goff BA, Nielsen PE, Lentz GM, *et al*. Surgical skills assessment: a blinded examination of obstetrics and gynecology residents. *Am J Obstet Gynecol*. 2002; 186: 613–17.

9. Nielsen PE, Foglia LM, Mandel LS, Chow GE. Objective structured assessment of technical skills for episiotomy repair. *Am J Obstet Gynecol*. 2003; 189: 1257–60.

10. VanBloricom AL, Goff BA, Chinn M, *et al*. A new curriculum for hysteroscopy training as demonstrated by an objective structured assessment of technical skills (OSATS). *Am J Obstet Gynecol*. 2005; 193(5); 1856–65.

11. Swift SE, Carter JF. Institution and validation of an observed structured assessment of technical skills (OSATS) for obstetrics and gynaecology residents and faculty. *Am J Obstet Gynecol*. 2006; 195(2): 617–21.

12. Lentz GM, Mandel LS, Goff BA. A six-year study of surgical teaching and skills evaluation for obstetric/gynecologic residents in porcine and inanimate surgical models. *Am J Obstet Gynecol*. 2005; 193(6): 2056–61.

13. Bodle JF, Kaufmann SJ, Bisson D, Nathanson B, Binney DM. Value and face validity of objective structured assessment of technical skills (OSATS) for work based assessment of surgical skills in obstetrics and gynaecology. *Med Teach*. 2008; 30: 212–16.

14. Setna Z, Jha V, Boursicot KA, Roberts TE. Evaluating the utility of workplace-based assessment tools for speciality training. *Best Pract Res Clin Obstet Gynaecol*. 2010; 24(6): 767–82.

15. Homer M, Setna Z, Jha V, *et al*. Estimating and comparing the reliability of a suite of workplace-based assessments: an obstetrics and gynaecology setting. *Med Teach*. 2013; 35: 684–91.

16. Crossley J, Davies H, Humphris G, Jolly B. Generalisability: a key to unlock professional assessment. *Med Educ*. 2002; 36(10): 972–8.

17. Landau A, Reid W, Watson A, McKenzie C. Objective Structured Assessment of Technical Skill in assessing technical competence to carry out caesarean section with increasing seniority. *Best Pract Res Clin Obstet Gynaecol*. 2013; 27(2): 197–207.

18. https://stratog.rcog.org.uk/tutorial/workplace-based-assessment-elearning-resource/summary-6327 (accessed 15 May 2016).

19. www.rcog.org.uk/en/careers-training/about-specialty-training-in-og/assessment-and-progression-through-training/workplace-based-assessments (accessed 15 May 2016).

20. www.gmc-uk.org/Workplace_Based_Assessment___A_guide_for_implementation_0410.pdf_48905168.pdf (accessed 15 May 2016).

21. Jackson S, Brackley K, Landau A, Hayes K. Assessing non-technical skills on the delivery suite: a pilot study. *Clin Teach*. 2014; 11: 375–80.

Chapter 33

Non-Technical Skills to Improve Obstetric Practice

Kim Hinshaw

Introduction and Background

The importance of ensuring patient safety in obstetrics, by minimizing harm and optimizing the outcome for both mother and baby, are end points that all maternity providers must aim to achieve. Historically, training on the labour ward has relied on the development of technical skills for individual practitioners and more recently a new emphasis on the importance of leadership and multidisciplinary team working [1]. Non-technical skills (NTS) include individual cognitive skills (situation awareness and decision making), social or behavioural skills (communication, teamwork, leadership, followership and assertiveness) and personal resource skills (management of stress and fatigue) [2–5]. Good NTS complement technical skills and are critical to safe and efficient performance, particularly relevant in safety-critical environments such as the labour ward. The various components of NTS will be described and related to obstetric care. Non-technical skills do not sit in isolation. The term 'human factors' describes the relationship between the 'system' (i.e. environmental, organizational and job factors) and the human/individual characteristics described above, and how that interaction can influence behaviour at work, affecting both health and safety outcomes. Throughout the chapter, training methods are discussed which can help to develop non-technical skills for the individual and the team. Table 33.1 defines the elements of non-technical skills which will be reviewed individually in this chapter. The main aim of the author is to introduce the reader to the concept of NTS in obstetrics. Introductions similar to this are a common point of entry in formal NTS training programmes in other safety-critical industries (including oil/gas exploration, nuclear, aviation, etc.) [2].

Patient Safety and Error

Healthcare is potentially hazardous and iatrogenic error or injury crosses national and international borders and affects all specialist areas. Hyman and Silver reviewed the risks of healthcare in the USA and presented data suggesting 180 000 people might die annually because of iatrogenic injury. Drug error accounted for up to 770 000 injuries or deaths each year at a cost of approximately $5.6 million per hospital, with unnecessary surgery accounting for up to 12 000 deaths per annum [6]. Patients are particularly at risk in 'safety-critical' environments where complex or emergency procedures occur (e.g. surgical operations) and in situations where patients may destabilize acutely, often without warning (accident and emergency, labour ward, etc.). Surgeons reviewing 146 critical surgical incidents noted that 33% resulted in permanent disability. Communication breakdowns between personnel were contributory in 43% of cases and fatigue/excessive workload in 33%. Errors were reported significantly more often with emergency procedures. Cognitive errors by individuals contributed in 86% of cases [7].

The Keogh report investigated 14 NHS hospitals in England that had all been outliers for the previous two consecutive years on either the 'Summary Hospital-Level Mortality Indicator' or the 'Hospital Standardised Mortality Ratio' [8]. Ninety per cent of mortality occurred in those admitted on an emergency basis. Human factor issues underpinned most of the key findings: lack of appropriate leadership (inadequate involvement of senior clinical staff/Trust Boards in monitoring quality performance), inadequate staffing or poor staff-mix within teams, excessive workload in the urgent care pathway and poor use of safety checks (including early warning scores, escalation

Best Practice in Labour and Delivery, Second Edition, ed. Sir Sabaratnam Arulkumaran. Published by Cambridge University Press. © Cambridge University Press 2016.

Table 33.1 Non-technical skills: elements and definitions

Element	Definition
Cognitive skills	
Situation awareness	The sensory perception of elements in the environment, the ability to understand their meaning and the prediction of their status in the near future.
Decision making	The process of reaching a conclusion and choosing a course of action to meet the needs of a given situation.
Social or behavioural skills	
Teamwork	A collaborative and dynamic process involving two or more people, engaged in one or multiple activities, with the aim of completing a shared goal/task.
Communication	The exchange of information, requests, ideas or suggestions, and feelings or concerns.
Leadership	A team leader has delegated authority to direct and coordinate the work of other team members. However, leadership skills (maintaining standards, planning, prioritizing, managing workload/resources) may be shared within teams.
Followership	The active ability of individual team members to perform delegated tasks, to cooperate, to support the leader and to offer constructive challenge when appropriate.
Assertiveness	The quality of being appropriately self-assured and able to express an opinion confidently without aggression.
Personal resource skills	
Managing stress and coping with fatigue	Awareness of the detrimental effects of stress and fatigue and the ability to implement coping strategies.

policies and inadequate Clinical Incidence Reviews, etc.).

Using an 'Adverse Outcome Index', about 1 in 12 women will experience an adverse event in labour. However, the range is wide (4–16.5%), implying that in some units *up to 1 in 6 women* are exposed to a significant safety risk [9]. The Confidential Enquiry into Stillbirths and Deaths in Infancy reports (CESDI) found that 52% of 873 intrapartum fetal deaths were likely to have received suboptimal care [10]. Recurrent themes in the series of CESDI reports were: failure to recognize (situation awareness), failure to refer (communication) and inappropriate delegation (leadership/teamwork). Maternal mortality reports have also reported that suboptimal care was contributory in up to 50% of cases of maternal death. The recent MBBRACE-UK report confirmed that human factors remain highly relevant in maternal deaths. System factors meant more than two out of three women who died did not receive the nationally recommended level of antenatal care; one-quarter did not receive a minimum level of antenatal care [11]. In intrapartum care, recurrent NTS factors included: basic observations not recorded/responded to (situation awareness, communication), delayed involvement of senior staff by junior staff (situation awareness, communication, follower-

ship, team working) and lack of involvement of specific specialist help (leadership, team working).

If we reflect on our own obstetric practice, most obstetric adverse events relate to non-technical (rather than technical) skills errors. A critical analysis of obstetric serious untoward incidents (SUIs) in two London hospitals confirmed that 82.6% involved human factor errors (with multiple factors apparent in 78.9%) [12]. The 'Human WORM' classification was used to analyse cases and NTS errors were the most common underlying cause: 'Omissions' in 61.6% of cases (situational awareness, decision-making errors), 'Relationship' issues in 47.7% (communication, team working errors) and *Mentorship*' in 31.2% (lack of senior presence, etc.). 'Workmanship' errors were involved in 44.2% of SUIs (i.e. knowledge or technical skills issues). There were no differences in the contribution of the various elements in the two neighbouring units (one was a general hospital and the other a tertiary referral centre).

Human and Systems Error

In medicine, as in other safety-critical industries, errors that compromise patient safety are due to a combination of *human* and *organizational* or *system*

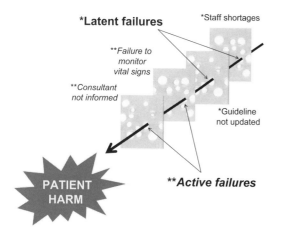

Figure 33.1 Hazards in obstetrics leading to harm.

factors [13]. The importance of both human–human and human–system interactions leading to error needs to be appreciated. In many medical situations where error has occurred, it is historically the nurse, doctor or midwife who is 'blamed', i.e. the *individual* at the so-called 'sharp end'. The subsequent follow-up often involved a punitive or disciplinary approach. However, without addressing both the human *and* systems errors, the potential for patient harm will remain. The 'Swiss cheese' model of barriers, defences and failures described by Reason shows how patient harm can result when several minor failures link together [14].

Figure 33.1 shows an obstetric version of the Reason model with a series of 'holes' in the defences/barriers made up of a combination of 'latent failures or conditions' and 'active failures'. The former are described by Reason as the 'resident pathogens' in our systems (e.g. understaffing, inexperience, equipment lack/failure, inappropriate guidelines). Latent conditions may lie unrecognized for months or years and only lead to harm in combination with a specific set of active failures. The latter are 'unsafe acts' by personnel in direct contact with the patient or with the system/equipment. The situation described in Figure 33.1 will be familiar to all personnel who have worked on a busy labour ward.

Vignette: due to staff sickness the levels required on a particular shift are less than adequate, and the skill mix may also be inappropriate for the busy workload (perhaps too many relatively inexperienced midwives, with more high-risk patients in labour than expected). Three high-risk inductions were started during the afternoon shift. A patient has developed pyrexia in

labour but the recently updated sepsis guideline has not been uploaded so is not available. Her vital signs confirm a rising early warning score (EWS), but the significance is not recognized and therefore not acted on with appropriate escalation. By the time the consultant is called, the patient has developed signs of septic shock and an acute emergency has arisen, compromising both maternal and fetal safety. In the subsequent critical incident review (CIR), the report only focused on the staff member who did not recognize or act on the deteriorating EWS.

Inadequately conducted CIRs will contribute to continuing risk to patients, particularly if systems errors are ignored while concentrating on single errors by individual practitioners. The most important objectives in a high-quality approach to risk management in obstetrics are to delineate *all* contributory factors (individual, team and system) and to produce appropriate 'actions' that are implemented and disseminated widely, in a timely fashion [15].

Errors and Violations

Reason published a useful taxonomy which describes the various types of human error and violation which may compromise patient safety [13]:

Errors

- *Execution errors*: these include slips, lapses, trips or fumbles which can occur even in the presence of an appropriate plan. Error in these cases results from an action failure.
- *Mistakes*: these occur because a plan was inherently faulty or inadequate. Error in these cases results from a higher level failure involving poor planning or judgement, and occurs even when execution of specific actions is done correctly.
- All errors are associated with some form of *deviation* away from the norm.

Execution Errors

Slips tend to be associated with attention errors, either failure to select correctly or failure to recognize when undertaking a task. These often occur during routine procedures when the individual (or team) is distracted or perhaps working in an unfamiliar environment. An example on the labour ward would include surgical error during abdominal entry for an elective third repeat caesarean section, when unexpected patient discomfort/movement leads to distraction and inadvertent bladder damage. *Slips* also occur when operating in inadequate settings, for example a second theatre in a converted delivery room – cramped, with backup equipment and an inexperienced assistant. *Lapses* relate to failures of memory or attention and again lead to error during execution of a task. Both slips and lapses tend to occur when there is attentional capture – i.e. when the individual is distracted and/or preoccupied or when changes are made to a pre-defined plan.

Mistakes

Mistakes are either *'rule-based'* or *'knowledge-based'* and occur after a problem has been confirmed. In medicine, these often occur with unexpected complications that require a change in approach or deviation away from the agreed plan. *'Rule-based'* mistakes occur when an individual uses a management approach with which they are familiar, in an inappropriate circumstance (e.g. giving intravenous ergometrine during a large postpartum haemorrhage to a patient with underlying severe pre-eclampsia). Alternatively, they may approach a specific complication incorrectly (e.g. giving 2 l of crystalloid rapidly for reduced urine output in severe pre-eclampsia, leading to fluid overload and pulmonary oedema). *'Knowledge-based'* mistakes occur in new situations which are unfamiliar to the individual or team, often in the absence of agreed or available guidance to direct care. This type of mistake is less likely to occur with direct input from an experienced clinician. Managing these cases requires critical assessment so that a clear 'mental model' is formed which will help to clarify the most appropriate action. However, if the available information is incomplete, incorrect decisions may be made. Any subsequent error may be compounded by various *biases*. In unfamiliar, safety-critical situations, the tendency is to look for those bits of information that support a pre-determined cause and action. This can lead to a 'blinkered' view, with the individual or team excluding information that may be vital in reaching a correct plan of action. This is known as *confirmation bias* and leads to a loss of situational awareness. Mistakes can result from: relative inexperience (but not exclusively), inadequate challenge from within the team, poor communication or decision making, lack of senior supervision, tiredness and fatigue. These factors will be explored in subsequent sections.

Violations

Deliberate violations imply an intended action with deliberate deviation away from evidence-based guidelines, safe operating procedures (SOPs), etc. 'Routine' violations occur when guidance is only partially followed, often to save time or effort. 'Optimizing' violations may result from boredom, where moving away from defined guidance is a form of 'risky' behaviour undertaken by an individual to compensate. *'Situational'* violations occur when the action proposed, although not in keeping with agreed procedure, is felt to be a better (or possibly the only) option to follow. Deliberate violations may be related to underlying motivational or team issues which can stem from organizational issues such as poor leadership, inadequate support, failure to correct poor performance, etc. Senior clinicians may deviate from a labour ward guideline based on prior experience and the individual patient's circumstance. This may be viewed by some as a violation, but can be justified and the reason for deviating from guidance should be clearly recorded. A 'protocol' is defined as 'a system of rules that explain the correct conduct and procedures to be followed in formal situations'. By implication, a protocol does not imply flexibility and violations should not occur – in the labour ward situation this would encompass drug regimens (e.g. magnesium sulphate and intravenous antihypertensive treatment in eclampsia).

Maxfield *et al.* assessed the frequency of four safety concerns among labour ward teams in the USA: dangerous shortcuts (violations), missing competences, disrespect and performance problems [16]. In total, 3282 participants completed surveys, with 92%, 93% and 98% of physicians, midwives and nurses respectively reporting at least one concern in the previous 12 months. They reported: serious patient harm by a dangerous shortcut/violation (8.4%); performance problems which undermined patient safety (55.3%). It is clear that human error is as relevant in labour ward practice as it is in other safety-critical environments.

Managing Error in Health Systems

Historically, the 'person approach' process has been used to manage error in medicine. This often led to blame levelled against one or more individuals. The 'system approach' accepts that error is an inevitable consequence of the human state, even in the most expert and aware organizations. 'High-reliability' organizations aim to minimize risk and use a system approach for handling error. They acknowledge that 'to err is human' and accept that while 'error is inevitable, harm is not'. Nuclear power plants, nuclear-powered aircraft carriers and air traffic control are three examples [14]. These organizations have developed 'resilient systems' and maintain error reduction by addressing issues with individuals, teams, systems, equipment, environment and the totality of the organization. These safety-critical environments, like the labour ward, must maintain reserve capacity to deal with significant and unpredictable peaks of activity. Keogh confirmed that understanding the causes of high mortality in the NHS was not about finding a rogue surgeon, but required a 'whole-system' approach [8].

In the following sections we will explore NTS in more detail, highlighting the fallibilities of human cognition and interactions. We will discuss methods which can be used to minimize error to benefit patient safety.

Non-Technical Skills: Cognitive Components

The cognitive components of NTS are situation awareness and decision making. Human cognition ('thinking' or 'reasoning') describes the mental processes dealing with information gathering, interpretation and use of knowledge. Cognition relies on complex brain interactions involving three types of memory: sensory storage, short-term (or working) memory and main (or long-term) memory. Between 70% and 80% of human errors relate to problems with cognition. In medicine we train in technical skills but the importance of cognitive and non-technical skills training is only now being realized.

A simple 'dual process model' can be used to describe the differences between 'automatic' (unconscious) and 'analytic' (conscious) cognitive processes [3]. These are at play in every aspect of our lives and clinical practice; we switch between them without conscious effort. Undertaking an elective caesarean in a primiparous patient of low BMI is usually a relaxed affair for the middle-grade registrar and conversation will often take place between the operating team and with the patient and partner – 'automatic' cognition is in use. However, the situation changes if there is an atonic haemorrhage following delivery of the placenta. The registrar and team focus on the problem, considering options and outcomes as well as appropriate management. Noise levels in the operating room

drop to allow the surgeon, anaesthetist and team to concentrate, with a seamless switch to 'analytic' thinking. Distractions may lead to error and conversation will be minimal and focused. This is similar to expectations in the aviation industry when an emergency occurs. The 'silent cockpit' refers to an environment where unnecessary or irrelevant conversation is prohibited. In many airline disasters, 'black box' recordings reveal episodes of distracting conversation, resulting in loss of situation awareness with few routine checks and cross-checks occurring. The development of NOTECHS (non-technical skills training) led to improvement in pilots' cognitive skills and reduction in air disasters [17].

The 'automatic' part of the system is intuitive and does not involve working or short-term memory. Overall active 'awareness' is low and actions/skills are undertaken in a reflexive way using honed skills. There is a high degree of 'automaticity', with fast thought processes and activity conducted speedily using minimal effort. The process is relatively 'unreliable' because of the high degree of automaticity, and the potential for error can be quite high and susceptible to biases. The 'analytic' system that we switch to in crisis or emergency situations uses short-term memory, requires conscious effort and awareness, and a deliberate/rule-based approach. It is 'slow' and effortful, but less liable to bias with relatively few errors. We use both systems and neither is necessarily better or worse than the other. The automatic part is more primitive biologically, but both systems are required for efficient and effective function, dependent on the clinical scenario at the time. We will often use a more 'automatic' approach in busy antenatal clinics, switching to an analytic approach when dealing with a complex obstetric case where there are multiple risk factors. Errors in both elective and emergency situations can arise if the switch from automatic to analytic cognition does not occur at the correct point.

Situation Awareness (or *Situational Awareness*)

Situation awareness (SA) is a cognitive skill and is the way we maintain awareness of our environment. Endsley defines SA as 'the perception of the elements in the environment within a volume of time and space, the comprehension of their meaning, and the projection of their status in the near future' [18]. Three levels are described:

- Level 1 is perception of information from the environment using all of our senses. 'Sensory storage' will only hold information very briefly –between 0.5 s for visual and 2.0 s for auditory memory [2].
- Level 2 is assimilation and interpretation of the information we receive. This occurs in short-term memory which is where we are 'consciously aware'. Storage in working memory is limited, holding up to seven 'bits' of information only and is easily overloaded. External distractions or interruptions can interrupt cognitive processing and lead to error. Over time, 'expert tasks' become automatic and are embedded in long-term memory (e.g. managing operative vaginal delivery). This is an advantage for the more experienced accoucheur, as it frees up 'bits' within working memory, allowing better SA.
- Level 3 is the ability to predict the 'near future state'. This relies on experiential learning which is stored in long-term memory and uses 'pattern recognition'. This is a primitive but well-developed process in humans which happens automatically, with minimal conscious processing. However, it is prone to error if the pattern is misinterpreted. If no pattern is recognized then automatic cognition does not function effectively and the process can be distorted by pre-existing biases. More experienced practitioners build up a series of 'mental models' or 'schema' which are stored in long-term memory and consist of specific patterns or sensory cues which are associated with a particular meaning. This anticipatory function feeds directly into decision making and is prone to error in the presence of distractions or interruptions.

The three levels of SA are shown in Figure 33.2; the mnemonic 'CIA' may be a useful reminder.

The importance of maintaining SA cannot be over-emphasized in safety-critical environments. Between 80% and 90% of all aviation disasters involving human error are caused by SA errors and 70–80% of these were level 1 (perception) errors. These errors can affect both individuals and teams. When allocated a specific task that requires concentration and focus, it is possible to miss what may be a very obvious deterioration in the overall situation. Task focus can be likened to putting on a pair of 'blinkers' which restrict one's wider vision. In their classic psychology experiment,

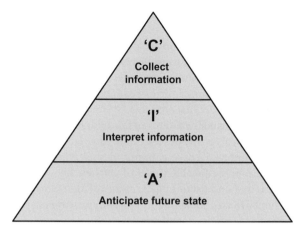

Figure 33.2 The three levels of situational awareness (after [18]).

Chabris and Simons arranged two teams of students in white or black T-shirts. Each team passes a basketball to each other, while the audience is asked to count the exact number of times the white team passed the ball, ignoring the black team passes. Despite this occurring in a space no larger than a small labour room, *half of the subjects missed an adult in a full-sized black gorilla suit crossing the room!* [19]. This error of perception is known as 'inattentional blindness' and demonstrates the need to learn how to maintain SA, particularly in the presence of multiple distractions and interruptions.

In a situation in which an obstetric team are managing a large atonic postpartum haemorrhage after a forceps delivery, the registrar will be focused on managing the atonic uterus. While applying fundal and possibly bimanual pressure, he or she will also be examining the genital tract to exclude trauma. Their SA will be compromised and they may miss the fact that the patient has developed cardiovascular instability. This requires someone to 'step back' from all the other required tasks (e.g. airway management, checking vital signs, siting IV access, sending bloods to labs, etc.). They need to take the lead, keeping a careful eye on the patient's overall condition and watching for the 'gorilla in the room'. This may be a senior midwife, particularly if the anaesthetist is occupied with airway management or securing IV access. Effective teams do not rely on hierarchy but ensure a nominated person is keeping an eye on the bigger picture. In an emergency, all team members will have specific roles and tasks to perform, but the ability to watch for overall deterioration using any spare cognitive capacity should be encouraged throughout the team. 'Cross-checking' is a tool that can facilitate safety. Each member should feel able to challenge others confidently and constructively, checking that planned interventions are correct. This was one of three NTS identified by Bahl *et al.* which were *specific* to conducting operative vaginal delivery (the two other *procedure-specific* skills were maintaining professional behaviour and a professional relationship with the woman) [5,20].

The following vignette demonstrates how SA errors can arise in labour. A primiparous patient with a twin pregnancy was admitted in labour at 37 weeks; both presentations were cephalic. Monitoring was via fetal scalp electrode and abdominal transducer. Four hours into labour the trace on twin 1 was pathological and a fetal scalp pH was undertaken which was normal. As the trace did not improve, two further samples were taken before full dilatation. The registrar and consultant reviewed regularly. Progress in the second stage was rapid – twin 1 delivered normally in good condition, followed within five minutes by twin 2. Twin 2 was asphyxiated and required prolonged resuscitation: arterial cord pH 6.95, base excess –16 mmol/l. No-one in the team had noticed that the transducers were crossed – the pathological CTG had been from twin 2 for the last four hours. This is a classic level 1 SA error – once missed, the error was not picked up by any of the experienced team.

Various methods are described for maintaining SA, but the following summary could be usefully adopted in obstetric practice [2]:

- Consider fitness to work (health, tiredness, fatigue).
- Start with a structured, relevant briefing.
- Minimize interruptions or distractions.
- Prohibit all non-essential activities (maintain a 'sterile cockpit').
- Regularly update (compare real clinical data with the 'mental model').
- Monitor (self and others, and vice versa).
- Encourage good followership (ask others to cross-check and 'challenge').
- Good time management (leaves maximum time for critical decisions).

Decision Making

In safety-critical environments, the 'naturalistic decision making' (NDM) process has been adopted to assess how experts reach decisions in the real-life work environment, with all its associated stresses [2]. Four decision-making processes are described:

1. *Intuitive* (or 'recognition-primed'): this is 'automatic', involves rapid access to prior memories or patterns and is classically used by experienced clinicians.
2. *Rule-based*: this involves more cognitive effort and is classically used by learners based on recognized 'rules'. With experience, rule-based scenarios become embedded in long-term memory and can be used 'automatically' as part of intuitive decision making (e.g. an experienced clinician will use an eclampsia protocol intuitively).
3. *Analytical* (or 'choice-based'): this requires review of several options and experienced operators will use mental models to facilitate this approach. Error can occur if 'models' are missed during options appraisal.
4. *Creative*: this is rarely used in safety-critical environments except in very unusual circumstances. The author used this process in a case of unresponsive, intractable atonic haemorrhage in a 20-year-old primigravid patient. The decision to *combine* a B-Lynch suture with intrauterine balloon tamponade allowed uterine conservation.

The four approaches are subject to differing errors and the practitioner must be aware of the weaknesses of each. 'Rule-based' is not ideal when a 'rule' does not exist or cannot be recalled and may lead to a cognitive 'freeze'. This can be avoided by involving the team, as well as the individual, in ongoing review. Actions can be modified as the situation changes.

Improving Decision Making

Decision making is influenced by external and internal factors. External factors include input from the wider team (i.e. 'team cognition') but also maintaining situation awareness and aiming for a calm environment. Internal factors include prior experience and individual cognitive expertise or personality traits. Yee *et al.* confirmed that obstetricians with high levels of 'reflective coping' had a 30% reduction in operative vaginal delivery (OVD) rates with no differences in outcome – OR 0.70; 95% CI (0.50–0.98) [21]. *Reflective coping* is a measure of coping, self-efficacy and proactive attitude with the ability to tolerate uncertainty.

In medicine we have relied on 'years of experience' to move trainees from analytical towards intuitive decision making. With training time reduced, we need to appreciate that this can be accelerated using formal training techniques such as *critical task analysis* (CTA) and *tactical decision aids* (TDAs). These are already used to develop decision-making skills in the armed forces [22]. A CTA of how experts approach decision making in OVD highlighted clinical steps and processes which could be used to accelerate trainees' learning [23].

Non-Technical Skills: Social Components

The social or interactive components of NTS are vitally important. The present pyramidal structure in health systems (i.e. with the leader at the top and team below) is based on hierarchy and does not always allow good communication. Constructive challenge may not be encouraged or accepted by the leader and this can be detrimental to patient safety. Each of the social components of NTS will be reviewed.

Teamwork

In obstetrics we function in multidisciplinary teams; the importance of team working and how this can be optimized is covered in Chapter 30. The TeamSTEPPS™ Teamwork Attitudes Questionnaire (T-TAQ) is a useful starting point and can be used in your own teams to assess attitudes towards components of teamwork and to determine training needs [24]. Leadership, followership, communication and assertiveness contribute to overall team performance and each will be described.

Leadership, Followership and Assertiveness

NICE intrapartum guidance suggests that effective leadership from senior staff is key to ensuring high-quality care within maternity services [25]. Francis recommended strong *organizational leadership* to promote safety culture [26] and the King's Fund described *collective leadership* with improved cross-organization collaboration [27].

Leadership

Good leadership requires a breadth of knowledge, skills and attitudes, as listed in Table 33.2.

Table 33.2 Leadership: skills, knowledge and attitudes

Element	Descriptor
Experienced	Good leadership requires appropriate experience of the specific situation. Does not always require the most senior clinician.
Visible	Present, supportive but not controlling.
Communicates	Confirms team roles, tasks, responsibilities and expected normal behaviour.
Listens	Uses 'active listening'. Encourages 'shared leadership'.
Anticipates	Exhibits strong situation awareness. Manages workload in elective and emergency situations.
Decisive	Decisive, not 'bossy'. Consistent. Uses intuitive decision making to reach rapid decisions in urgent situations.
Delegates appropriately	Delegates specific tasks to team member(s) ensuring they have the appropriate skill set.
Collaborative	Recognizes strength of individual team members. Collaborative ethic develops team strength.
Understanding and empowering	Listens and supports. Respectful. High emotional intelligence quotient.
Models appropriate behaviour	Encourages same in other team members.
Motivational	Work ethic, enthusiasm, behaviour and support for others, encourages strong desire to achieve.
Resilient	Able to adapt and mount a robust response in unexpected and unpredictable circumstances.
Other qualities:	
Aware of legal responsibilities	High-level management awareness.
Manages resources	Ensures appropriate resource for effective and safe team function.

Effective leaders exhibit a range of styles dependent on the clinical situation (i.e. 'situational leadership'). They may be more 'democratic' in elective situations where there is time to seek wider opinion or more 'autocratic' in critical situations where the team is stressed and they have prior experience. In many safety-critical labour events, the most senior obstetrician will be the team lead. However, if their focus is required for a specific task where situation awareness may be compromised (e.g. managing severe intra-abdominal haemorrhage), then emergency leadership should be allocated to the person who can step back and assess the situation as a whole. Leadership may change through a developing scenario, but the change in leadership must be explicit and clear to all team members.

Exemplary leaders have a high *emotional intelligence quotient* and this means the ability to recognize, understand and manage not only your own but others' emotions [28]. Effective leaders recognize patterns of behaviour that indicate others' intentions, they encourage questions and use 'active listening' (where listening is not a passive act, but requires acknowledgement and feedback). The effective leader promotes 'shared decision making' within the team, but makes critical decisions in acute situations. By developing skills including active listening, feedback, empowerment and motivation, a leader provides an environment for continuous team development: 'minds are like parachutes, they only function when open' (Thomas Dewar, 1864–1930). Teaching leadership skills is complex, requiring knowledge of leadership concepts and tools, observation of exemplary leadership, followed by 'supervised' leadership training in simulated and real scenarios. The NOTSS tool developed to assess leadership/non-technical skills in surgery has been modified and piloted successfully for obstetric trainees [29,30].

Followership and Assertiveness

Followership is the role undertaken by other members of a team to *actively support* the leader to accomplish an agreed goal. It requires mutual understanding and a high degree of interaction and teamwork. Exemplary followers will look for relevant roles and function effectively. They will offer ideas and maintain a positive attitude, while being prepared to raise concerns when needed (i.e. 'positively challenge'). This positive relationship encourages the use of shared decision making, cross-monitoring for safety and shared leadership.

Members of many healthcare teams adopt a 'passive' approach and will not challenge the leader's decisions, perhaps expecting a demeaning response. Failure to challenge the leader appropriately can compromise patient safety and was the cause of many aviation accidents in the past. The mnemonic PACE uses staged assertiveness to engender a response. The recipient should react to concerns at the 'Alert' stage:

- *Probe* – 'Do you know that ...'
- *Alert* – 'I'm more concerned now because ...'
- *Challenge* – 'Please stop what you're doing and ...'

Table 33.3 The SBAR handover tool

Situation	• states the current problem succinctly • gives relevant signs/symptoms only • summarizes relevant observations
Background	• reviews relevant immediate past or long-term history • states relevant drug history • gives relevant positive or negative investigation results
Assessment	• states interpretation of the findings (i.e. gives diagnosis) • includes whether stable/unstable
Recommendation	• states clearly if immediate or delayed action is required • recommends specific action(s)

- Emergency – 'I need you to take action right now and ...'

Communication

NICE guidance states that good communication is *crucial* between all those involved in the care of women during the process of childbearing [25]. Communication with patients and relatives is particularly important during labour interventions, and regular updates should be the norm. Clear and focused team communication is a vital first step in maintaining patient safety. To be effective, communication must also be complete, brief, timely, direct, explicit and respectful [31]. We will review some of the tools that are useful in obstetric care.

Handover Tools

The 'SBAR' tool offers a simple framework for effective handover and can be used in both elective and emergency situations (see Table 33.3).

The aim is to construct a brief, structured handover [32], and many hospitals have embedded SBAR as the single tool for use between *all* professional groups. To improve effectiveness, handovers themselves should ideally take place at the same time for each shift and in an environment without interruption or distraction. Printed summary sheets are a useful adjunct to effective handover and various mnemonics have been designed to facilitate good communication between teams, which include review of patients on antenatal and gynaecology wards, as well as 'outliers' (including emergency admissions) [32,33] – see Table 33.4.

Table 33.4 'SHARING': a handover tool for use in obstetrics and gynaecology (after [32])

Staffing	• review named senior staff and team • review support staffing • summarize relevant observations
High Risk	• review all 'high-risk' cases in all obstetric areas
Awaiting Theatre	• review both potential emergency and elective
Referrals-Recovery	• include 'outliers' in other parts of the hospital
Inductions	• review risk status of all inductions/augmentations • consider all other workload
Neonatal Unit	• check cot/ventilator availability
Gynaecology Ward	• check bed state/staffing • review emergencies and case mix

Closed-Loop Communication

In safety-critical emergencies, many tasks arise simultaneously. The team leader is responsible for ensuring specific task allocation to individuals, but as labour ward teams change every few hours, it is not uncommon for people to be unfamiliar with the names of all staff attending an acute emergency. In an attempt to avoid embarrassment, tasks are often allocated using requests like '*Will someone get the blood from the labs?*' This may result in no blood products appearing, which is not a surprise – who is 'someone'? The use of closed-loop communication ensures *effective* communication. The sender must not only ensure that the message has been received, but closing the loop ensures that the message has been *interpreted correctly* [34] (see Figure 33.3).

The use of these *information exchange strategies* improves team effectiveness in obstetric emergency

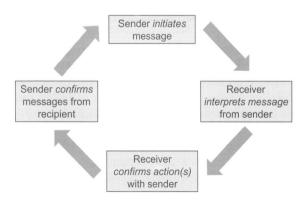

Figure 33.3 Closed-loop communication.

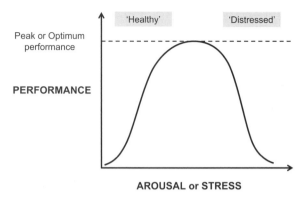

Figure 33.4 Stress–response curve.

simulations, with reduction in decision-to-delivery intervals in cord prolapse and faster administration of magnesium sulphate in eclampsia.

Non-Technical Skills: Coping with Tiredness and Fatigue

Excessive tiredness, fatigue, ill health and stress may have a detrimental effect on performance. The classic inverted-U stress–response curve is shown in Figure 33.4 [35,36]. The curve demonstrates that some degree of stress is positive and will lead to improved performance. The rising part of the stress–response curve aligns with a 'healthy' state for the individual as arousal increases. The classic Yerkes–Dodson curve shows a persistent decline in performance with increasing levels of stress. However, there are alternative theories which incorporate the effects of 'cognitive anxiety'. It is proposed that individuals with low levels of 'cognitive anxiety' (i.e. better coping mechanisms related to cognitive function) can maintain performance even in the presence of increasing physiological stress. That may relate to specific personality traits but also clinical experience.

One strategy to help maintain personal awareness of potential performance issues is to consider the mnemonic 'HALTS' when arriving at a safety-critical situation. Ask yourself if your performance is likely to be affected because you are:

- *Hungry*
- *Angry*
- *Late*
- *Tired*
- *Stressed*

All of these factors make it difficult to switch into analytical thinking mode. However, switching into analytical mode is in itself 'calming', and may be of benefit in dealing with stress within a team during an acute emergency.

Conclusion

In this chapter we have described the cognitive and social elements of NTS and their relevance to healthcare and obstetrics. We have outlined the significant contribution of NTS and 'human factor' errors to poor outcome and the risks to patient safety. Knowledge of the fallibility of human cognition allows us to consider strategies to maintain our 'situation awareness'. Effective communication between and within teams is vital. Strong leadership supported by active followership will add to the synergy of the team. We should embrace strategies, including shared decision making, cross-monitoring ('watching each other's backs') and shared leadership, and must be aware of the weaknesses of the hierarchical systems which have historically underpinned our healthcare practice. We have a responsibility to manage our own personal resource skills and maintain patient safety on the labour ward. Training in technical and non-technical skills is vital for safe obstetric practice and is available on courses such as ALSO, MOET, PROMPT and ROBuST. They are also being incorporated within core training in obstetrics and gynaecology in the UK.

References

1. RCOG. *Tomorrow's Specialist: Lifelong Professional Development for Specialist in Women's Health: Working Party Report*. London: RCOG Press; 2014.

2. Flin R, O'Connor P, Crichton M. *Safety at the Sharp End: A Guide to Non-Technical Skills*. Burlington, VT: Ashgate Publishing Company; 2008.

3. Mitchell P (ed.). *Safer Care: Human Factors in Healthcare Training Manual*. Argyle & Bute, Scotland: Swan & Horn; 2013.

4. Jackson K, Hayes K, Hinshaw K. The relevance of non-technical skills in obstetrics and gynaecology. *TOG*. 2013;15: 269–74.

5. Strachan B, Bahl R. Non-technical skills. In Gale A, Siassakos D, Attilakos G, Winter C, Draycott T (eds), *ROBuST Course Manual (RCOG Operative Birth Simulation Training)* (pp. 31–43). Cambridge: Cambridge University Press 2014.

6. Hyman DA, Silver C. Speak not of error. *Regulation*. 2005;Spring: 52–7.

7. Gawande AA, Zinner MJ, Studdert DM, Brennan TA. Analysis of errors reported by surgeons at three teaching hospitals. *Surgery*. 2003;133(6): 614–21.

8. Keogh B. Review into the quality of care and treatment provided by 14 hospital trusts in England: overview report; 2013. www.nhs.uk/NHSEngland/bruce-keogh-review/Documents/outcomes/keogh-review-final-report.pdf (accessed 16 May 2016).

9. Nielsen PE, Goldman MB, Mann S, *et al*. Effects of teamwork training on adverse outcomes and process of care in labor and delivery: a randomized controlled trial. *Obstet Gynecol*. 2007;109(1): 48–55.

10. Weindling AM. The Confidential Enquiry into Maternal and Child Health (CEMACH). *Arch Dis Childhood*. 2003;88(12): 1034–7.

11. Knight M, Kenyon S, Brocklehurst P, *et al*. (eds). *Saving Lives, Improving Mothers' Care: Lessons Learned to Inform Future Maternity Care from the UK and Ireland Confidential Enquiries into Maternal Deaths and Morbidity 2009–12*. Oxford: National Perinatal Epidemiology Unit, University of Oxford; 2014.

12. Coroyannakis C, Chandraharan E, Matiluko A. Comparative analysis of the human 'WORM': role of human factors on adverse incidents in two adjacent obstetric units in London. *BJOG*. 2013;120(1): 413.

13. Reason J. Understanding adverse events: human factors. *Qual Health Care*. 1995;4(2): 80–9.

14. Reason J. Human error: models and management. *BMJ*. 2000;320: 768–70.

15. Singhal T, Harding K. Risk management in obstetrics. *Obstet Gynaecol Reprod Med*. 2014;24(12): 357–64. http://dx.doi.org/10.1016/j.ogrm.2014.10.001.

16. Maxfield DG, Lyndon A, Kennedy HP, O'Keeffe DF, Zlatnik MG. Confronting safety gaps across labor and delivery teams. *Am J Obstet Gynecol*. 2013;209(5): 402–8.

17. Flin R, Martin L, Koerters KM, *et al*. Development of the NOTECHS (non-technical skills) system for assessing pilots' skills. *Human Factors Aerospace Safety*. 2003;3(2): 95–117.

18. Endsley M. Toward a theory of situation awareness in dynamic systems. *Human Factors*. 1995;37(1): 32–64.

19. Chabris C, Simons D. *The Invisible Gorilla and Other Ways Our Intuition Deceives Us*. London: HarperCollins Publishers; 2011.

20. Bahl R, Murphy DJ, Strachan B. Non-technical skills for obstetricians conducting forceps and vacuum deliveries: qualitative analysis by interviews and video recordings. *Eur J Obstet Gynecol Reprod Biol*. 2010;150(2): 147–51.

21. Yee LM, Liu LY, Grobman WA. The relationship between obstetricians' cognitive and affective traits and their patients' delivery outcomes. *Am J Obstet Gynecol*. 2014;211: e1–6.

22. Committee on Improving the Decision Making Abilities of Small Unit Leaders; Naval Studies Board; Division on Engineering and Physical Sciences; National Research Council. *Improving the Decision Making Abilities of Small Unit Leaders*. Washington, DC: National Academies Press; 2012.

23. Bahl R, Murphy DJ, Strachan B. Decision-making in operative vaginal delivery: when to intervene, where to deliver and which instrument to use? Qualitative analysis of expert clinical practice. *Eur J Obstet Gynecol Reprod Biol*. 2013;170(2): 333–40.

24. US Dept of Health & Human Services – Agency for Healthcare Research and Quality (AHRQ). *TeamSTEPPS™ – Teamwork Attitudes Questionnaire Manual*; 2016. www.teamstepps.ahrq.gov/taq_index.htm (accessed 16 May 2016).

25. NICE. Intrapartum care: care of healthy women and their babies during childbirth: clinical guideline 190; 2014. www.nice.org.uk/guidance/CG190 (accessed 16 May 2016).

26. Francis R. *Report of the Mid Staffordshire NHS Foundation Trust Public Inquiry*. London: The Stationary Office; 2013.

27. West M, Eckert R, Steward K, Pasmore B. Developing collective leadership for healthcare. King's Fund, 2014. www.kingsfund.org.uk/sites/files/kf/field/field_publication_file/developing-collective-leadership-kingsfund-may14.pdf (accessed 16 May 2016).

28. Hasson G. *Emotional Intelligence*. Chichester: Capstone; 2014.

29. Yule S, Flin R, Maran N, *et al*. Surgeons' non-technical skills in the operating room: reliability testing of the NOTSS behaviour rating system. *World J Surg*. 2008;32: 548–56.

30. Jackson S, Brackley K, Landau A, Hayes K. Assessing non-technical skills on the delivery suite: a pilot study. *Clin Teach*. 2014;11(5): 375–80.

31. US Dept of Health & Human Services – Agency for Healthcare Research and Quality (AHRQ). TeamSTEPPS 2®. Video training tools – Inpatient surgical hand off; 2014. www.ahrq.gov/professionals/education/curriculum-tools/teamstepps/instructor/videos/ts_ISHandoff/INPTSURG-768.html (accessed 16 May 2016).

32. Toeima E. SHARING: improving and documentation of handover – mind the gap. *J Obstet Gynecol*. 2011;31: 681–2.

33. Edozien L. Structured Multidisciplinary Intershift Handover (SMITH): a tool for promoting safer intrapartum care. *J Obstet Gynecol*. 2011;31: 683–6.

34. US Dept of Health & Human Services – Agency for Healthcare Research and Quality (AHRQ). TeamSTEPPS 2®. Video training tools – Inpatient surgical check back; 2014. www.ahrq.gov/professionals/education/curriculum-tools/teamstepps/instructor/videos/ts_checkback/checkback.html (accessed 16 May 2016).

35. Easterbrook JA. The effect of emotion on cue utilization and the organization of behavior. *Psychol Rev*. 1959;66(3): 183–201.

36. Hanoch Y, Vitouch O. When less is more: information, emotional arousal and the ecological reframing of the Yerkes–Dodson Law. *Theory Psychol*. 2004;14(4): 427–52.

Index